IMMUNOBIOLOGY

Adapted from

Hospital Practice

with illustrations by

Irving Geis

(except as noted)*

Designed by

Robert S. Herald

**Other Illustrators*

Bunji Tagawa, Chapters 1, 22, 23

Robert S. Herald, Chapter 4

Carol Woike, Chapters 20, 27, 29

Dan Todd, Chapters 26, 30

Albert Miller, Chapter 28

IMMUNOBIOLOGY

Current Knowledge of Basic Concepts in Immunology and Their Clinical Applications

Edited by

Robert A. Good, M.D.

Professor and Chairman, Department of Pathology, and Regents' Professor of Pediatrics, University of Minnesota Medical School

and

David W. Fisher

Executive Editor, Hospital Practice

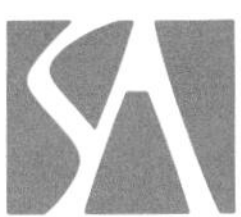

Sinauer Associates, Inc. • Publishers • Stamford, Connecticut

First printing July 1971
Second printing October 1971
Third printing February 1972

IMMUNOBIOLOGY

Printed in the United States of America.

Sinauer Associates, Inc.
20 Second Street
Stamford, Conn. 06905

SBN 0-87893-201-1

Library of Congress Catalog Card Number 77-155366

Table of Contents

Section V

CLINICAL APPLICATIONS OF IMMUNOLOGY IN PROPHYLAXIS AND IN THERAPY

Contributing Authors

K. FRANK AUSTEN	Professor of medicine, Harvard Medical School; physician-in-chief, Robert B. Brigham Hospital; and physician, Peter Bent Brigham Hospital, Boston.
SOLOMON A. BERSON	Murray M. Rosenberg professor of medicine and chairman of the department, Mount Sinai School of Medicine, New York City.
JOHN R. DAVID	Associate professor of medicine, Harvard Medical School; visiting physician, Robert B. Brigham Hospital; and senior associate in medicine, Peter Bent Brigham Hospital, Boston.
FRANK J. DIXON	Chairman of the department of experimental pathology, Scripps Clinic and Research Foundation, La Jolla, Calif.
VINCENT J. FREDA	Assistant clinical professor of obstetrics and gynecology, College of Physicians and Surgeons, Columbia University, and assistant attending obstetrician and gynecologist, Presbyterian Hospital, New York City.
H. HUGH FUDENBERG	Professor of medicine and director of the section of hematology and immunology, University of California San Francisco Medical Center, and professor of bacteriology and immunology, University of California, Berkeley.
HENRY GEWURZ	Professor of immunology and chairman of the department, Rush Medical College, Chicago.
ROBERT A. GOOD	Professor of pathology and head of the department, American Legion Memorial research professor, and Regents' professor of pediatrics and microbiology, University of Minnesota Medical School, Minneapolis.
JAMES L. GOWANS	Director of the cellular immunology unit, Medical Research Council, Sir William Dunn School of Pathology, Oxford University, England.
BEULAH HOLMES GRAY	Assistant professor of microbiology, University of Minnesota Medical School, Minneapolis.
INGEGERD HELLSTRÖM	Research associate professor of microbiology, the University of Washington School of Medicine, Seattle.
KARL ERIK HELLSTRÖM	Professor of pathology, the University of Washington School of Medicine, Seattle.
DAVID M. HUME	Stuart McGuire professor of surgery and chairman of the department, Medical College of Virginia, Virginia Commonwealth University, Richmond.
KIMISHIGE ISHIZAKA	Professor of medicine and microbiology, the Johns Hopkins University School of Medicine at the Good Samaritan Hospital, Baltimore.

C. HENRY KEMPE — Professor of pediatrics and chairman of the department, University of Colorado School of Medicine, Denver.

ARTHUR KORNBERG — Professor of biochemistry, Stanford University School of Medicine. Corecipient of the 1959 Nobel Prize for medicine for investigations leading to the synthesis of DNA.

EUGENE M. LANCE — Associate professor of surgery in orthopedics, Cornell University Medical College at New York Hospital and Hospital for Special Surgery, New York City.

H. SHERWOOD LAWRENCE — Codirector of New York University medical services, professor of medicine, and head of the infectious disease and immunology division, department of medicine, New York University School of Medicine, New York City.

GEORGE B. MACKANESS — Director of the Trudeau Institute at Saranac Lake, N.Y.

PETER B. MEDAWAR — Director of the National Institute for Medical Research, Mill Hill, London, England. Corecipient of the 1960 Nobel Prize for medicine for the discovery of acquired immunologic tolerance.

THOMAS C. MERIGAN JR. — Associate professor of medicine and head of the division of infectious diseases, Stanford University School of Medicine, Stanford, Calif.

MICHAEL E. MILLER — Assistant professor of pediatrics, the University of Pennsylvania School of Medicine, and director of the laboratory of clinical immunology, the Children's Hospital of Philadelphia.

ALFRED NISONOFF — Professor of biological chemistry and head of the department, University of Illinois College of Medicine, Chicago.

ROBERT P. ORANGE — Postdoctoral fellow of the Helen Hay Whitney Foundation; associate in medicine (immunology), Harvard Medical School; and research associate, Robert B. Brigham Hospital, Boston.

OSCAR D. RATNOFF — Professor, department of medicine, Case Western Reserve University School of Medicine, Cleveland, and career investigator, American Heart Association.

ROBERT S. SCHWARTZ — Professor of medicine, Tufts University School of Medicine, and chief of the clinical immunology service, New England Medical Center Hospitals, Boston.

THOMAS E. STARZL — Professor of surgery, University of Colorado School of Medicine, and chief, surgical service, Veterans Administration Hospital, Denver.

THOMAS B. TOMASI — Professor of medicine and director of the immunology and rheumatology service, department of medicine, State University of New York at Buffalo School of Medicine.

BYRON H. WAKSMAN — Professor of microbiology, Yale University School of Medicine, New Haven.

WILLIAM O. WEIGLE — Department of experimental pathology, Scripps Clinic and Research Foundation, La Jolla, Calif.

GERALD WEISSMANN — Professor of medicine, New York University School of Medicine, and career research scientist, Health Research Council of the City of New York.

ROSALYN S. YALOW — Chief, nuclear medicine, Veterans Administration Hospital, The Bronx, New York, and research professor of medicine, Mount Sinai School of Medicine, New York City.

Introduction

In assembling IMMUNOBIOLOGY, we have attempted to bring together, selectively but with representative completeness, the serious thoughts, experimental studies, and clinical applications that have characterized and that underlie the surging influence of immunology and immunobiology upon medicine in the present period.

The central position that immunobiology and its applications to the treatment of the sick now occupies has its roots in the evolution of our species. The very existence of man as a consequence of our development in a veritable sea of potentially hostile fungi, bacteria, and viruses is necessarily dependent on recognition of foreignness. Our heritage of ever-increasing cellular complexity has, on one hand, demanded a continuing cellular thrust toward individuality and, on the other, a vital need for powerful mechanisms of homeostasis. The requirement for containment and management of these two powerful countercurrents places immunobiology in the center of all biology. This, in turn, assures its significance for student and practitioner alike.

This conviction has guided the selection of contributions to this volume. They range from such fundamental considerations as the synthesis of functional DNA, the molecular nature of antibodies, and the cellular and developmental bases of immunity to the highly practical applications of immunology in prevention, diagnosis, and treatment of human disease.

Major attention is paid to mediators and effectors of immunity, to the relationships of immunity and inflammation and of immunity and coagulation, and to the pathogenesis of immunologic injury. The growth of our understanding of immunologic processes has permitted us to include here a number of models of obvious clinical importance, such as that for the immunopathology of glomerulonephritis. We are also able to discuss the nature of autoimmunity, progress in organ transplantation, the developing understanding of delayed and immediate allergy, and to give special attention to the exciting relationship between immunology and cancer.

The combination of the theoretical and the pragmatic is as old as the science of immunobiology, dating in fact from Jenner's first publication in 1798. Appropriately, every effort is made here to emphasize the clinical utility of immunologic knowledge. Applications considered in detail include the control of Rh disease, current practices related to vaccination and immunization, immunosuppression encompassing the background and potential of antilymphocyte serum and its variants, and the uses and abuses of gamma globulin for therapy and prophylaxis. The diagnostic revolution, employing immunohistochemistry and radioimmunoassay, is similarly represented.

Finally, we have sought to glimpse the shadow being cast by immunobiology into the future by inclusion of chapters on immunologic reconstitution, on the synthesis of DNA, and on the clinical potential of interferon.

In terms of the organization of IMMUNOBIOLOGY, it should be noted that we have not tried to offer a detailed documentation of the entire field, with the massive intrusion of footnotes and references that such an effort would mandate. Rather, we have striven for maximum readability while providing those readers who wish it an opportunity for further penetration of the vast storehouse of knowledge that exists. To the latter end, each of the authors has provided a selected list of readings appropriate to the chapter. These references are contained in a separate section at the end of the main body of the text.

Most of the chapters here were first published as articles in the immunology series of HOSPITAL PRACTICE. Each of these has been appropriately brought up to date by the authors. In addition, several new chapters have been added to assure a fully rounded presentation of current knowledge in the field.

While on the subject of the preparation of this volume, we would be most remiss if we did not give a measure of recognition to the organization that in so many ways contributed to making publication of IMMUNOBIOLOGY possible, that of HOSPITAL PRACTICE. Certainly, the publication of the original series of articles on which this text is based was only possible because of the enthusiastic encouragement and guidance provided by the publisher, Blake Cabot. Throughout the period when the material was appearing in the journal, and then during the performance of the complex job of adapting the material for book publication, we were uniquely fortunate in having the benefit of the remarkable editorial judgment and skills of HOSPITAL PRACTICE's managing editor, Gertrude Halpern. The task of integrating necessary revisions and preparing the material for the book was ably and uncomplainingly undertaken by Charles Ryberg, with the very competent collaboration of Norma Goodman, Evelyn Gottlieb, and Doris Ross. We are also indebted to Mary Johnstone for her skillful preparation of the index.

In designing the book, Robert Herald, art director of HOSPITAL PRACTICE, displayed a versatility and resourcefulness that solved many problems that at first seemed insurmountable. In fulfilling his responsibilities, he had invaluable assistance from Adele Spiegler and Joan Dworkin, as well as from Ronald Aya, who followed through on so many of the hundreds of details involved in getting it all together. Finally, our special gratitude goes to Samuel C. Bukantz, M.D., whose knowledge, derived from the continuous application of immunobiology to clinical medicine, was continually available to us.

In preparing this book for publication, we have been motivated by the evidence at every hand that immunobiology is not only expanding as a discipline but also penetrating into more and more areas of clinical medicine and biology. It seems certain that in the coming years this logarithmic growth will continue. With this in mind, we have done our best to make this work of special value to students of biology and medicine. At the same time, we have recognized that the most critical test of the validity of the work of the immunobiologists occurs at the interface between this work and that of the men and women whose daily work is the treatment of human disease. Therefore, we have organized this volume in an effort to assure its value to the general physician and to specialists and specialists-in-training in pediatrics, medicine, and surgery.

We are confident that from the taproots extended and the fruits already harvested modern immunobiology will continue to yield dividends in the form of both interim and complete solutions to human disease. There can be no doubt that the advancing understanding of immunobiology can and will contribute to maintenance of the prime of health and to the alleviation of misery and suffering. We hope that our readers will find this book as rewarding as it has been, in its assembly, for its editors.

ROBERT A. GOOD, M.D.
DAVID W. FISHER

Minneapolis and New York,
April 1971

Section One

The Development of the Immune Systems; Cellular Mechanisms of Immune Response

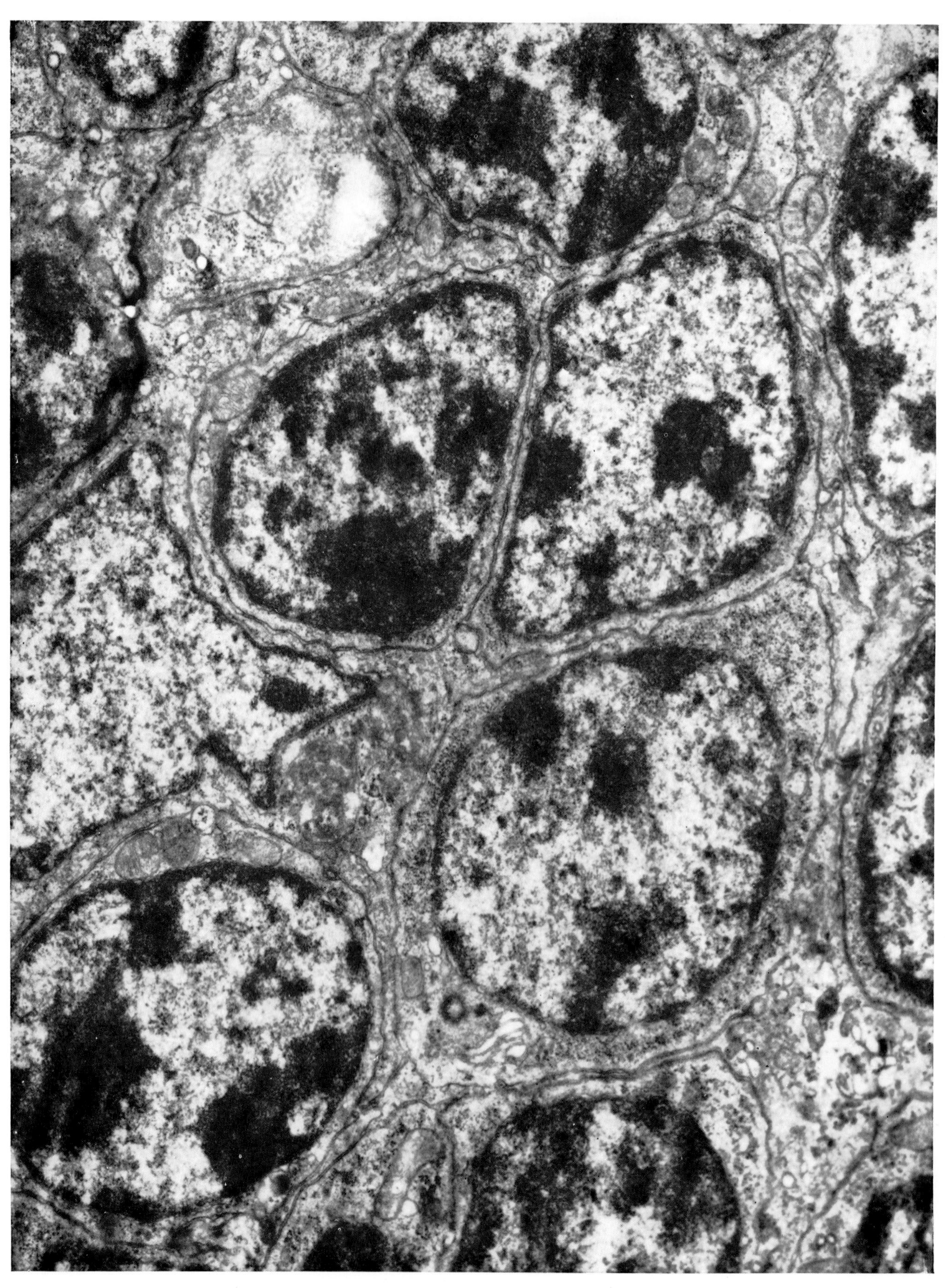

Electromicrograph of chicken thymus reveals the fine structure of this lobular organ, with its profusely vascularized cortex and medulla. At 16,000x magnification the organ's rich supply of lymphocytes can be clearly seen.

Chapter 1

Disorders of the Immune System

ROBERT A. GOOD
University of Minnesota

This is an exciting moment in research on the nature of immunity. Recent developments are adding up to nothing less than an entirely new picture of how the immune system works. It is as though we had been viewing things out of focus for years and now, suddenly, they have become sharply defined.

Progress has been achieved as a direct consequence of establishing a bridge between the clinic and basic science, a bridge carrying increasingly heavy traffic. A series of experiments and observations is bringing order to phenomena that not long ago seemed terribly confused. For example, in immunobiology the role of the thymus, one of the most stubborn problems of the recent past, is being clarified. Continuing studies are pointing to a previously unsuspected and subtle division of labor in the immune system.

This work has already had an impact at the clinical level, helping to explain certain negative and apparently contradictory observations in connection with the immunodeficiency diseases. There is also new evidence illuminating the relationship between disorders of lymphoid mechanisms and the so-called autoimmune diseases or certain types of malignancy. Moreover, evolutionary studies of immunity are providing a theoretical framework for the basic understanding of such disorders.

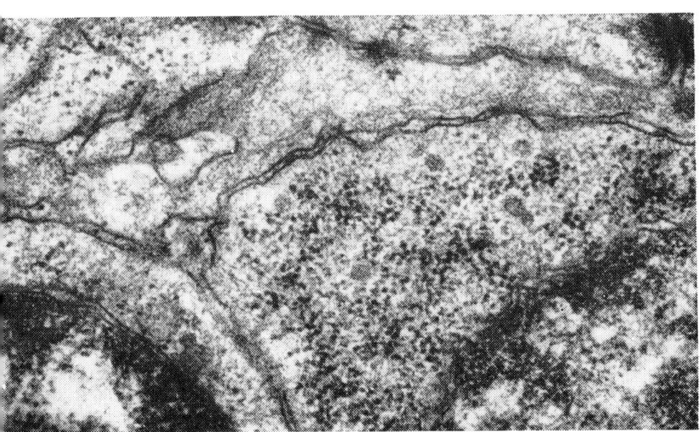

At 55,000x magnification, ribosomes in cytoplasm of thymic lymphoid cells become visible as black dots.

My own involvement with immunobiology goes back more than 27 years, when, as a student at the University of Minnesota Medical School, I was pursuing an interest in the viruses that affect the central nervous system. It was not until 1953, however, that a chance clinical observation aroused my interest in the thymus.

The patient was a 54-year-old man who had developed a series of severe bacterial infections after a lifetime of excellent health. He also happened to be the first patient in whom agammaglobulinemia and thymoma had been seen together. Given this hint, this provocative experiment of nature, Richard Varco and I—like others before us—decided to investigate the possibility that the thymus had something to do with adaptive immunity, for we were convinced that the association of two such infrequently encountered conditions could hardly be a matter of chance. The findings we came up with were negative. We found that thymectomy had no demonstrable effect on the antibody response of either adult or young rabbits.

Not long afterward the reason for our inconclusive results became clear. It was primarily a matter of timing. Bruce Glick, then a graduate student at Ohio State and now at State College, Mississippi State University, and his associates showed that marked effects could be obtained if experiments were performed on very young rather than adult animals. They used chicks and found that if soon after hatching they removed the bursa of Fabricius – a strange thymus-like organ at the tail end of the gastrointestinal tract—the immune mechanisms did not develop normally.

Glick's findings were confirmed and extended by Harold Wolfe and his colleagues at the University of Wisconsin and later by Ben Papermaster in our laboratories. By 1960 Olga Archer, James Pierce, and I had demonstrated that extirpation of the thymus of neonatal rabbits interfered with antibody production; Carlos Martinez, John Kersey, and I showed that in newborn mice it impaired transplan-

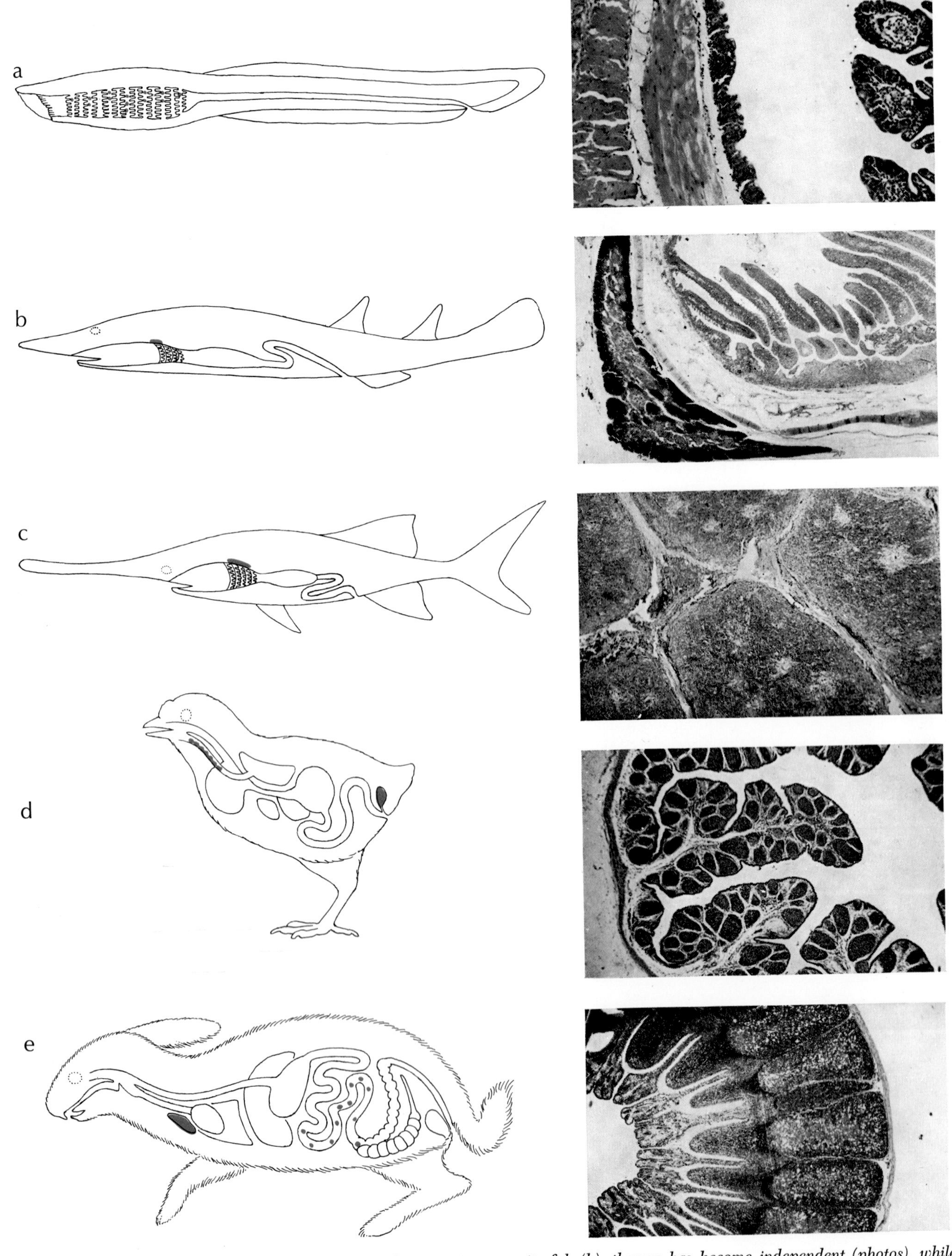

Phylogenesis of the immune system shows that the primitive thymus of the lamprey (a) consists of a few lymphocytes in the gills (photos show two levels of magnification). In the guitarfish (b), thymus has become independent (photos), while the paddlefish (c) has a lobular thymus and more varied cells (photos). In addition to the thymus, chicken (d) has a

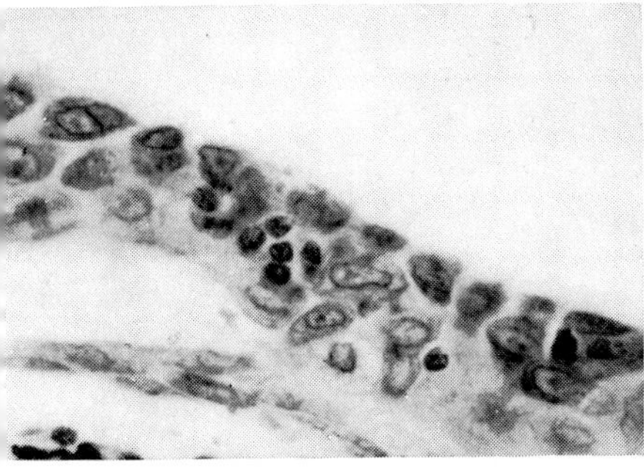

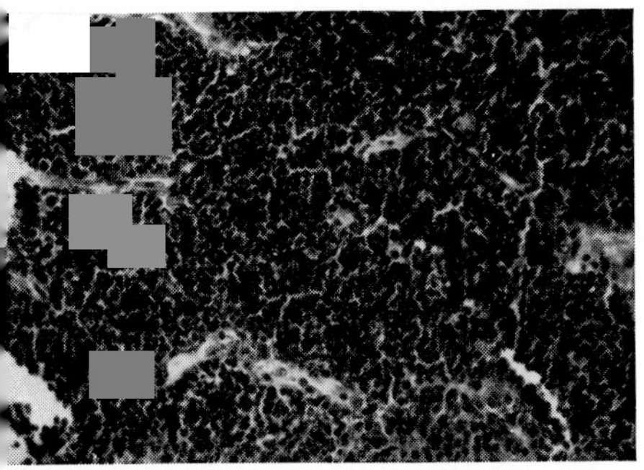

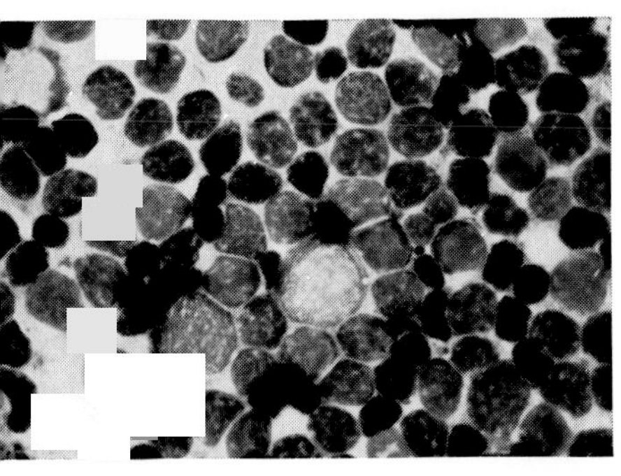

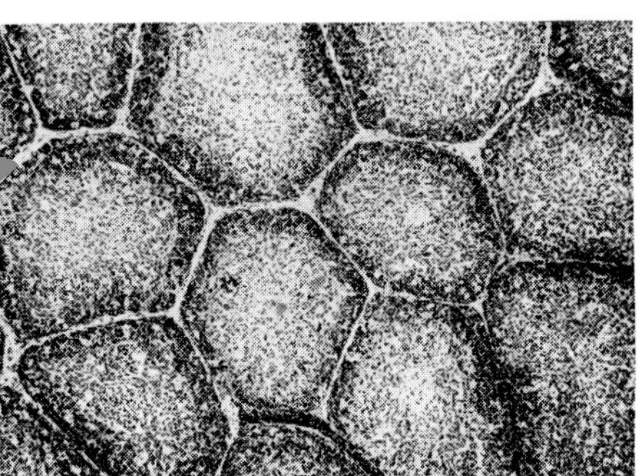

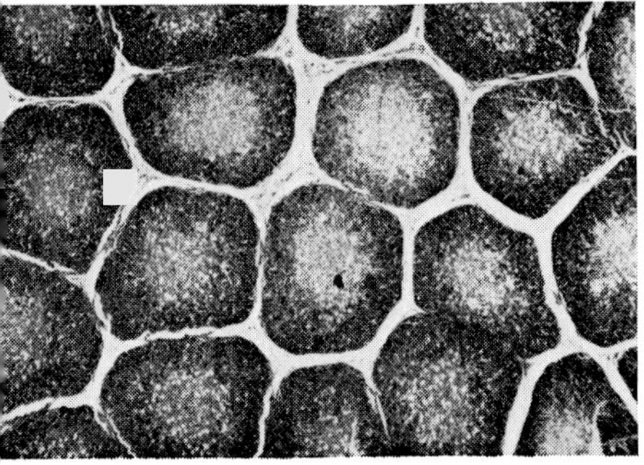

bursa of Fabricius, rabbit (e) has Peyer's patches, which are microscopically almost identical (photos).

tation immunity and development of all the cell-mediated immune responses, even antibody formation to some antigens like sheep red blood cells. Jacques Miller at the Chester Beatty Research Institute in London reached the same conclusion at about the same time. A core concept had been established: The crucial period during which thymus and bursa influence immunologic development occurs during early life, when the lymphoid tissue is forming and immunologic capacity is maturing.

But fruitful research always seems to generate fresh problems and paradoxes as well as fresh insights, and this work was certainly no exception. For example, many neonatally thymectomized animals were immunologically deficient, yet they contracted autoimmune diseases and other conditions that have always been associated with excessive immunologic activity. In view of such conflicting observations we decided to have another look at the chicken, which promised to be particularly useful for further experiments since it has a thymus as well as a bursa. The existence of two distinct lymphoid organs implied a difference in function and a possibility that more precise and delicate manipulation of immune responses could be achieved. Then, at our thymus conference in 1962, the Australian investigators Noel Warner and Alexander Szenberg presented results of experiments in chickens. The studies seemed to indicate that interference with development of the bursa affected antibody production primarily, while interference with thymus development affected homograft immunity.

The next year Max Cooper started a long series of experiments in our laboratories. He removed either the thymus or bursa from some newly hatched chicks, and both from others. Then, to destroy all peripheral lymphoid components, he subjected the chicks to intense x-irradiation just below the lethal level. His results were beautiful, because they clarified things so incisively.

Cooper showed that a clear-cut separation of immunologic function does indeed exist in the chicken. The thymus represents the body's recognition system, the lymphoid mechanisms whereby alien elements are distinguished from "native stock." It produces and is necessary for the development of a widespread population of highly specialized cells, consisting chiefly of small lymphocytes, that play a vital part in cellular immunity—graft-vs-host reactions, delayed hypersensitivity, and homograft rejection. But its influence on antibody response has not been clearly defined, antibody formation to some, but not all, antigens being reduced in thymectomized chicks.

The thymus in the chicken functions exactly as does the thymus in the mouse. It represents the site of differentiation of a population of lymphocytes that subserve largely the functions of cell-mediated immunity. Thus, the thymus is essential to development of those lymphocytes involved in delayed allergic reactions, in allograft rejection, and in the initiation of graft-vs-host reactions. This population seems to represent a major bulwark of bodily defense against many bacteria such as certain gram-negative coliform organisms, salmonella, typical and atypical acid-fast bacteria, listeria, and brucella. In addition, this population of lymphocytes represents a major defense against fungi and certain viruses, including chickenpox, measles, vaccinia, and others. Since our initial discovery of the role of the thymus involved demonstration of a deficit of ability to produce circulating antibodies in neonatally thymectomized rodents, the thymus-dependent, or T cell, system also seems to play a role in humoral antibody response to selected antigens like sheep red blood cells and bovine serum albumin. Nevertheless, neonatally thymectomized rodents, like chickens thymectomized in the newly hatched period, develop normal concentrations of all known immunoglobulins. Further, production of immunoglobulins and some natural antibodies seem to progress at a normal rate.

The bursa can be regarded as executive headquarters of the chick antibody-producing system. It goes into action once recognition has been effected, setting up the same defenses that in man have been taken advantage of in the form of immunization techniques ever since the time of Jenner. This system is represented morphologically by the larger lymphocytes of the germinal centers and plasma cells and functionally by the immunoglobulins. Bursectomized irradiated chicks reject homografts and exhibit all other normal "thymic" cellular immunity responses. But they produce no gamma globulins and no circulating antibodies, no matter how intensively or how often we stimulate them, even when we repeat intramuscular and intravenous injections of bovine serum albumin and *Brucella abortus* organisms, with or without complete Freund's adjuvant. So the chick also has a bursa-dependent, or immunoglobulin-producing, system.

Elimination of the bursa (B) cell system can be accomplished by means other than bursectomy at hatching. When extirpation is carried out on the egg, fascinating results are obtained. If the maneuver takes place on the 15th or 16th day of embryonation, the result often includes a total inhibition of development of the antibody-producing system of cells and elimination of both plasma cells and germinal centers. Chicks bursectomized and irradiated at hatching fail to develop either IgM or IgG classes of immunoglobulins and cannot make antibodies. They represent a clean experimental model of an animal developing without a B system of cells.

Two other models for selective prevention of development of the B cell system include those developed by Weidanz in Philadelphia and Cooper at Alabama. Weidanz discovered that agammaglobulinemia can be produced in chickens by giving them large doses of cyclophosphamide shortly after hatching. Although this treatment damages cells of the thymus and T system as well as cells of the B system, the T system recovers completely while neither the bursa nor the B system cells recover from the insult. Such animals grow up as severe immunologic cripples unable to form antibodies and many are agammaglobulinemic. By contrast, their cell-mediated immune functions seem entirely normal.

Cooper, a former associate in our laboratory, his associate Lawton, and a student, Kincaid, have come forward with studies that may be the most telling of all. They have found that injection of specific antibody against the μ (IgM) immunoglobulin chain into the developing chick embryo at the precise moment of appearance of IgM-staining cells in the bursa prevents the development of both IgM- and IgG-producing cells in the chicken. Their further studies employed immunofluorescent techniques. When specific goat antiserum directed against μ chains was tagged with fluorescein isothionate and specific antiserum against gamma chains was tagged with Rhodamine, it was clear that the bursa of Fabricius was the first site to develop both IgM- and IgG-producing lymphocytes. Further, the bursa of Fabricius was the only site where cells that stained both for IgM and IgG were to be found. The immunoglobulin-producing cells of the lymph nodes, the spleen, the "cecal tonsils," or the gastrointestinal lamina propria did not contain dual-staining plasma cells. Rather, the immunoglobulin-containing cells at such peripheral lymphoid sites stained only with antisera directed against one or the other of these immunoglobulins.

These findings are entirely consonant with observations that bursectomy at 17 to 19 days of embryonation regularly prevented development of a population of IgG-producing plasma cells.

A very important contribution to our understanding of ontogenic development of the immunologic system came from studies by Moore and Owen and their colleagues, first at Oxford, later in Australia. These studies in mice and chickens showed that stem cells originate in yolk sac and subsequently are to be found in fetal liver and then in the bone marrow. These stem cells, we believe, then give rise to cells that can enter the thymus or the bursa and in turn spawn the immunologically competent populations at these special sites of differentiation.

Both Tyan and his associates working in San Francisco and Stutman and his associates working with us at Minnesota following up the lead of Ford and associates at Harwell have presented compelling evidence that establishes that proliferation in the thymus is associated with development of an immunologically competent population of cells that can then leave the thymus and exercise the functions of cell-mediated immunity.

All of these findings can now be confidently incorporated into a scheme for development of immunologically competent cells, illustrated on pages 8 and 9.

According to this view a basic hematopoietic stem cell is differentiated to a lymphoid stem cell that has capacity to enter alternatively the thymus or the bursa (or its equivalent differentiative site in mammals). In the thymus, through a process involving a series of repeated and apparently wasteful replications, the cells are differentiated to a population of cells that resides in the thymic medulla and can leave the thymus to enter a recirculating pool of lymphocytes in the peripheral lymphoid system. It is this thymus-dependent cell system that subserves the functions of cell-mediated immunity. In the bursa of birds an alternative differentiation is accomplished, which takes the cells through a succession of developments to B cells capable of leaving the bursa and producing and secreting one or another of the immunoglobulins. First to develop is a capacity to produce IgM molecules. Later differentiation makes possible alternative production of IgG or still other kinds of immunoglobulin molecules. These are the B cells. The development is not basically different in mammals than it is in other animals, with the exception of birds with their unique, highly developed bursa of Fabricius.

Another distinct area of basic research reinforces and illuminates many of the recent findings made in our laboratories and at other centers. While the chick experiments were going ahead, I put my muscle into a

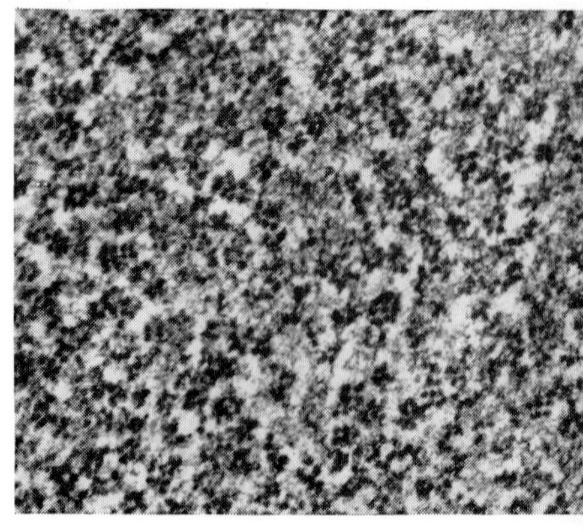

Polyribosome mosaic (55,000x) in young plasma cell is where antibodies will form.

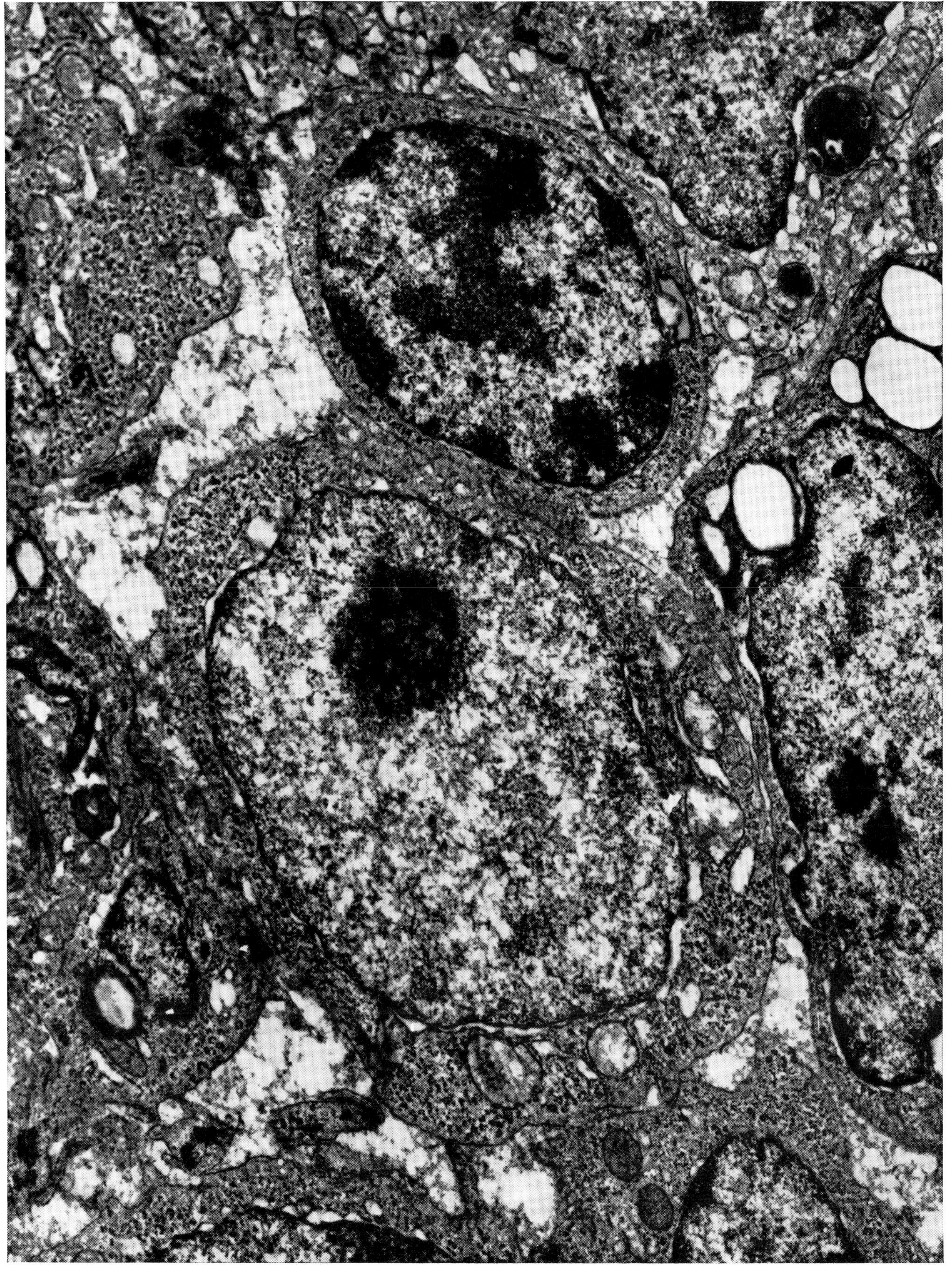

Lymphoid cells (16,000x) are from chick's bursa of Fabricius, the second component of its immunologic mechanism, corresponding to mammalian Peyer's patches. These cells manufacture immunoglobulins and antibodies.

broad problem that has been nagging me ever since my student days, the problem of understanding how the lymphoid system evolved through eons of history, the meaning of its evolution, and the selective forces that shaped it. So a continuing investigation was initiated, involving many of my associates—Papermaster (who rekindled my interest in the subject about nine or 10 years ago), Henry Gewurz, Joanne Finstad, Bernard Pollara, Dominique Frommel, Andreas Rosenberg, and Gary Litman – and about 30 species of fish, amphibians, reptiles, and mammals, as well as several invertebrates.

According to what has been learned to date, the thymus-dependent system developed at a relatively early stage in the evolution of vertebrate forms. The first faint trace seems to have appeared some 400 million years ago among primitive marine vertebrates and perhaps among some of the invertebrates as well. We could not find evidence of adaptive immunity in the most primitive of vertebrates, the hagfish, or in any of several invertebrates we studied. In the hagfish, however, we did find lymphocyte-like cells that seem to participate in chronic inflammation.

The lamprey, a somewhat better developed species, possesses the most primitive known thymus, not a single organ but a number of scattered foci of five to 20 lymphoid cells, and a primitive spleen. We find in the lamprey the five responses associated with adaptive immunity (delayed hypersensitivity, homograft immunity, antibody production, gamma globulins, and immune memory), but all in feeble form. For example, the lamprey responds to only two of the 22 antigens we use in our tests. A still more advanced species, the guitarfish, produces antibodies to six of 20 experimental antigens and has a thymus organ that can be distinguished from that of a mammal only with difficulty.

A fully developed immunoglobulin-producing system comparable to man's probably arose about 250 million years ago with a great upsurge of immunologic capacity in the higher sharks and the paddlefish. These species show the first well-defined plasma cells in spleen, pericardial tissue, kidneys, and gonads; they also produce complex gamma globulins, and tests on sharks and paddlefish showed that these formed antibodies to all the antigens we used.

Another step forward occurred among the dipnoid fish, an offshoot of forms ancestral to the amphibians. Both the dipnoid lungfish and the amphibians have two separate immunoglobulin classes with molecular features very similar to those of mammalian IgM and IgG. In none of the sharks, paddlefish, or teleost fish that we have studied could we find an immunoglobulin similar to IgG of mammals. Both high- and low-molecular-weight immunoglobulins are to be found in circulation, but the low-molecular-weight form has characteristics of a monomer of the high-molecular-weight form. In all of the placoderm-derived vertebrates (sharks, paddlefish, dogfish, etc.) the basic structure of the immunoglobulins includes a composite polypeptide chain structure based on both high- and low-molecular-weight (heavy and light) polypeptide chains. Lamprey immunoglobulin by contrast seemed to be a very different molecule. Indeed, the antibodies of the lamprey have proved to be unique thus far in the phylogenetic analysis. The fully functional molecule is comprised of four equal-sized polypeptide chains. Its physicochemical characteristics distinguish it sharply from the immunoglobulins of higher forms. Particularly, it is a much more rigid molecule than any of the immunoglobulins of the placoderm-derived vertebrates.

In our as yet far from complete studies of those molecules in invertebrates that are capable of specific cellular interactions such as the hemolysis or agglutination of red cells, none have primary, secondary, or tertiary structural characteristics that permit us to link them with vertebrate immunoglobulins. Perhaps the immunoglobulins of the lamprey or even the hagfish will help us bridge this gap in the chemical evolution of the immune responses. Recent studies by E. Cooper of UCLA and Duprat of France indicate that invertebrate earthworms can recognize and reject heterografts and homografts, with evidence of memory. This intriguing finding will ultimately also need to be analyzed in molecular perspective.

Another major step forward among amphibians was the appearance of plasma cells in the lamina propria of the intestinal tract—cells that in this location in mammals are specialized in the production of gamma A globulins and antibodies designed specifically to combat external invaders of the gastrointestinal tract. The latest stages of this phylogenetic process are represented by the development of bursa-like tissues, true lymph nodes, and other refinements of both the thymus-dependent and immunoglobulin-producing systems in reptiles, birds, and mammals.

Viewed from the broad aspect of these studies, several points stand out. For one thing, the studies emphasize the fundamental importance of the lymphoid system to the survival of vertebrates. Nature knows a good thing when she sees it, and every animal form phylogenetically distal to

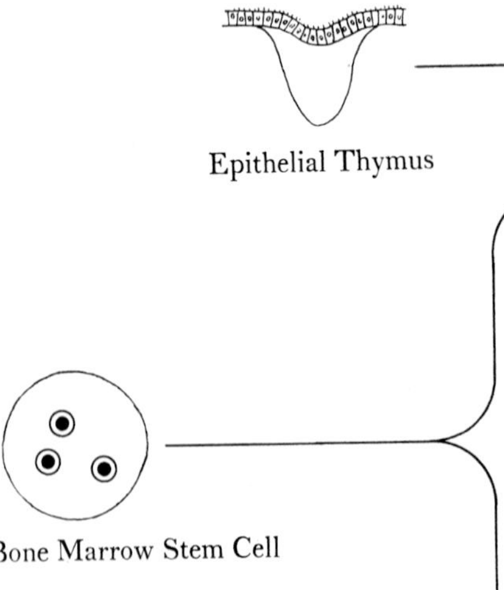

The two branches of the immune mechanism are believed to develop from the same lymphoid precursor. The central thymus system starts as an epithelial

the lamprey has a thymus. The same thing goes for plasma-cell structures, including those found in the lamina propria, and for the spleen, which, incidentally, is one of the two organs in man whose function continues to elude us (the other is the pineal).

The most intriguing question is why these structures appeared in the first place. Finstad, Ragnar Fänge, and I recently found that although the hagfish and many invertebrates have little or no lymphoid tissue they can tolerate fantastic amounts of total body radiation, more than 10 times as much as the lamprey. So something was lost as well as gained, which suggests that the selective pressures favoring the development of the lymphoid system must have been enormous. I doubt very much that the system originally had primarily to do with defenses against infection because, among other things, invertebrates have no such defenses—yet compete successfully with vertebrates in every ecologic niche.

My guess is that lymphoid development was definitely connected with the appearance of more and more elaborate species during the course of evolution, that it reflected the survival value of having improved control over proliferation in increasingly complex tissues among the vertebrates. Structures like the hematopoietic tissues and the lining of the gastrointestinal tract involve rapidly multiplying cells and tremendous opportunities for somatic variation. But you simply cannot have somatic variation and still have genetically stable species. So there had to be a kind of police system that, in the event of somatic variation, could distinguish "self" from "nonself" cells and destroy the latter. In other words, lymphoid mechanisms probably first developed as much to defend against inside as against outside antigens, to eliminate the unwanted insiders that "bore from within" and threatened the integrity of the individual and the survival of the species.

Phylogenetic research, descriptive and theoretical, has had a strong influence on our thinking about the immune system in man. It provided a most valuable perspective on the chick studies, for example, underlining the fact that the bursa is not an anomalous "freak" organ representing a quirk of avian evolution but is indeed the main control organ of a system represented in all classes of vertebrates — the immunoglobulin-producing system. Furthermore, it points up the importance of identifying the ana-

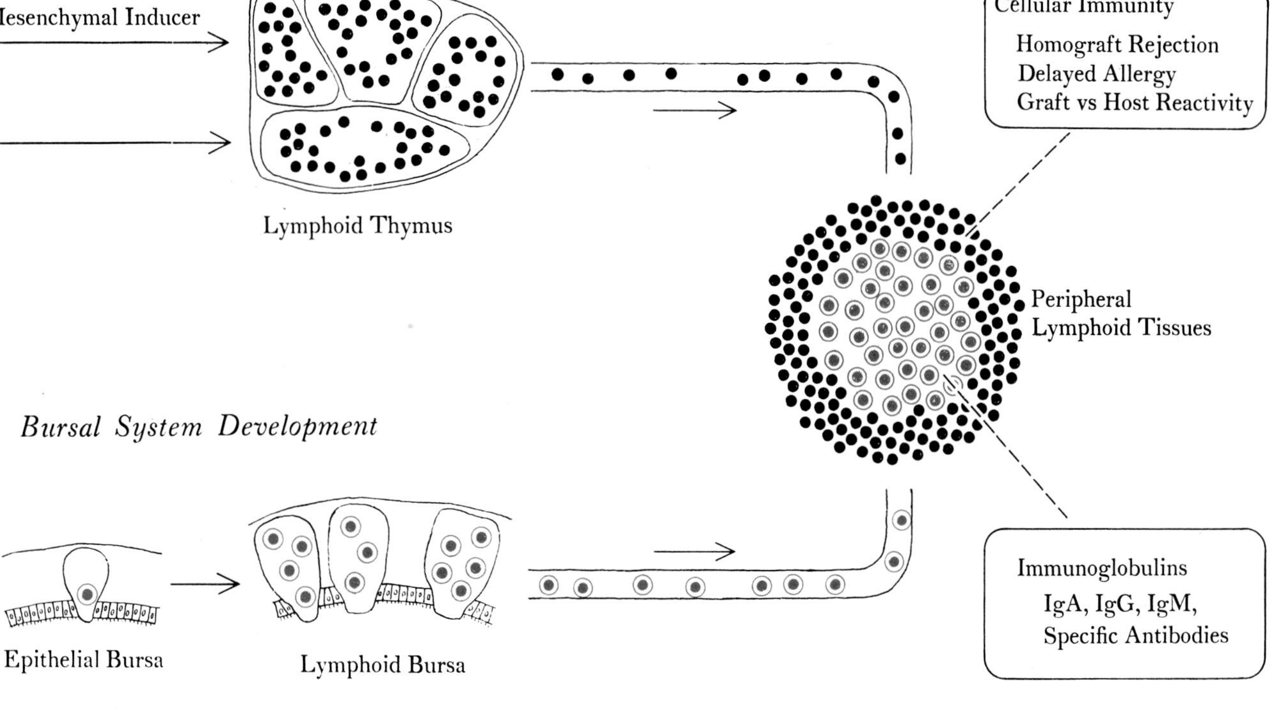

structure arising from third and fourth embryonic pharyngeal pouch and becomes a lymphoid organ under stimulation by a mesenchymal inducer. The bursal system develops by budding from the intestinal epithelium. After release from the central organs into the bloodstream, the lymphoid cells reassemble in peripheral lymphoid tissues. Here the lymphocytes – thymus-dependent in origin – control cellular immunity, while bursa-dependent plasma cells synthesize serum antibodies.

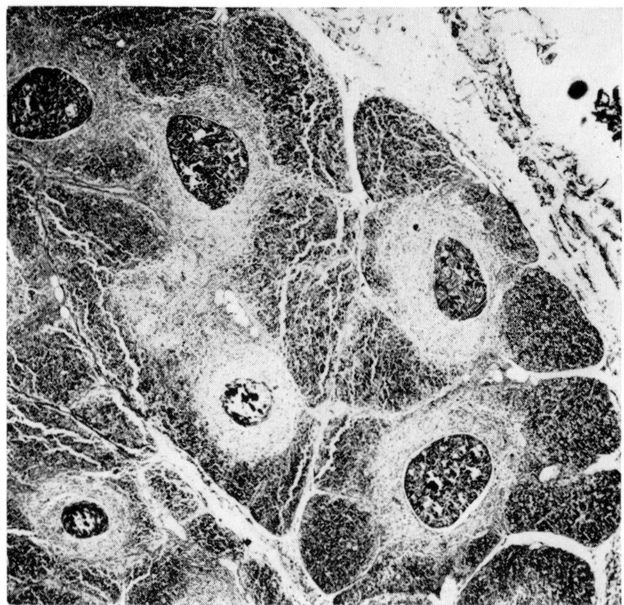

Photomicrograph of a thymus section from a child with myasthenia gravis reveals giant Hassal's corpuscles in the medullary portion of the organ.

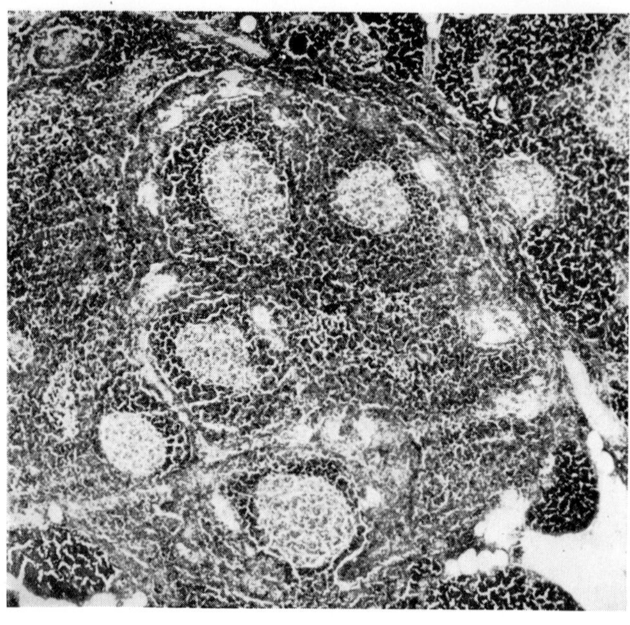

Characteristic of this thymus from an adult with myasthenia gravis are the many nests of germinal centers. Lymphocytes are also present in large numbers.

logous system in man, a problem not yet solved, although we have clues.

The Bursa Equivalent

Studies in the rabbit suggest that along its intestinal tract are to be found follicular lymphoepithelial structures that may, indeed, subserve functions exercised by the bursa of Fabricius of birds. Such lymphoepithelial follicular structures have been found in many sites along the gastrointestinal tract throughout phylogeny, but proof that any of them is the equivalent of the bursa of Fabricius is lacking. It now seems possible to define the bursa of Fabricius in sufficiently precise terms so identification of its equivalent site in both ontogeny and phylogeny will be possible.

It should be the site where IgM- and IgG-containing cells first appear. In addition, it should be the only anatomic location in which cells contain both IgM- and IgG-type immunoglobulins and the only site where antigenic stimulation by a number of routes does not expand the population of immunoglobulin- or antibody-producing cells. Using such criteria, Dr. Y. S. Choi, Bernard Pollard, Eliot Trask, and I are seeking to define the bursa for mice, man, and amphibians.

Some of our research seems to direct attention to the Peyer's patches, oval areas of densely packed lymphoid nodules found at the lower end of the intestines. The evolutionary record shows that all animals having an immunoglobulin-producing system also have these plate-like elements, as well as an appendix and other gut-associated tissues. Moreover, in rabbits Peyer's patches resemble the bursa so closely that in some views it takes a highly skilled histologist to tell the two structures apart. Further evidence comes from rabbit experiments conducted by Max Cooper and Daniel Perey, a young surgeon from Montreal, who have been studying immunobiology in our laboratories. They removed the half dozen or so Peyer's patches from irradiated animals, together with the sacculus rotundus (the "intestinal tonsil") and appendix, and produced a condition strikingly like that found in bursectomized irradiated young chickens—a depression of antibody-producing capacity without any effect on the cellular immunities.

Interaction of T and B Cell Systems in Immune Responses

As mentioned earlier, the initial discovery in Minneapolis of the role of the thymus in development of immunity related to its role in development of capacity of the animal to produce circulating antibodies. Yet the experiments in chickens and mammals and man indicate that production of immunoglobulins and their antibody molecules is the business of a separately differentiated system of cells – the B cell system. Apparent resolution of this paradox came with studies by Claman and associates in Colorado, Miller and associates in Australia, and Davies in England. These investigators all showed that thymus-derived cells act synergistically with bone-marrow-derived cells that are independent of thymus to achieve antibody responses to certain antigens like sheep red blood cells. Antibody synthesis even to such thymus-dependent antigens is not, as we and others have pointed out, the function of T cells. The role of the T cells in such thymus-dependent antibody responses, many of which have now been described, has not yet been elucidated, but it seems likely to us that it is a secondary consequence of the capacity of T cells to express cell-mediated immunity. The real question as to a major direct T and B cell interaction in achieving effective antigenic stimulation of the antibody-producing B cells is why animals completely lacking T cells have normal

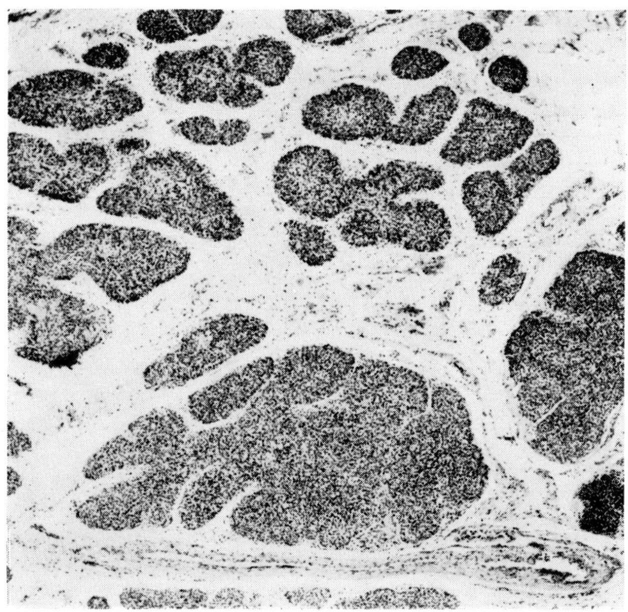

In Swiss-type agammaglobulinemia the abnormality of the stem cell leads to various types of developmental failure, but a poorly formed epithelial organ is typical of all.

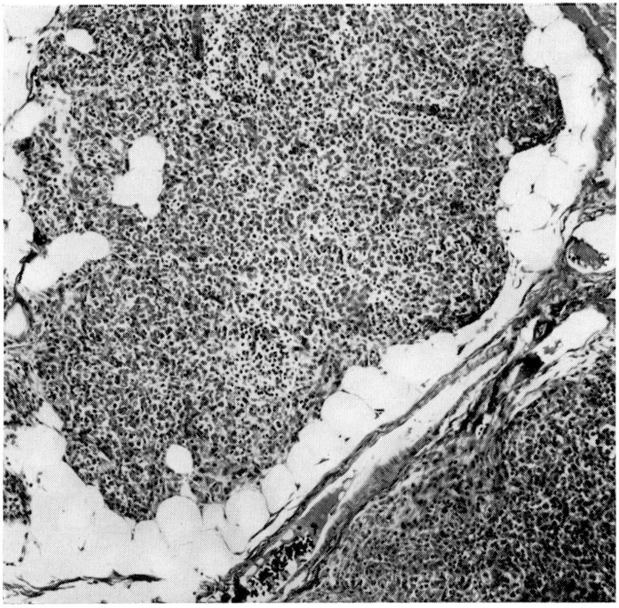

No cortex or Hassal's corpuscles and very few lymphocytes are seen in this thymus from a patient with ataxia-telangiectasia. Abnormal stem cell is characteristic.

numbers of plasma cells, normal levels of all immunoglobulins, and normal antibody responses to many antigens.

Involution of Immunity with Aging

Finally, in considering the development of the immune response in its entirety it is essential to think of the involution of the central lymphoid organs, the two lymphoid systems, and immune responses. Throughout the entire range of phylogeny the thymus of older animals tends to be small and fibrous rather than succulent and lymphoid as in young animals. In all these species the thymus seems to reach relative maximal development early in life and absolute maximal development at the onset of sexual maturity. Thereafter the thymus begins apparent programmed involution, which is followed in turn by involution of functions of the T cell system. The involution of the latter, however, lags considerably behind the thymic involution itself.

Edmond Yunis, Glen Rodey, and O. Stutman, studying this basic question with us at Minnesota, have shown that the involution of the thymus-dependent system seems to involve progressive inadequacy of the thymic stroma. The bursa, like the thymus, begins to involute at sexual maturation and in all orders of birds a striking involution occurs. The bursa-dependent system, at least with respect to capacity to maintain immunoglobulin levels, seems to persist more adequately than does the thymus-dependent system. Extensive studies, authoritatively reviewed by Walford, Yunis et al., and Makinodan, have shown that both cellular and humoral immune responses reach their zenith at the prime of life and a functional as well as anatomic involution is experienced. Associated with this involution is emergence of a variety of autoimmune diseases and phenomena and some malignancies.

One is pressed to raise the question of why the lymphoid system, which clearly has such major survival advantage, involutes and why this involution is programmed in a broad way to begin at the time of sexual maturation in many if not all forms. One way to visualize these relationships is to consider the involution to be in keeping with many of nature's schemes for placing restrictions upon numbers in the various species. There seems distinct survival advantage in nature to get individuals to the point of maximum and most efficient reproduction but after that point no great advantage to maintaining individuals that have reproduced themselves. This can be seen in many control mechanisms observable in nature, ranging from the programmed destruction of the lemmings to the territorial phenomena so widespread in mammals and birds. All other things being equal, there is no advantage in nature to long life or excessive numbers, which can threaten the adequacy of the ecologic niche.

This is where the bridge to the clinic comes in. In providing a new outlook on the normal workings and pathology of the immune system, laboratory experiments offer new approaches to many diseases, notably the 20-odd immunologic deficiency diseases. In a sense we move backward in time and deal successively with diseases representing different types of deprivation, interferences affecting structures formed at earlier and earlier stages in development. These conditions have been classified by the World Health Organization. The specific defects and their relationships to the thymic dependent (T) and the bone marrow or bursal dependent (B) cells and to abnormalities in stem cell populations are recorded in the table on page 12.

First there is Bruton's congenital,

Classification of Primary Specific Immunodeficiency States

TYPE	SUGGESTED CELLULAR DEFECT		
	B Cells	*T Cells*	*Stem Cells*
Infantile sex-linked agammaglobulinemia (Bruton type)	A	N	N
Selective IgA deficiency	A (some)	N	N
Transient hypogammaglobulinemia of infancy	A	N	N
Sex-linked immunodeficiency with IgM elevation	A	?	N
Thymic hypoplasia (pharyngeal pouch, Di George syndrome)	N	A	N
Episodic lymphopenia with lymphocytotoxin	N	A	N
Immunodeficiency with normal or elevated gamma globulins	A	A (sometimes)	?
Immunodeficiency with ataxia-telangiectasia	A	A	?
Immunodeficiency with thrombocytopenia and eczema (Wiskott-Aldrich syndrome)	A	A	?
Immunodeficiency with thymoma	A	A	?
Immunodeficiency with short-limbed dwarfism	A	A	A
Immunodeficiency with generalized hematopoietic hypoplasia	A	A	A
Severe combined immunodeficiencies			
(a) autosomal recessive	A	A	A
(b) sex-linked	A	A	A
(c) sporadic	A	A	A
Variable immunodeficiency (common, largely unclassified)	A	A (sometimes)	?

Classification is based on the recommendations of investigators on primary immune deficiencies at a meeting that was sponsored by the World Health Organization in June 1970. It was agreed that underlying cellular defects would be divided among the three cell types participating in immunoresponse mechanisms – the bone marrow or bursal dependent (designated as B cells), the thymic dependent (designated as T cells), and the stem cells. In the table, A indicates the absence or abnormality of the particular cell population, N stands for normality. For purposes of this tabulation, primary specific immunodeficiency is considered to result from failure to produce effectors of immune response, either antibodies or sensitized lymphocytes. States resulting from enhanced destruction of the effectors or from their destruction by exogenous immunosuppression are excluded as are these associated with lymphopenia due to intestinal lymphangiectasia or neoplasia, or to defects in complement activation or phagocytosis. The specific classifications encompass only a minority of patients with immunodeficiency. Despite great strides forward in our understanding, the majority still cannot be unequivocally classified and must be grouped as having "variable immunodeficiency."

sex-linked agammaglobulinemia, originally described by Ogden Bruton in 1952. It is chiefly a disease of the immunoglobulin-producing system, which, in ontogeny as in phylogeny, develops after the thymus and thymus-dependent system. As one might expect, children with this condition generally have a normal-appearing thymus, produce normal quantities of blood lymphocytes, and can exhibit delayed hypersensitivity and homograft rejection. But they have virtually no ability to form plasma cells and gamma globulin, and several patients with Bruton's syndrome have never produced detectable antibodies.

Ontogenetic studies indicate what has apparently happened. The immune system arises from stem cells that come from either gut epithelium or closely associated developing lymphoid tissues. Their differentiation to functional lymphoid cells is induced by mesenchyme. A further differentiation, or branching, of the lymphoid cells then takes place—first involving the appearance of thymus tissue and the thymus-dependent system at about the sixth or seventh week of embryonic life. Plasma cells and the immunoglobulin-producing system appear later.

So Bruton's disease is probably the result of a genetic defect, perhaps a missing enzyme that interferes with the development of the immunoglobulin-producing system after the branching point. Monthly gamma globulin injections, administered intramuscularly, help compensate for the deficiency by maintaining circulating levels of about 150 mg/100 cc (normal levels range from 700 to 1,400). But patients, since they depend on others for their antibodies – particularly for antibodies against streptococcal, pneumococcal, hemophilus, and meningococcal infections – are walking on a frayed tightrope. Attempts have been made to provide better protection by injections of live plasma cells as well as gamma globulins, but since these patients can "recognize" the foreign cells and eliminate them, the cellular treatment has only short-lived effects.

Another immunologic deficiency disease, ataxia-telangiectasia, which is characterized by progressive cerebellar ataxia, oculocutaneous telangiectasia, and frequent sinopulmonary infections, provides a fascinating and most significant contrast to Bruton's disease. It also involves interference with the differentiation of lymphoid cells, but in this case the defect clearly occurs in the earlier developmental branch that leads to formation of the thymus-dependent system. The disease is extraordinarily variable from case to case but, largely as a result of insights offered by ablation and phylogenetic studies, a pattern has begun to emerge. Autopsies and biopsies reveal that many patients have either no detectable thymus or a small, histologically abnormal one. Most of them show deficient transplantation immunity. Although gamma globulin levels are generally normal, a few of the patients lack IgG, and almost half have either complete absence of IgA or show only a very low level of this immunoglobulin.

Standard treatment for this condition includes antibiotics and drainage of the pulmonary tract to combat infections. But nothing can be done about the progressive ataxia and neurologic failure, and children usually live for only 4 to 12 years. Recently we proposed a transplantation procedure that may offer a better prognosis. We would obtain normal adult thymus epithelium—perhaps a piece of the thymus removed from a patient during cardiac surgery—and irradiate it to destroy lymphocytes with the immunologic capacity to bring about graft-vs-host reactions. We would then implant it under the renal capsule or in the peritoneal cavity. This operation may be attempted as soon as we find a suitable case.

Defects that appear to be the mirror image of Bruton-type agammaglobulinemia have been described by Nezelof in France and Angelo Di George, a Philadelphia endocrinologist. The patients produce the normal amounts of all the immunoglobulins but fail to produce cellular immunities. They possess germinal centers and plasma cells, Peyer's patches and tonsils, but either have a vestigial embryonic thymus or lack the thymus completely, consequently lacking the thymic-dependent system of lymphocytes. This disease now seems to be correctable by transplant of a thymus.

Another immunologic disease, the so-called Swiss type of lymphopenic agammaglobulinemia, involves a still earlier stage of development. A genetic factor is at work here, and, according to our model, the deficiency arises at the stage where stem cells normally differentiate to lymphoid cells. Infants afflicted with this condition fail to develop any primordial lymphoid tissue and have neither a thymus-dependent nor an immunoglobulin-producing system. The thymus in these babies is a small vestigial organ, plasma cells are lacking, and there is no delayed hypersensitivity, homograft rejection, or any detectable antibodies.

Although no one has ever cured this condition, we can now report encouraging results via cellular replacement in other immunologic deficiency diseases [see Chapter 23, "Immunologic Reconstitution: The Achievement and Its Meaning"]. In this condition the infants regularly die in six months to a year of overwhelming fungus or virus infections. But Richard Hong, Cooper, and I had encouraging, if only temporary, results in an eight-month-old boy suffering from a massive candida infection, which produces only a very mild thrush in most normal babies. His lymphocyte count was down to 500, and homograft rejection was severely impaired. In fact, a skin graft obtained six weeks before from a medical technician was taking quite as beautifully as if it were the child's own skin.

Since death was imminent, we decided to try to treat the baby with a transplantation procedure designed to reconstitute the thymus-dependent system. We figured that if this worked, deficiencies of the immunoglobulin-producing system might be controlled with gamma globulin injections. A supply of primordial stem cells was needed, so we telephoned the world's leading lymphoid tissue bank, under the direction of Dr. H.E.M. Kay at the Royal Marsden Hospital in London, and obtained by air a fragment of fetal liver, a rich source of stem cells. Ten days or so after intraperitoneal implantation of the liver tissue and a small bit of fetal thymus, the patient's infection was clearing up, lymphocyte counts had tripled, circulating antibodies appeared, and the homograft was beginning to slough off. Then a sudden and lethal reaction set in as the child developed severe anemia and an extensive gen-

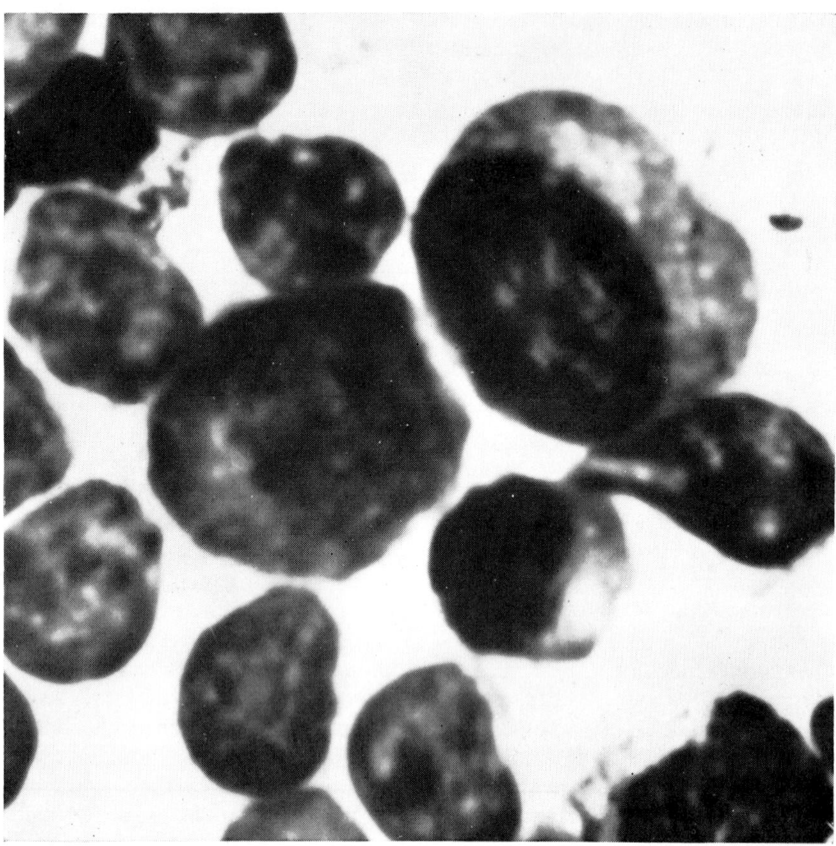

In the Bruton type of agammaglobulinemia, the bursal system is absent, the thymic system normal. Large plasma cells can be seen (above) in a normal child after antigenic stimulation. These cells are absent and only lymphocytes are found (below) when a child with Bruton's disease is similarly challenged.

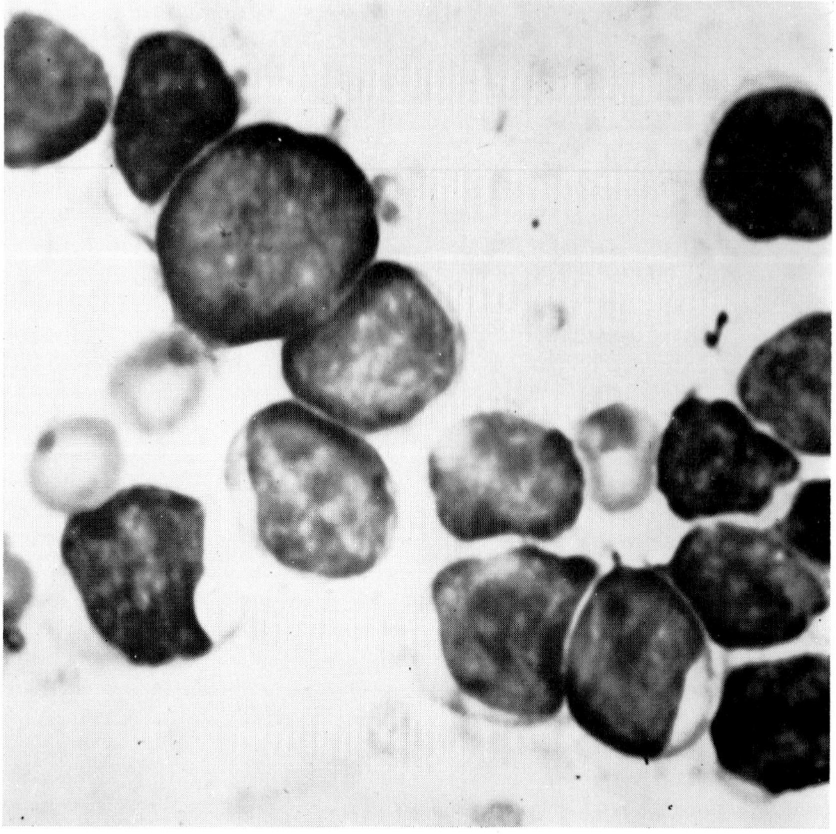

eralized skin rash—signs of an acute fulminating graft-vs-host reaction. This experience, disappointing as it was, proved valuable in the later development of what we now refer to as "cellular engineering" techniques for immunologic diseases incompatible with life. The reader is again referred to Chapter 23 for one development of these concepts.

Evidence is growing that basic defects of the immune system underlie many other conditions. Defects of immune function have long been regarded as factors in the etiology of such autoimmune diseases as rheumatoid arthritis, which is characterized by the frequent presence in the serum of a macroglobulin antibody, the "rheumatoid factor," directed against the patient's own gamma globulin. And rheumatoid arthritis is often associated with agammaglobulinemia; its incidence is about 30 times higher among patients with Bruton's syndrome than among the general population, and it commonly occurs in primary "acquired" agammaglobulinemia, which most often develops in adult life. (The agammaglobulinemic patient we saw back in 1953 developed moderate-to-severe arthritic attacks.) The frequent occurrence of rheumatoid arthritis together with immunologic deficiencies, as well as the periods of high fever and leukocytosis experienced by some patients, seems to suggest that an infective agent may be present.

Morphologic abnormalities in the thymus and in other lymphoreticular tissues are also common in systemic lupus erythematosus (SLE), the prototype of all other autoimmune diseases. The serum of many SLE patients presents a dramatic example of a breakdown in the body's ability to distinguish "self" from "nonself," since their serum contains autoantibodies that react with almost every imaginable tissue. Furthermore, SLE and another autoimmune disease, myasthenia gravis, sometimes occur simultaneously. Another interesting correlation in this highly complex network of associations is that thymectomy sometimes brings about clinical improvement in myasthenia patients and even produces occasional cures. In addition, we have already mentioned the appearance of autoimmune diseases in neonatally thymectomized experimental animals. Rabbits have turned up with autoimmune hemolytic anemia and mice were observed by Marco DeVries in Holland and Yunis in our laboratories to develop hemolytic anemia and lupus-like lesions in the kidneys and blood vessels.

A further set of associations is of special interest in cancer research. Lymphoreticular malignancies, among the most common neoplastic diseases of man, often occur together with immunologic deficiency syndromes and autoimmune diseases—lymphatic leukemia, lymphosarcoma, Hodgkin's disease, and reticulum cell sarcoma being the morphologic types most frequently diagnosed. A form of acute lymphatic leukemia is a common cause of death among patients suffering from Bruton's syndrome, while many ataxia-telangiectasia patients die of lymphoreticular malignancies. It seems a reasonable hypothesis, then, that the same lymphoreticular cell defect that underlies the immunologic deficiencies predisposes the patient to lymphoreticular malignancies.

New knowledge concerning the two specialized types of lymphoid tissue found at least in higher animals may be useful in the study and classification of these neoplastic diseases. For example, in Hodgkin's disease there is an impairment of the mechanism for cellular hypersensitivity, the thymus-dependent system, while the immunoglobulin-producing system seems to be intact. On the other hand, in myeloma we may be seeing, in bold relief, evidence of disorders in the latter system. The immunoglobulin-producing system, incidentally, may also prove to be involved in benign follicular lymphoma.

The key to our concepts of the relationship between malignancies of the lymphoid system first came from experimental studies carried out in chickens by Raymond Peterson of our laboratories and Ben Burmester and his collaborators of East Lansing, Mich. These investigators showed that one virus-induced malignancy of the lymphoid system can be prevented by removal of the bursa of Fabricius but not by removal of the thymus. This lymphoid malignancy involves only the bursa-dependent lymphoid system and, as Peter Dent, Cooper, and the East Lansing group have now demonstrated, it first appears in the bursa. Jacob Furth and his associates had long ago shown that, in mice, lymphomatous diseases are dependent on the presence of a thymus, and Richard Siegler in Philadelphia, Henry Kaplan at Stanford, and Henry Rappaport in Chicago have found that at least some of them begin focally in the thymus. Thus in experimental animals malignancies of the lymphoid system were shown to involve either the thymus-dependent system or the bursa-dependent system and to start in the central organ of the system that is involved.

A good possibility exists that lymphoreticular malignancies, like immunologic deficiency diseases, will eventually be recognized as expressions of basic developmental flaws. One highly probable result of the deficiency diseases may be the continuing and persisting presence in lymphoid tissue of appreciable numbers of immature, relatively undifferentiated lymphocytes, and this is a most dangerous situation when the nature of the malignant process is considered. The fundamental idea is that four major factors must operate together for the initiation of lymphoreticular neoplasia: an oncogenic agent, probably a virus; genetic susceptibility, probably related to cell receptor sites; a population of immature cells that can be induced to proliferate and become malignant; an appropriate environment, often attributable to hormones.

What are we to make of all this? In a general way these and many other points serve to reinforce the concept that neoplastic and autoimmune phenomena may essentially be side effects of either induced or genetic abnormalities in the lymphoreticular system. Specifically, the abnormalities lie in the relationship between the thymus-dependent and immunoglobulin-producing systems. It is interesting, too, that the work that led to these concepts provided one more example of the unpredictability of research; certainly in the beginning we did not expect that studies of diseases of the immune system, diseases that generally appear early in life, would apply in a most important way to the understanding of widespread diseases that tend to appear later.

Moreover, there is a deep biologic significance in the notion that immune-system disorders may be at the root of certain types of cancer and such degenerative conditions as rheumatoid arthritis and other expressions of autoimmunity. What probably happens is that the immune system tends to become increasingly disorganized as we grow older, which makes some sense from an evolutionary point of view. After all, nature is not basically interested in individuals who have passed the age of maximum reproductive efficiency. The coming of language and brains capable of intricate learning and long memories, factors that helped make old people important as bearers of tradition, is a very recent development in evolution.

Therefore, involution of adaptive immunity is a kind of evolutionary hangover, a reminder of prehuman times, when natural rather than cultural selection was the main determinant of species survival. With this involution, the body in effect lowers its guard. It is no longer as competent as it once was in distinguishing friend from foe, in recognizing the normal cells of its own tissues. And one consequence may be the production of destructive autoantibodies and autoimmune syndromes. Malignancy may represent a related type of failure of lymphoid "policing" systems, because with the breakdown of recognition mechanisms, somatic variation is no longer under precise homeostatic control. Cancer or potential cancer probably arises in every one of us every day of our lives in the form of mutant cells. But they are promptly and effectively eliminated by lymphoid cells, which recognize the "foreignness" of the mutants and act accordingly. When the policing cells are defective, however, such mutants may gain a foothold.

I should like to emphasize that the central role of genetic and evolutionary factors does not in any way imply a negative attitude toward therapeutic possibilities. On the contrary, if our theories are correct there is all the more reason for optimism. Leukemia provides a case in point. For years it was thought that a major factor in this disease is an excessive and abnormal proliferation of leukocytes—this was the belief, that is, until some investigators had the audacity to check it. It then became evident that there is no excessive proliferation at all. To be sure, leukocyte counts increase. But this is not because certain controls are off, thus permitting a wild process of cell multiplication.

The real problem involves just the opposite effect, the arrest rather than the release of a process—specifically, an arrest in the normal development of lymphocytes, which, instead of maturing and dying and being disposed of, simply stop differentiating and tend to accumulate. This, of course, puts a new light on the observation that a large proportion of patients who have chronic lymphatic leukemia also have hypogammaglobulinemia. According to the old explanation based on the excessive proliferation idea, the overwhelming flood of rapidly multiplying cells squeezed out the plasma cells associated with the immunoglobulin - producing system. Today we believe antibody deficiencies reflect the same phenomenon that accounts for the leukemic state, an essential arrest or retardation of development.

So it appears that something is lacking, that missing factors may affect the process whereby lymphoid cells differentiate into cells specialized for adaptive immunity. We have already pointed to the possibility of isolating such factors, perhaps hormones and other inducing agents, in connection with the future treatment of immunologic deficiency diseases. Now it is clear that the very same therapeutic principle may apply to lymphoreticular malignancies and to autoimmune conditions. An analogous situation existed during the early 1920's with respect to pernicious anemia, which appeared to be just as malignant as acute lymphatic leukemia seems today. It was later recognized as a deficiency disease involving the arrested and abnormal development of erythrocytes in the bone marrow.

Animal experiments also furnish a basis for long-run optimism. To cite only one example, Perry Teague, working with Dr. George Friou, has been using mice of the so-called A strain to study factors affecting involution of the immune system. The animals spontaneously develop autoimmunity in their old age, including antinuclear antibody. Yunis has found that animals of this strain and four other Minnesota inbred strains, but not others, such as CBA, develop severe hemolytic anemia early in life and other evidence of the autoimmune process if their thymuses have been removed. But the appearance of autoimmune phenomena can be postponed by transplanting young lymphoid cells. Maybe we will be able to achieve indefinite postponement by successively transplanting fresh thymuses before the previous transplants involute. In other words, a young thymus in an old animal may make an immunologically young animal.

Such transplants are made possible only because this is a highly inbred strain, and that raises what has become the main obstacle confronting surgery today—the problem of transplant rejection. The rekindling of interest and use of Waksm. n's antilymphocytic serum in animals by Anthony Monaco and Paul Russell of Harvard, and now in man by Thomas Starzl of the University of Colorado School of Medicine, and by John Najarian and his Minnesota group, represents the latest effort to overcome homograft immunity, and results have been most encouraging. But I believe that we do not yet have the precision tools we need. We must look for agents that enable us to manipulate the thymus-dependent system primarily, the system involved in most homograft rejections. In some cases, though, such as the occasional very rapid rejection of renal grafts observed by David Hume at the Medical College of Virginia [see Chapter 19, "Organ Transplants and Immunity"], involvement of the immunoglobulin-producing system is also indicated. We must be able to temporarily suppress the lymphoid function and establish a specific negative adaptation, such as tolerance or immunologic paralysis or even immunologic enhancement.

A key problem is to learn how the system works at the molecular level. Immunologic recognition requires that information be transmitted, perhaps through the membranes to the nuclei of specialized lymphoid cells, and the information is somehow embodied in highly specific chemical structures. So we must, in effect, discover the nature of the fundamental biochemical language of recognition. Ultimately we may learn that it signals to and operates through the basepair language of DNA-RNA mechanisms—which in the last analysis represents the very basis of biologic individuality.

Chapter 2

Immunobiology of the Small Lymphocyte

JAMES L. GOWANS
Oxford University

Hematologists are familiar with the small lymphocyte as one of the white cells that circulate in the blood. It makes up about 20% of the blood leukocytes in man and variable proportions in other mammals. Small lymphocytes, however, are not restricted to the blood; they are the major cellular type in the lymph nodes, spleen, and Peyer's patches, and they are also distributed diffusely through other tissues, for example, bone marrow and intestinal submucosa. Taken in aggregate the small lymphocytes of an animal would add up to an organ of impressive size, and it was therefore rather surprising that until a few years ago ignorance of the function of the small lymphocyte was almost complete.

It is true that the cell has no striking morphological features. It measures about 8 μ across in fixed preparations, has very little cytoplasm, and in the electron microscope it can be seen to lack endoplasmic reticulum and a Golgi apparatus, structures normally associated with protein synthesis and secretion. It is unlike other leukocytes in that it is neither phagocytic nor chemotactic. Unlike large lymphocytes, small lymphocytes are not dividing when freshly isolated from blood or lymph, although, as we shall see later, they can be provoked to divide under special circumstances. Until a few years ago the only known activity of small lymphocytes was motility, and pathologists were fond of lamenting our ignorance of the function of these cells. Thus, the distinguished Johns Hopkins pathologist Arnold Rich described the small lymphocytes as "phlegmatic spectators watching the turbulent activities of the phagocytes."

Long before any precise knowledge of the function of small lymphocytes existed, their participation in various inflammatory and immunologic reactions had been suspected from their abundance in chronic inflammatory lesions such as those of syphilis and tuberculosis, in the tuberculin reaction, and in the stroma of certain tumors. Recent knowledge owes much to the advent of such modern techniques as radioactive tagging and analysis of chromosome patterns, as well as to the rapid development of the fields of transplantation immunology and radiobiology.

The lack of experimental techniques did not prevent classical hematologists from proposing a wide variety of theories about the fate and function of small lymphocytes. Most of these theories suggested that small lymphocytes did not themselves perform physiologically but that they served as precursors of other cell types. The older literature is filled with controversies as to whether small lymphocytes can give rise to erythrocytes, granulocytes, monocytes, fibroblasts, plasma cells, and so on. In fact, a cynic once remarked that every cell in the human body outside the nervous system has at some time or other been credited with lymphocytic ancestry!

Our own studies began with an effort to solve one of the most striking problems posed by the small lymphocyte. It is known that lymphocytes enter the blood by way of the major lymphatic trunks in the neck; indeed, Blalock suggested that lymphocytes probably enter the blood exclusively by this route, since if the big lymphatic trunks are occluded the blood lymphocyte level falls to virtually zero. The striking fact about the flow of lymphocytes from the lymphatic trunks is the number of cells involved. It has long been known that the number of lymphocytes entering the blood by way of the main lymphatic vessels was sufficient to replace all those in the circulating blood several times daily. This is true of all the mammals investigated so far, including man, with the curious exception of the pig. The problem can be highlighted by refer-

The Recirculation of Small Lymphocytes

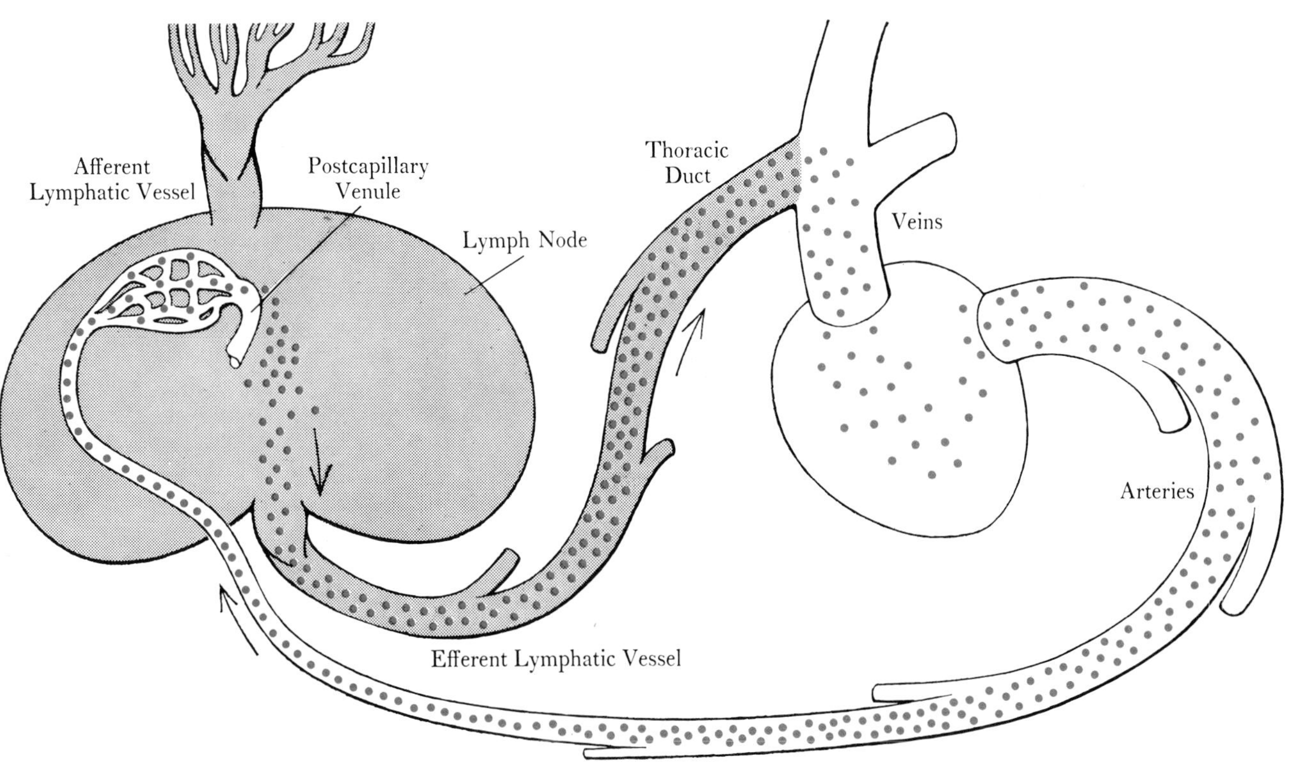

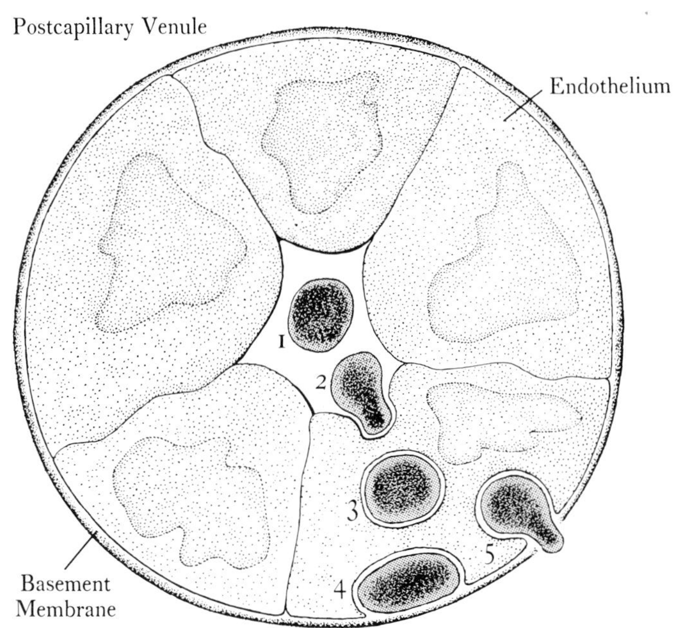

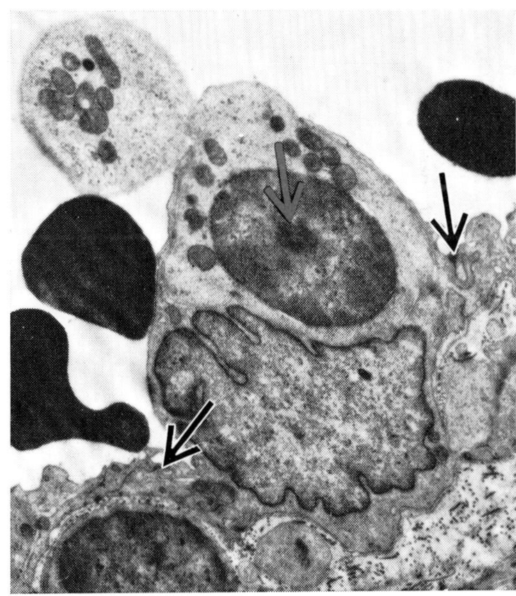

The pathway of small lymphocyte recirculation is represented in the schematic drawing above. Starting within the lymph node the lymphocytes pass through the substance of the node by a route still to be defined. They leave the node via an efferent lymphatic that leads into one of the major lymphatic vessels, exemplified in this case by the thoracic duct. From there they are tipped into the blood circulation through the veins in the neck region. The short residence time of the cells in the bloodstream is completed as they enter the arterial circulation and are carried back to the lymphoid tissue. All lymphoid structures except the thymus appear to be on this recirculation route. In the detail drawing (bottom) the structure of the postcapillary venule, with its high-walled endothelium, is depicted. The unique passage of the lymphocytes directly through the endothelial cytoplasm is shown. The lymphocyte starts in the lumen of the venule, invaginates the endothelial cell, enters the cytoplasm and then comes out at the basement membrane. Here it is briefly held back by the connective tissue bed on which the venule rests and it then enters into the substance of the node. The EM (15,800x) shows the lymphocyte (red arrow) partially enclosed in the cell cytoplasm, while the cellular junctions (black arrows) remain intact. A second small lymphocyte is seen at top left.

ence to the rat. In the rat it is simple to cannulate the major lymphatic vessel, the thoracic duct, with a fine plastic cannula and to collect lymph and lymphocytes over a period of days without an anesthetic. During the first 24 hours after cannulation, about 10^9 cells can be collected from the duct.

Since the number of lymphocytes in the blood remains more or less constant it is necessary to account for the disappearance of this huge number of cells. We studied this problem by removing small lymphocytes from the thoracic ducts of rats, labeling them with a radioactive tag, and then determining their fate by autoradiography after their reintroduction into the animal or into other animals of the same inbred strain. We hoped by this means to obtain important clues to their function. But we were disappointed. We found that the lymphocytes that were infused into the blood could be recovered in large numbers from the thoracic duct lymph. In other words, the cells had no particular fate but recirculated continuously from the blood into the lymph and thence back into the blood. The autoradiographic study showed that the route from blood to lymph lay in the lymph nodes and Peyer's patches and that, perhaps not surprisingly, the lymphocytes "homed" accurately into all those areas of the animal's lymphoid tissue that are normally occupied by small lymphocytes. Thus, they were identified in high concentration in the cortex of all the lymph nodes and in the white pulp of the spleen. However, they did not enter the thymus.

A recirculation of lymphocytes explains not only the high output of cells from the lymph ducts but is consistent with recent observations suggesting that the great majority of small lymphocytes in the lymph have an extremely long life span. At one time, because of the rapid cell turnover in the blood and because of the difficulty of keeping lymphocytes alive in vitro, it was widely thought that their life span could be measured in hours. However, with the development of methods for following the incorporation and persistence of radioactive labels in DNA our concepts of lymphocyte life span have been radically altered. Ottesen in Denmark was the first to show that labeled DNA persists in blood lymphocytes for a considerable period; indeed, the decay curves of radioactivity suggest that some of the cells live for more than a year in man. This work was extended in experimental animals by a number of workers, among them Brecher at NIH and Everett at the University of Washington. Both these investigators noted a biphasic curve of declining radioactivity in small lymphocytes tagged with tritiated thymidine. At first the decline in radioactivity is steep, but it then levels off and the remainder of the loss occurs over a prolonged period. From this it was deduced that the small lymphocyte population is actually heterogeneous and includes both short-lived and long-lived cells. In the rat the long-lived small lymphocytes, with life spans of a year or more, make up about 90% of the small lymphocytes emerging from the lymphatic ducts. The short-lived cells, which disappear after a week or two, are relatively more frequent in blood and spleen.

It is not known what the relationship is – in terms of function or origin – between these two, or possibly more, classes of small lymphocytes in the blood and lymph. The possibility that the two types play different roles in immunologic processes is currently being investigated by a number of workers. Before we leave the subject of lymphocyte life span we must mention some indirect but striking evidence that small lymphocytes in man may actually survive for more than a decade. The evidence rests on the discovery by Nowell in Philadelphia that blood leukocytes will divide in vitro when they are incubated in a bean extract, phytohemagglutinin. It was later shown by Brecher and by Roberts in London that the cell in blood which was stimulated to divide was a small lymphocyte. Roberts actually isolated single small lymphocytes and filmed them at all stages of their enlargement and division. The use of phytohemagglutinin enables the pattern of the chromosomes of lymphocytes to be observed, and the technique was applied by investigators in

Sensitization to Homografts

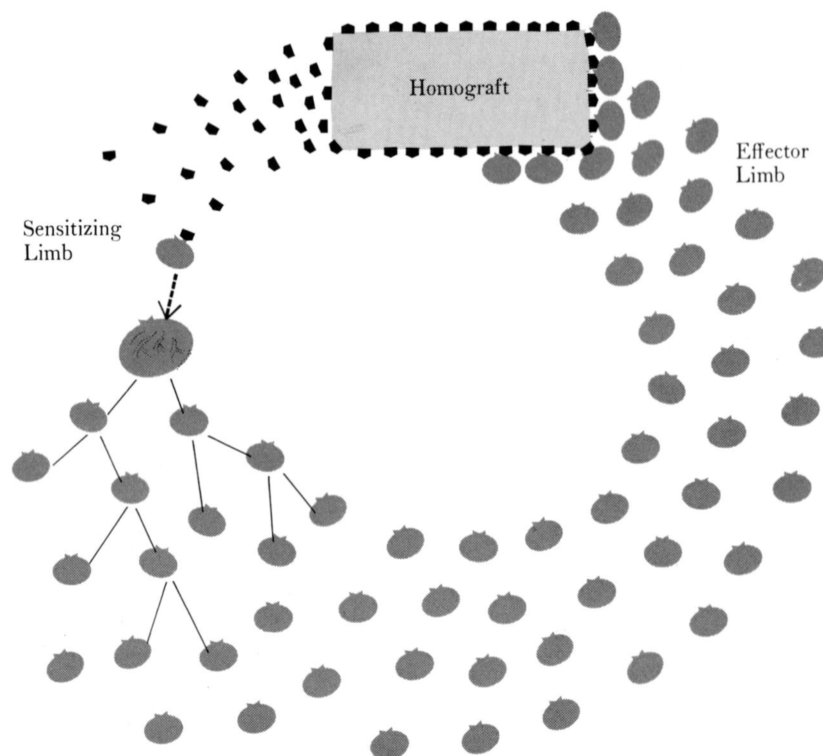

In the homograft reaction, sensitization may take place peripherally in the tissues. Antigen from the graft interacts with small lymphocytes that are thought to carry specific receptors on their surfaces. This interaction causes the small lymphocytes to grow and divide, so that the number of specifically instructed lymphocytes is increased and the effector mechanism of rejection is primed. Antibody-bearing lymphocytes then enter the graft and destroy it, possibly with the assistance of macrophages.

Edinburgh to the study of patients who 10 to 15 years before had received therapeutic x-irradiation for ankylosing spondylitis. It was observed that the karyotypes of some of these patients were grossly abnormal. In fact, some of the chromosomal abnormalities were so severe that it could be inferred that the lymphocytes were entering their first division since x-irradiation 10 years previously.

Having characterized a large population of long-lived small lymphocytes that divide their time between the blood and lymph circulatory systems, the next problem was to pinpoint the exact anatomical route followed by the cells in passing from one circulation to another. We have already mentioned that the small lymphocytes enter the bloodstream from the lymphatic vessels. There is no good evidence that lymphocytes pass directly from lymphoid tissue into the blood except in the spleen. This is a natural exception, of course, since the spleen is, in effect, a large lymph node positioned on the blood circulation and it is percolated by blood rather than by lymph. The exact way in which cells gain entrance into the lymphatics is not clear but they must somehow migrate across the lining wall of the lymphatic sinuses. The passage from blood back into the lymph nodes is more thoroughly understood, and here the key structures are small vessels called postcapillary venules. This is a somewhat overelaborate designation since almost all venules are necessarily "postcapillary." However, it is the name applied by the histologists who first described these structures and it has persisted. The unusual feature of these venules is a high-walled endothelium, which gives them a glandular appearance when the lumen is empty and the opposing walls are touching. When radioactively labeled small lymphocytes are infused into the blood they can be detected after a few minutes in the walls of the postcapillary venules. They can then be followed as they pass through the walls and accumulate under the endothelium. Here they appear to be held back temporarily by the periendothelial connective tissue before they finally enter the substance of the lymph node in the mid- and deep cortical regions. The areas in the spleen and lymph nodes through which lymphocytes recirculate are those areas that remain atrophic in animals thymectomized around the time of birth. This observation is part of the considerable body of evidence that suggests that the long-lived, recirculating lymphocytes originate in the thymus.

An electron microscope study by Marchesi and the author has emphasized the uniqueness of small lymphocytes' transit through the postcapillary venules. They pass through the endothelium not by prizing open the intercellular junctions as do other leukocytes in venules elsewhere, but by invaginating endothelial cells on one side, entering and traversing the cytoplasm, and emerging from the endothelial cell on the other. This strange phenomenon suggests that some type of structural complementarity exists at the molecular level between the lymphocyte and the endothelial cell. The nature of this relationship is not now known, but Gesner at New York University produced some evidence that sugar groupings on the lymphocyte surface may be involved. The possibility that some important transaction takes place between the lymphocyte and the endothelial cell during the intracellular phase must not be ignored.

There is now good evidence for the existence of lymphocyte recirculation in species other than the rat, for example, in mice, sheep, and calves. However, although recirculation explains the high output of lymphocytes from the lymphatic ducts, we do not yet know what proportion of an animal's total lymphocyte population recirculates and what proportion remains permanently or temporarily fixed in lymphoid tissue. And there is little information about the regulation of this process. Hall at Cambridge, England, has shown that in sheep there is a transient shutdown in the exit of lymphocytes from the efferent lymphatic vessel following the injection of antigen into the leg. It has been suggested that the lymphocytosis that occurs following injection of pertussis vaccine may be due to a dis-

The Kinetics of Sensitization

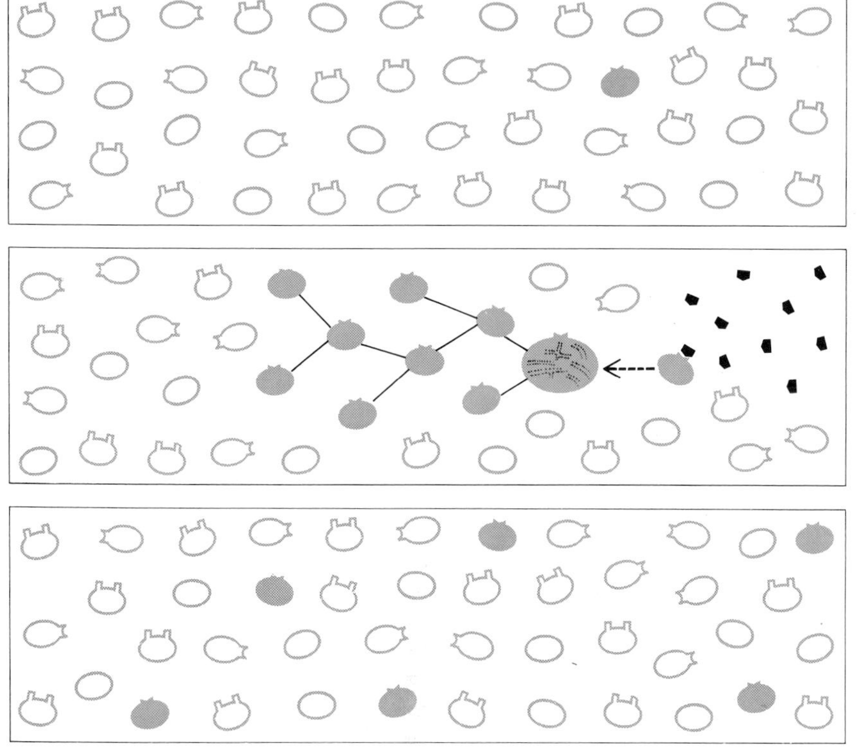

Rejection cycle shown on facing page has led some investigators to suggest that the "naive" or nonsensitized small lymphocytes (top panel) are qualitatively identical with sensitized lymphocytes. What changes after sensitization is the concentration of cells bearing specific antibody (bottom panel), resulting from the division following interaction between antigen and the appropriate small lymphocyte (center panel).

turbance in the mechanisms regulating recirculation, and it is also possible that the lymphopenia induced by small doses of corticosteroids may have a similar basis.

What then is the functional significance of small lymphocyte recirculation? Ideas on this must rest on what is known about the function of small lymphocytes, to be discussed later.

Heterogeneity of Lymphocytes

We have defined the small lymphocyte in the terms used by hematologists, that is, as a small cell with a densely staining nucleus and scanty cytoplasm when observed in smears of blood or lymph. It is now becoming clear that cells with this gross appearance make up a heterogeneous collection with respect to their life span and also with respect to their origin and function. We have already discussed the short- and long-lived small lymphocytes that are present in the blood and lymph. The small lymphocytes in bone marrow are almost certainly a distinct population, formed continuously and rapidly in the bone marrow and having functions different from small lymphocytes in lymph and lymphoid tissue. Hints that further subclasses of "small round cells" may exist are emerging from current studies on the origin of macrophages and fibroblasts, though matters here are still of a controversial nature.

The complexity of the subject is illustrated by some recent studies on the origin of macrophages. For example, Volkman and the author showed that macrophages that emigrate onto glass coverslips placed on or under the skin of rats arise from a rapidly dividing precursor in the bone marrow; no evidence could be obtained that such cells originate from lymphocytes in the lymph or in lymphoid tissue. On the other hand, studies by Howard in Edinburgh suggest that lymphocytes may sometimes give rise to large phagocytic cells.

Howard studied the origin of Kupffer cells in the liver in two experimental situations. In one, large numbers of new Kupffer cells arose in the livers of mice that were undergoing a graft-vs-host reaction as a consequence of an injection of foreign thoracic duct lymphocytes. By employing a chromosome marker that was present in the donor but not present in the tissues of the host animal, it was shown that the new Kupffer cells unequivocally had a donor origin. However, there is still another way of inducing formation of new Kupffer cells. This is by removing part of the liver, which is followed by rapid compensatory regeneration of the remaining portion. When mice treated this way were given injections of chromosome-marked bone marrow cells and lymphocytes it was found that the new Kupffer cells had taken origin from the bone marrow and not from lymphocytes. Howard's experiments make out a case for a lymphocytic origin of Kupffer cells in certain special circumstances. However, the case is not proved because rare, dividing macrophages, possibly from the peritoneal cavity, may have contaminated the donors' thoracic duct lymph.

We have already mentioned that the long-lived, recirculating lymphocytes probably arise in the thymus. After a heavy dose of x-irradiation the lymphoid tissue and circulating lymphocytes can be restored to normal by injecting suspensions of bone marrow cells, and workers at Harwell, employing chromosome markers, have shown that as such animals recover, their thymus glands and their nodes become filled with cells of marrow origin. Thus, the "thymus-derived" cells are, in fact, derived ultimately from the bone marrow. A second variety of small lymphocyte in normal lymphoid tissue is thought to come directly from the bone marrow without undergoing a period of development in the thymus. The relation, if any, between these "marrow-derived" lymphocytes and the small lymphocytes that can be identified in histologic preparations of bone marrow is not known; nor is anything known about the origin and function of the short-lived small lymphocytes. We shall return to the problem of thymus- and marrow-derived lymphocytes when discussing the cellular basis of immune reactions.

Function of Lymphocytes

The reaction to foreign tissue grafts: Chronologically the first link in the chain of evidence implicating the small lymphocyte in rejection of solid tissue homografts was the discovery by Simonsen in Denmark and Billingham, now at the University of Pennsylvania, that if animals are injected with foreign lymphoid cells they will under certain circumstances waste and die. The circumstances under which such graft-vs-host reactions can be initiated amount to a list of the different conditions under which animals will accept a graft of foreign tissue, i.e., newborn mice or rats which have not yet developed their immunologic rejection capacity, heavily irradiated animals, or animals of a particular genetic constitution.

When members of two different inbred strains of rats or mice are mated it is found that the progeny, the F_1

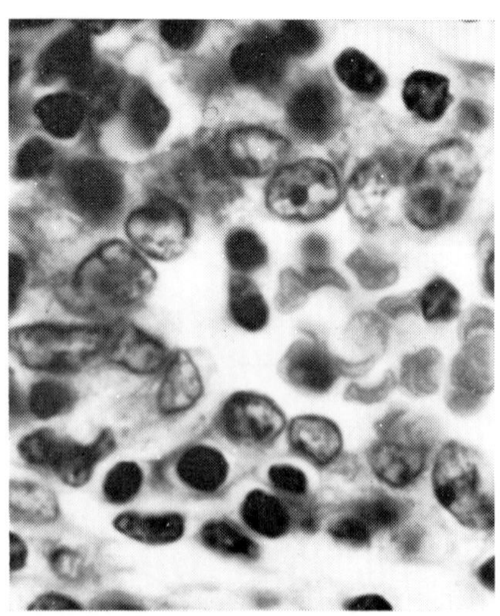

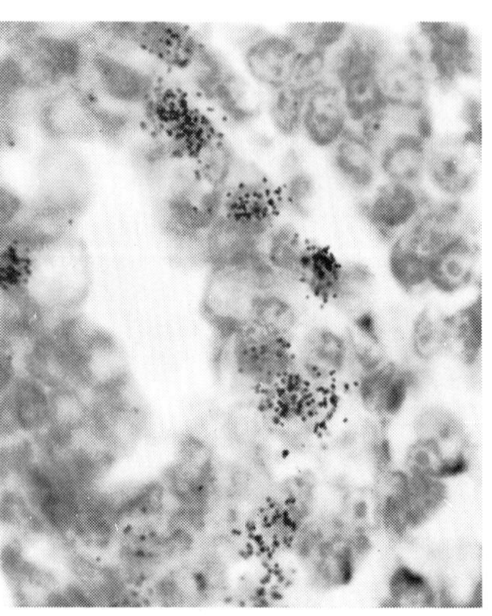

Postcapillary venules are shown in both photos. On left is venule in rat lymph node. Lumen is lined by endothelial cells with large, pale nuclei; many small lymphocytes are under endothelium. On right, venule is seen 15 minutes after transfusion of labeled lymphocytes which are in endothelium but have not yet penetrated node.

Genetic Demonstration of Graft-vs-Host Reactions

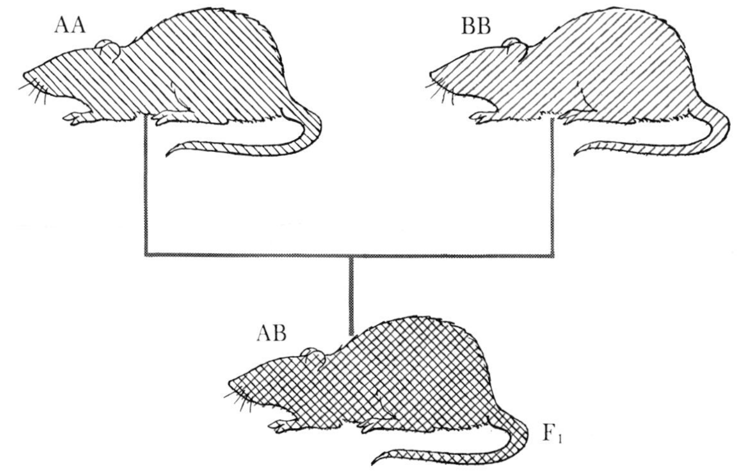

A genetic technique for demonstrating the role of the small lymphocyte in graft-vs-host reactions is shown. When two inbred rat strains (AA and BB) are crossed, the F_1 hybrid offspring will accept small lymphocytes from either of the parent strains. But the accepted cells will then mount an attack on the host tissues that bear antigenic determinants from the other parent. The wasting syndrome and death will result. The specificity of this reaction is demonstrated by using as the lymphocyte donor an animal made tolerant to the cells of the other strain. Now the lymphocyte injection will be accepted without any immunologic reaction taking place.

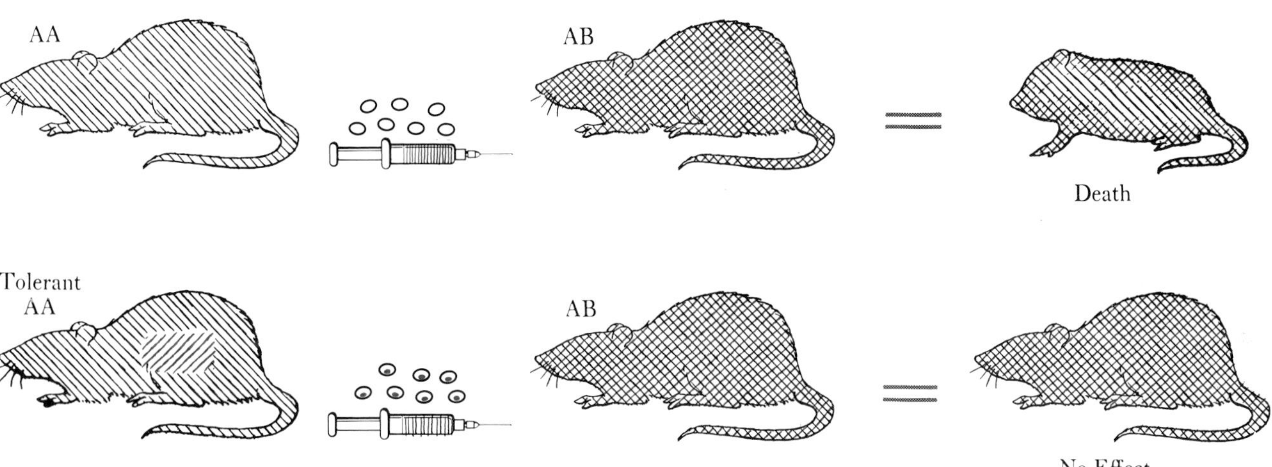

hybrid generation, will accept grafts of tissue from either parental strain. The grafts are accepted because the F_1 hybrid recipients possess all the antigens of both parents, and the grafts will not be recognized as foreign. Thus if lymphoid cells from one parent are injected into F_1 hybrids they will be accepted, but they are confronted in the tissues of the host with the antigens inherited from the other parent and proceed to mount a graft-vs-host reaction against them. In effect, as Simonsen and Billingham demonstrated, the roles of graft and host become reversed. The whole animal becomes the graft. It is attacked by the parental lymphocytes and "rejected," that is, killed.

Billingham and Medawar showed that cells capable of causing graft-vs-host reactions are present in the peripheral blood of mice. Working separately but more or less simultaneously, Billingham, Hildemann at the University of California, and our group pinned responsibility to the small lymphocyte. In our laboratory, for example, this was done by cannulating the thoracic duct of rats, drawing off lymphocytes, and then eliminating the large dividing cells in the lymph so that what remained was essentially a population of small lymphocytes. When such parental-strain small lymphocytes were injected into normal adult F_1 hybrid rats a vicious graft-vs-host reaction occurred and the animals wasted and died. There is only one interpretation of this experiment: The small lymphocyte reacts with the foreign antigens in the host and initiates an immunologic response against them. It can be shown that the antigens involved are the histocompatibility antigens, since no disease is caused by lymphocytes from an animal rendered immunologically tolerant of the recipient's antigens. Thus, a convincing argument can be built up that small lymphocytes are not only responsible for graft-vs-host reactions but that they also initiate the reaction of animals against foreign grafts such as skin and kidneys. Small lymphocytes recognize the foreign antigens and initiate processes leading to rejection.

There is some evidence that the interaction of small lymphocytes with graft antigens occurs not centrally in the regional lymph nodes but peripherally within the graft itself. The experimental evidence was obtained by Strober in the author's laboratory in investigations in which lymphocytes were perfused through isolated foreign kidneys. When such lymphocytes were injected back into the animal that had provided them, the animal was found to possess a heightened reactivity against skin grafts taken from the kidney donor. In other words, the lymphocytes had been triggered during their passage through the isolated kidney, and the animal into which they were returned behaved as if it itself had been sensitized with a graft. It is not known whether this process of peripheral sensitization is important for all kinds of grafts; indeed, Billingham has some evidence that it may not be important in skin grafts. But when the graft is a large organ with a large blood supply the opportunities for contact between circulating lymphocytes and graft antigens may be so great that effective sensitization may occur peripherally.

The way in which lymphocytes recognize foreign antigens is not known, but the most popular idea is that it depends upon specific receptors on the lymphocyte surface. Since the only agent known to combine with antigen is antibody, the assumption is that the receptor is a special kind of specific antibody on or in the surface of the cell. Following the clonal selection views of Burnet, one might expect almost as many different lymphocytes as there are antigens, assuming one specificity per lymphocyte.

The immunologic response to foreign grafts may conveniently be considered to possess two limbs: the afferent, or sensitizing, limb and the efferent, or effector, limb. We have considered the sensitizing limb but have said nothing about the way in which the graft is actually destroyed. A further piece of evidence, obtained from studies on graft-vs-host reactions, can now be considered. By following the fate of small lymphocytes in F_1 hybrid rats it was shown that a proportion of them enlarged and started dividing. Further analysis showed that the dividing cells produced lymphocytes of progressively decreasing size, ending with small lymphocytes. These dividing cells have strongly pyroninophilic cytoplasm and one or two prominent nucleoli, and they are also found in the regional lymph nodes of animals rejecting foreign skin grafts. A simple hypothesis is that these new lymphocytes constitute the efferent, or effector, limb of the response and that they emigrate from the regional node, circulate in the blood, invade the graft, and in some unknown way destroy it. John David has shown that when sensitized lymphocytes interact with antigen they liberate a substance that immobilizes macrophages [see Chapter 15, "The Lymphocytic Factors"]. The individual components of the cellular infiltrate in homografts undergoing rejection are very difficult to identify, but they are usually thought to include both lymphocytes and macrophages. It seems plausible to suggest that the new lymphocytes which were formed in the regional node and which invade the foreign graft initiate the rejection mechanism. This may then be aided and abetted by macrophages recruited into the tissue by the kind of mechanism David described. Other activities have recently been identified in supernatants from suspensions of sensitized lymphocytes exposed in vitro to the specific antigen. These include a factor that will kill some varieties of mammalian cells in vitro (lymphotoxin), a chemotactic factor, a factor inducing mitosis in other lymphocytes, and another that increases the permeability of skin blood vessels. Much work will be needed to establish whether these factors have importance in vivo as mediators of delayed hypersensitivity or graft destruction. Finally, it should be emphasized that

Small Lymphocytes and Immunologic Memory

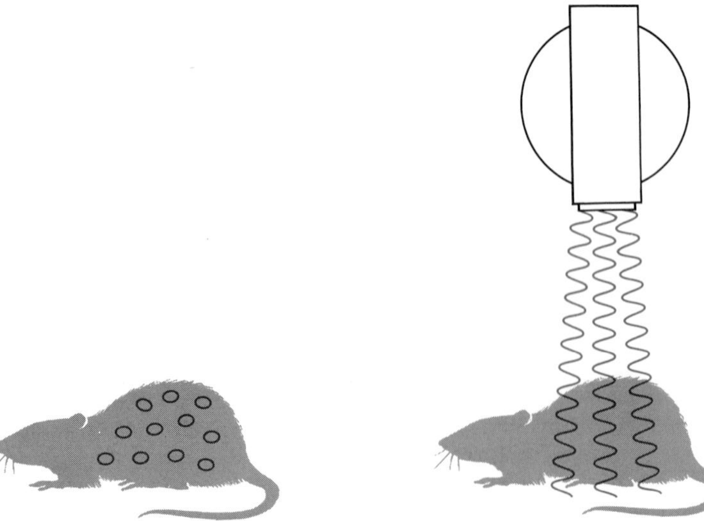

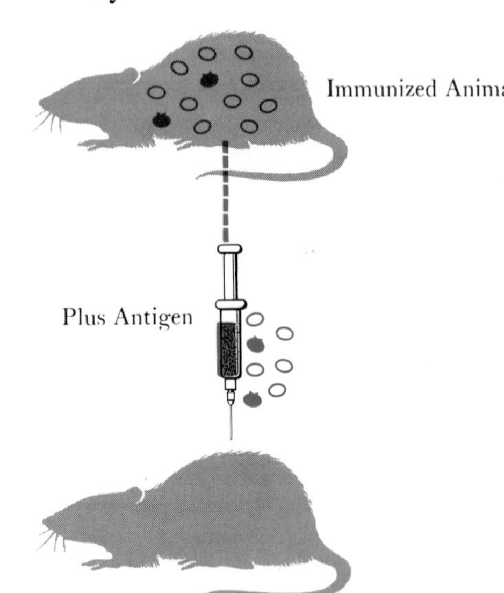

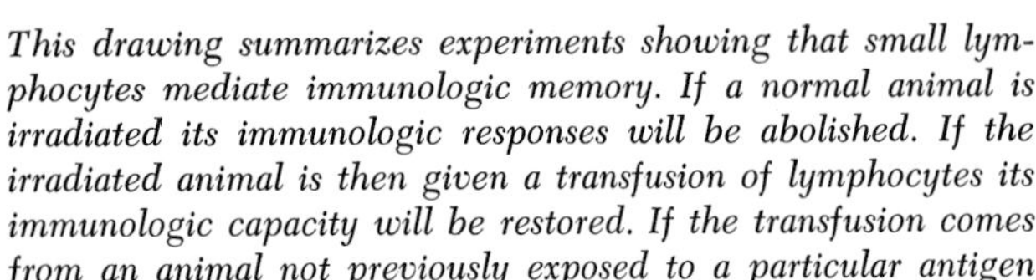

This drawing summarizes experiments showing that small lymphocytes mediate immunologic memory. If a normal animal is irradiated its immunologic responses will be abolished. If the irradiated animal is then given a transfusion of lymphocytes its immunologic capacity will be restored. If the transfusion comes from an animal not previously exposed to a particular antigen the animal will react to the antigen on a primary response level. But if an immunized animal is used as the source of restorative lymphocytes (as in drawing) the previously nonimmunized recipient reacts in a secondary manner. The transferred memory cells (shaded) provide the precursors of the antibody-forming cells that develop in the irradiated recipient.

the precise mechanism of tissue destruction in homograft reactions varies depending upon the nature of the target organ. Gorer pointed out many years ago that homografts form a spectrum from dissociated target cells (for example, bone marrow or lymphoid cells), which can be destroyed by circulating antibody to solid grafts with a stroma and a blood supply into which antibodies penetrate with great difficulty and where the destruction is initiated by infiltrating lymphocytes.

The antigen-triggered enlargement and division of small lymphocytes to produce more small lymphocytes raises the question of whether the original and new small lymphocytes differ in any way. Medawar suggested that they may not and that immunization consists simply of the generation of more cells with the same specificity. Thus the nonimmune animal is assumed to possess lymphocytes that are capable of recognizing the homograft but are too few in number to destroy it. Antigen stimulates these lymphocytes to divide until sufficient numbers are available to destroy the graft. Consequently there may be no difference between the "naive" cell and the "sensitized" cell in transplantation reactions; there may simply be a shift in the proportion of a particular kind of lymphocyte. On the other hand, some believe that lymphocytes from sensitized animals acquire new properties as they develop from their precursors in the naive animal. It will be clear that much remains to be learned about the mechanism of the homograft reaction.

The homograft reaction is, of course, a matter of great practical importance since it places a barrier to the free and successful transplantation of organs and tissues between human individuals. From a theoretical point of view, however, the fact that small lymphocytes initiate homotransplantation reactions does not really illuminate their function. Grafting, after all, is not a normal biologic hazard. Thomas at New York University was the first to suggest that the homograft reaction might normally function as a surveillance mechanism for destroying cells carrying antigenic mistakes and that it might consequently provide a defense against tumors in those cases where the tumor cells carried new antigens. There is some evidence for Thomas' intriguing idea. For example, there is an increased incidence of experimental and spontaneous tumors in animals thymectomized at birth or treated for prolonged periods with antilymphocytic serum and in human patients receiving immunosuppressive drugs or suffering from certain immunologic deficiency diseases.

Antibody Formation

Up to this point we have been considering the role of small lymphocytes in immunologic mechanisms whose effector limb is thought to involve the activity of cell-bound antibodies. Classical circulating antibody is synthesized mainly by plasma cells, which possess a well-developed endoplasmic reticulum and are quite unlike small lymphocytes morphologically. Is there any evidence that small lymphocytes may be involved in the inductive processes leading to antibody formation in the same way as they are involved in the initiation of homotransplantation reactions?

The first point to make is that an animal depleted of small lymphocytes by chronic drainage of cells from a thoracic duct fistula loses much of its ability to respond to a first injection of certain antigens, for example, tetanus toxoid or sheep erythrocytes. But if immunized animals are depleted of lymphocytes the secondary response is relatively unaffected. This suggests that the primary antibody response may involve the activity of small lymphocytes and that secondary responsiveness can be mediated by a system of fixed cells in lymphoid tissue which cannot be withdrawn from the animal by thoracic duct drainage.

Further support for the idea that small lymphocytes play a part in humoral antibody responses comes from two simple experiments involving rats immunologically crippled by a high dose of x-irradiation. One set of experiments showed that the ability of such rats to make antibody against sheep erythrocytes can be restored very efficiently simply by injecting small lymphocytes from normal, nonimmune, donors. Moreover, if the small lymphocytes are derived from a donor made immunologically tolerant of sheep erythrocytes, then no restoration is achieved in the irradiated recipient. These findings argue rather strongly that the small lymphocyte may initiate the antibody response against sheep erythrocytes, presumably by interacting with the antigen or with antigen that has been "processed" by macrophages.

The second experiment was conducted in precisely the same manner as the first except that the small lymphocytes were obtained from immunized donors. After cell transfer, the irradiated recipients were able to respond to their first injection of antigen in a typical secondary manner. Secondary responsiveness to bacteriophage ϕX174, to tetanus toxoid, and to hapten-protein conjugates has been conferred on heavily irradiated rats in this way. The small lymphocytes transferred the faculty of "immunologic memory."

There seems little doubt that small lymphocytes can restore either primary or secondary responsiveness to a variety of antigens in irradiated animals when the donors are either normal or immune respectively. Further, it has been shown in the experiments with rats that the antibody-forming cells that develop in the irradiated hosts are the descendants of the injected small lymphocytes. These experiments lead to a simple view of the cellular basis of antibody formation: The antigen stimulates certain small lymphocytes that enlarge, divide, and differentiate to form antibody-secreting plasma cells. This is probably an oversimplified view. Miller in Melbourne, who has been responsible for most of our current knowledge of the function of the thymus, has shown that the induction of antibody formation to sheep erythrocytes in mice involves collaboration between two different kinds of lymphocytes, one derived from the thymus and the other derived from the bone marrow; it is the latter that develops into the antibody-forming cell.

It has been suggested that certain antigens may become attached by one of their determinants to the surface of thymus-derived lymphocytes, allowing another determinant to be presented to the bone marrow lymphocytes. The idea is that thymus-derived lymphocytes may concentrate antigen on their surface and present the relevant antigenic determinants to the bone marrow lymphocytes. This notion does not explain why lymphocytes should like having antigen presented to them on other lymphocytes; nor is it claimed that all antibody responses involve a collaboration of this kind. In the context of the experiments with rats all that can be said is that if the responses in the irradiated recipients involve cellular collaboration then the collaborating partners are both small lymphocytes and are both present in the thoracic duct lymph. The problem of cellular interactions in the immune response is of very considerable interest but there are, as yet, too few solid facts for generalizations to be made.

It will be noted that two cellular mechanisms have been proposed to explain secondary immune responsiveness in animals. One involves cells in lymphoid tissue that were not depleted by thoracic duct drainage, the other, recirculating small lymphocytes. These are not mutually exclusive mechanisms. The fixed cells may comprise the dividing elements in germinal centers, which many workers believe give rise to plasma cells after secondary antigen stimulation, or they may be nonrecirculating small lymphocytes.

The lymphocytes that initiate the reactions of delayed hypersensitivity and graft rejection are thought to be derived from the thymus. We have already noted that the lymphocytes giving rise to plasma cells are derived from the bone marrow and that under certain circumstances the thymus-derived lymphocytes may collaborate with them during the induction of antibody formation. The idea that lymphocytes of different origin mediate these two broad categories of immunologic response has been put forward by Good at the University of Minnesota on the basis of observations on human immune deficiency states and of experiments in birds that showed the homograft reaction depends upon the presence of the thymus, while the ability to make antibodies depends upon a lymphoid organ associated with the hind end of the gut called the bursa of Fabricius.

While there is no good evidence in mammals for an equivalent of the avian bursa, the current view is that all lymphocytes in mammalian lymph nodes and spleen have a remote origin in the bone marrow: Those that have undergone an intermediate cycle of proliferation in the thymus mediate the "cellular" immunities, while those that seed directly into lymphoid tissue probably provide the precursors of antibody-forming cells. It is quite unclear whether there are two different lymphoid precursors in the bone marrow or only one whose final activity is determined by the chance of whether it settles first in the thymus or in peripheral lymphoid tissue. So although it may be possible to prepare, for example, from thoracic duct lymph, suspensions of "pure" small lymphocytes in the sense of the classical hematologist, there is little doubt that such small lymphocytes are, in reality, a heterogeneous collection of cells with respect to origin and immunologic activity.

Having considered the evidence that small lymphocytes can initiate immunological responses we may now return to the problem of the functional significance of lymphocyte recirculation. One obvious possibility arises if one accepts Burnet's idea that the extraordinarily wide repertoire of immunological response is underwritten genetically. If each small lymphocyte is genetically restricted to respond to one or only a few specific antigens then the problem facing an animal is to muster at any particular regional site as many of the appropriate lymphocytes as possible. The same sort of argument could be applied to the secondary immune response. Lymphocyte recirculation could serve this requirement admirably. There is a scattered distribution of lymph nodes linked by a large pool of lymphocytes recirculating continuously among them. Thus if an antigen gained access to the arm, all the recirculating lymphocytes in the body would have an opportunity to confront the antigen, and not just those within the regional node in the armpit. A second possibility turns on the idea that if too much antigen reaches a lymph node it may paralyze the lymphocytes rather than stimulate them into immunological activity. Thus the first lymphocytes to confront the antigen will not respond. But if these are continuously replaced by a recirculating population, other lymphocytes will be stimulated after the antigenic concentration has fallen to nonparalyzing levels.

A final suggestion concerns an area of cellular immunology which is outside the province of this article — the possible immunological role of macrophages in the earliest stages of antibody formation. If the processing of antigens by macrophages is an essential preliminary to the induction of antibody formation then any mechanism that increases the number of contacts between macrophages and lymphocytes would be expected to enhance the efficiency of the immune response.

There is no decisive evidence for any of the three possibilities just outlined, but some recent work by Ford in our laboratory has shown that the efficiency of an antibody response by the isolated, perfused spleen is greatly enhanced if lymphocytes are present in the perfusate. In other words, the spleen's own lymphocytes are not sufficient to enable it to mount a maximal antibody response, but if a traffic of lymphocytes is passing through the spleen much more antibody is made.

Although a considerable amount of knowledge has accumulated about the activities of small lymphocytes since the days when they were described as "phlegmatic spectators of inflammatory reactions," many of the ideas about lymphocyte activity are still speculative and there is still much to be learned. But clinical practice is not waiting for the gaps in knowledge to be filled. This is shown by the widespread interest in the use of antilymphocytic serum (ALS) as an immunosuppressive agent. The current interest in ALS stems from work by Woodruff in Edinburgh, who first showed that ALS was effective in prolonging the survival of homografts in experimental animals. Antilymphotic serum is the subject of another chapter in this book [Chapter 25, "Antilymphocytic Serum: Its Properties and Potential," Eugene M. Lance and Peter B. Medawar] so it will not be discussed at any length here.

There is a strong suggestion that ALS is much more effective in suppressing homograft reactions than reactions involving the synthesis of circulating antibody. Medawar has suggested that this is because both the afferent and efferent arcs of the homograft reaction are mediated by circulating lymphocytes particularly susceptible to the action of injected ALS. However, it is somewhat paradoxical that the degree of immunosuppression brought about by ALS does not seem to be related in any simple way to the degree of lymphopenia that it produces. Indeed, an equally severe depletion of recirculating lymphocytes can be achieved by other measures, for example by chronic drainage from the thoracic duct or by irradiating lymphocytes as they circulate through the blood, and yet the resulting immunosuppression is less than that given by ALS. ALS certainly depletes the pool of recirculating lymphocytes, but it must have additional effects that account for its dramatic activity in prolonging the survival of homografts.

These uncertainties once again emphasize that cellular immunology is likely to provide a rewarding field for study for many years to come.

Chapter 3

Delayed Hypersensitivity: Immunologic and Clinical Aspects

BYRON H. WAKSMAN
Yale University

In recent years, with the tremendous concentration of effort in the field of organ transplantation, there has been a resurgence of interest in delayed or cellular hypersensitivity. This is understandable in view of the critical role of delayed hypersensitivity mechanisms in graft rejection. What is less understandable is the relative lack of interest in this branch of immunobiology during the years prior to the "transplant era."

Such investigational indifference to delayed hypersensitivity is especially baffling when one looks at all the areas in which it represents a critical factor — including not only transplantation immunity but also the pathogenesis of various autoimmune diseases and host defense against disease. The latter involves natural resistance to cancer and is central for defense against most viral, fungal, protozoal, and many bacterial diseases.

There are, it should be stressed, types of infection in which humoral antibody is the predominant mediator of immunity. Most prominent of these are acute bacterial infections such as those caused by streptococci, pneumococci, staphylococci, and such viral diseases as hepatitis. Yet patients with agammaglobulinemia, who may be incapable of making any measurable humoral antibody, maintain good protection against almost all other viral, fungal, protozoal, and bacterial diseases. In general, humoral antibodies have only limited efficacy against those pathogens that are capable of intracellular survival and proliferation. In such infections, cellular hypersensitivity mechanisms are the major participants in host defense.

Much more can be said of clinical situations in which delayed hypersensitivity is unequivocally significant. Before doing so, however, we might summarize what is now known about the mechanisms of delayed hypersensitivity and about the course of histologic events occurring in reactions of this type.

Delayed hypersensitivity reactions evolve slowly, often taking days to develop. This sets them apart from anaphylactic reactions, which occur within minutes, and Arthus-type reactions (lesions produced by antigen-antibody complexes), which evolve over a period of hours. The antigens that provoke delayed reactions are usually protein or conjugated molecules containing protein. The antibody appears to be produced by and to remain fixed to a cell, specifically a lymphocyte, the so-called sensitized cell.

Although much work is still to be done before the exact character of either antigen or antibody can be defined, a number of principles related to each have been elucidated. As noted, the antigen must have a protein constituent. In some situations, delayed hypersensitivity may be elicited by very small proteins at the level of simple polypeptides. In others, complex molecules are involved. For example, the strong transplantation antigen in the mouse, known as H-2 (H = histocompatibility), has been shown to be lipoprotein. In contact allergies — an example is poison ivy sensitivity — the antigen is another kind of complex formed by an exogenous, simple molecule, the allergen, which combines in vivo with protein of the epidermis. In fungus infections, e.g., those produced by trichophyton species, although the antigen includes both polysaccharide and protein moieties, the antigenicity is destroyed when the protein portion is removed.

This brings us to a concept which is clinically significant. The delayed hypersensitivity reaction is concurrent with the presence of antigen. Again, poison ivy is an example. Once the eliciting allergen in or on the skin is destroyed, the disease process ceases. Similarly, with a tuberculin reaction, a previously sensitized person will have a reaction to injected bacillary protein which lasts for several days or until the protein is destroyed.

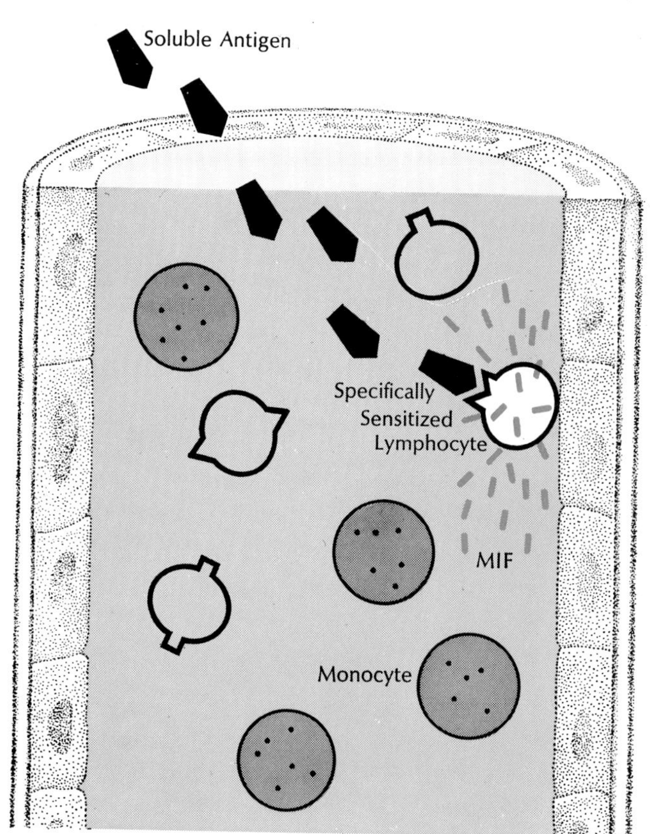

The steps in a delayed hypersensitivity reaction: Soluble antigen encounters sensitized lymphocyte in a venule. The antigen combines with cell-bound antibody and protein "migration inhibitory factor" (MIF) is released (above).

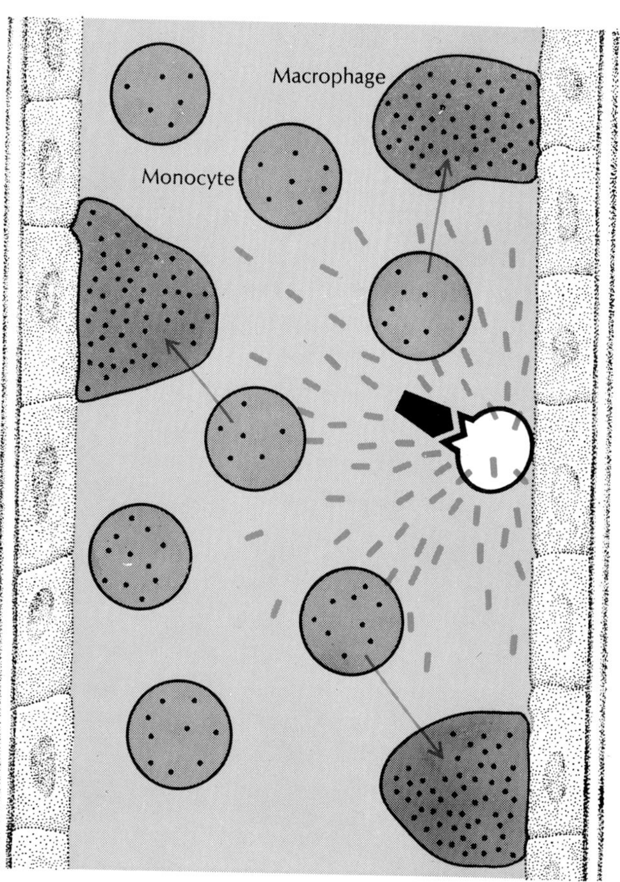

MIF stops the migration of monocytes by making them sticky and it may also affect the endothelial lining of the venule. As a result monocytes adhere to endothelium. These monocytes are activated by MIF and are gradually transformed into macrophages.

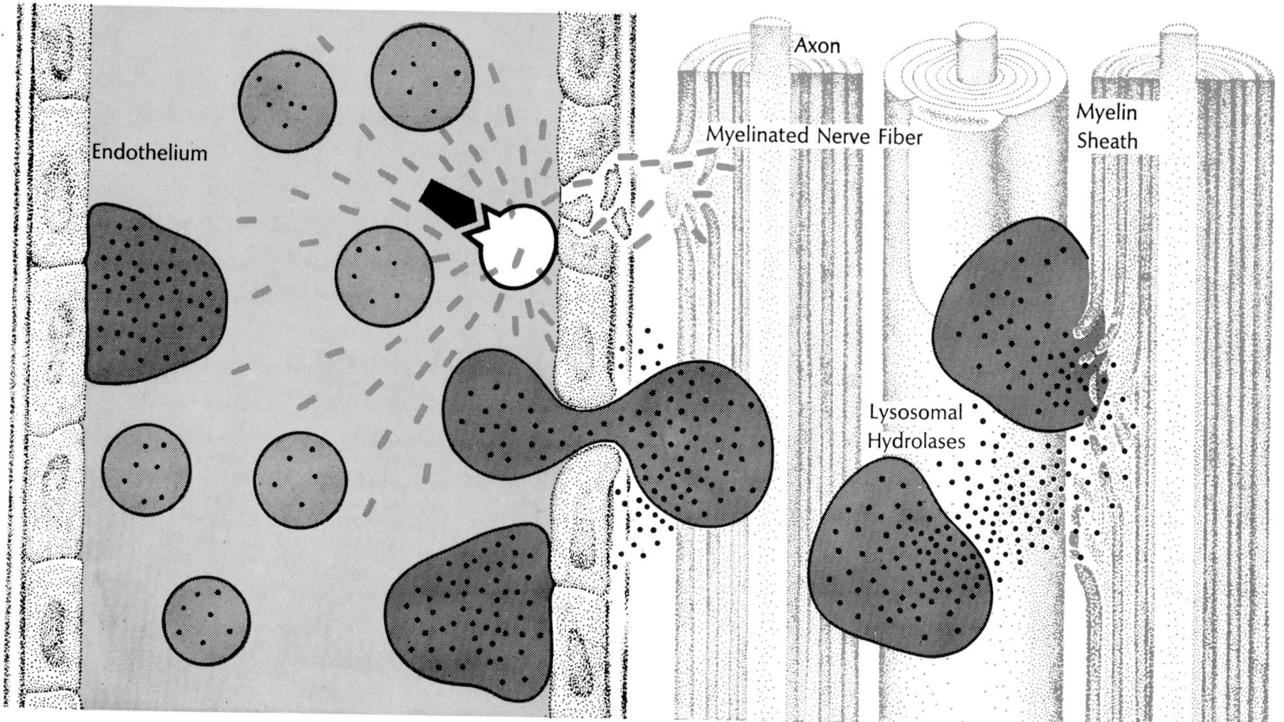

Macrophages force themselves through the endothelium and vessel wall and release lysosomal hydrolases which attack both vessel wall and parenchymal elements. The parenchymal target is represented by the myelin sheath, as in experimental neuritis and encephalomyelitis. MIF may possibly affect the parenchyma directly; the macrophages clearly do so (see photo on next page).

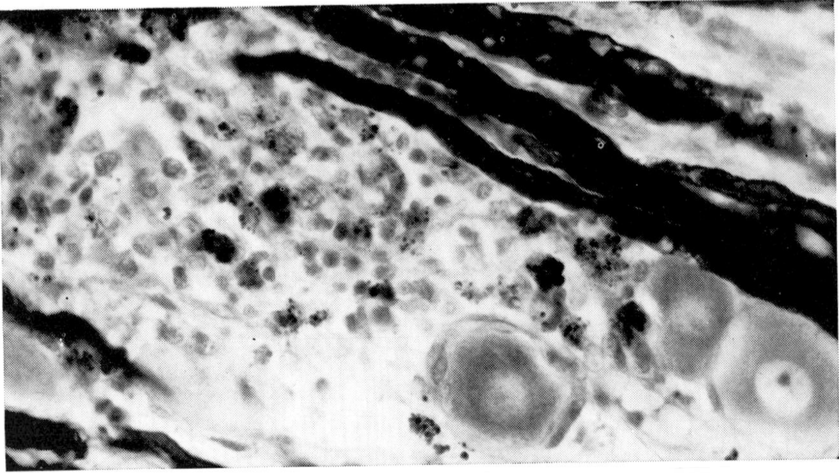

Photomicrograph shows the end result of the events schematized on preceding page. One can see the actual breakdown of myelin in a sensory ganglion in a rabbit with autoallergic neuritis, a model for Landry-Guillain-Barré syndrome in man.

In contrast to these self-limited hypersensitivity responses are the reactions occurring in the granulomatoses and in autoimmune disease. The granulomatoses are interesting illustrations of the relationship between antigen persistence and duration of disease. In berylliosis, for example, it is known that beryllium oxide or phosphor, once introduced into the body, persists in the lungs and other tissues for 20 years or more. In an individual who becomes sensitized to the metal, lesions appear and persist so long as beryllium remains in the tissues. The available evidence suggests that such a granulomatous lesion is initiated by and evolves in a like manner to a short-lived delayed hypersensitivity reaction, although the long-lasting lesion subsequently develops somewhat different histologic characteristics. Similarly, autoimmune diseases are likely to have long, fluctuating courses consistent with the hypothesis that they result from hypersensitivity to an antigen that is a normal constituent of the body and thus remains present.

Delayed hypersensitivity states may be characterized by lesions with some variety of histologic features. As a prelude to discussing the histology, it is important to present some facts with regard to the distribution of lesions. The hypersensitive state itself depends on the presence of sensitized lymphocytes in the circulation, that is to say, of lymphocytes with cell-bound antibody to a specific antigen. Lesions can therefore occur anywhere that an eliciting antigen is introduced, provided the site is accessible to the bloodstream. In general, the distribution of lesions is determined by the distribution of eliciting antigen.

Let us use the tuberculin reaction as an example. The test antigen (tuberculoprotein) is injected into the dermis and diffuses slowly from there. The resulting lesions occur throughout the zone of diffusion. One can obtain disseminated lesions by injecting a large amount of tuberculoprotein, which diffuses through the body.

In contact allergy the eliciting antigen is a complex of exogenous allergen and epidermal constituents. Lesions occur in the upper dermis where vessels are in close proximity to the epidermis containing antigen. In beryllium disease, lesions occur wherever beryllium is deposited. In autoallergic diseases, such as autoallergic encephalomyelitis, the antigen is a constituent of normal tissue, in this case the myelinated nerve fibers of central nervous system white matter; the lesions therefore are distributed throughout the white matter.

The role of the vasculature is equally critical in determining the distribution of lesions in delayed hypersensitivity diseases. Not only are the lesions restricted to sites accessible to the circulation, but they are primarily perivenous lesions and will occur only where there are veins of a certain size range. This is well demonstrated in the disease called experimental autoallergic neuritis, which is a delayed hypersensitivity response to a myelin antigen in the peripheral nervous system.

This antigen is present throughout the dorsal and ventral spinal roots, the sensory ganglia, and the nerves themselves. But the distribution of the lesions is limited and varies from species to species. In the guinea pig, lesions are found almost exclusively in the peripheral nerves, sparing the roots and ganglia. Rabbits, on the other hand, show autoallergic lesions in the ganglia and dorsal roots and only an occasional large focal lesion in the peripheral nerves. Now if one looks at the circulatory system of the guinea pig, one sees capillary networks in the roots and ganglia but very few veins; in contrast there are large and complex venous plexuses in the peripheral nerves. In the rabbit, conversely, there is an extensive venous network in the sensory ganglia and dorsal roots, but only an occasional vein within the peripheral nerves.

The same rule of perivenous distribution prevails for tuberculin reactions in rats and guinea pigs. The former species is characterized by a relative lack of venous pathways in the upper dermis. The tuberculin reaction elicited by the usual skin test will therefore occur only in deep dermal and subcutaneous connective tissue. But in guinea pigs there are many veins throughout the dermis, and the tuberculin reaction will manifest itself very well in superficial layers of the skin. By the same token, contact allergies can be elicited consistently in guinea pigs, almost not at all in rats.

The histology of the delayed hypersensitivity reaction is still subject to some disagreement. However, a number of facts are universally accepted and form the foundation for a discussion of mechanism. Many of these facts are based on in vitro experiments that have produced some of the newest and perhaps potentially most significant findings in this field.

A delayed hypersensitivity reaction begins with perivenous accumulation of sensitized lymphocytes and other mononuclear cells. These infiltrative lesions enlarge and multiply with time, and there is cellular invasion and destruction of tissue elements. The importance of this "invasive-destructive" lesion is well shown in the example considered above of autoallergic encephalomyelitis. Destruction of myelin in the zone of cell infiltration is a major element in the lesion and is, in fact, responsible for most of the symptoms of this "demyelinative" disease. This myelin destruction may also be responsible for the release of antigen which elicits new lesions, giving the disease its chronic character.

Conventional histologic techniques, which were all that were available to us for many years, gave no hint as to the actual sequence of events. It was widely assumed that parenchymal tissue was first damaged by antibody and that the mononuclear cell infiltration was secondary to this damage; the cells were thought to be activated local histiocytes. It is now quite clear both from careful, sequential histologic studies and from experiments in which cells are tagged with radioactive tritiated thymidine, that most, if not all, of the cells participating in the delayed hypersensitivity reaction come from the bloodstream and that they are capable of tissue destruction. This has importance because it refutes the early conception and permits a meaningful discussion of mechanism.

Labeling techniques have also confirmed that two distinct cell types participate in the delayed hypersensitivity reaction. The antibody carrying lymphocyte is one. This cell is almost certainly formed in the lymph nodes and is immunized or sensitized there [see Chapter 2, "Immunobiology of the Small Lymphocyte," by James L. Gowans]. The second cell type is the monocyte, which originates in the bone marrow and arrives at the lesion directly via the blood. When the monocyte first comes to the lesion, it morphologically resembles a lymphocyte, but it evolves rapidly and, depending on the type of lesion, may either remain lymphocytic in appearance or become a typical histiocyte or a macrophage full of phagocytosed material. In chronic granulomatous lesions, the monocytes evolve into epithelioid cells, accompanied by an occasional giant cell. (One should note that in the literature discussing these cells, terms such as reticuloendothelial cell, monocyte, histiocyte, and macrophage are used virtually as synonyms, but all describe the same cell type at different stages of its evolution. Even epithelioid and multinucleate giant cells are known to derive from the same cell.)

Cells of the monocytic line are, as far as we know, devoid of antibody and devoid of specificity. They are secondary participants in the immunologic reaction. Moreover, recent research has shown that cells of the same type are evoked by toxic or traumatic agents and participate in the nonspecific inflammatory processes induced by such irritants. But the number of such cells attracted to a delayed hypersensitivity lesion is many times greater than the number participating in nonspecific reactions. In the delayed lesions investigated so far, monocytes constitute 80% to 90% of the cells mobilized to the lesion.

Even more interesting than the quantitative relationship between the monocytes and the sensitized lymphocytes are the functional relationships between these two cell types. To trace these functional relationships, let us recall the origins of the cells involved. After arising in bone marrow, the small lymphocyte migrates to the thymus. Here it undergoes rapid differ-

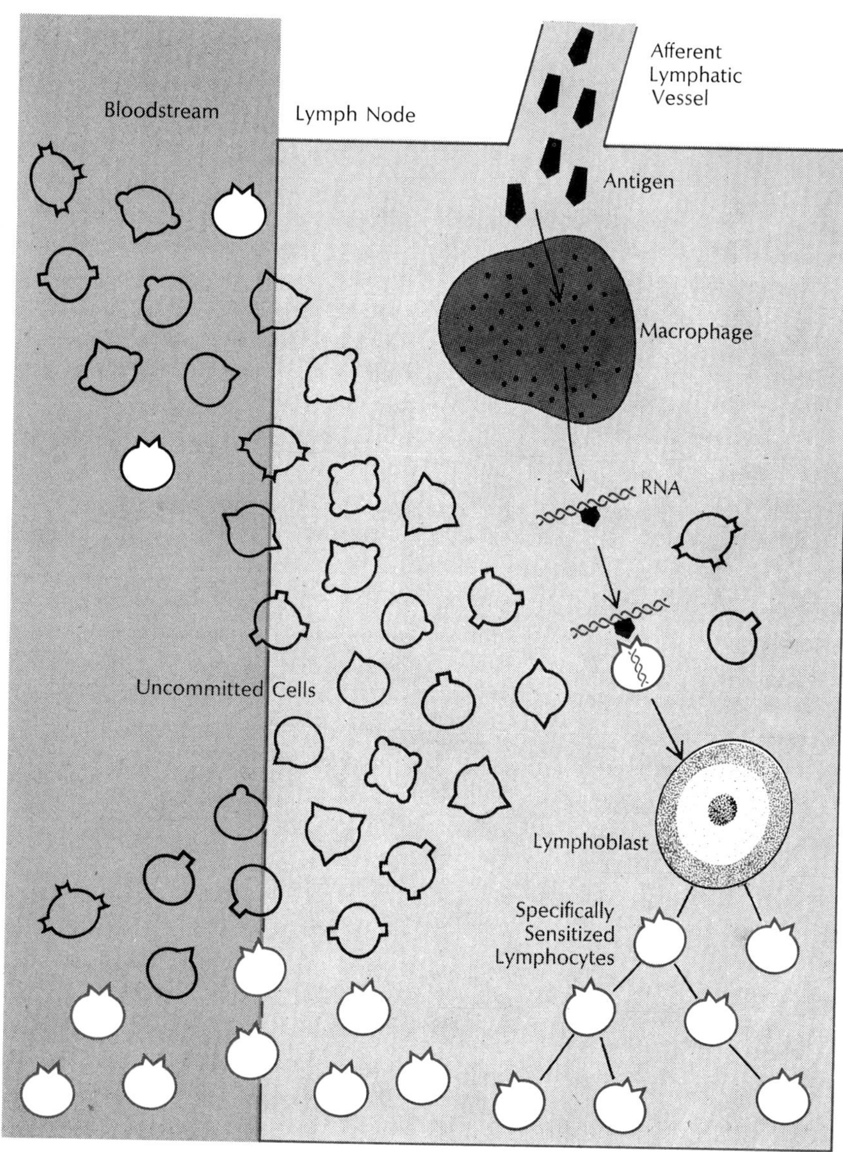

Drawing offers a hypothesis for the mechanism of sensitization of the small lymphocyte, and also suggests the possible mechanism of induction of specific tolerance. After interacting with a macrophage in the lymph node, the antigen acquires RNA or some other cellular component, which is then transferred to the "uncommitted" lymphocyte. This causes enlargement of the lymphocyte into a large pyroninophilic cell (lymphoblast) that divides repeatedly, giving rise to many sensitized lymphocytes. Theoretically, tolerance can be produced if the antibody combining site on the lymphocyte is preempted by antigen not processed by the macrophage and lacking the cellular component.

entiation and, in the view of some investigators, acquires specificity — that is, it becomes precommitted to the making of one type of antibody. The small lymphocyte then enters the peripheral pool and begins a cycle of recirculation, described by J. L. Gowans, which includes the lymph nodes, the lymphatic vessels, and the bloodstream. When an antigen is injected to induce immunization, each small lymphocyte which is precommitted to that antigen responds by becoming a large, rapidly dividing cell and gives rise to many committed, or sensitized, lymphocytes.

At this point one can correctly speak of the animal (or person, of course) as being sensitized, with subsequent exposure to antigen likely to provoke a hypersensitivity reaction. In this sense, hypersensitivity is analogous to the "memory" phenomenon encountered with humoral antibodies; hypersensitivity reactions are in effect anamnestic, or "booster," responses. Whether the sensitive state consists simply of an increase in the relative numbers of small lymphocytes specifically committed to a particular antigen, or whether there is also some qualitative change in the committed small lymphocytes — perhaps the acquisition of more antibody combining sites — is still open to question.

What about the other "end cells" in the hypersensitivity reaction — the monocytes? These too arise from the stem cell population of the bone marrow. The weight of evidence is that they do not undergo further differentiation in the thymus or peripheral lymphoid organs, but enter the blood in their reactive form.

Having accounted for the development of the two major cell types participating in delayed hypersensitivity responses, we can begin to detail the events in which they interact.

Many years ago, Rich and Lewis demonstrated that specific antigen could markedly inhibit the migration of fibroblasts or macrophages from spleen or lymph node explants taken from sensitized animals and placed in tissue culture.

J. R. David, now at Harvard, and B. Bloom and B. Bennett at Albert Einstein College of Medicine have worked out the mechanism of this phenomenon. These investigators have shown that when the sensitized lymphocytes interact with antigen they release a protein factor which has profound effects on other cells involved in the reaction. This protein may in fact be a new type of antibody, or it may act as a nonspecific mediator. Working with peritoneal exudates from sensitized guinea pigs, they demonstrated that the cells from these exudates are inhibited by specific antigen from migrating out of capillary tubes in tissue culture. The peritoneal exudates contain both sensitized lymphocytes and macrophages; these workers have shown conclusively that the inhibition of migration is due to the substance released by the sensitized lymphocytes, which is now known as MIF (migration inhibitory factor). What's more, one sensitized lymphocyte is enough to inhibit migration of 99 or more macrophages.

Employing a similar culture system Dr. Nancy Ruddle in our laboratory has shown that MIF kills fibroblasts, which show a rapid and marked increase in their content of lysosomal hydrolases such as acid phosphatase. Previously, in our laboratory Mrs. M. Matoltsy had observed that macrophages become markedly activated over a period of 24 to 48 hours.

The temporal sequence of these events is interesting. Inhibition of migration is seen within the first 24 hours, killing of fibroblasts in two to three days. One can therefore distinguish three steps in this process: the antigen-antibody reaction takes 30 minutes; the production of MIF, a matter of hours; and the effect of MIF on the target cells, a few hours to a day or more.

These in vitro observations permit a fairly complete interpretation of what happens at the site of the local delayed hypersensitivity reaction. A circulating sensitized lymphocyte reacts with antigen and releases its product, MIF, and this in turn affects the adjacent endothelium, the passing monocytic cells, or both. The monocytic cells stick to the endothelium, either because of their increased stickiness or because the endothelium has been damaged, and ultimately pass through the vessel wall. The fact that the monocytes become activated over a 24- to 48-hour period permits them, in turn, to destroy adjacent elements of the parenchyma. This, for example, would explain the myelin destruction discussed earlier.

Two additional factors may contribute to the destructive processes in delayed reactions. The sensitized lymphocytes when they release MIF may damage or destroy a variety of cells. Thus when sensitized lymphocytes from animals that have been transplant recipients are layered in tissue culture on epithelial, fibroblastic, or tumor cells of donor type, they directly kill these cells. Secondly, when coated with a specific cytophilic antibody macrophages have direct cytopathogenic effects. Now, in in vivo situations it appears almost certain that there are some circumstances in which the lymphocytes directly destroy the target cells, others in which activated macrophages secondarily destroy some parenchymal cells, and still others in which the lymphocytes release a cytophilic antibody that permits the macrophages to adhere to the target cells. These cytotoxic effects are not mutually exclusive, and investigations to date have not been successful in disentangling one effect from another.

It is obvious that in this account of the lesion-producing processes of delayed hypersensitivity there are still significant gaps. However, the knowledge achieved thus far is formidable. Unfortunately, there is one major area of basic understanding where facts are as yet almost completely lacking. I refer to the structure of the cell-bound antibody of delayed hypersensitivity. As previous articles in this series have shown, considerable detail is available on the structure of various classes of serum antibody; indeed a partial sequence of amino acids has been defined for one such class — IgG.

No such information is available on the antibody of delayed hypersensitivity. The sensitized lymphocytes have been found to carry cell-bound light chains like those in other immunoglobulins. There are also a few tenuous links to the IgA class.

In experiments performed some years ago, it was shown that neonatally thymectomized mice and rats had as their principal defects in adult life the inability to produce an immunoglobulin analogous to IgA and a failure in delayed hypersensitivity responses. There is an interesting human coun-

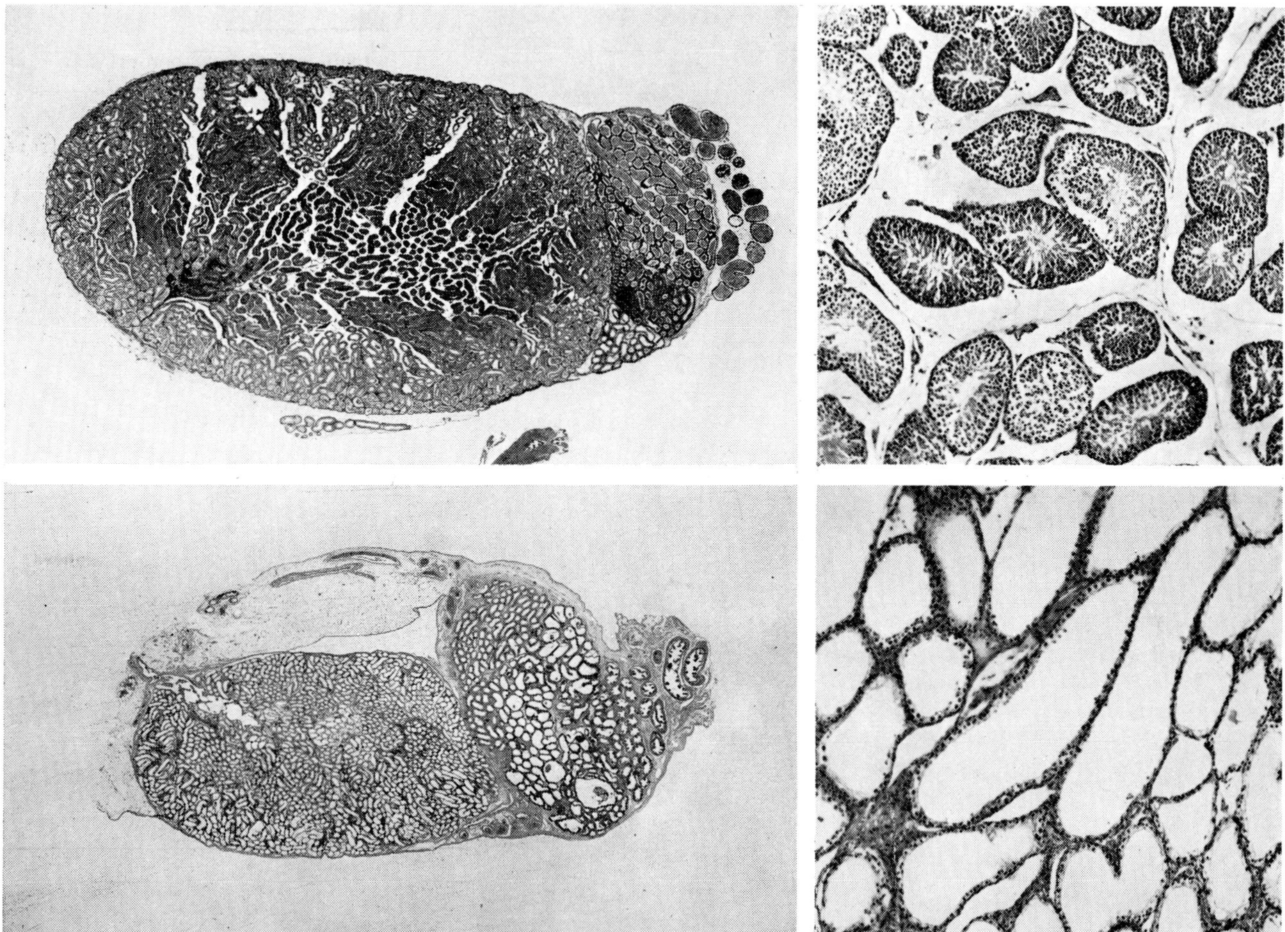

The progression of the inflammatory lesion caused by delayed hypersensitivity in experimental orchitis is illustrated above. One can see the testis still containing sperm and then the testis emptied of sperm (left, above and below) as well as the seminiferous tubules as they appeared before and after the autoimmune reaction had been induced (right, above and below).

terpart. Patients with ataxia telangiectasia, who have severe thymic abnormalities, are deficient in IgA and in delayed hypersensitivity antibody formation.

The direct relationship between the thymus and the antibody of delayed hypersensitivity leads to another subject which may prove to be of major clinical importance — that of tolerance as it applies to delayed hypersensitivity. It is hardly necessary to stress the significance that would attach to any success in inducing a specific tolerance to one antigen responsible for delayed hypersensitivity in one of the autoimmune diseases or the antigen(s) of a specific homograft, while leaving the basic mechanisms of cellular immunity otherwise intact. To date, all clinical efforts to control graft rejection mechanisms have relied on immunosuppression, and by definition such immunosuppression is relatively general. Therefore the patient who is "unprotected" against the graft is almost equally unprotected against infection. With antilymphocyte serum, for example, which is a powerful immunosuppressant of delayed reactions in particular, the patient is also "unprotected" against development of spontaneous tumors. For this reason, it is my conviction that the best hope for overcoming immunologic barriers to transplantation, without crippling the recipient's ability to respond to infection and neoplasia, lies in the induction of specific tolerance.

Experimentally, tolerance has been effectively induced for delayed hypersensitivity by pretreatment with antigen in a form not readily phagocytosed. An example is bovine gamma globulin from which particulate, aggregated, or denatured material is removed. The remaining BGG is not phagocytosed, and a large intravenous dose produces specific tolerance to the protein. One can also produce tolerance with smaller doses of antigen, provided these are injected directly into the thymus. This effect can be greatly potentiated by irradiating the animal while shielding the thymus, thus destroying the peripheral lymphocyte pool. The animal's thymus must therefore regenerate a complete new lymphocyte pool. And if antigen has been injected directly into the thymus, the animal will be completely tolerant for this antigen, both with regard to delayed hypersensitivity and formation of some immunoglobulins.

In discussing tolerance and the possibility that it may soon be feasible to induce such clinically advantageous tolerance, one is confronted with the more fundamental problem of uncovering the mechanism by which an immunizing dose of antigen triggers changes in a lymphocyte that it encounters within the lymph node. In other words, what happens to cause the lymphocyte to proliferate and perhaps to change qualitatively — for example, into an antibody-forming plasma cell or a sensitized cell of delayed hypersensitivity? A good deal of recent research suggests that the sensitization process involves the uptake of antigen by phagocytic cells and the attachment of either whole antigen or an antigenic fragment to some undefined cellular component, such as RNA. The attached antigen can now react with those lymphocytes that have a combining site of the correct specificity on their surface.

This hypothesis implies that the purpose of the processing is merely to bring the RNA into the lymphocyte where it triggers proliferation and differentiation to a protein-synthesizing end cell. Some indirect support for this suggestion comes from a line of work initiated by J. A. Mannick and R. H. Egdahl. These investigators were the first to show that RNA from sensitized cells has the ability to endow nonsensitized cells with the property of transplantation immunity. This work parallels that of Marvin Fishman on humoral antibody.

All this relates to tolerance because, according to our present picture, most brilliantly drawn by N. A. Mitchison of the National Institute for Medical Research, London, tolerance consists of the same antigen-lymphocyte interaction as does sensitization, but without the little bit of attached RNA. Again the event occurs at the specific combining site on the lymphocyte. This site may be blocked or damaged, or the lymphocyte may be launched into an aberrant pathway. If this concept can be confirmed, it would obviously open up significant new possibilities for selective induction of tolerance. Mr. David Scott, a graduate student in our laboratory, has shown within the last few months that a processing step may be necessary in this process as well and has thus focused attention on the nature of the initial uptake of the antigen.

In the course of this article we have mentioned several autoallergic diseases. There are now about 18 experimental autoallergic diseases; almost without exception, they depend on the mechanisms of delayed hypersensitivity. These experimental diseases involve the central and peripheral nervous systems, the lens and uvea of the eye, the testes, the thyroid, and other endocrine organs. Most serve as models for one or more human diseases and as such have great clinical potential. One of the most recently described, a very interesting and typical example, is the experimental autoallergic disease affecting the islets of Langerhans, developed through the work of Renold and Le-Compte, which may be a model for some types of diabetes. Almost all the autoallergic diseases are produced by immunizing animals with normal tissues from different species, usually with the aid of Freund's adjuvant or similar preparations. In the autoallergic "diabetes," the immunizing agent was insulin, and the effects of the destructive lesions within the islet tissue appeared to resemble closely those of juvenile diabetes in man.

There is one other clinical area in which delayed hypersensitivity promises to provide a potent tool for investigation, namely, cancer. From the experimentalist's point of view, many tumors can be regarded as foreign tissue grafts in or on the body. Tumors that are induced by viruses or chemical carcinogens very frequently have antigens not present in the host. In such cases — and we are talking here only of solid, vascularized tumors — immunologic rejection, when it occurs, depends on the delayed hypersensitivity mechanisms. There are many immunologists and oncologists who regard the primary role of delayed hypersensitivity as the cleaning up of tumors arising throughout life.

It is in fact fully established in animal studies that many virus-induced tumors persist and grow because of the induction of specific immunologic tolerance. Clearly, then, a fuller understanding of the tolerance mechanisms as applied to delayed hypersensitivity might open an important new approach to the prevention of cancer by inhibiting or breaking tolerance.

This discussion has attempted to underscore the importance of delayed hypersensitivity to experimental and clinical medicine and to pinpoint some of the vital areas in which knowledge is still to be gained. It is therefore appropriate to close by noting that intensive research is now in progress to gain an answer to what may well be the central question in all immunology. This is the nature of the original differentiation of the stem cell that gives rise to a cell with immunologic specificity; for delayed hypersensitivity this "generation of diversity" may take place in the thymus.

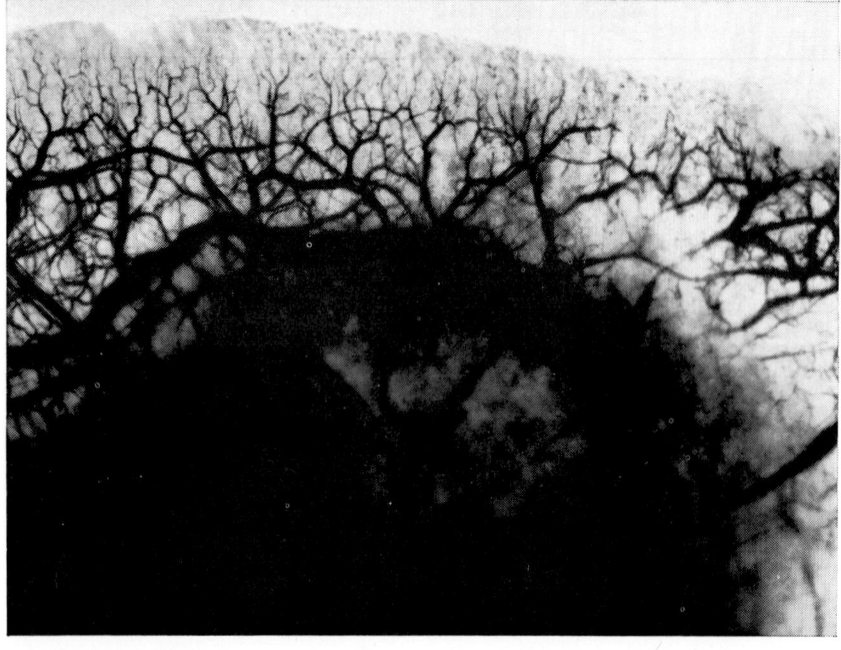

An early tuberculin reaction is visualized in a guinea pig ear. A few minutes after dye injection, the vessels are well filled; dark reaction is caused by leakage of dye into inflammatory zone. Pale center shows almost no dye in vessels with no leakage. Stasis is seen in zone which will become necrotic due to infarction.

WOW IF TRUE *

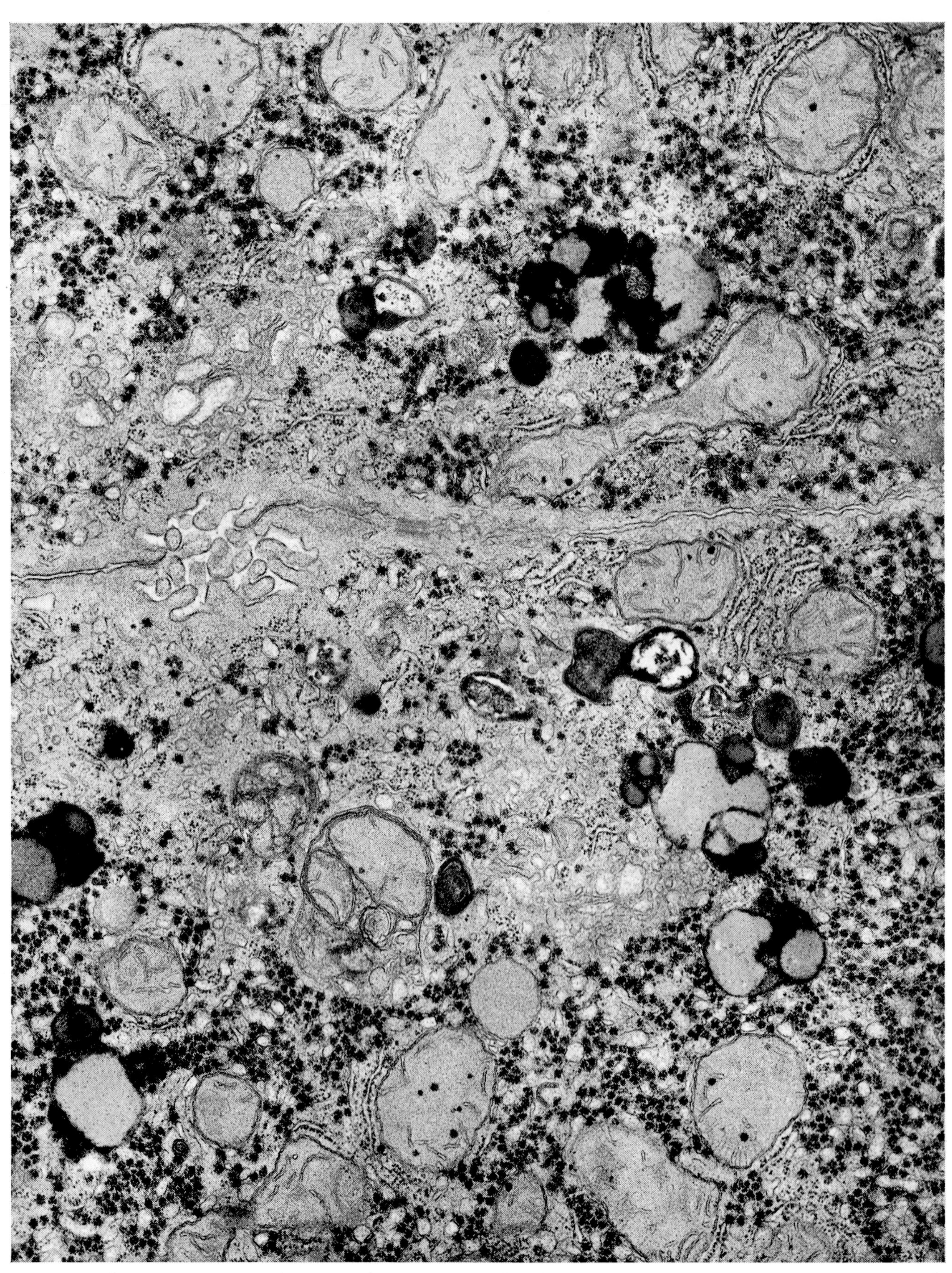

Two types of lysosome are present in this 22,000x electronmicrograph of a pair of human hepatocytes. Below the bile canaliculus, between the two cells, is an autophagic vacuole inside of which mitochondria and other cytoplasmic structures are undergoing degradation (see drawing, opposite). On both sides of the canaliculus are "dense bodies" in which lipofuscin is deposited. This pigment, often associated with lysosome-like particles in hepatic cells, and more abundant in aged specimens, is thought to reflect

Chapter 4

The Many-Faceted Lysosome

GERALD WEISSMANN
New York University

When Christian de Duve postulated the existence of the lysosome some 15 years ago, he described it as a bag of acid hydrolases exhibiting structure-linked latency and he nicknamed it the "suicide sac," suggesting that the lytic enzymes in this organelle would leak from its ruptured membrane and digest the cell after its death. His hypothesis was based on biochemical considerations.

Very shortly afterward, Alex B. Novikoff demonstrated that with a modification of the Gomori technique of localizing acid phosphatase activity, lysosomes could be identified within intact cells by either light or electron microscopy. The particles have since been observed in most vertebrate tissues, as well as in invertebrates and unicellular organisms.

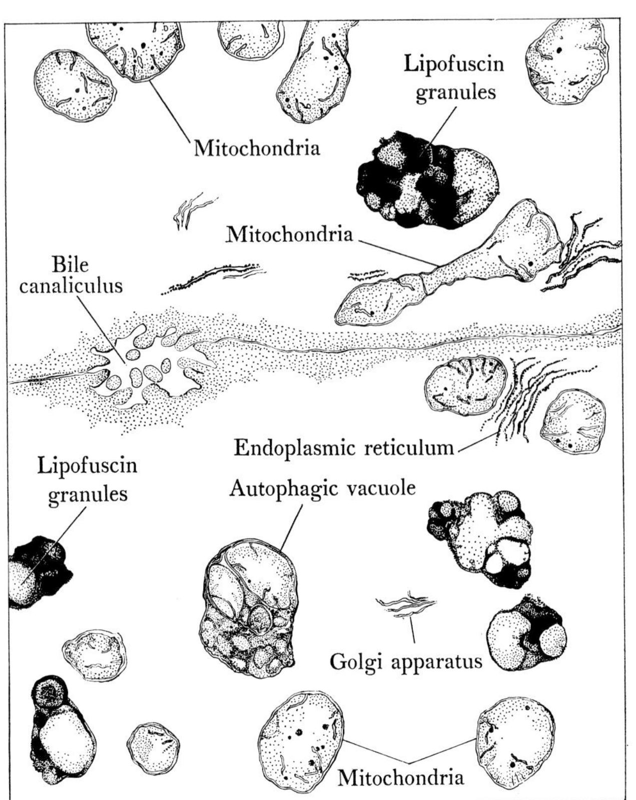

the relative absence of lipolytic enzymes from the liver lysosome's armamentarium. The lipofuscin may originate in indigestible cell components ingested by the lysosome, since few enzymes acting on lipid substrates have been identified within lysosomes.

Nowadays we realize that the "suicide sac" activity is only one of the lysosome's functions. Its others, in normal physiology as well as in pathologic states, though still early in the process of documentation, appear to be heading for pivotal importance. For instance, what we already understand about the lysosome has made it possible to defend the thesis of a "final common pathway" to joint injury in connective tissue diseases. There are hypotheses that link lysosomes to the inflammatory manifestations of acute rheumatic fever, and there is evidence that lysosome-like structures abound in the myocardium of patients with congestive heart failure, especially that caused by mitral stenosis. Lysosomes appear to be involved in hepatitis and cholestatic jaundice, while abnormal amounts of two lysosomal enzymes have been found in the urine of patients with pyelonephritis. Lysosomal function has been associated with such heritable storage diseases as Pompe's disease and Hurler's syndrome, as well as the Chediak-Higashi syndrome and other disorders of leukocyte formation. The role of lysosomes in fever has not yet been elucidated, but there are indications that this is a potentially fruitful area of research. Finally, recent work in A. C. Allison's laboratory, and our own, implicates lysosomes in triggering widespread gene activation, such as that accompanying mitosis or neoplasia.

My involvement with the lysosome began with an interest in connective tissue diseases. I was working with Dr. Lewis Thomas at New York University on a phenomenon he had discovered: When an exogenous protease, papain, was injected into rabbits, their ears became droopy like those of spaniels. We discovered that papain acted as a protease by breaking the protein-to-polysaccharide bond of cartilage. We were rather excited about this, since it was a model for tissue destruction in a living animal.

At about the same time, both Dr. Thomas here and Dame Honor Fell at the Strangeways Research Laboratory in Cambridge, England, discovered that an excess of vitamin A had a similar effect: it rendered the anionic polysaccharide bond free to diffuse away, and cartilage lost

The Structures and Activities Involved in Lysosomal Function

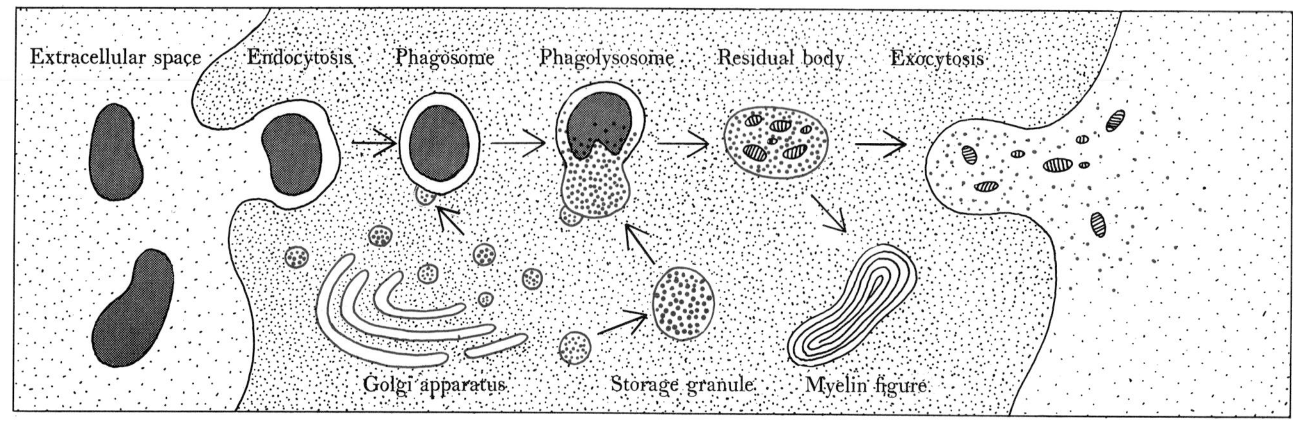

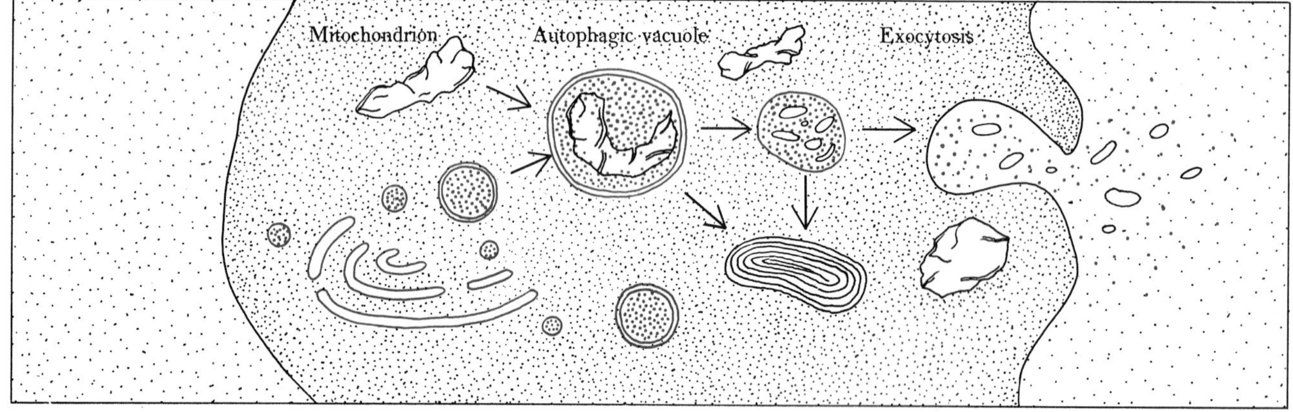

Degradation of both extracellular and native substances is major function of lysosomes (after packaging in the Golgi apparatus they become organized in the primary storage granule form). Following endocytosis, the membrane of the storage granule merges with the membrane of the phagosome, which now incorporates foreign body, to form phagolysosome (top drawing). After lysosomal enzymes have finished digestion, residual body is filled with debris, mainly lipid, which is ejected in exocytosis. Autophagic vacuole exercises similar degrading function on intracellular material and structures such as mitochondrion (bottom drawing).

its rigidity. If you gave a lot of vitamin A to a rabbit, its ears would fall down.

We had demonstrated that an excess of vitamin A was damaging to connective tissue; next we wanted to find out the effect of some substance that seems to benefit connective tissue. So we injected vitamin A into rabbits and at the same time gave them cortisone. We found that the cortisone prevented the vitamin-A effect completely. We then postulated that vitamin A might act to release from cells a papain-like enzyme.

As I was finishing my postdoctoral research training here in 1960, Dr. Thomas suggested that I go to England and work on the problem at Cambridge, which I did. At the Strangeways, John Dingle and I read de Duve's papers, and Dingle suspected vitamin A might act on lysosomes. There was at that time no strong reason to connect de Duve's hypothesis and the papain-like effect, but as we speculated on where in the cell the papain-like enzymes were concentrated, it occurred to us that they might be in lysosomes. We framed a hypothesis that vitamin A might rupture lysosomes, and that cortisone might stabilize them to prevent the release of the enzymes.

It then occurred to us that we might be dealing with a general mechanism of tissue damage in connective tissue diseases. Perhaps lysosomal enzymes were released not only in cellular death but in cellular life as well, and cortisone might prevent this release by stabilizing the lysosomes.

The fact that ultraviolet irradiation aggravates lupus suggested a method of testing our hypothesis. We exposed two samples of lysosomes to UV irradiation; one was from a normal animal, the other from an animal that had been treated with cortisone. We were elated to find that in the normal sample the UV ruptured the lysosomes and that in the cortisone-treated sample the effect was significantly reduced. Here was a new way in which an enzyme could be activated to produce tissue damage.

As reports on the structure, function, and natural history of lysosomes were published by investigators here and abroad, the enormous potential role of this "new" organelle began to be appreciated. But each new finding seemed to introduce a new complication, not the least being the question of what is and what is not a lysosome. De Duve characterized lysosomes as strikingly pleomorphic particles, physically and chemically heterogeneous, and cautioned that "an acid phosphatase–positive particle is not by definition a lysosome; it is only likely to be one."

We now recognize that the term "lysosome" includes a group of organelles more pleomorphic than such cell structures as nuclei or mitochondria. Their state in tissue varies with the physiologic or pathologic state of the cell in which they are found, but there are four principal varieties: the storage granule, the digestive vacuole, the autophagic vacuole, and the residual body.

The storage granule, or the primary lysosome, is one that has not yet participated in acts of digestion. It is best exemplified by the specific granules of polymorphonuclear leukocytes, or eosinophils. The membranes of these primary lysosomes can merge with those of the vacuoles formed as invaginations of the cell surface when cells take in proteins, microorganisms, or inert particles. The vacuole before it has merged with the lysosome and received the lysosomal hydrolases is a "phagosome." After union the resultant structure is termed a "phagolysosome" or, more simply, a secondary lysosome.

Whenever a cell must sacrifice a portion of its own cytoplasm as a result of fasting, anoxia, or active catabolism, a vacuole forms, bounded by a single membrane and enclosing such structures as mitochondria, Golgi vesicles, and bits of endoplasmic reticulum. This is the "autophagic vacuole." It was first described in the kidney after ureteral ligation, and later in the liver after perfusion by glucagon, and is also a secondary lysosome.

Finally, when lysosomes have carried out digestive functions — either as phagolysosomes or as autophagic vacuoles — they appear filled with debris, generally lipid. These structures are the "residual body" lysosomal form.

Much lysosomal activity is associated with the cell's engulfing processes — phagocytosis, pinocytosis, and micropinocytosis, to name only the most frequent. In order to make discussion more convenient, de Duve suggested that all these processes be grouped in the term "endocytosis." G. E. Palade has pointed out that this is an unusual usage of the prefix "endo-", which usually means "in" or "within," but seldom "inward," as in this case. "The ideal solution to this terminology problem," he said, "would be a pair of words meaning 'import-' and 'export in bulk'!" However, "endocytosis" has been accepted. It has even been joined by the elegant term "exocytosis" — extrusion into bile or urine of the contents of residual bodies whose outer membranes abut on excretory chan-

Lysosomes, Cell Injury, and Immunity: Three Theories

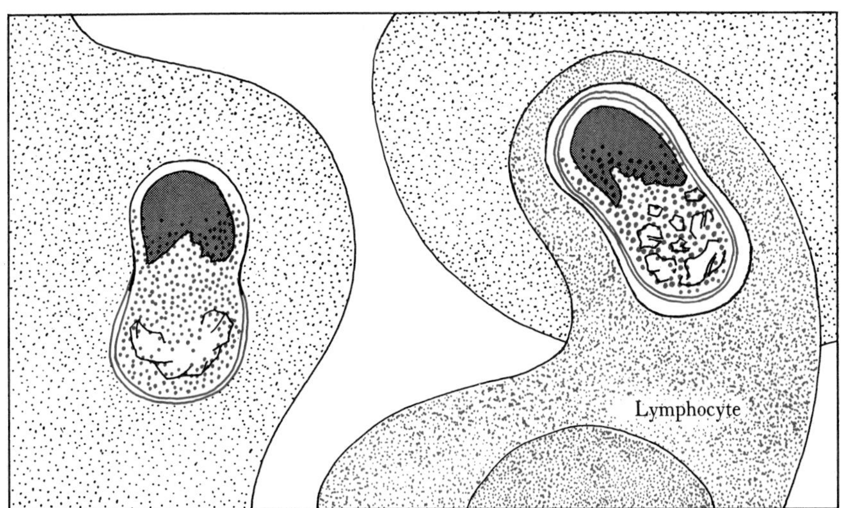

Fragmentation of antigens within phagolysosome (left) or autophagic vacuole may render them more immunogenic. Lymphocyte, attracted in some way, receives these antigenic fragments (right), leading to antibody formation.

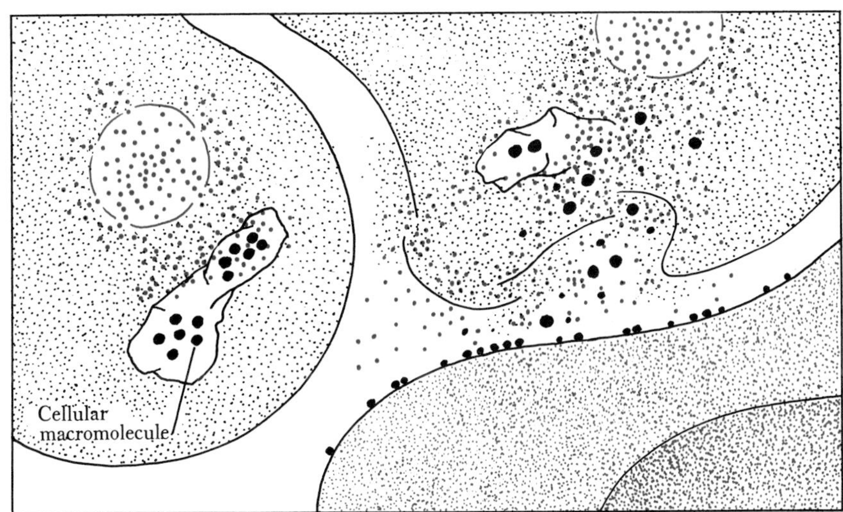

Autoantigenic fragments (left) may arise consequent to the leakage of enzymes from lysosomes made fragile by exposure, for example, to exogenous toxins. This process is thought to occur most often in the neighborhood of antibody-forming cells.

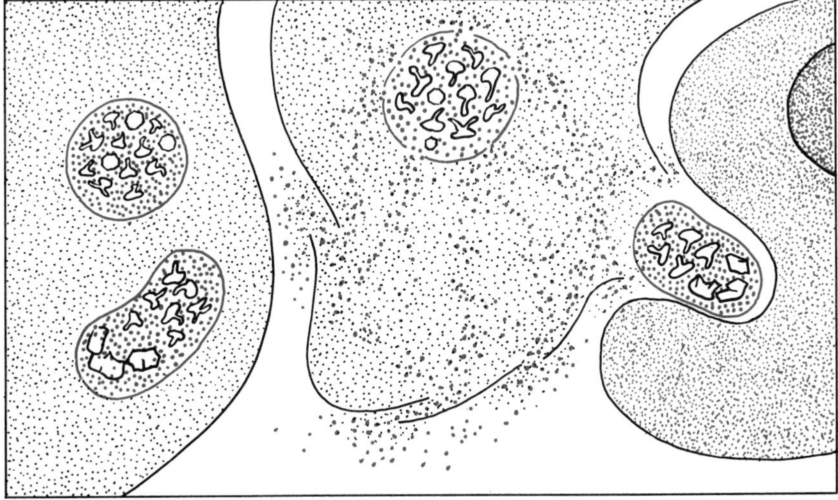

There is evidence that phagolysosomes may be weaker than parent bodies. Degradation of connective tissue components might be hastened by leakage of enzymes from phagolysosomes (center) overloaded by indwelling viruses, bacteria, or bacterial L forms.

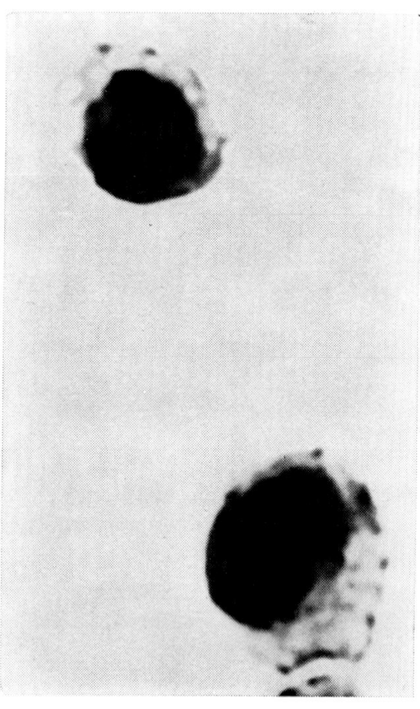
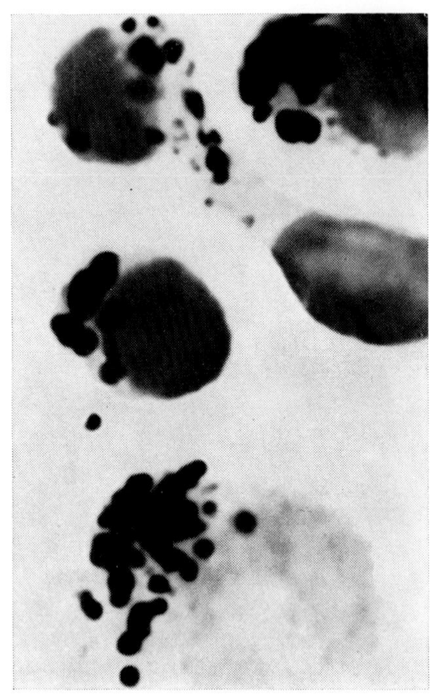

Possible lysosomal role in immune response is suggested by finding that phytohemagglutinin-treated lymphocytes (right) produce more lysosomes than do control cells.

nels, as they do in the liver or kidney.

Some 25 enzymes, and several other substances that have not been thoroughly characterized and may not even be enzymes, have been biochemically localized to the lysosome. Some or all of these may be present in any of the four forms of the organelle. Histochemically, electron microscope studies have identified only a few of the enzymes within the lysosome. Acid phosphatase, of course, is one; the others are arylsulphatase, organophosphorus-resistant esterases, and β-glucuronidase.

Discovery of the lysosome has turned our attention away from the confusing array of cell types involved in the various connective tissue diseases and focused our interest on those cellular organelles and mechanisms that might mediate the tissue injury common to all members of this group of disorders. When lysosome activity is considered as a factor, it appears that the disease processes, however diverse their points of origin, all arrive at local injury of the joint via a final common pathway.

Whether the initial insult is provided by microorganisms, crystals, or the offending agent or agents of rheumatoid arthritis, the final common pathway is composed of a sequence of events that begins with endocytosis, which leads to the formation of new and fragile lysosomes. From the fragile lysosomes there is inappropriate release of inflammatory materials, followed by leukocytic infiltration, joint injury, and cartilage degradation.

Certainly the presence of lysosomes within the cells involved in these diseases is no longer questioned. They have been found in synovial lining (type A) cells, in cartilage cells, in wandering and fixed macrophages, in the pericytes of blood vessels, and in the polymorphonuclear leukocytes that enter joint spaces from the blood.

Also amply documented is the ability of substances within the lysosome to produce cutaneous and joint inflammation. These substances are: a cationic protein that disrupts mast cell granules, a protease — inhibited by ϵ-aminocaproic acid and the mucoprotein inhibitor trasylol — that induces capillary permeability, and one or more proteases that act like cathepsin D and can break down the protein polysaccharide of cartilage. These substances have been localized to leukocyte lysosomes (which have been shown to consist of at least two subgroups), but cartilage lysosomes also contain an acid protease capable of degrading cartilage matrix.

Degradative enzymes released from lysosomes may denature the native constituents of cells or connective tissue. The denatured products could trigger the formation of circulating antibodies as part of the normal immune response in normal individuals as well as in patients with connective tissue diseases. In rheumatoid arthritis, as in systemic lupus, circulating antibodies to denatured gamma globulin or DNA have been found, but these autoantibodies have not been conclusively shown to bring about tissue damage in organs other than the kidney.

Three possible mechanisms have been suggested through which release of lysosomal products into cell sap or surrounding tissue may initiate inflammation and tissue destruction and thereby produce autoantigens, which in turn lead to autoantibody production. None has been demonstrated so far in any human disease, but each has been documented in the production of experimental rheumatic lesions in laboratory animals.

First, it is thought that by endocytosis antigens of high molecular weight are taken up by phagocytes and degraded by hydrolytic enzymes within the phagolysosomes. In a manner still poorly understood, antigenic fragments, perhaps of enhanced immunogenicity, appear in the phagocytic cell. This "processed" antigenic material is transferred to antibody-forming lymphocytes. While no similar mechanism has been described for the degradation of autoantigens, what is true for the phagolysosome may hold true for the autophagic vacuole. Probably, fragments of degraded macromolecules, whether native or foreign, are treated by the phagocytic cell as antigen fragments.

In the second hypothetical sequence of events, leakage of enzymes from lysosomes rendered fragile by repeated exposure to exogenous toxins or inborn error may lead to synthesis of partially degraded autoantigenic fragments. This process is particularly likely to take place in the neighborhood of antibody-forming cells, as, for example, in the lining cells of synovium, in pericytes of vascular endothelium, and in the reticuloendothelial system.

Finally, an excess of phagolysosomes within synovial lining or similar tissues might be brought about by intracellular residence of various microorganisms, viruses, or bacterial L forms. Accelerated degradation of connective tissue components might follow, since there is evidence that phagolysosomes are more fragile than the parent lysosomes, and leakage of enzymes might be expected.

Lysosomal membranes bear close resemblance to the unit membranes that surround erythrocytes, and most of the substances that rupture lysosomes in vitro are hemolytic.

Few of the agents that disrupt lysosomes in vitro can be shown to produce the same effect in living cells. Among those agents that do affect lysosomes in vivo and in vitro are vitamin A, streptolysins O and S, ultraviolet and x-rays, staphylococcal alpha-toxin, and polyene antibiotics.

On the other hand, bacterial endotoxins, 2,4-dinitrophenol, oxygen excess, and heterologous antibody with complement labilize the lysosomes of living cells but are apparently ineffective with the isolated granules.

The roster of agents that labilize lysosomes is far longer than that of lysosome-stabilizing substances. Chief among the agents that stabilize lysosomes are the anti-inflammatory steroids (except for corticosterone): cortisone, cortisol, prednisolone, and betamethasone. These substances appear to act both in vitro and in the living cell, which points to the hypothesis that they exert their pharmacologic action on the membranes of lysosomes. Just as some labilizing agents can affect mitochondria and other organelles, cortisone and cortisol protect the membranes of hepatocytes, erythrocytes, and mitochondria. It appears likely that the effect of these agents on the permeability of lysosomes is an example of their ability to interact with the lipids that are common to various membrane-bound structures.

It is significant that several of the agents known to disrupt lysosomes — in vitro and in vivo — can also be used

Lysosomal Disruption and Joint Injury

Filipin, a polyene antibiotic, induces arthritis when injected into rabbit joints. In vitro, filipin has been shown to disrupt lysosomes by reacting with the phospholipids of their membranes. It may thus be assumed that filipin attacks the lysosomes of chondrocytes, releasing enzymes capable of degrading the cartilage matrix itself.

Rabbit joint in photomicrographs has been injected with filipin in dimethyl sulfoxide (DMSO), while injections of the vehicle alone serve as control. Top left: DMSO alone maintains regular columnar arrangement of chondrocytes and does not disturb anionic polysaccharide of matrix. In superficial layer of transitional area (bottom left) filipin induces disappearance of polysaccharide, which persists in deeper layers. In more advanced stage (top right) there is clustering of chondrocytes and polysaccharide is scant. Finally, polysaccharide disappears and fibrillar strands divide cartilage with clustered chondrocytes into irregular islands (bottom right).

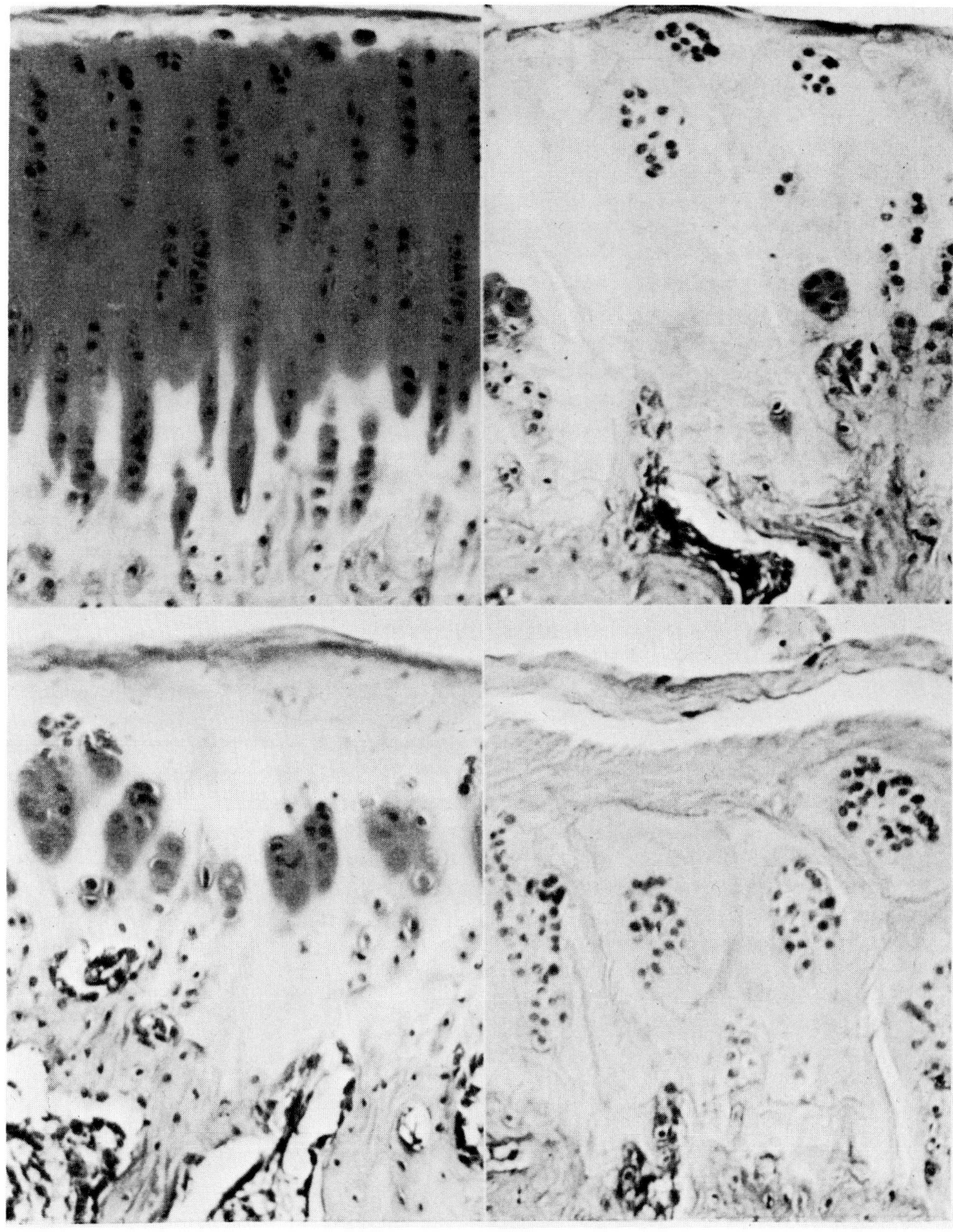

Possible Sources of Lysosomal Enzymes in Joint Injury

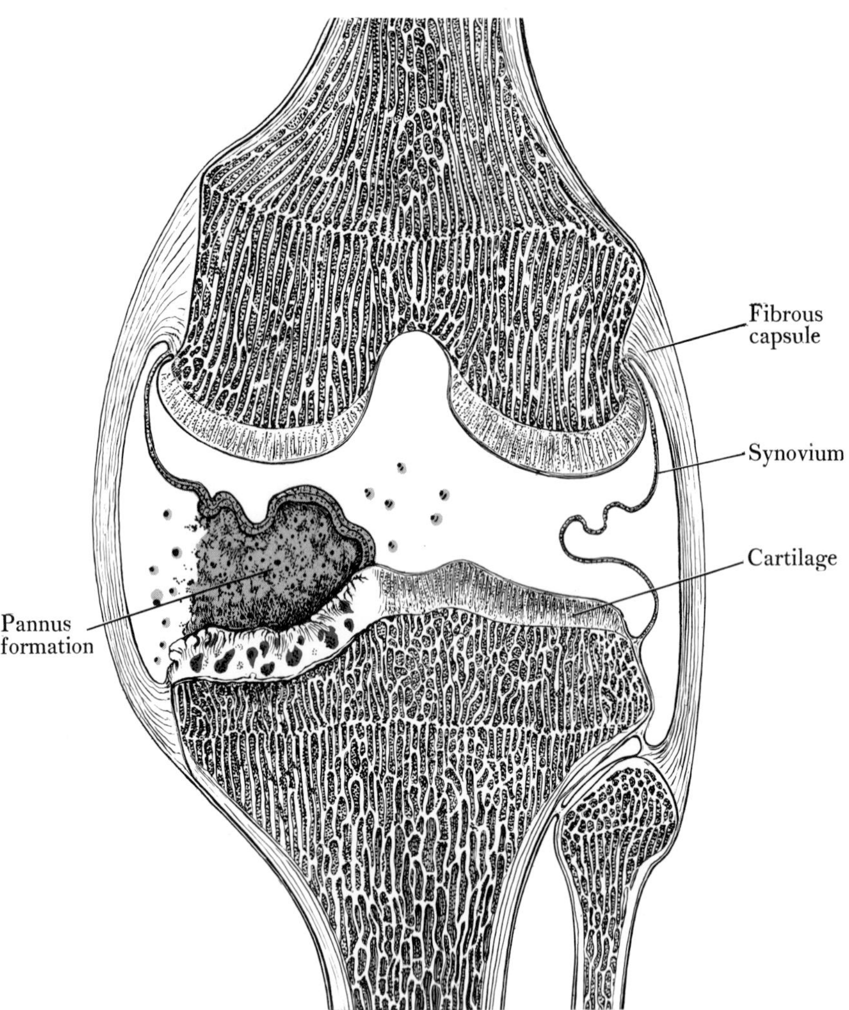

Cells believed to participate in inflammatory changes of arthritis by releasing lysosomes include the chondrocytes, whose normal arrangement becomes distorted (red), synovial lining cells, and infiltrating mono- and polymorphonuclear cells (pink).

to produce experimental rheumatic lesions or aggravate existing rheumatic diseases. Conversely, agents that relieve the rheumatic diseases have been shown to stabilize lysosomes.

Streptolysin S repeatedly injected into laboratory animals produces a chronic arthritis characterized by synovial hyperplasia, focal collections of lymphocytes, and pannus formation with cartilage destruction and joint erosion. This effect has been traced to the lysin's action on the lysosomes, and the lesions resemble those of rheumatoid arthritis. Injection of the polyene antibiotic filipin — which has less effect on the lining cells but acts on the cartilage cells — produces cartilage degradation closely resembling the acute lesions of osteoarthritis. Finally, injections of purified lysosomes (when lysed to sucrose) can provoke local changes in rabbit joints that closely resemble those of rheumatoid arthritis. Hypervitaminosis A has been extensively studied as a condition in which proteases released from lysosomes degrade cartilage. Urates disrupt the membranes of lysosomes after crystals are fed to leukocytes. This is borne out by the observation that the level of circulating polymorphonuclear cells is a crucial factor in the experimental production of crystal-induced arthritis in dogs. Immune reactions, too, have been shown to labilize lysosomes.

The agents that, almost empirically, have been found of value in the treatment of joint inflammation have, each in its own way, a stabilizing effect upon lysosomes. The adrenal glucocorticoids and their synthetic analogues, as has been seen, directly stabilize the lysosomal membrane. However, although acetylsalicylic acid, in doses which can be used clinically, has been claimed to stabilize lysosomal membranes in vitro, we have not found this to be so.

Gold salts are selectively taken up by the lysosomes of macrophages. There is evidence suggesting that gold inhibits lysosomal enzyme activity. Phenylbutazone has not been shown to have any direct effect on lysosomes, but it appears to inhibit the release of lysosomal enzymes into the circulation. Indomethacin inhibits the migration of leukocytes. Thus, lysosomal products of these cells might be kept from reaching inflammation sites.

Colchicine has no effect on the lysosomal membrane. It permits leukocytes to engulf crystalline and particulate matter, but inhibits the merger of the phagosomes thus formed with lysosomes, owing to its action on microtubules.

The relationship of lysosomes to disorders other than those of connective tissue has been established, and there are several that can definitely be attributed to a lysosomal defect. Pompe's disease, glycogen storage disease type II, has been traced to a lack of the enzyme α-1, 4-glucosidase in liver lysosomes. Activity of the other lysosomal enzymes is normal. Electron microscopic examination of livers from victims of this fatal disease of small children shows segregation of a large proportion of glycogen in vacuoles surrounded by a single membrane. It is thought that this segregation of the polysaccharide may be the cause of this deposition disease. Presumably the enzymes of the phospholytic pathway have been inactivated by lysosomal protease in the vacuoles.

Deficiency of the lysosomal enzyme β-D-galactosidase has been advanced as a factor in Gaucher's disease. The serum level of acid phosphatase is increased in patients with this disorder, while their spleens show increased activity of other lysosomal hydrolases. In metachromatic leukodystrophy there is a significant diminution of arylsulphatase A, while other lysosomal enzymes stay within the normal range. Cerebroside sulfate collects in several organs, principally in the nervous system. In Tay-Sachs disease, the abnormal ganglioside is stored within membrane-bounded organelles that stain positively for acid phosphatase. Indeed, most of the common lipid, or polysaccharide, storage diseases are turning out to be due to the deficiency of a lysosomal enzyme specific for that disease.

According to one hypothesis, the Chediak-Higashi syndrome of children may be considered a general disorder of organelle formation. Among other subcellular abnormalities, patients' leukocytes contain deformed granules, which have been shown to be abnormally large and fragile lysosomes. Similar lysosomal fragility has been demonstrated in Aleutian mink suffering from an analogous autosomal recessive trait.

The deficiency of an as yet unidentified bactericidal product of the lysosomes may be responsible for the lethal granulomatous children's disease that has been studied by B. H. Gray and R. A. Good [Chapter 6], in which leukocytes cannot kill some pyogenic bacteria after phagocytosis. Leukocyte lysosomes of these children appear morphologically intact and merge properly with phagosomes to form phagolysosomes, but phagocytosed bacteria within the vacuoles appear to escape degradation. These children react to every infection as though it were caused by intracellular parasitism, that is, with the formation of necrotizing granulomata. Moreover, since the bacteria are surrounded by the phagolysosomal membrane, they are unaffected by the usual levels of antibiotics.

Tantalizing evidence of significant lysosomal involvement in hypertension and in diseases of the liver, kidney, and heart continues to mount. Lysosomal hydrolases were found to be released into the coronary sinuses of dogs after experimental ligation of the coronary arteries. The aging pigment of myocardium can be detected in the abnormally large number of autophagic vacuoles and residual bodies found in the heart muscle of patients with congestive heart failure, particularly that due to mitral stenosis.

Juxtaglomerular cell granules have been shown to be lysosomes. In ischemia they appear to release the protease renin, just as other substances are released from lysosomes, and may play a role in hypertensive disease. Beta-glucuronidase and muramidase, two lysosomal enzymes, have been detected in abnormal concentrations in the urine of pyelonephritis patients. There is good evidence that these enzymes originate from renal parenchyma or inflammatory cells in the kidney, not in plasma or the leukocytes of urine. Newly formed lysosomes appear in the renal papillae of patients with chronic potassium deficiency. The periodic acid–Schiff positive granules found within tubules have been identified as lysosomes or phagolysosomes. Similarly, PA–S positive structures in the livers of patients who have hepatitis or cholestatic jaundice have been found to be autophagic vacuoles.

Lysosomes were found to be labilized in hepatitis, but not in chronic cirrhosis. In the lysosomes of hepatocytes of patients with Wilson's disease, both copper and the reaction product of acid phosphatase activity have been found. Lipofuscin and many hepatocellular pigments, especially those of Dubin-Johnson syndrome, have been found to be deposited in lysosomes.

Our present work is concerned principally with the substances and circumstances that rupture lysosomes, and those that stabilize them. We are also looking into the role of lysosomes in the production of fever — which we have shown can be related to substances that damage lysosomes. Among these are pyrogenic steroids such as etiocholanolone and the other 5-β-hydrogen steroids. We think that they may produce fever in man by releasing endogenous pyrogen, which has been shown to be present in some lysosomes. It appears that these steroids act on membrane-bounded structures, because cortisone antagonizes their effect both in vitro and in vivo.

Our studies have been aided by the fact that it is possible to make in the laboratory synthetic lipid bodies resembling natural membrane-bounded cells or organelles. These artificial "liposomes" are made of lecithin, dicetylphosphate, and cholesterol, and form as concentric lamellar spherulites. The lipid layers can be made to surround marker molecules at the time of membrane formation. Agents that disrupt lysosomes bring about leakage of the marker molecules, while the presence of cortisone, cortisol acetate, or chloroquine retards the leakage. We have found that if 1% of cortisone is preincorporated into the liposome membrane, the liposome will prove to be more resistant to subsequent disruption.

In our future work, my associates and I expect to continue our study of the role played by lysosomal hydrolases in the mitosis of lymphocytes. We hope this research, which we started recently, may shed more light on the problem of how and whether, in immune conditions, damage can be produced by lymphocytes. Recently we were able to show that a lymphocyte stimulated by antigens or phytohemagglutinin contains more lysosomes than a nonstimulated lymphocyte and is thus potentially capable of tissue injury. This has been clearly observed in cultured cells and remains to be studied in the living organism.

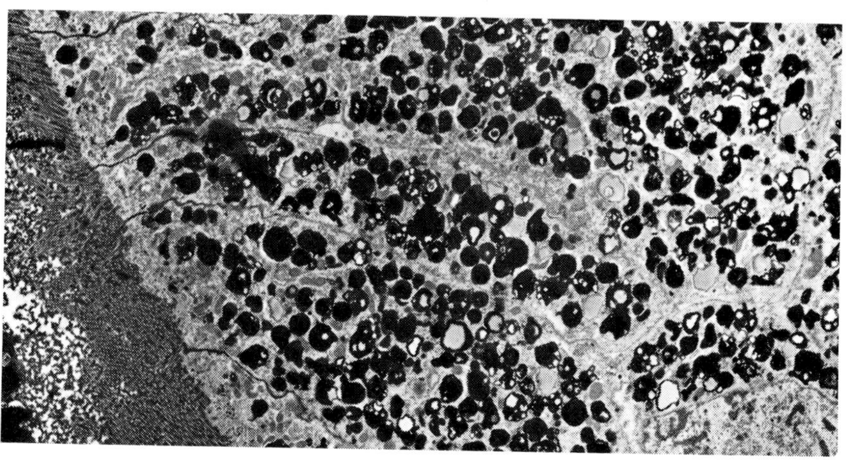

Autophagic vacuoles almost fill gut cells of flesh fly Sarcophaga bullata *during histolysis accompanying insect's metamorphosis to pupal stage. Magnification is 6,000x.*

Chapter 5

Cell-Mediated Immunity to Infection

GEORGE B. MACKANESS
Trudeau Institute

Acquired immunity to some infectious agents differs from the classical mechanisms in which specific antibody interferes with infectivity or pathogenicity by combining with the invading organism or its toxic products. There is no evidence, for example, that viruses, bacteria, or protozoa are influenced in any way by antibody while they are protectively accommodated within the cytoplasm of host cells. It is true that some intracellular parasites are subject to rapid inactivation by antibody while in transit from one host cell to the next. Plasmodial parasites, for example, are highly susceptible to humoral antibody during the merozoite stage of their life cycle. But there are many pathogenic bacteria and several protozoan parasites that are quite unaffected by antibody, even during the extracellular phases of their existence. Parasites with properties such as these obviously present a special problem of defense that can be met only by measures that drastically alter the intracellular environment from one in which the parasite normally prospers to one that will not support its continued survival. A mechanism of this sort has become widely recognized only in recent times, even though Metchnikoff believed immunity normally operates in just this way.

It was Lurie who first marshalled evidence suggesting that acquired resistance against tuberculosis is expressed through the phagocytic cells of reactive lesions. He thought that monocytes mature into epithelioid cells in response to the presence of ingested organisms. The mechanism of macrophage activation is now known, however, to be a more complex event than this, for it involves the necessary participation of immunologically committed lymphocytes. It depends, in fact, upon a very formal response on the part of the host's immunologic apparatus.

Helmholtz was the first to suggest, on rather equivocal evidence published in 1909, that living cells were necessary for the passive transfer of tuberculin sensitivity. The subject remained controversial until Landsteiner and Chase showed in 1942 that contact sensitivity could be transferred with exudate cells from sensitive donors [see Chapter 11, "Transfer Factor and Cellular Immunity," H. Sherwood Lawrence]. This marked the beginning of concept of a cell-mediated form of immunity, but the real significance and functional potential of an immune mechanism conveyed by cells rather than serum antibodies did not dawn for a further decade, when Mitchison showed that the rejection of grafted tissues depends upon immunologically committed lymphoid cells created in response to the presence of the graft.

The predominating importance of cells in the rejection of foreign tissue is now a well-established fact, but the existence of a similar mechanism of defense against infectious disease is a much more recent discovery. This is surprising, for the classical manifestation of cell-mediated immunity is delayed-type hypersensitivity, and this is so commonly associated with infection it was once known as bacterial allergy. A role for hypersensitivity in resistance to infection might have been recognized sooner had it not been the obvious cause of pathologic changes such as caseation. Moreover, hypersensitivity is only a superficial manifestation of an immunologic process that seemed to have no functional meaning until Medawar recognized that graft rejection and a tuberculin reaction are very similar events.

Within the last decade, a few isolated reports have suggested that some degree of resistance to certain bacterial infections (tuberculosis and tularemia) can be adoptively transferred to normal recipients with lymphoid cells from donors whose serum is inert in passive protection tests. But the protection conferred with cells was not impressive, perhaps because immunity to organisms that do not provoke the formation of protective antibodies is seldom incisive, though often quite efficient in the long run. Indeed, the problem of demonstrating clear-cut protection against the tubercle bacillus has impeded the search for better vaccinating procedures. Fortunately, there are a few intracellular infections in which acquired immunity is efficient enough to make the mechanism easier to study. *Listeria monocytogenes*, though unimportant as a human pathogen, provides an excellent model of an acute bacterial infection in which acquired resistance depends upon a cell-mediated form of immunity. This model has been used by several investigators, beginning with Osebold in 1962. It will be mentioned frequently in the following account of what is known about the way in which cellular immunity operates. The topic begins most logically with a description of the activated macrophages that represent the final step through which immunity is expressed. This will be followed by an account of what is known of the manner in which the macrophage becomes activated and acquires its enhanced antimicrobial properties.

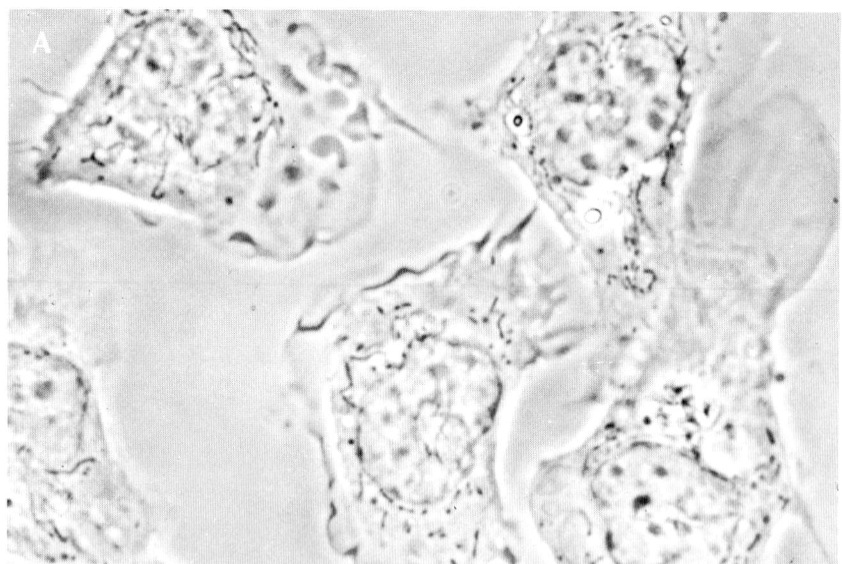

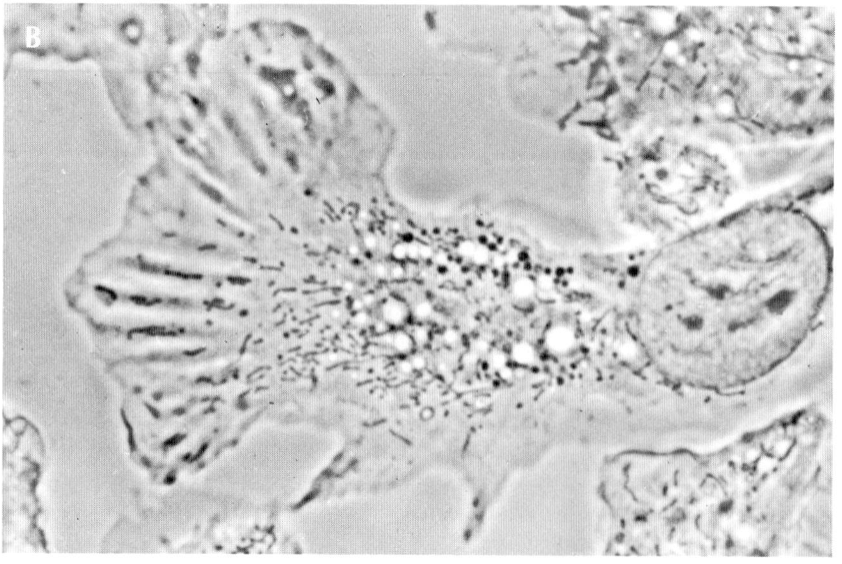

In phase-contrast micrographs of peritoneal macrophages from normal (A) and BCG-infected mice (B) after 12 hours in culture at 37°C a difference in size, tendency to spread, and content of cytoplasmic organelles is clearly apparent. The most distinctive features of activated macrophages are their increased content of mitochondria (filamentous phase-dense bodies) and of lysosomes (spherical phase-dense granules) and their pinocytotic activity. The latter is revealed by the phase-lucent vesicles; in living cultures these can be seen to arise in the cell periphery and migrate toward the center where they fuse to form larger vesicles and acquire hydrolytic enzymes.

When the host has to deal with organisms that flourish within its mononuclear phagocytes, it is obviously cells of this general class that must undergo modification in the defense of the host. There is abundant evidence that both the free and fixed mononuclear phagocytes of the reticuloendothelial system come under the influence of an intense stimulus during certain infections. They become morphologically and functionally altered. The photomicrographs at the left demonstrate increased size and structural complexity of peritoneal macrophages obtained from tuberculous mice. Their enormously enriched content of mitochondria is a morphologic expression of the added metabolic activity characteristic of activated macrophages. A striking feature of these activated cells is their ability to spread rapidly on charged surfaces (see next page). This is no more than a manifestation of their greatly enhanced capacity to ingest particulate material. There are, however, a number of less obvious changes that are nonetheless indicative of a response to stimulation that may extend to every free and fixed mononuclear phagocyte in the body of an infected animal.

During the course of a listeria infection in mice, a wave of mitosis passes over the whole reticuloendothelial system (see page 48). In a series of carefully detailed studies, R. J. North has demonstrated that this division of host phagocytes is followed immediately by evidence that activation has occurred in the responding cells. From the viewpoint of a host infected with living microorganisms, the most important sign of activation is an increase in the cells' microbicidal ability. It has been demonstrated, however, that mitosis is not the event that creates an activated macrophage. It is more likely that the stimulus that causes activation also leads to cell division if sufficiently intense. The immediate stimulus to activation and cell division will be discussed later. For the present, it suffices to say that it is probably applied at the

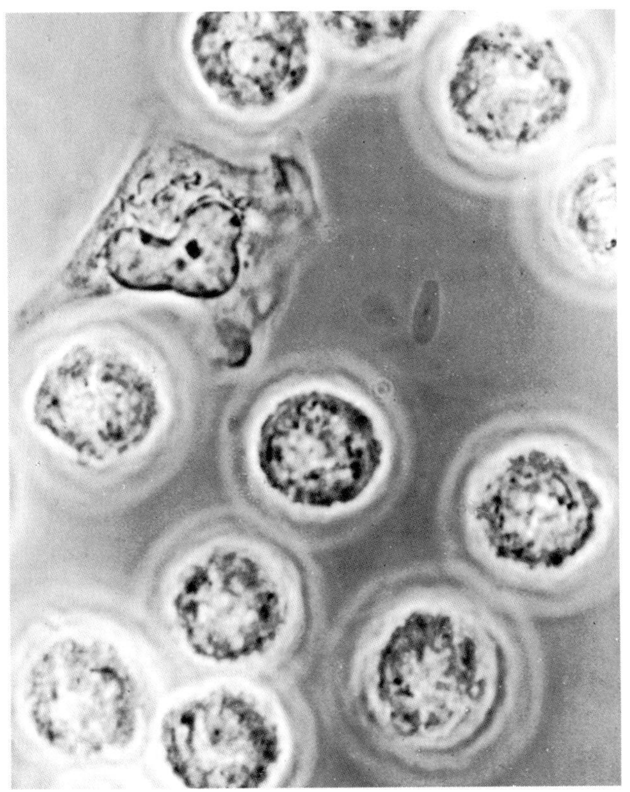

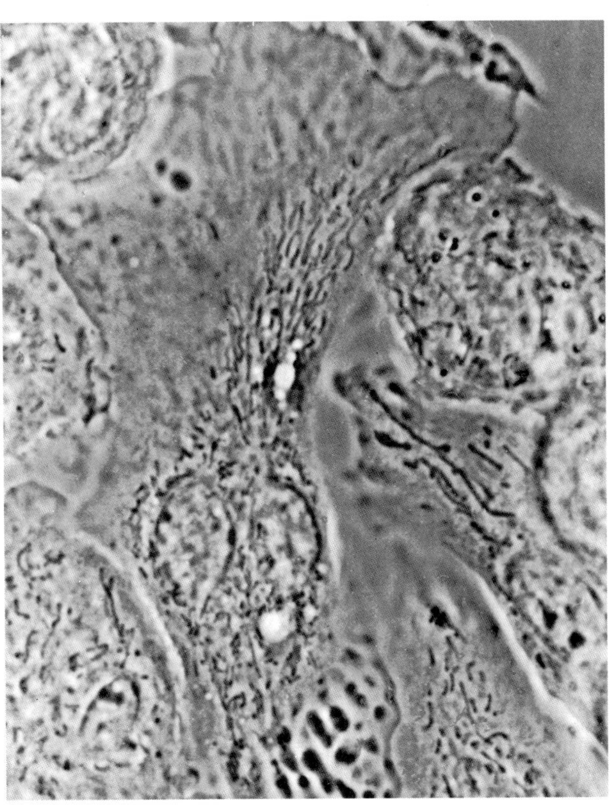

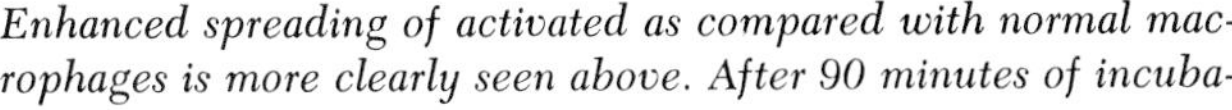

Enhanced spreading of activated as compared with normal macrophages is more clearly seen above. After 90 minutes of incubation only one normal cell (photo at left) had begun to spread, whereas after 15 minutes most activated cells had done so.

cell surface, for there is ample evidence that increased pinocytotic activity occurs in stimulated cells. Cohn and his colleagues at the Rockefeller University have shown that a stimulus applied to the surface of macrophages results in increased pinocytosis and that vigorous pinocytosis consistently leads to an increased formation of lysosomes with their content of acid hydrolases. An increased enzyme content is another characteristic feature of activated macrophages, but we do not know whether the enlarged armamentarium of degradative enzymes is related to the enhanced killing capacity of activated macrophages. It could account for their greater digestive capacity, a property first noted by Delazenne in the last century. But there are several reasons for thinking that ingested organisms are killed by a mechanism much more subtle than mere digestion. Whatever its nature, it, too, is greatly augmented in the activated macrophage.

Included in the evidence pointing to the defensive importance of activated macrophages was the close parallel between an animal's ability to inactivate a second inoculum of bacteria in vivo and the capacity of its macrophages to perform the same act in tissue culture. Most infectious diseases have a characteristic time course, which shows a gradual mounting of host resistance until bacterial populations in the tissues cease to increase and begin to disappear. This stage is reached at a time that depends mainly upon the biologic properties of the infectious agent. Organisms that grow rapidly tend to produce a faster onset of resistance than do those that proliferate more slowly. In all cases, however, curtailment of the infectious process usually does not occur until host macrophages show their most striking signs of activation. While the host's tissues remain populated by such cells, it is virtually impossible to reinfect it.

Nothing has been said so far of the immunologic processes involved in the creation of activated macrophages. It has been mentioned, however, that resistance against organisms such as *L. monocytogenes* cannot be passively transferred with the serum of convalescent animals. If the spleens of animals that have survived a sublethal infection are dissociated into single cells and filtered to eliminate preformed phagocytes, the resulting suspension will protect recipients against a listeria challenge (see graph on page 49). The protection conferred by the cells of a single spleen is almost equal to that enjoyed by the donor. The transferred cells must be alive and metabolically active or they fail to immunize the recipient. Since their protective activity is abolished by treating the cells or the recipient with antilymphocyte serum, the cells involved are lymphoid in nature.

This inference was recently confirmed in studies by McGregor and Koster, who found that the thoracic duct lymph of subcutaneously infected rats contains at least as many protective cells as does the spleen of intravenously infected donors. The very fact that protective cells are present in the main lymphatic duct is reason enough to call them lymphocytes; but this does not tell us all we wish to know about the nature of the mediators of cellular immunity. One of their most important characteristics is specificity. Cells obtained from the spleens of animals that have been

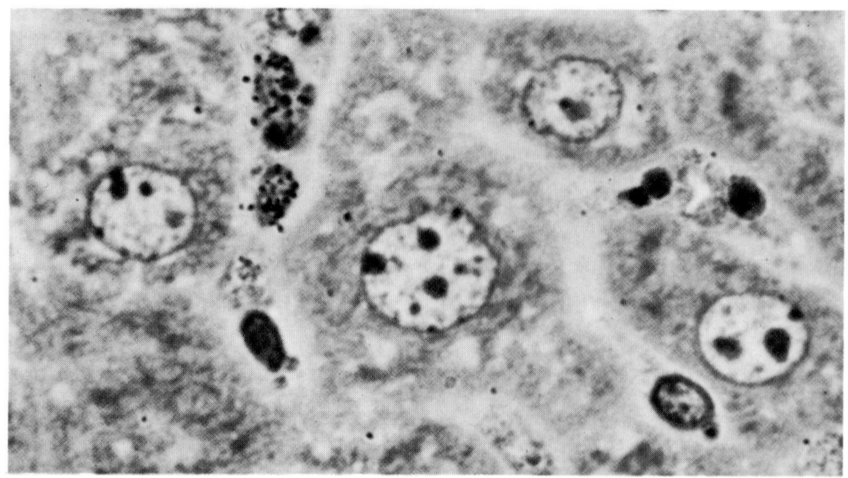

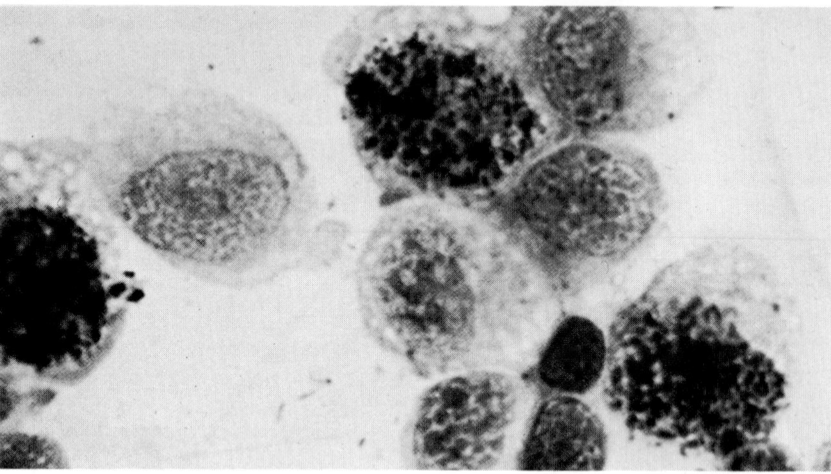

Mitotic response that occurs in reticuloendothelial system of mice infected with listeria is demonstrated: Phagocytes from liver sinusoids (top) were labeled with carbon (yellow granules) two weeks before infection, and pulse of tritiated thymidine was given on second day of infection. Granules overlying nuclei identify dividing cells that incorporated labeled precursor into their DNA (photomicrograph by Dr. R. J. North). Peritoneal macrophages (lower photo), taken on second day of infection, were incubated for 15 minutes with tritiated thymidine. Three heavily labeled cells can be seen.

immunized with tubercle bacilli can confer tuberculin sensitivity upon normal recipients, but they do not afford protection against a listeria challenge. Yet the tuberculous donor can be highly resistant to a listeria challenge because of the activated macrophages it possesses.

The failure of lymphoid cells to transfer this nonspecific resistance could mean that specific and nonspecific immunity are totally unrelated phenomena. It seems much more likely, however, that nonspecific resistance is an inadvertent by-product of specific resistance. This notion has been tested in studies that revealed that immune spleen cells from tuberculous mice will protect against a listeria challenge if the cell recipients are also injected with a small dose of tubercle bacilli. In this circumstance, the macrophages of the adoptively sensitized animal become activated within 24 hours, and host resistance to a listeria challenge rises. The obvious conclusion is that interaction between bacteria and specifically reactive lymphoid cells sets off the events that lead to the activation of macrophages. Again, we must leave discussion of the mechanism of stimulation, this time to deal more fully with the origin and nature of the immunologically committed lymphocyte.

The findings cited and other evidence make it clear that the specificity typical of humoral immunity is equally characteristic of the mediators of cellular immunity. This is one reason for calling them *immunologically committed cells.* Their presence in thoracic duct lymph and their susceptibility to inactivation by antilymphocyte globulin imply that they are lymphocytes. The process of their formation is a fascinating problem. North and his associates have shown that a second population of cells, in addition to the dividing macrophages, becomes mitotically active during the course of a listeria or a tuberculous infection. DNA-synthesizing cells are seen conspicuously in the spleens of intravenously infected animals. They become most numerous on the third day in an acute, rapidly moving listeria infection; but it is not until the 14th day that mitotic activity reaches its peak in the spleens of mice infected with the tubercle bacillus. In both cases, however, very large numbers of cells become involved, as the autoradiographs on the opposite page show. This intense proliferative response appears to be the process by which a population of immunologically committed lymphocytes is formed, for immunosuppressive drugs prevent the development of immunity in infected mice.

The dividing cells, which resemble lymphocytes in various states of maturity, do not contain immunoglobulins in amounts sufficient to be revealed by the fluorescent antibody technique. Labeling studies indicate that the newly formed cells are rapidly released into the circulation, where they are presumably available to mediate both hypersensitivity to the organism and protection against it. The argument for linking these two modalities rests mainly on the finding that the amount of hypersensitivity is proportional to the amount of protection that can be conferred with any given population of immune spleen cells.

The cells we have been discussing are the presumptive mediators of cellular immunity. We can only recognize them, however, through the immunologic function of the population as a whole. Even as a group, their identity remained obscure until this year. It has been mentioned already that representatives of the population are present in thoracic duct lymph of listeria-immune rats. Lymph-borne cells are mainly small lymphocytes.

Most of them have a long circulating life-span, which they spend in constant motion through lymphoid tissues to the blood and back again. These are the immunocompetent cells that can initiate an immune response; they are not the cells that serve an immediate role in protection against infections. To learn more about cells that do, McGregor and Koster studied the delivery of cells into the thoracic duct lymph of animals infected subcutaneously with *L. monocytogenes*. They found that a large number of newly formed cells are added to the lymph of infected rats. Their recent origin by cell division was shown by the incorporation of a radioactive marker in the form of tritiated thymidine. The most numerous addition was found to be a small lymphocyte that could not recycle from blood to lymph in the manner of the long-lived, immunocompetent small lymphocyte. The cells that confer protection against infection were found to belong among the newly derived cells that do not recirculate. This presumably makes them members of the short-lived small lymphocyte population that shows the largest percentage increase in response to infection. No function has previously been ascribed to cells of this category.

It is interesting to relate, therefore, that Koster and McGregor have uncovered another distinguishing property of short-lived small lymphocytes. They are predisposed to enter areas of inflammation. When a cellular exudate is induced in the peritoneal cavity of the rat, it is constituted mainly of mononuclear phagocytes; but a small proportion of the immigrant cells are nonphagocytic elements from the blood that do not adhere to charged surfaces. This property permitted the latter to be separated from the rest. They were found to be small lymphocytes of the short-lived variety only. It is not surprising, therefore, that lymphocytes recovered from a peritoneal exudate in listeria-immune rats were more highly protective for listeria-challenged recipients than were an equivalent number of thoracic duct cells. The selective process that brings these immunologically committed lymphocytes into an inflammatory exudate points to a

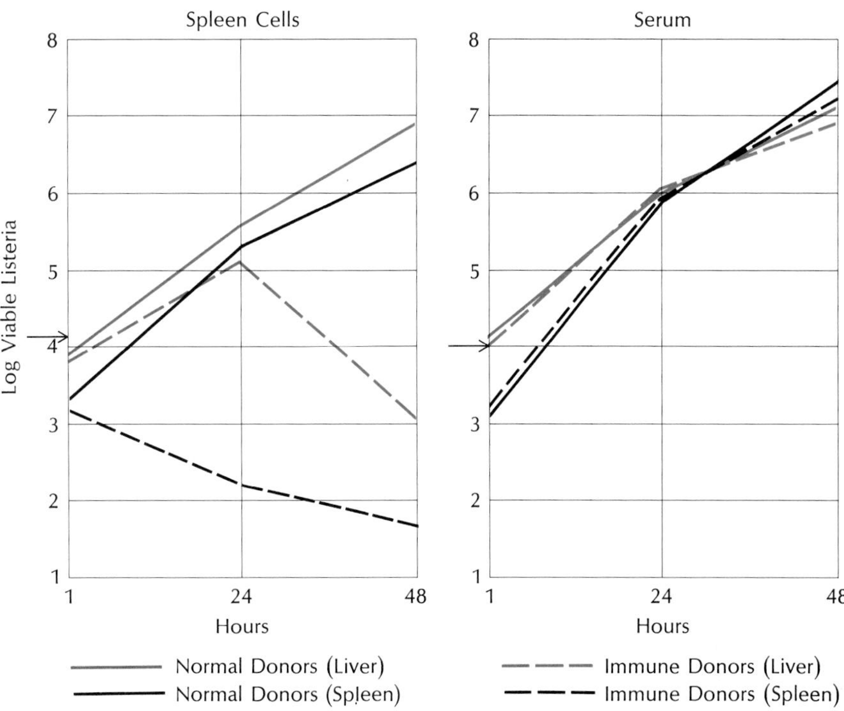

In contrast to those from normal donors, dissociated spleen cells from listeria-immune mice protect against growth or survival of Listeria monocytogenes *in spleen and liver of recipient mice. Serum from the same donors, either immune or normal, does not protect.*

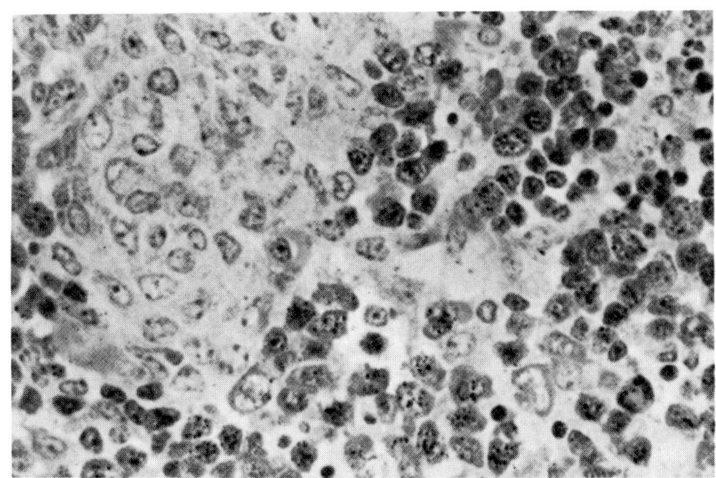

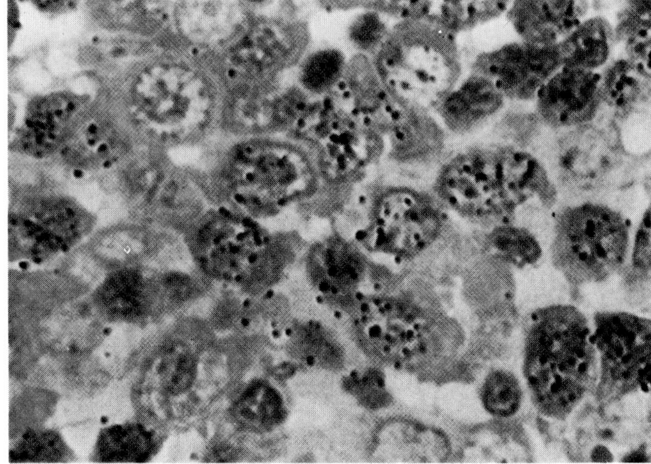

In section of mouse spleen excised 30 minutes after injection of tritiated thymidine given on 12th day of infection with virulent tubercle bacilli, rapidly dividing lymphoid cells of varying size and appearance can be seen surrounding a prominent tubercle composed of epithelioid cells (left). The structure of the lymphoid cells is better seen in autoradiograph at right. Cells range in appearance from blasts with prominent nucleoli to small lymphocytes with a narrow rim of pyroninophilic cytoplasm.

functional trait that may compel cells of this type to participate in any inflammatory process, thus ensuring the presence of specifically committed cells in areas where they may be needed. Some years ago, Polak and Turk drew attention to the fact that the cells that mediate tuberculin sensitivity also belong among the nonadhering cells of an exudate. This points again to the conclusion that hypersensitivity and antimicrobial protection are vested in the same cell population.

From the foregoing observations it seems fair to conclude that cell-mediated immunity is vested primarily in cells that look like small lymphocytes but are created in response to the infection and have a short circulating life-span. They do not recycle from blood to lymph, and show a marked proclivity to become engaged in inflammatory processes. The last two properties might easily explain their short life-span in circulation. Cells that are prone to migrate into a mildly irritated peritoneal cavity might find many suitable exits from the circulation. The gut would be a very likely portal through which such cells could be enticed to leave the circulation.

It must be known to most readers that lymphocytes are not physiologically equipped to make a direct attack on microorganisms. In a previous article in this series [Chapter 21, "Immunologic Defenses Against Cancer"], the Hellströms reviewed the evidence that committed lymphocytes can attack specific target cells, thereby accomplishing the destruction of a tumor by interacting directly with its constituent cells. A similar process of interaction between lymphocytes and bacteria is hard to visualize in the case of cell-mediated immunity against a microbial infection. The intervention of a phagocytic element would seem to be essential. Direct evidence is in fact available to prove that cell-mediated immunity involves collaboration between committed lymphocytes and phagocytic cells.

The photo on page 54 illustrates a lesion in liver of an animal that was infected three days earlier with *L. monocytogenes*. Immediately prior to infection the animals were injected twice with tritiated thymidine to introduce a radioactive label into the dividing precursors of blood monocytes in bone marrow. During the intervening days, labeled monocytes would have entered the circulation to reach infective foci. The illustration shows that by the third day the lesions had become populated exclusively by cells of this type. Since a majority of the participating cells display the radioactive label, they must have originated three days previously from cells that were dividing during the brief period when tritiated thymidine was available for

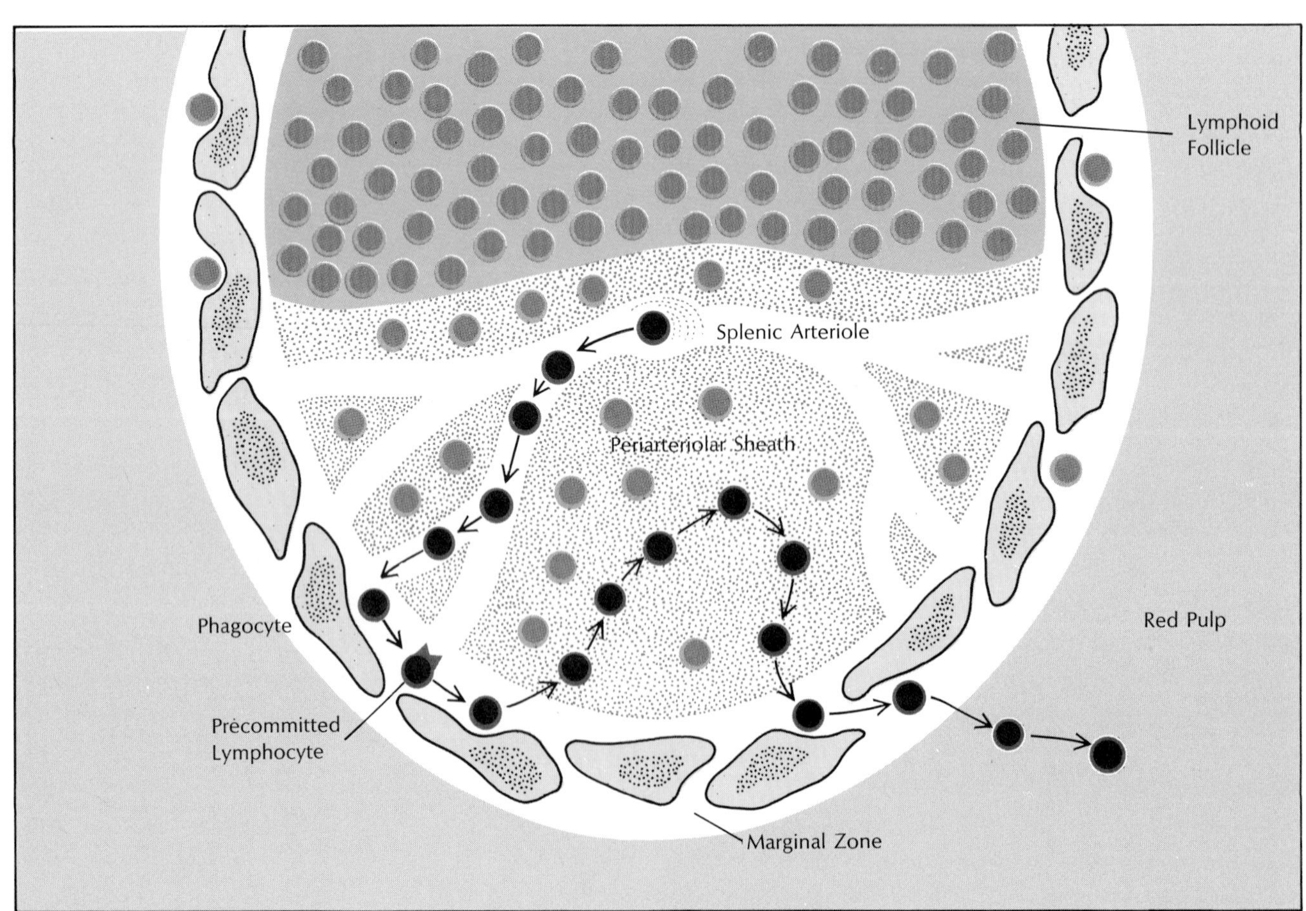

Transformation of uncommitted to committed small lymphocytes is depicted schematically on these pages. Periarteriolar sheath is visualized as lying adjacent to a lymphoid follicle in the mouse spleen. Small lymphocytes enter the splenic white pulp by way of the central arteriole and its capillary offshoots; the latter empty into the marginal zone, rich in phagocytes, that borders the red pulp. Cells entering red pulp are free to recirculate, but if any are induced to respond immunologically they return to the peri-

incorporation into DNA. They could not therefore have been members of the special population of committed lymphocytes that would not have been created until much later in the infection. Their indispensability to the host's defense is nonetheless absolute, as the following observations show. If a prospective recipient is x-irradiated prior to the adoptive transfer of listeria-immune spleen çells, it is no longer able to benefit from the protection that immune cells normally confer. Drugs that damage dividing cells can also interrupt the supply of monocytes from bone marrow precursors and render animals incapable of defending themselves against a listeria infection, even after adoptive immunization.

If committed lymphocytes and circulating monocytes are *both* needed for defense against organisms that can survive ingestion by phagocytic cells, there must be some provision for the two cell types to interact. A clue to the nature of the event was obtained when spleen cells from tuberculous donors were given to normal recipients. They had no overt effect on the functional state of recipient macrophages unless tubercle bacilli were injected along with the reactive spleen cells. When this was done, activated macrophages appeared in the peritoneal cavity within 24 hours, and the animals became resistant to a listeria challenge.

Additional evidence has since accumulated that committed lymphocytes can influence the behavior and activity of mononuclear phagocytes only in the presence of the infectious agent used to immunize the host or sensitize the donor in the case of adoptive immunization. Thus, the wave of macrophage mitosis that precedes the onset of resistance during a listeria infection peaks 24 hours earlier in adoptively immunized animals, suggesting that donor lymphocytes render recipient phagocytes sensitive to listeria antigen.

The marshalling of circulating monocytes at an infective focus is another influence that can now be attributed to committed lymphocytes. It has long been known that epithelioid tubercles form more rapidly in tuberculin-sensitive animals. The counterpart of accelerated tubercle formation is seen in a listeria infection when immune spleen cells are given prior to a challenge infection. Adoptive immunization causes a manifold increase in the rate at which labeled monocytes accumulate in lesions. Cell-mediated immunity to infection thus involves at least two separate operations: one that ensures the mobilization of cells at sites of bacterial implantation and another that causes the activation of individual cells to produce an environment in which the organisms cannot

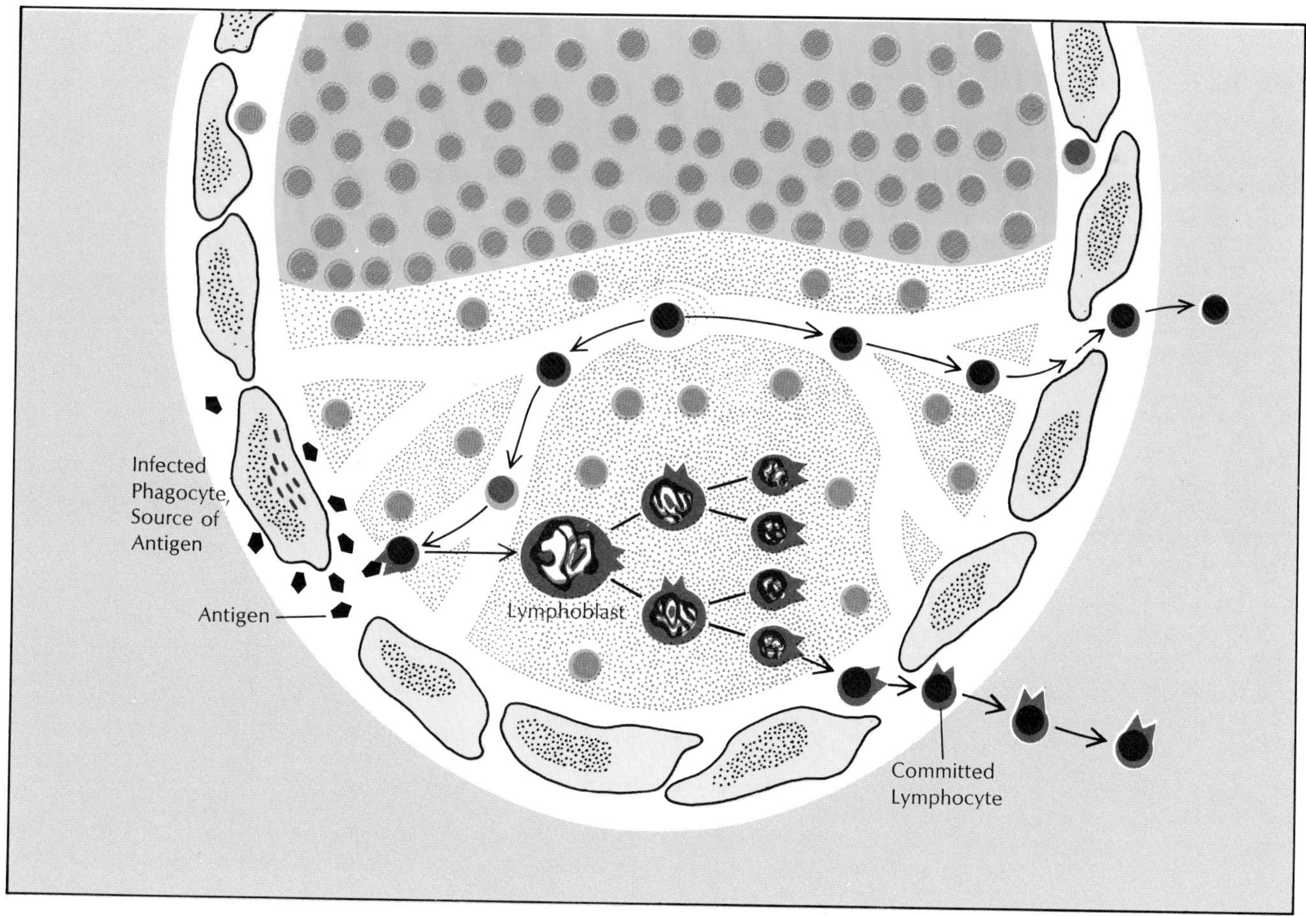

arteriolar sheath, there to undergo blast transformation and a succession of divisions that yield cells of diminishing size. Small pyroninophilic cells are the last stage that can be recognized morphologically in the development of a population of immunologically committed lymphocytes. These leave the white pulp and enter the systemic circulation by way of venous sinuses in the red pulp, whereupon they become available to mediate immunologic reactions specific for their corresponding antigens.

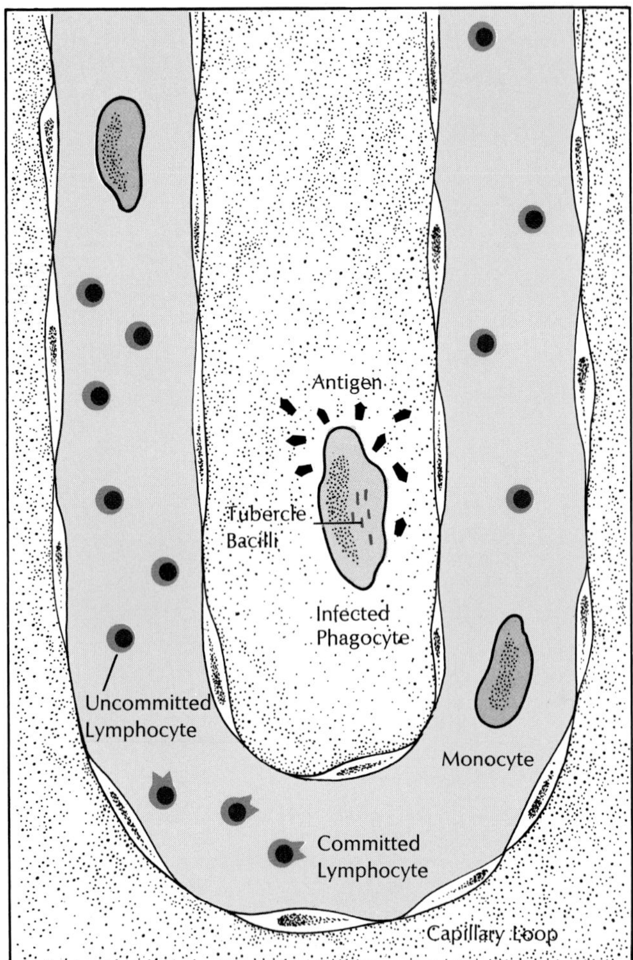

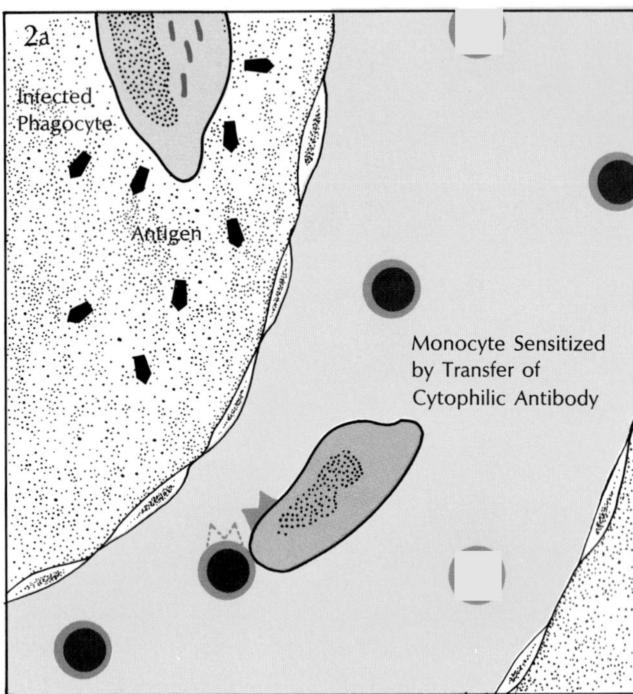

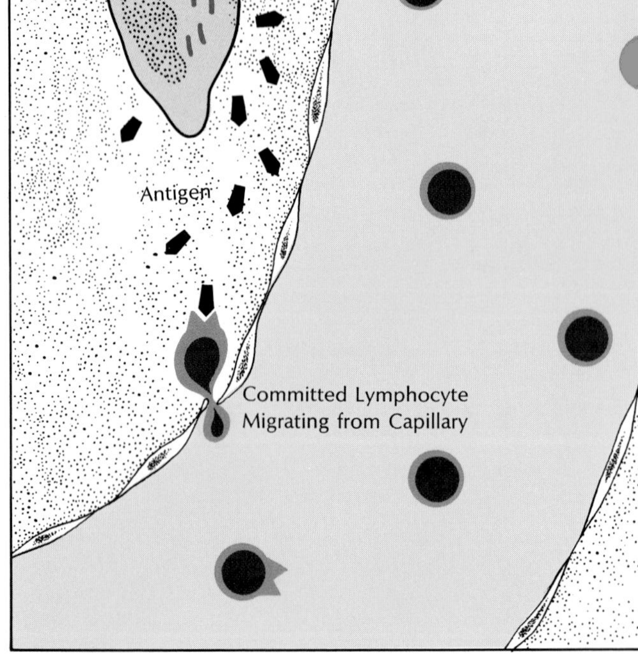

Two hypothetical mechanisms that could explain how tubercles are formed are presented schematically. The participating elements in both are depicted in panel 1. Their involvement in the first mechanism envisages the transfer of specific reactivity from committed lymphocytes to circulating monocytes (2a) which, in response to mycobacterial antigens emanating from the infected phagocyte, leave the circulation (3a) to become consolidated into a tubercle (4a). The second mechanism is based on substantial evidence that when committed lymphocytes encounter specific antigen (2b) they release biologically active molecules (3b) which attract monocytes to the infective site where they become immobilized by migration inhibitory factor (4b). The occurrence of such encounters between committed lymphocytes and antigen would be greatly enhanced by the tendency of these cells to leave the circulation in response to any form of mild irritation.

survive. This second step in the development of cellular immunity will be discussed later.

In the ultimate analysis, a chemical explanation must be found for the various effects that committed lymphocytes produce. One plausible explanation for their influence on macrophages postulates the production of a cytophilic antibody that binds to the surface of the macrophage with an affinity sufficient to explain its absence from serum. If macrophages were rendered sensitive to antigen by a cytophilic antibody, microbial antigens would then become the immediate stimulus that acts on the cell surface to increase pinocytotic activity and raise the metabolic level. There is evidence from the work of Cohn and his colleagues and of North at the Trudeau Institute that an antigen-antibody reaction at the macrophage surface has a stimulatory effect on the cell; but there is no good evidence for the existence of a macrophage-sensitizing antibody in cell-mediated immunity.

An alternative explanation for macrophage activation is based on the concept of molecular mediators. These are substances produced by committed lymphocytes under the stimulating influence of specific antigen. The first to be described was the migration inhibitory factor (MIF),

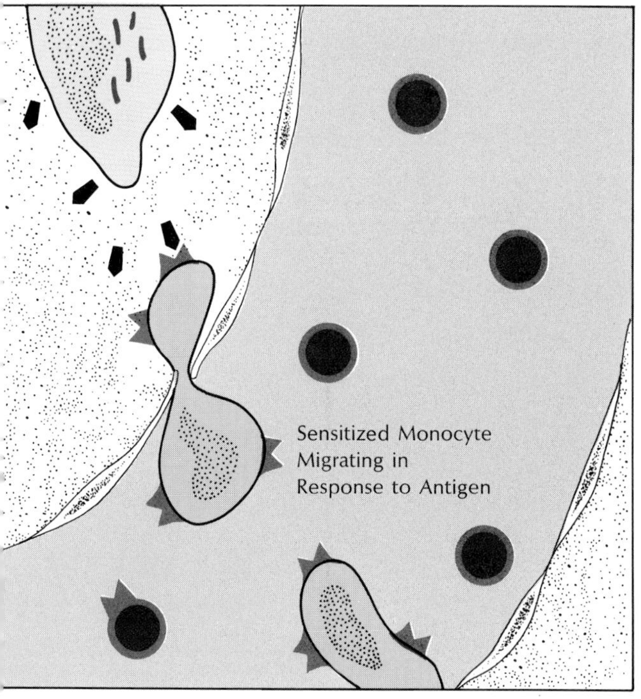

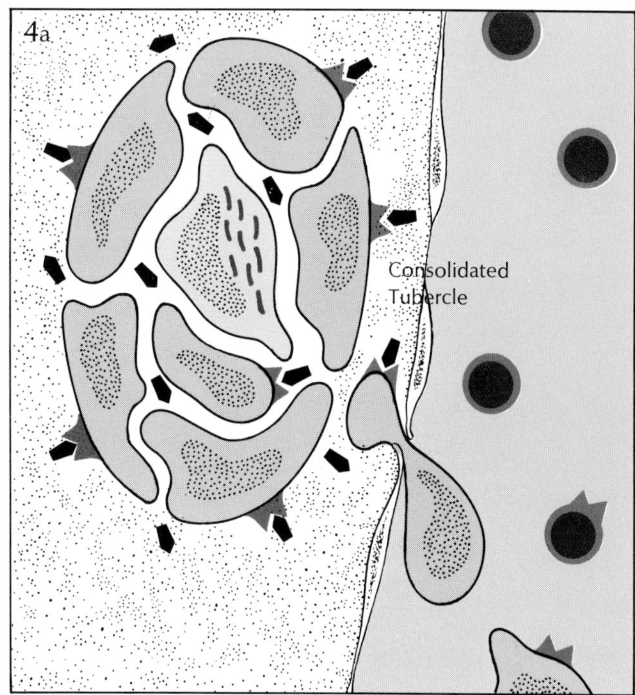

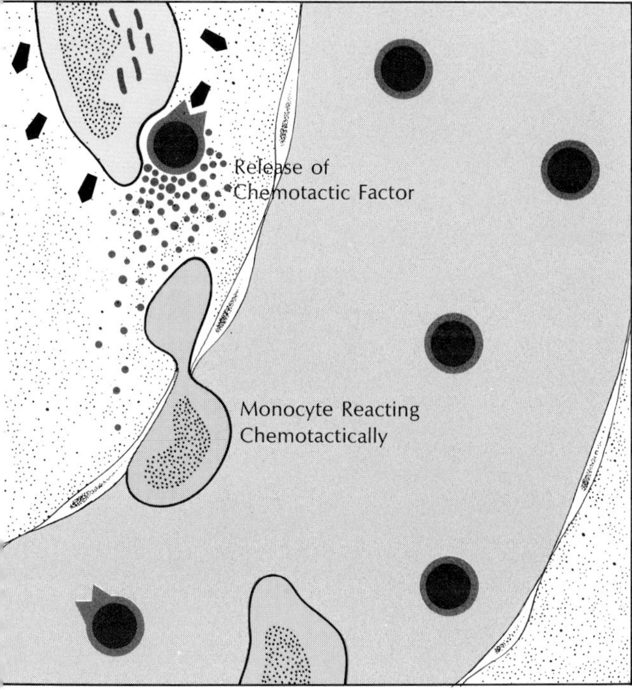

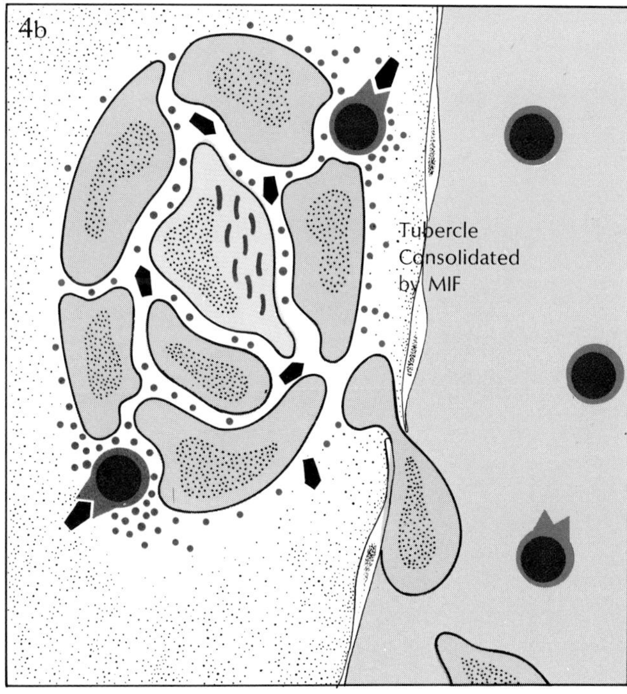

which has been studied by David and Bloom. The nature of MIF is still the subject of dispute. There is little doubt, however, that specifically committed lymphoid cells release biologically active substances when incubated in the presence of specific antigen. A molecule that could immobilize macrophages at sites of bacterial implantation would have a useful function to fulfill in any mechanism of antimicrobial immunity. There may be little difference between the inhibition of migration from a capillary tube in vitro and the trapping of bloodborne monocytes at infective foci in vivo. It is even possible that MIF or a related substance could operate on macrophages at a distance, influencing them to migrate into a focus of infection. Ward and David have, in fact, described a factor that is chemotactic for monocytes. It, too, is produced when committed lymphocytes are incubated with their specific antigen.

The idea that local release of a substance can influence monocyte movement in the vicinity presupposes that the source of the active factor is present within the locus. When a tuberculin reaction is enacted at the center of the avascular cornea, the site becomes populated by mononuclear cells that originate at the limbus. One can imagine that monocytes sensitized by ad-

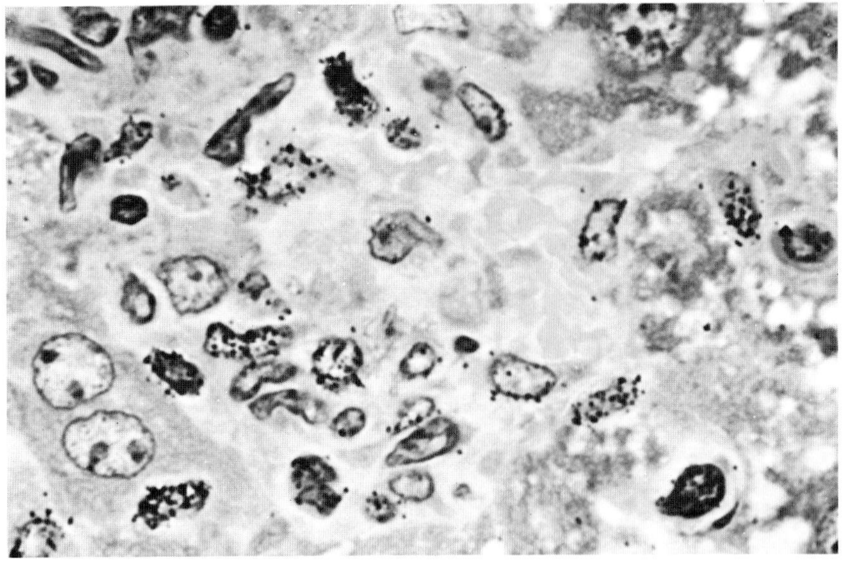

Before infection with virulent listeria, mice were injected with tritiated thymidine to label dividing precursors of blood monocytes in the bone marrow. Three days after infection, this lesion in the liver was populated almost exclusively by mononuclear phagocytes, many of them labeled, indicating that these cells arise from blood monocytes.

sorbed antibody would move into the cornea in search of a higher concentration of antigen to which they have become vicariously sensitized. But if this concerted movement of cells depends on a chemotactic substance released when tuberculin acts on committed lymphocytes, it would first be necessary to explain the presence of committed lymphocytes at the center of the cornea. Problems like this make the concept of molecular mediators in cellular immunity no more difficult to accept but they do raise a number of questions for which we still lack answers.

When we have found how cells are directed to a particular locus, we may also learn what gives them the functional capacity to inactivate bacteria. Since we do not know how susceptible bacteria are killed within *normal* phagocytes, we are in no position to speculate about the killing of resistant organisms within *activated* macrophages. There are indications, however, that the process is metabolically determined. This means that the microbicidal mechanism is not merely a digestive process involving nothing more intricate than an enzymatic attack upon constituents of the bacterial cell wall: It probably exists as a byproduct of an ongoing metabolic event. If so, the elevated metabolic rate of activated macrophages would confer a distinct advantage. Whatever the mechanism, it is greatly enhanced in the activated macrophage. But like the mitotic response of macrophages and accelerated tubercle formation, the process of macrophage activation is poorly understood. We do know, however, that it also depends upon the mediating cell that arises in response to infection. The evidence for this was mentioned earlier.

In summary, cellular immunity to infection has been depicted as a process involving two cell types. The mediating cell is a committed lymphocyte that belongs in the category of short-lived small lymphocytes. It is produced specifically in response to certain infectious agents. In the presence of specific antigen, committed lymphocytes can influence macrophage function in various ways. Whether they do so through the elaboration of chemical mediators or by the production of a sensitizing antibody remains uncertain. It is established, however, that beneath the whole process there are molecular events that are analogous to those of an antigen-antibody reaction, for the element of specificity is conspicuously present in the system: Immunologically committed lymphocytes created for defense against the tubercle bacillus do not function against unrelated organisms. Once the activation process has been set in train, however, activated macrophages appear. Through their enhanced metabolic properties these cells can protect effectively against microbial agents that are unrelated to those that brought them into existence. In other words, we have been discussing an immunologically specific mechanism of defense that creates a population of defensive phagocytes with quite nonspecific antimicrobial properties. Cellular immunity is nonetheless impressive as a mechanism of acquired resistance, for the range and magnitude of the protection it has been shown to provide is often quite remarkable.

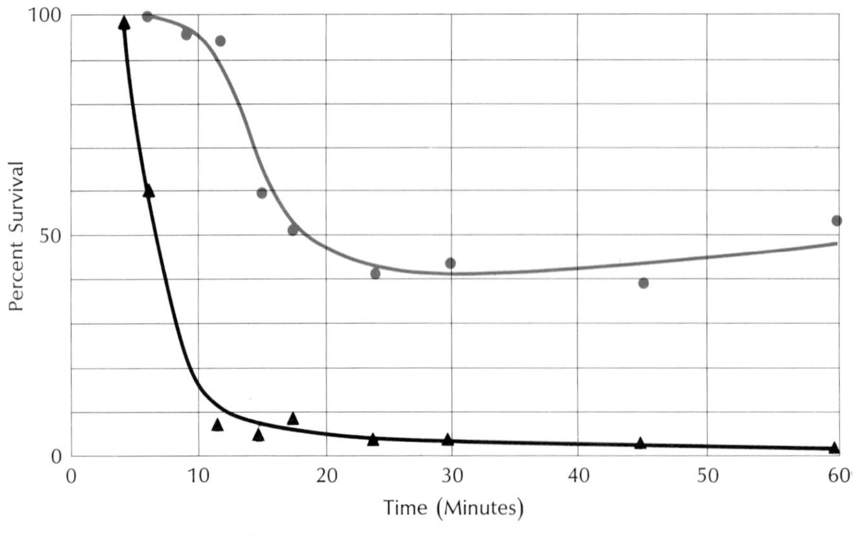

Faster onset of killing and greater bactericidal capability of activated vs normal macrophages was demonstrated in experiment with opsonized Salmonella typhimurium.

Chapter 6

Chronic Granulomatous Disease of Childhood

BEULAH HOLMES GRAY *and* ROBERT A. GOOD
University of Minnesota

Chronic granulomatous disease is a syndrome of paradoxes: Its victims are completely competent in handling such virulent organisms as streptococci, meningococci, pneumococci, and *Hemophilus influenzae* but are likely to succumb to microorganisms of low virulence such as staphylococci, aerobacter, *Escherichia coli*, and even to such semisaprophytes as *Serratia marcescens*, candida, aspergillus, and nocardia. This disease is a deficiency of bodily defense and may be considered to be an immunodeficiency disease but is usually characterized by hypergammaglobulinemia. The leukocytic defect central to the syndrome results in the subversion of normally defensive phagocytes to "protective capsules" that harbor pathogens and make them inaccessible to antibody and antibiotics, allowing dissemination and chronic infection.

Finally, it now seems clear that those pathogens that seem to be handled efficiently and normally by the host defense mechanisms of the child with CGD actually are not killed by the host cells but commit a form of metabolic "suicide."

Taken together, these paradoxes add up to a clinically tragic situation. The child with CGD, usually a boy, rarely survives to adolescence; in our experience and that of Landing and coworkers at the University of Southern California the average age at death has been seven years. At the same time, the paradoxes cited above have provided a means of dissecting many of the most puzzling aspects of normal bodily defense mechanisms, particularly those that relate to the phagocytosis and destruction of bacteria and other disease-causing organisms. And because CGD is inherited – most commonly as an X-linked recessive trait in the male offspring of female carriers but also (it now appears) as an autosomal recessive in female infants – it may also cast at least a ray of light upon some of the genetic bases of bodily defense.

How does the disease manifest itself clinically? As has been noted, the repeated severe infections seen from the first weeks of life are most often related etiologically to bacteria of low virulence. The presenting signs may be those of chronic suppurative and granulomatous lymphadenitis with scrofulous erosions on the surface. Skin lesions frequently progress from granulomatous to suppurative, and in our experience with some 32 cases we have found the simultaneous occurrence of granulomatous and suppurative purulent inflammation to be strongly suggestive of a CGD diagnosis, particularly in patients with leukocytosis and hypergammaglobulinemia. This last phenomenon is probably simply a consequence of repeated infection.

Visceral involvement characteristically includes hepatosplenomegaly with parenchymatous granuloma often associated with purulent inflammation. Septic and granulomatous osteomyelitis frequently develop as well as liver abscesses and pericarditis. Lipochrome-laden macrophages in the reticuloendothelial organs are a prominent feature of the disease. The progressive destructive processes in the lungs involving both sepsis and the proliferation of granuloma are most often the immediate cause of death in these children.

Probably the outstanding characteristic differentiating this disease from other diseases involving immunodeficiency or cellular defects is the granulomatous response to inflammation in the lymph nodes, spleen and liver, skin, and lungs. While the explanation for this response is not yet completely elucidated, many of the steps from phagocytosis to granuloma formation parallel pathogenetic features of tuberculosis in which the virulent organism, *Mycobacterium tuberculosis*, is not normally killed by polymorphonuclear leukocytes, and a second defensive effort leads to the localization of the organism by the granulomatous process. The susceptibility of the patient with chronic granulomatous disease to infection with low-grade pathogens is now known to be a consequence of a defect in polymorphonuclear leukocyte function. Bacteria are in-

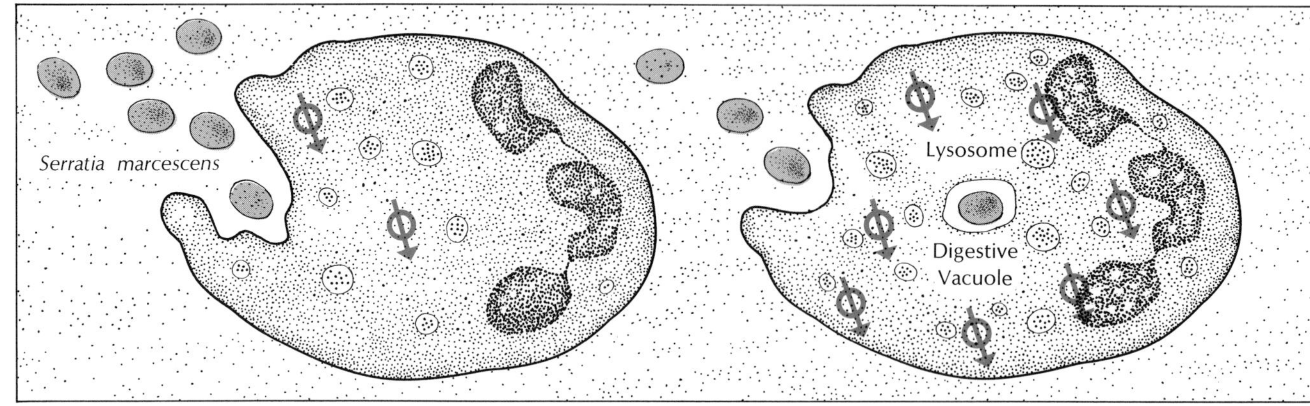

The handling of Serratia marcescens *by the normal polymorphonuclear leukocyte begins with phagocytosis. Oxidative metabolism (arrow-circle symbol) is enhanced and large quantities of hydrogen peroxide are produced through* O_2 *consumption as the*

gesteu by the leukocytes but are not subsequently killed. A review of these steps from phagocytosis to intracellular destruction of bacteria provides a useful device for discussing the main features of the disease.

In the normal sequence, neutrophils, or polymorphonuclear leukocytes, ingest bacteria and then proceed to destroy the ingested bacteria by a process that involves an enhancement of their oxygen consumption and hexosemonophosphate (HMP) shunt activity. In addition, it has been found that the leukocyte will produce two to four times more H_2O_2 when it is engaged in phagocytosis than it will at rest, and, as has been shown by Klebannoff at the University of Washington and by Sbarra and coworkers at Tufts, this hydrogen peroxide plays a key role in the killing of ingested bacteria. The ingested bacteria are contained within a vacuole, surrounded by the cell membrane, pinched off by the process of phagocytosis. Hirsch and Cohn, working at the Rockefeller University, first observed that the vacuoles fuse with cytoplasmic granules (lysosomes) containing many enzymes that are emptied into the vacuole. Many of the enzymes are responsible for the digestion and re-

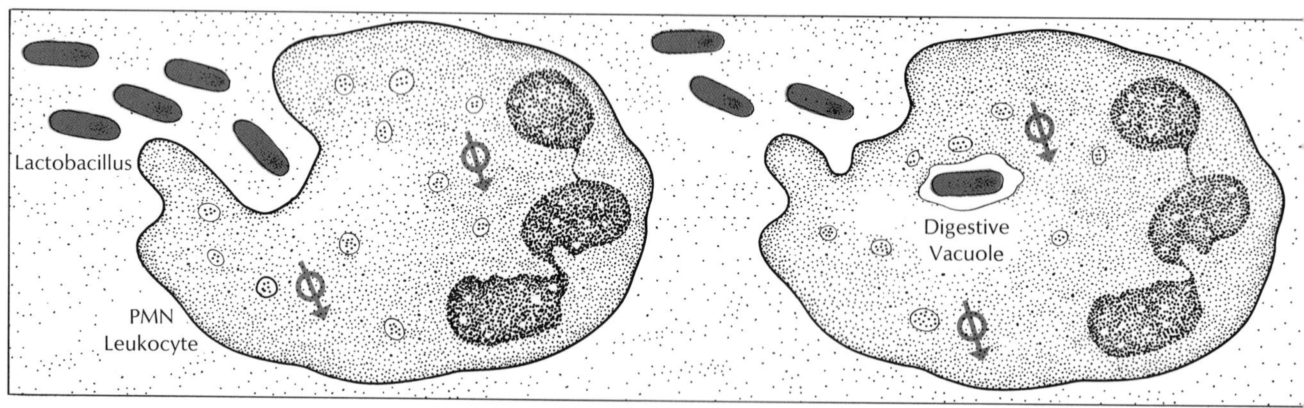

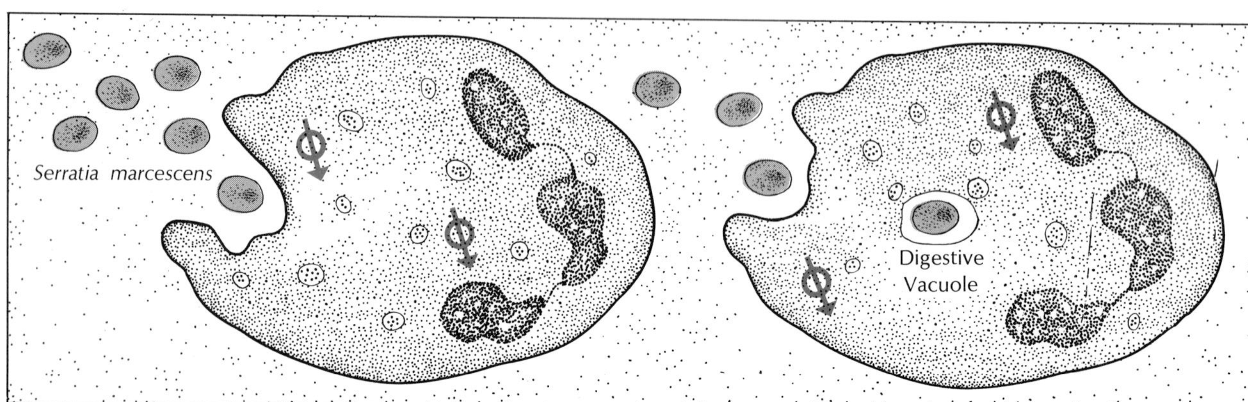

CGD leukocytes are not normally stimulated by phagocytosis of either lactobacillus or serratia. HMP shunt activity and H_2O_2 *production are not enhanced. However, the killing of the catalase-negative lactobacillus appears to proceed normally since the*

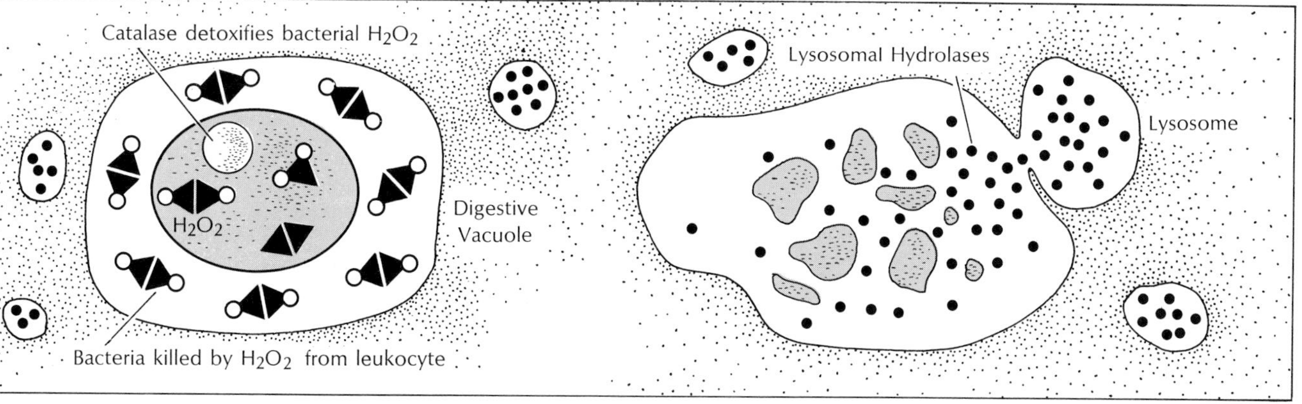

hexose monophosphate shunt is stimulated. Since serratia is catalase-positive, this enzyme detoxifies the bacterial H_2O_2. However, peroxide produced by leukocyte kills the serratia and lysosomal hydrolytic enzymes disrupt and digest it.

moval of bacteria, but the initial event, the killing of bacteria, is associated with the action of hydrogen peroxide and myeloperoxidase, an enzyme present in high concentration in the granules of polymorphonuclear leukocytes.

It is well established that CGD leukocytes are not able to respond during phagocytosis with a burst of oxidative metabolism. While the bactericidal defect may be due to the inability of the cells to produce hydrogen peroxide, it may also be related to an abnormal release of myeloperoxidase from leukocyte granules, at this time a matter of controversy.

The work of Baehner and Nathan at Harvard involved the incubation with nitroblue tetrazolium (NBT) of leukocytes from both normal individuals and from patients with CGD. During phagocytosis, the normal leukocytes reduce NBT and produce a dark blue precipitate but CGD leukocytes do not. This failure is unique among leukocytes capable of normal phagocytosis. It is thus a histochemical abnormality peculiar to CGD leukocytes and can be correlated with the failure of the cells to enhance their oxidative metabolism and H_2O_2 formation during phagocytosis.

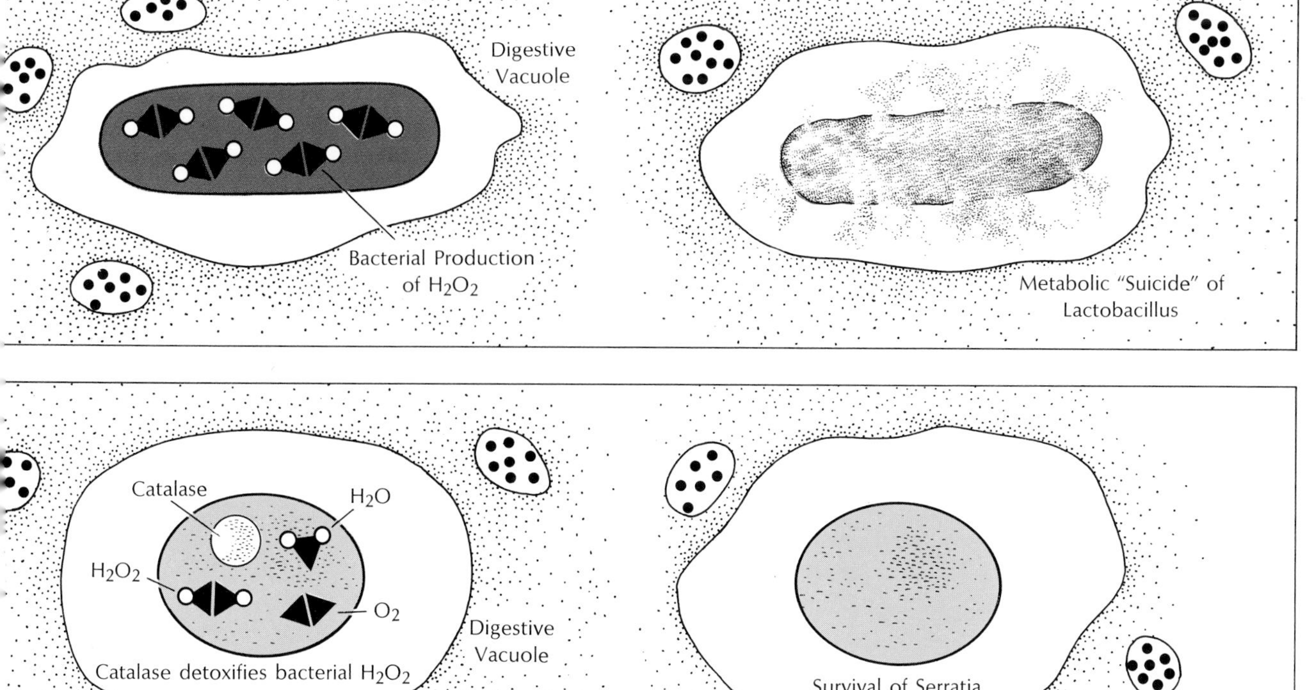

bacillary production of H_2O_2 is not detoxified, and this peroxide is sufficient for the killing of the bacterium. With the serratia the deficiency in leukocyte H_2O_2 is critical since the catalase detoxifies the bacterial peroxide and the organism survives.

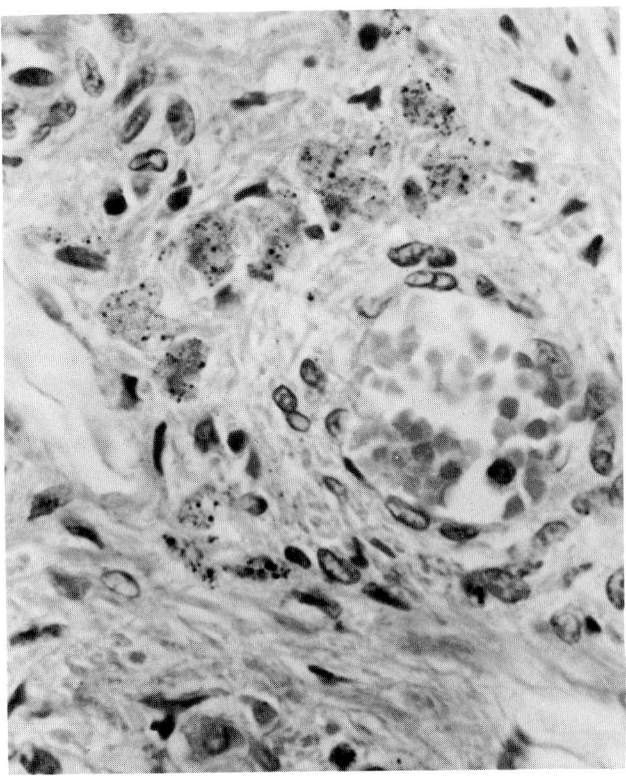

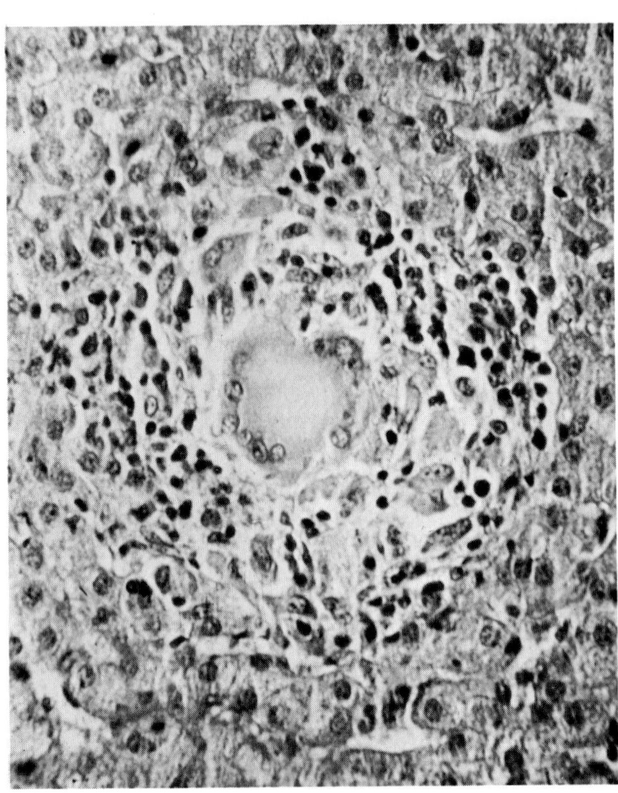

Illustrations above and on facing page show some of the typical histologic and radiographic abnormalities seen in chronic granulomatous disease in children. Shown (from left to right) are: (1) lipochrome pigmentation of histiocytes, a characteristic finding in reticuloendothelial organs; (2) microscopic granuloma in the liver, probably an end product of the defective handling of

Chronologically, the next step in the development of our understanding came with the work of Klebanoff and White. Earlier work by Klebanoff had shown that the halides are bactericidal in the presence of hydrogen peroxide and of the enzyme myeloperoxidase. The investigators therefore took lactobacillus as a representative of the organisms that are killed by CGD leukocytes and serratia as an example of those that are not. They incubated each of the microbial species with the CGD leukocytes and with radioactive iodine-125 and found that the iodine was bound by the lactobacilli but not the serratia. Furthermore, when killed lactobacilli were substituted for live bacteria, iodine binding was inhibited. Klebanoff and White concluded that it was the hydrogen peroxide being produced by live, metabolically active lactobacilli that allowed the iodine to be bound.

It was this elegant work that initiated our speculation about the catalase involvement. Work by Quie and coworkers at Minnesota (and others) showed that catalase-negative organisms were killed by the leukocytes of these patients. The organisms that plagued these patients clinically were all catalase positive. Specifically, bacterial killing occurred only for those organisms that produced hydrogen peroxide but not catalase to detoxify it. Many highly pathogenic bacteria are catalase negative, among them those of the lactic acid bacteria grouping that includes streptococci. In fact, although one defines CGD as a syndrome in which the patient is unable to handle some low-grade pathogens, the reality is that CGD leukocytes alone would be unable to kill any of the bacteria tested. The bacteria that do succumb after ingestion are suicides – their own elaboration of hydrogen peroxide substituting for a deficiency of the product in CGD leukocytes.

The inability of the patient with chronic granulomatous disease to defend himself against low-grade pathogens is in reality an expression of the absence of a mechanism to handle catalase-positive organisms. These microorganisms are only ingested by the leukocytes, they are not subsequently killed.

Such catalase-positive organisms include the *Staphylococcus aureus*, *Aerobacter aerogenes*, *Paracolon hafnia*, *S. marcescens*, and *Candida albicans*. These are all among the normally low-virulence organisms the CGD leukocytes are unable to handle.

Within the leukocytes, they can release their toxic products and initiate a granulomatous inflammatory process. The leukocytes not only provide the pathogens with vehicles for widespread tissue distribution within the body but also protect them against many normal host defenses and even against antibiotics. In a very real sense, then, the child with CGD is placed in a position vis-à-vis such organisms as serratia that is analogous to that of the normal individual versus the tubercle bacillus or a certain number of the facultative intracellular pyogenic pathogens.

While the metabolic defect of the CGD leukocyte has been identified as an inability to produce hydrogen peroxide in normal quantities because the pathways of oxidative metabolism are depressed, the specific enzymatic anomaly responsible for this functional deficiency remains in an area of unresolved controversy. Any abnormality must account for the failure in

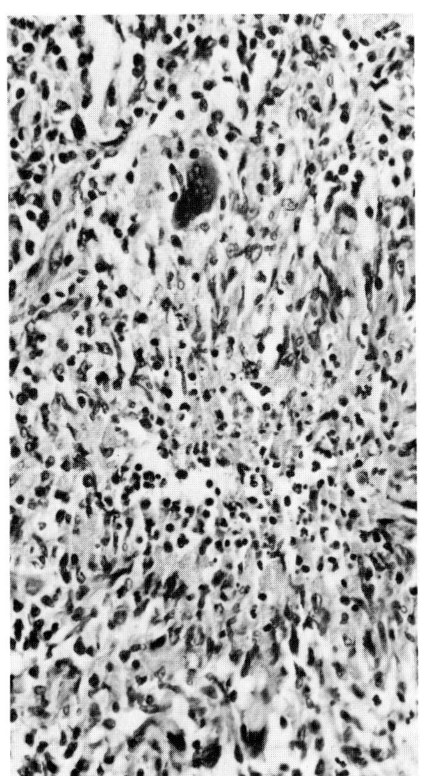

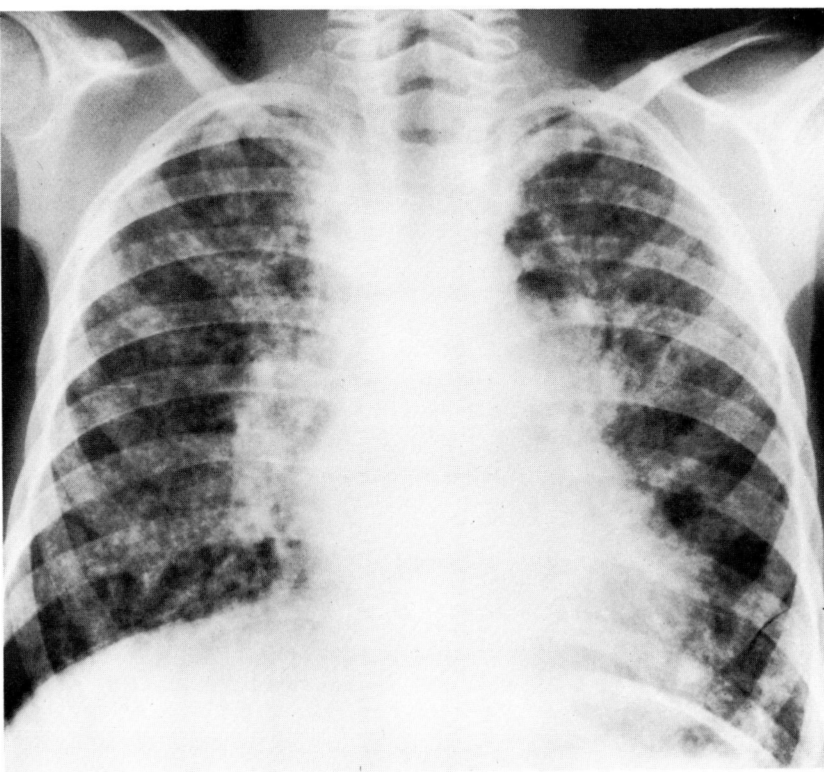

bacterial pathogens; (3) a diffuse pulmonary granuloma with a giant cell; and (4) x-ray of diffuse bilateral infiltration of the lungs. It is the progressive destructive processes in the lungs, involving both proliferation of granuloma and sepsis, that are most frequently the direct causes of death in children suffering from chronic granulomatous disease.

oxygen consumption, hexosemonophosphate shunt activity, and hydrogen peroxide production. A number of observations and hypotheses are worthy of review although no conclusions can yet be drawn.

One of the more intriguing of these findings is that of Baehner and Nathan, working with Karnovsky, at Harvard. They have reported a deficiency of NADH oxidase in CGD leukocytes of five patients, four boys and one girl. There is a special teleologic appeal to this finding since it would satisfactorily explain all of the metabolic peculiarities of the disease, if we assume a linkage to the oxidation of NADPH, making NADP available for stimulation of the HMP. And since one of the chief activities of NADH oxidase is the transfer of electrons to oxygen with consequent formation of H_2O_2, a lack of this enzyme could account for the complete constellation of metabolic defects in CGD.

However, in our laboratory we have measured NADH oxidase activity in eight patients, seven males and one female, with chronic granulomatous disease, and we have found them all to be normal in this respect. As far as we can determine, we have reproduced the methods of the Harvard group exactly and we can offer no explanation for the variance in the two sets of observations.

It is noteworthy that in the Harvard experiments implicating an NADH-oxidase deficiency in CGD, the one female patient tested had a more severe defect than any of the four males. Her enzyme activity level was reported as close to zero, as compared with a mean for the group of around 25% of normal. This may take on some significance in view of our finding of a possibly related metabolic defect in two of our female patients, specifically a glutathione-peroxidase deficiency. This anomaly could also explain the failure of the stimulation of the hexosemonophosphate shunt in CGD patients. Peroxide detoxification was shown by Reed at the University of Wisconsin to be linked to the HMP pathway through the glutathione-reductase and glutathione-peroxidase reactions that make NADP available to stimulate the shunt. Gluthathione-peroxidase deficiency would block stimulation of the HMP pathway but assumedly not affect oxygen uptake and formation of the product, hydrogen peroxide.

It is possible that a feedback mechanism might be operating in which a small amount of H_2O_2 would inhibit NADH oxidase, preventing the stimulation of oxygen consumption and the accumulation of peroxide. Without a feedback mechanism, one would have to postulate that the oxidase reaction in the female CGD leukocyte is normal, that oxygen consumption would have to be normal, and that peroxide would accumulate because it wouldn't be detoxified by the glutathione-peroxidase reaction. This, of course, is inconsistent with a number of the metabolic observations in CGD cells.

One other enzyme defect has been found in CGD and may prove to be the most fruitful enzymologic finding of all. Bellanti and Schlegel at George Washington University have reported, and we have confirmed, that glucose-6-phosphate dehydrogenase, the first enzyme in the hexosemonophosphate shunt, is more heat labile in the CGD leukocyte than in the cells of normal individuals. By heating the cytoplasmic fraction of the leukocyte at 38° C for 30 minutes they inactivated essentially all of the G-6-PD in CGD leukocytes, while normal enzyme remained relatively unchanged. In this case, of course, the lability was manifest at temperatures well within the range of the clinical febrile response to infection.

This finding in male patients with CGD would afford a very simple explanation for the failure of oxidative metabolism and of H_2O_2 formation. One major problem prevents our accepting this explanation. In patients in whose red cells G-6-PD abnormalities have been found, there is often an accompanying leukocyte deficiency. But we have not been able to detect bactericidal or metabolic abnormality during phagocytosis of leukocytes from our patients that contain only 25% of normal G-6-PD. Therefore unless we assume that the G-6-PD in CGD leukocytes is completely inactive in vivo – and there is no basis for such an assumption – we are faced with a continuing mystery.

However, we have reason to believe that this may be a mystery well worth solving. Not only is the G-6-PD deficiency a satisfactory explanation of the metabolic derangements in CGD, it also would jibe very neatly with what we know about the genetic basis of this disease. G-6-PD synthesis has been shown to be under the control of the X chromosome, and the predominant form of the disease, that seen in males, is almost certainly an expression of an X-linked defect. In addition, Baehner and coworkers have established the occurrence of leukocyte abnormalities of the CGD prototype in a middle-aged patient whose leukocytes were completely lacking in G-6-PD. A cyclic series of reactions has been proposed, which would explain all the metabolic abnormalities, starting with leukocytes with absent or nonfunctional G-6-PD.

When CGD was first described in 1957 by Berendes, Bridges, and Good and by Landing and Shirkey, it was suggested that it was a familial condition. This has since been confirmed and the mode of genetic transmission has been elucidated by Windhorst and in our laboratory. It should be stressed that we are now talking about the male cases, which represent more than 95% of CGD incidence. The pattern is completely consistent with that established for X-linked defects. Thus, all mothers of these children and about half of their female siblings have been demonstrated to be carriers. This was done by testing the mothers and sisters for the previously mentioned histochemical defect, the inability to reduce NBT. Intermediate values between normals and CGD patients were found in the presumptive carriers, i.e., the mothers and half of the sisters. The carriers were also found to have intermediate activity in killing those bacteria that CGD leukocytes fail to kill at all. In addition, all of the fathers of the affected boys were found to be normal and several maternal grandmothers were found to be carriers. Cytologic studies in the carriers revealed the mosaicism of normal and abnormal leukocytes that would be expected from the Lyon hypothesis. (This hypothesis suggests that there is a random inactivation of either of the two X chromosomes in females early in life so that one would expect 50% of cells to have a normal X chromosome and 50% to have the X carrier of the abnormal trait.)

By contrast, the genetic studies in the female patients have shown that the mothers and fathers are normal. None of the mothers are carriers nor, according to the functional, metabolic, and histochemical parameters that define the carrier in the X-linked disease, are any siblings thus far examined. Moreover, there is notable consanguinity in the parents of the female patients. The pattern here is consistent with transmission of the disease via an autosomal recessive gene.

Are there any other differences between male and female CGD patients? Other than the fact that the female patients seem to live longer – several have now lived into adolescence or young adulthood – no clear-cut differences have been discerned. The girls' disease is as severe. We do feel that there may be some clinical differences but these are too subtle to be definitely established. As far as we can determine, the leukocyte defect is identical in boys and in girls.

Turning now to an area that is, if anything, more controversial than the definition of the precise metabolic disorder – that of whether or not there is a defect in degranulation in CGD –

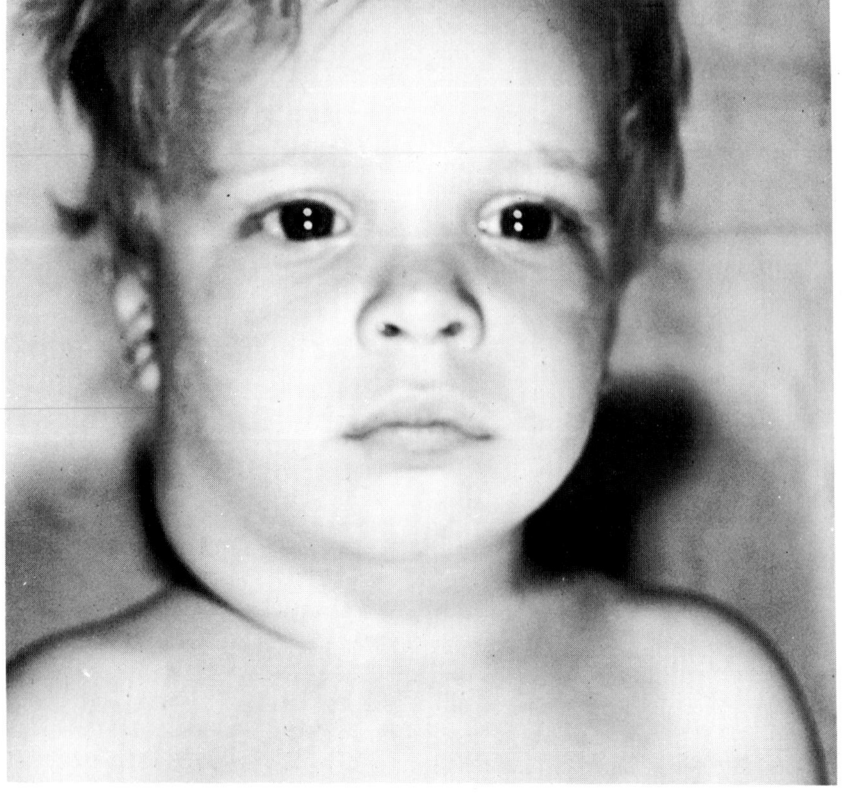

Child with chronic granulomatous disease had marked lymphadenopathy. With scrofulous and inflammatory skin lesions, lymphadenopathy is often a presenting sign of CGD.

it should be first stated that many laboratories have studied this question and concluded that granule lysis is normal. Our findings here are thus far unique. They are that lysosomal hydrolytic enzymes – specifically acid phosphatase and beta-glucuronidase – are not released during phagocytosis by CGD leukocytes in anything like the quantities seen in normal leukocytes. Similarly, the total quantity of enzymes in the CGD cell during phagocytosis does not change in the CGD cell but does in the normal leukocyte.

It is our belief that the failure by the polymorphonuclear leukocyte in CGD to digest phagocytized material is directly related to granuloma formation, and this could very well be the result of abnormal degranulation.

Two other disease entities have some similarities to CGD and must be accounted for in the differential diagnosis of chronic granulomatous disease. One is lipochrome histiocytosis, first described by Ford in three sisters. The susceptibility to bacterial infection, and indeed to the same low-virulence pathogens, is identical in lipochrome histiocytosis to what is seen in CGD. However, these three women all have rheumatoid arthritis, they all have survived into adult life, and, most important, none has had granuloma formation. Clinically, therefore, they are very different from patients with chronic granulomatous disease. However, when their leukocytes are studied by the methods already discussed, these cells appear identical by every parameter with those of the CGD patients. Leukocytes of such patients had normal glutathione peroxidase and did not have the labile G-6-PD that characterizes the leukocytes in the X-linked disorder.

The second syndrome is the leukocyte myeloperoxidase deficiency originally studied in one patient by Lehrer, Cline, and Klebanoff. Killing and iodination of both catalase-positive and catalase-negative organisms are abnormal since myeloperoxidase is required for both. However, there is a normal increase in oxidative metabolism during phagocytosis. The results of the studies of this interesting patient emphasize the importance of myeloperoxidase in the hydrogen peroxide bactericidal mechanism. However, they also reveal a possible compensatory mechanism: of the five reported cases, only the patient studied by Lehrer, Cline, and Klebanoff is known to have increased susceptibility to infection – and only as an adult. The condition is then certainly clinically unrelated to CGD.

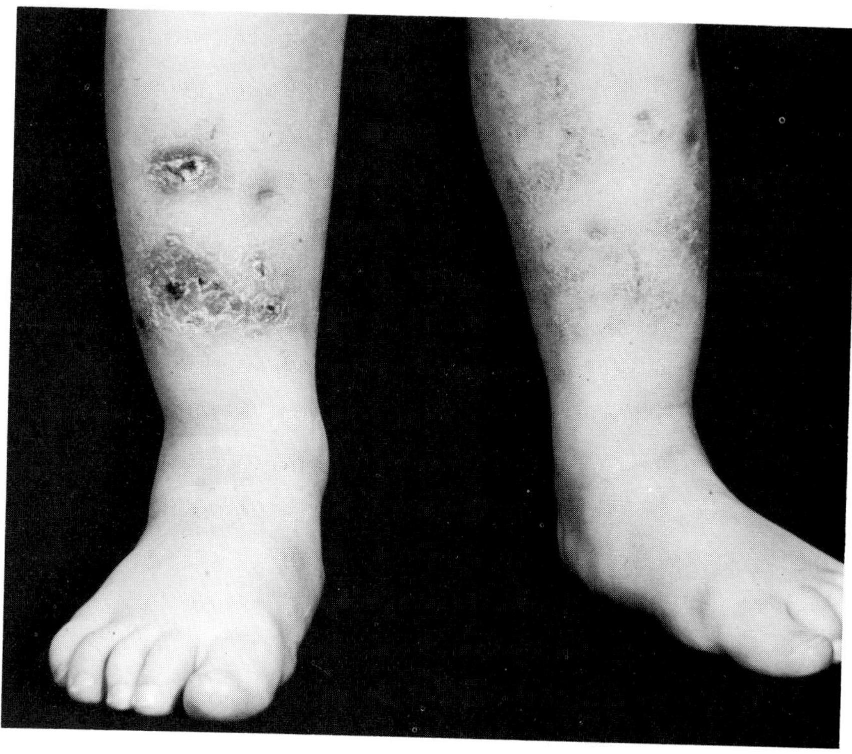

Scaling inflammatory lesions are seen on legs of child with CGD. Lesions were both granulomatous and purulent. Very often the skin erosions suggest lupus vulgaris.

Some have related to CGD a syndrome of cold abscess formation resulting from increased susceptibility to staphylococcal infection, the so-called Job syndrome, described by Wedgewood. However, the infections suffered by these patients are readily amenable to antibiotic therapy and there seems to be minimal threat to their lives. The leukocytes of these patients have been studied in a battery of functional tests by Klebanoff and Wedgewood and by us and have been found to be normal in every respect. It is our belief that there is no relationship between the Job syndrome and CGD.

As was stated at the outset of this discussion, chronic granulomatous disease in many ways serves as a model for studies to enlarge our understanding of the processes and mechanisms involved in the postphagocytic handling of pathogens. It has already brought major dividends in our understanding of the roles played by oxidative metabolism, peroxide, catalase, etc. It has focused attention on the part played by the invading organism in its own survival or demise; and it has made clear the need for better techniques and new information on various aspects of degranulation. The critical question is whether or not we can develop methods for treating these children. Although the disease is rare, its total lethality demands that some effort be made to save the lives of these patients. It seems probable that we are dealing with a single enzyme fault, a number of which could possibly account for the defect. One is likely to predominate as the pathogenesis of the disease in male patients. The enzyme will undoubtedly be difficult to replace directly. The more likely possibility exists that we may be able to correct the leukocyte defect by introducing a stem cell population that can be appropriately differentiated to permit the formation of normal leukocytes in the bone marrow. Coupled with the hopelessness of the disease, our previous successes with this type of "cellular engineering" argues for just such an attempt.

Section Two

The Humoral Antibodies

Chapter 7

Molecules of Immunity

ALFRED NISONOFF
University of Illinois

One of the central problems in immunology, indeed one of the central problems in the entire area of the life sciences, is the phenomenon of specificity. Reactions of great complexity are under way when the body mass produces antibodies in response to a new foreign antigen such as a bacterium or virus or, more exactly, in response to antigenic determinants – "markers" in the form of characteristic configurations of atoms on the bacterial or viral surface.

First of all, utilizing an elaborate system for distinguishing friend from foe, "native" agents from outsiders, the body recognizes the antigen as alien. Then the appearance of the foreign substance somehow influences genetic (DNA-RNA) mechanisms to bring about increased production of a special kind of protein, antibody designed to fit neatly with the unique configuration of the antigenic determinant. Furthermore, the same general events take place every time the body is exposed to a new antigen, so that each of us probably produces at least tens of thousands of different antibodies in a lifetime. (This is a very conservative estimate. The actual numbers could be considerably larger.)

A great deal remains to be learned about such processes. But knowledge is coming at a much faster rate than most of us would have believed possible less than a decade ago — and one reason is the outstanding success of the structural approach in biochemistry. More and more, experiments are yielding precise information about how antibodies are put together. And structure provides fundamental clues to function. Theories as to the operation of the defenses of the body in health and disease can be only as valid as our knowledge of the basic working parts of these defenses, a principle which applies with particular force to research on immunoglobulins.

There is a striking contrast between old and new models of the antibody molecule. It is as though we had seen a building only at a distance, through clouds, a building we can now see parts of close up, and in sharp detail. Less than 12 years ago, investigators recognized that antibody molecules of the predominant class are bivalent, that they include two small active sites capable of combining with the antigen which elicited formation of that antibody. But the location of the sites was obscure, and so was the general picture of the antibody, which was regarded simply as a kind of lengthy folded chain of amino acids.

Today's picture is far more precise. We are beginning to understand structure in terms of amino acid sequences and the arrangement of polypeptide chains in space. Recent studies are having an important effect on our thinking, for they indicate in broad outline a possible course of the evolution of the immune system at the molecular level and set definable limits to theories of antibody formation.

The modern era of antibody research began in 1959 with investigations conducted at the Rockefeller University by Gerald Edelman and his colleagues, particularly M. D. Poulik. Their chief finding, that the antibody molecule is made up of multiple polypeptide chains rather than of a single chain, holds for all the major human immunoglobulin classes – the gamma A globulin (IgA) found in serum as well as in saliva and other external secretions (where they are the predominant immunoglobulin class and are believed to be part of a special system for protecting body surfaces in contact with the external environment); the high-molecular-weight gamma M globulins (IgM), which tend to be present in higher proportions during the very early stages after challenge and may be designed for rapid protection; and the gamma G globulins (IgG). Two other classes, IgD and IgE, are present in relatively low concentrations in serum. The IgE class, which may be largely responsible for allergic reactions, is considered elsewhere in this volume. In this report, however, I shall confine the discussion to the IgG class, which makes up about 70 percent of normal human immunoglobulins and which has been most extensively studied.

Edelman's original experiments involved the use of a reducing agent which split disulfide bonds linking the chains in the antibody molecule, and a dissociating agent which caused separation of polypeptide chains. By treating molecules with these substances, he was able to obtain two types of subunit: heavy, or H, chains and light, or L, chains. His subsequent work, and parallel research by Rodney Porter's group, now at St. Mary's Hospital Medical School in London, was a first step toward a high-resolution picture of the immunoglobulins and has set the stage for continuing structural analysis, some of which was done in our laboratory.

According to present views, a molecule of gamma G globulin consists of two identical H chains and two identical L chains, linked by three disulfide bonds and by the so-called noncovalent interactions, such as hydrophobic bonds and electrostatic forces. The subunits are folded into a roughly cylindrical form some 35 Å in diameter and 200 Å in length – about one millionth the volume of a typical bacterium. The particle has a molecular weight of about 150,000 and is made up of about 1,400 amino acid residues. The molecular weight of each H chain is approximately 55,000, of each L chain 23,000.

In general, the main part of each active site seems to be embodied in an H chain. These chains, if isolated from the gamma G globulins of animals exposed to a particular antigen, will generally react specifically to that antigen and not to unrelated ones. Isolated L chains have little antibody activity, but they potentiate the activity of H chains on recombination, which proceeds spontaneously. So it turns out that both the H and L chains contribute to the active site, with the H chain the major contributor.

One interesting characteristic of the two active sites is that they make up such a small proportion of the total antibody surface. The "business" part of each site probably includes no more than a dozen amino acids on the average—that is, no more than a dozen amino acids actually make contact with the antigen—so it seems to take a relatively large number of amino acids to provide the framework for a pair of sites with precise contours and sufficient stability; here there is an obvious analogy to enzymes. At any rate, bivalence provides a good example of the relationship between structure and function. Aggregation of an antigen enhances its uptake by the macrophages—and the subsequent elimination of the antigen from the body. The bivalence of the antibody permits the

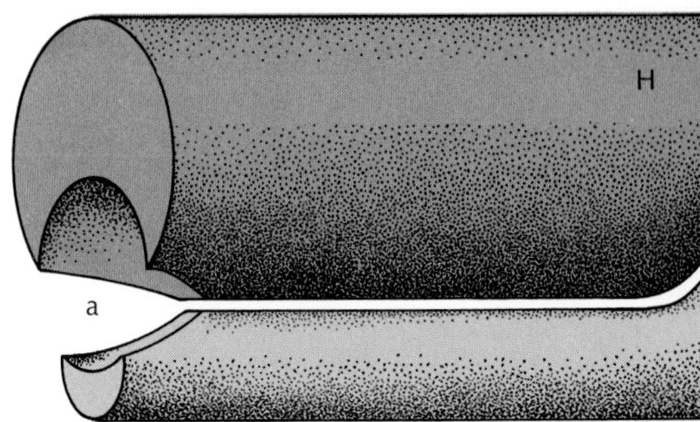

The Gamma G Molecule: A Theoretical Model

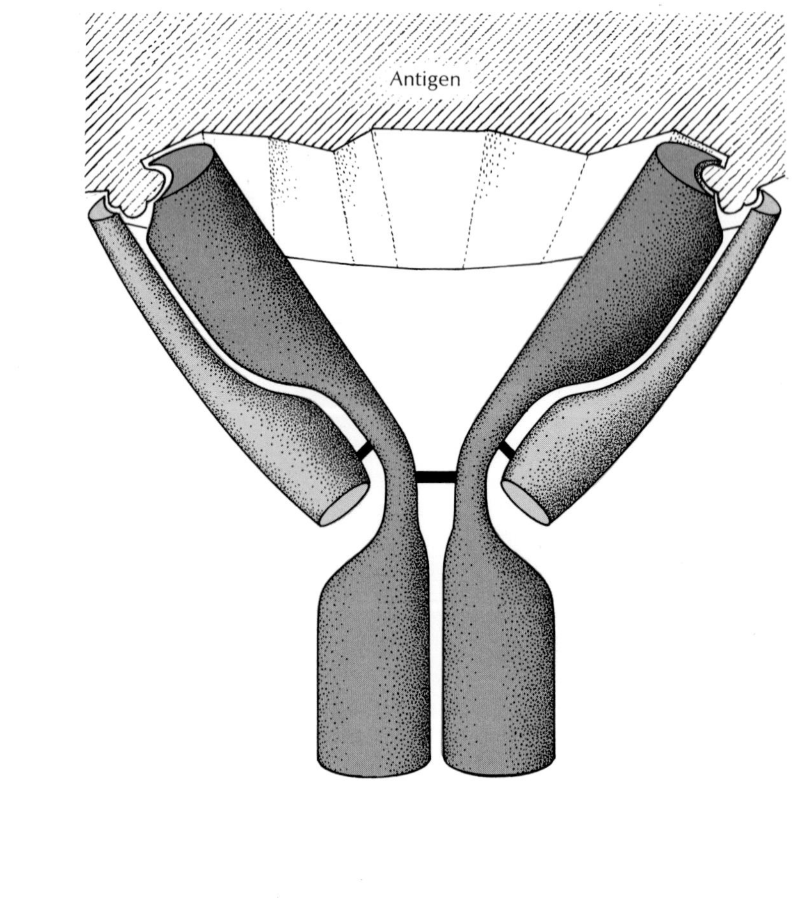

In model of IgG (top) both heavy (H) and light (L) chains contribute to the two antibody combining sites (a). Three interchain disulfide bonds (S-S) are seen. Flexibility of chains permits bivalent combination with a single antigen (lower left). When antibody is treated with papain, it splits into three parts. One (Fc) has two half H chains,

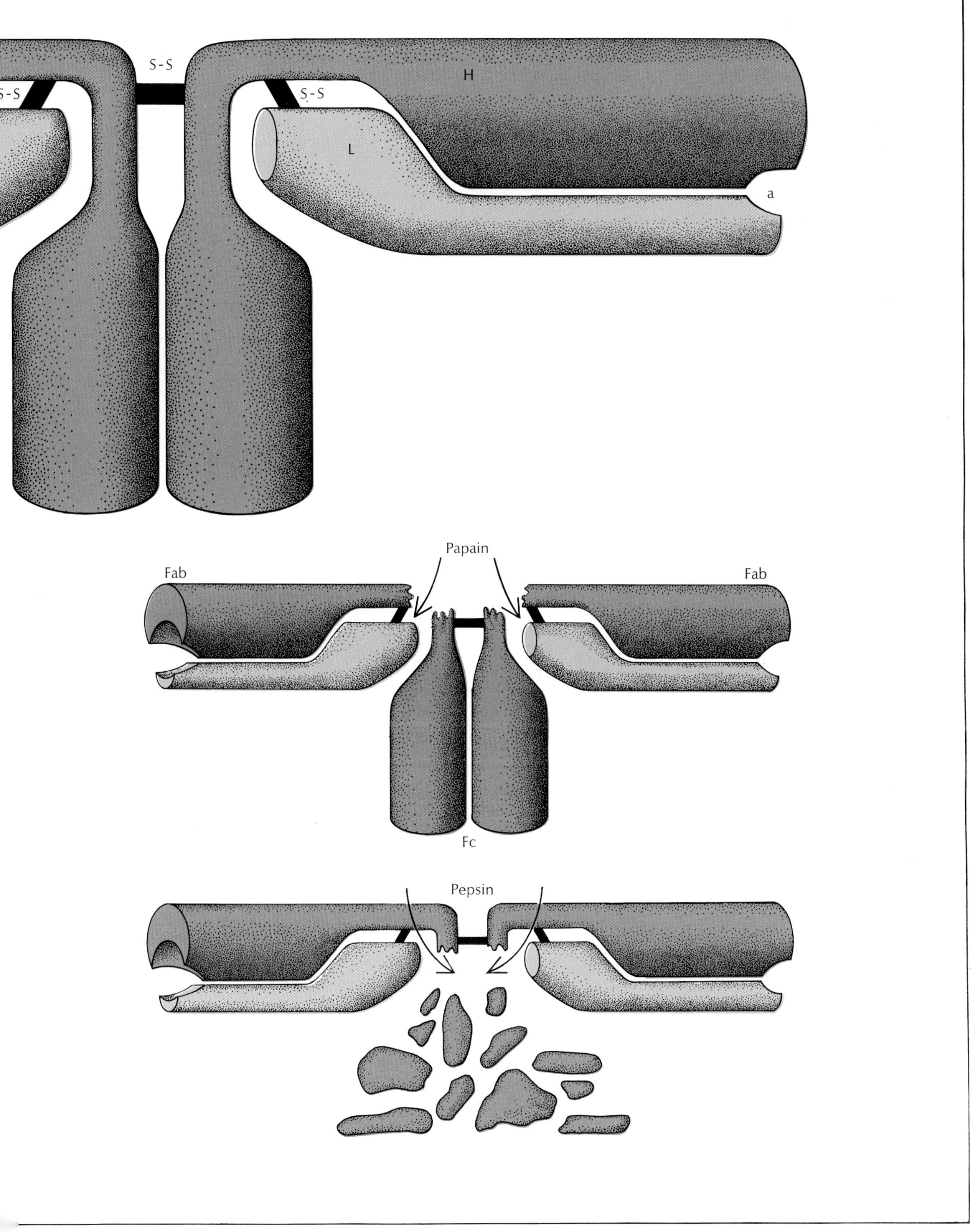

is crystallizable (homogeneous) and inactive. The others (Fab) each contain a combining site. It is believed that these are associated with the variable portion of the H and L chains and therefore with immunologic specificity. Pepsin treatment leaves the two Fab units united in a bivalent fragment including both combining sites, while "chewing up" the Fc fragment. A single disulfide bond joins the heavy chains in rabbit IgG (as shown above); there are two to five such bonds in human IgG.

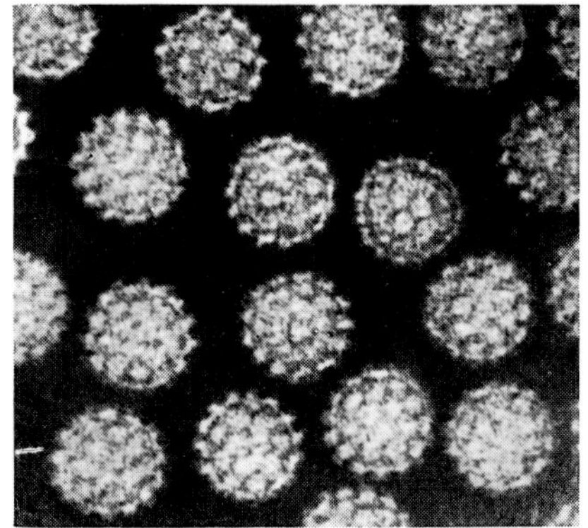

In this negatively stained preparation of human wart virus (300,000x), particles are randomly distributed and viral substructure may be clearly discerned.

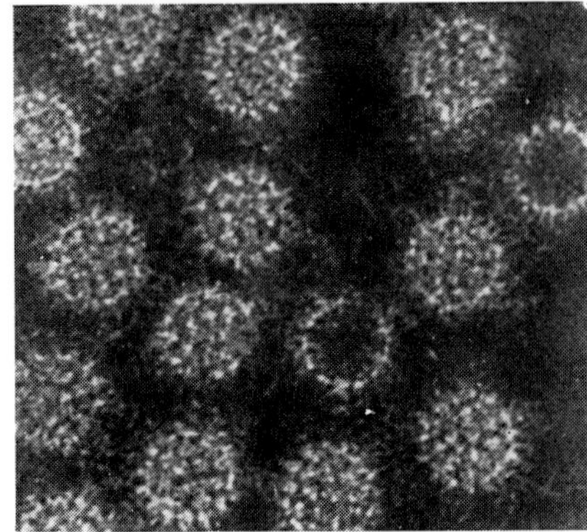

When specific antibody, obtained from rabbit, is added, clumping occurs and a halo of antibody is visible. Antibody also obscures viral substructure.

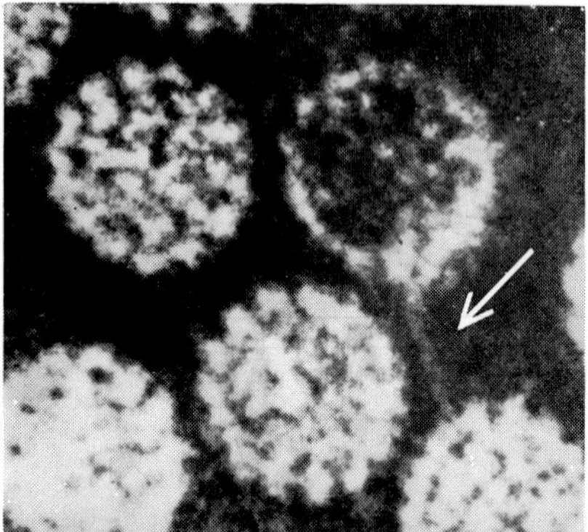

Linking antibody (arrow) is clearly defined in EM (400,000x) of polyoma virus particle. The four EM's in this group were made by Almeida, Cinader, and Howatson.

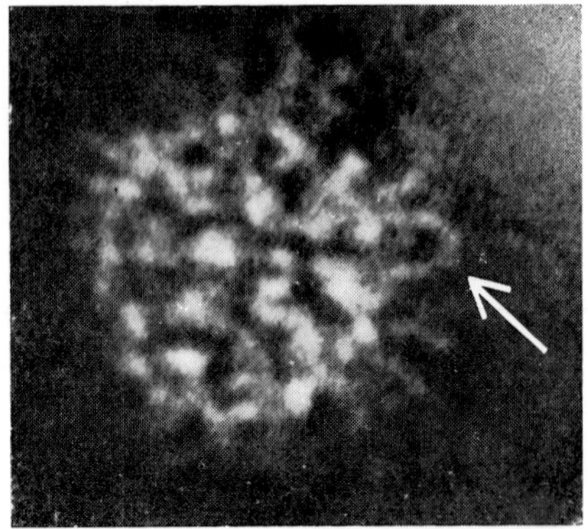

Here a horseshoe loop is visible when both combining sites of wart virus antibody become attached to the same particle of human wart virus (480,000x).

formation of a framework, or aggregate, with antigen and antibody alternating in the structure. The aggregation of antigen and antibody also activates the complement system and in this way facilitates lysis of many species of bacteria.

The combining sites are located at the extreme ends of the molecule, as indicated most directly by the electronmicrographs prepared by Bernhard Cinader and his collaborators at the Ontario Cancer Institute in Toronto, and also by Lafferty and Oertilis in Australia.

Antibodies are unique among all known proteins in that a vast array of specificities is associated with molecules that are otherwise very similar to one another (within a single class and subclass). Thus all molecules of the gamma G class are similar in size, shape, and many other significant properties. Yet within this class one can find antibodies capable of combining specifically with an almost unlimited assortment of antigens. What is the basis of this specificity? It now appears that each polypeptide chain is made up of a region that is invariable within that class of molecule, and a variable region. And it is highly probable that it is the region of variability that accounts for the specificity of antibodies.

This concept was first suggested by the work of Porter about eight years ago. He found that the proteolytic enzyme papain splits rabbit gamma G globulin molecules into three fragments. One of the fragments, consisting of two half H chains, is inactive in the sense that it does not combine with antigen. On the other hand, these fragments, when derived from a mixture of different antibodies, can crystallize together in large yields, suggesting a highly homogeneous structure. This region of the molecule is essential for certain biologic activities of gamma globulin, such as fixation to skin in passive cutaneous anaphylaxis and ability to cross the placenta in certain species; it also plays a significant role in complement fixation.

The other two fragments produced by papain digestion are probably identical to one another. Each consists of an L chain and half an H chain. They do not crystallize, which is consistent with other evidence for structural heterogeneity. Recent work has shown that the variable regions of both chains are associated with these fragments, which contain the two antibody-combining sites and thus are responsible for biologic specificity. Thus, variability of amino acid sequence can be directly associated with variability of specificity, or, to put it another way, with the presence in an immunoglobulin fraction of antibody to widely differing antigens.

Since each of the two noncrystallizable fragments is univalent, that is, each has only a single active site, it cannot serve as a coupling device to link antigen particles together. As a consequence, precipitation or agglutination do not occur. In point of fact, such fragments can actually inhibit precipitation or agglutination if they are exposed to antigen prior to the exposure to the bivalent antibodies. They do this by preempting the regions of the antigen which would otherwise combine with the bivalent antibody fragments.

Further structural insights, based on experiments with another proteolytic enzyme, were obtained shortly after Porter had announced his findings. At the time I was working with F. C. Wissler and L. Lipman at the Roswell Park Memorial Institute in Buffalo. As a part of a program to check certain aspects of Porter's results, we decided to investigate the effect of pepsin on rabbit gamma G globulin. Unexpectedly, the enzyme simply removed and partially digested a portion of the molecule, the part roughly corresponding to the inactive papain-produced fragment. This left essentially intact a single bivalent fragment with a molecular weight (100,000) that corresponded approximately to that of two of Porter's univalent fragments. As a matter of fact, by the reduction of a disulfide bond joining the fragments, this bivalent fragment could be dissociated into two univalent fragments very similar to (though slightly larger than) Porter's papain fragments. Furthermore, if the reducing agent was removed from the solution under proper conditions, a large proportion of the fragments recombined through re-formation of that disulfide bond.

These and later dissociation studies were continued and extended with William Mandy and Mercedes Rivers in our laboratories at the University of Illinois, and in cooperation with H. H. Fudenberg at the University of California. For one thing, we were able to produce antibodies of dual specificity in vitro. A pool of antiserum obtained from several rabbits hyperimmunized with ovalbumin yielded purified antiovalbumin, which was treated with pepsin and reduced to univalent fragments; univalent fragments of antibovine gamma globulin were produced in a similar manner. Then the fragments of the two antibodies were mixed in equal proportions and reoxidized. Random recombination of the fragments resulted in a mixture of three types of antibody: molecules containing two sites specific for ovalbumin, molecules containing two sites specific for bovine gamma globulin, and hybrid molecules with one site specific for each of the two antigens (in the approximate proportions of 1:1:2).

The existence of such antibodies can be demonstrated visually. (See illustrations on pages 70 and 71).

A detour into an area which is highly speculative suggests a possible clinical application of antibody hybridization. It is conceivable that we may be able to link a highly toxic antibiotic with a sensitive pathogen by hybridization of their respective antibodies. In this manner, a maximum amount of drug could be brought into contact with its pathogenic target at dosage levels low enough to obviate or minimize the antibiotic's toxic effects. A similar application might be made in the field of cancer chemotherapy, provided, of course, that specific antibodies to tumors can be prepared in sufficient yield.

Returning to investigations in our laboratory, the next development that can be cited came about quite serendipitously several years ago. In collaboration with J. L. Palmer and K. E. Van Holde, we were trying to arrive at the most gentle practical techniques for dissociating antibody molecules into their four constituent polypeptide chains. Porter and his coworkers had already shown that the chains could be separated, after reduction of their interchain disulfide bonds, by exposure to one-molar solutions of propionic acid (pH 2.5). We decided to omit the propionic acid but to maintain the same low pH, employing hydrochloric acid, which lacks the weak detergent action of propionic acid.

Examination of the products by ultracentrifugation, however, showed sedimentation patterns indicating we had obtained only one type of subunit rather than the two types that we would have obtained if we had separated H and L chains. Subsequent tests indicated that the antibody molecules had indeed been split into two halves, each consisting of a single L and a single H chain.

A large proportion of the separated halves recombine spontaneously at neutral pH to form complete molecules. Equally important is that this recombination occurs even though measures are taken to prevent reestablishment of the disulfide bonds. Thus, the noncovalent interaction between the H chains must be responsible for recombination. Furthermore, when one removes the blocking agents that have prevented reconstitution of the disulfide bonds, the liberated sulfur atoms come together to re-form the same disulfide bond that had existed in the native molecule.

It seems highly probable that in order for the interchain disulfide bond to re-form, the two sulfur atoms must be brought into very close proximity after reassociation of the half-molecules brought about by noncovalent interactions. This implies great precision in recombination and suggests that many or all of the atoms that are in contact prior to separation reestablish contact after recombination. Thus the H chain has within its architecture the information that will permit it to combine in a highly controlled and precise manner with another H chain on another half-molecule. It should be noted that Olins and Edelman at the Rockefeller University have demonstrated the same phenomenon with H and L chains as we have with half-molecules.

Half-molecules derived from different antibodies recombine at random; this provides an alternative method for preparing antibodies of mixed specificity in vitro. It should be noted that in this instance recombination occurs through noncovalent interactions in contrast to the reconstitution of two fragments after peptic digestion, which takes place through re-formation of a disulfide bond.

This brings us to the ultimate level, to the level represented by sequences of the 20 amino acid subunits of proteins. The current belief is that the three-dimensional structure of a polypeptide chain is determined by the sequence of its amino acids. Or to put it another way, a given amino acid sequence will arrange itself preferentially in one particular spatial pattern. Would it be possible to derive the architecture of a polypeptide from its amino acid sequence? Theoretically, yes. The job of establishing sequences has proved formidable but is now yielding to investigative efforts. It should be noted, however, that even

Amino Acid Sequences of Bence-Jones Light Chains

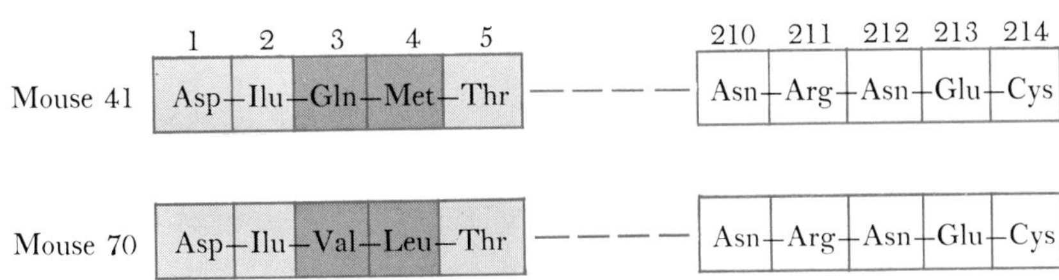

Diagram indicates amino acid sequences at the variable (left) and constant ends of the light chains of two mouse (above) and one human (below) Bence-Jones proteins. Notable are the interspecies similarities as well as the interanimal variations (Gray, Dreyer, and Hood; Putnam, Titani, and Whitley).

Human Ag — Asp-Ilu-Gln-Met-Thr ———— Asn-Arg-Gly-Glu-Cys

a knowledge of complete sequences would, practically speaking, leave us short of this goal, since great gaps still exist in understanding the forces that control the manner in which the polypeptide chain folds up.

Complete amino acid sequences have now been determined for a fairly substantial number of proteins of small to moderate size. These have been enzymes and other proteins that can be obtained in a homogeneous state. Such complete sequence studies have not been totally successful with antibodies, however, because antibodies of even a single specificity are heterogeneous with respect to amino acid sequence.

A highly significant advance in this direction was made six years ago by Norbert Hilschmann and Lyman Craig at the Rockefeller University. They circumvented the heterogeneity problem by going to the clinic for a source of material – patients suffering from multiple myeloma. Such patients have in their blood large amounts of a highly homogeneous immunoglobulin; and as noted more than 100 years ago by the English physician Henry Bence-Jones, they may also have a most characteristic urinary protein. In 1962, Edelman and J. A. Gally were able to identify the urinary proteins as the L chains corresponding exactly to the L chains of the complete myeloma globulin. In understanding the significance of this work, it is necessary to recall that L chains occur as one of two types, kappa and lambda. Bence-Jones proteins are characteristically either kappa or lambda, never both. Furthermore, both serum myeloma and Bence-Jones proteins are remarkable for their homogeneity. This probably reflects their biosynthesis from a single clone of malignant cells. From the point of view of this research, this homogeneity offered a unique opportunity to study the amino acid sequence of the molecule.

Hilschmann and Craig analyzed two Bence-Jones proteins of the kappa type. They arrived at an almost complete sequence analysis of one and derived a substantial portion of the amino acid sequence of the other. Subsequent sequence work on human and mouse L chains has also been done at a number of laboratories in the United States and England, notably those of F. Putnam at the University of Indiana, W. Dreyer at the California Institute of Technology, M. Potter at the National Institutes of Health, and C. Milstein at Cambridge University. All of these investigations confirm that L chains of a given class consist of variable and invariable parts, approximately equal in terms of the number of amino acid residues found in each part.

Thus, there are about 110 amino acid residues in the variable part and an approximately equal number in the invariant segment of the chain. Reading from the "amino-terminal" end of the polypeptide chain, the variable region comprises approximately the first 110 amino acid residues.

More recent investigations, notably by Edelman, F. W. Putnam, and W. Konigsberg, have demonstrated that the heavy chain is constructed on a similar principle, that is, with a variable and invariant region. The variable (amino-terminal) segment is slightly longer than that of the light chain, but the invariant segment is about three times as large. The presence of a variable region in both the heavy and light chain is consistent with other data indicating that both chains contribute to the function of one active site. Thus, variability of immunologic specificity can be associated with differences in amino acid sequence.

The nature of this variability is of some interest. It is now known that there are at least three subgroups of kappa light chains and four of lambda chains. Within a subgroup there are positions in the amino acid sequence of the variable segment in which sub-

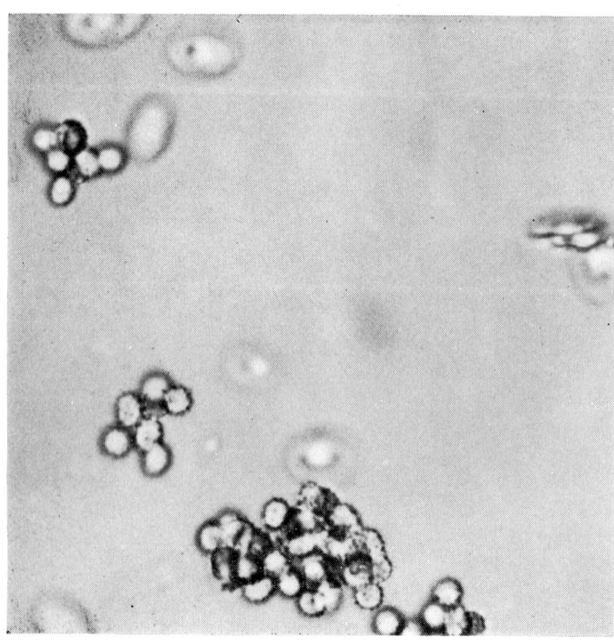

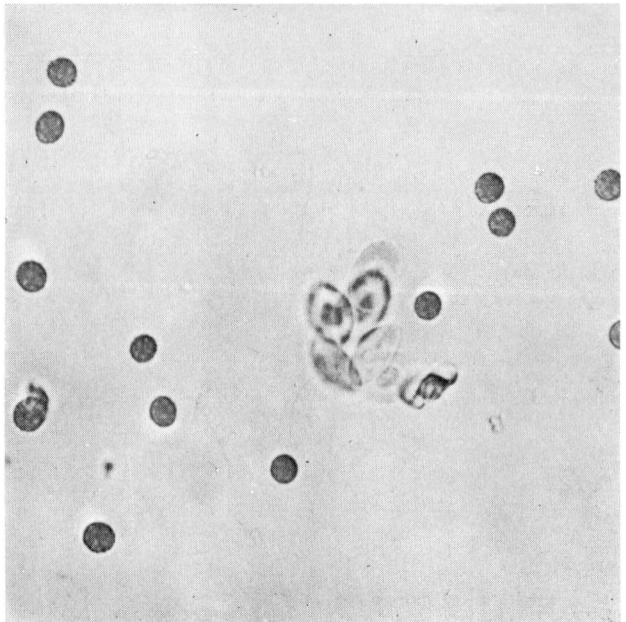

*Visual demonstration of hybrid antibodies with dual specificity: 1) Round human erythrocytes coated with ovalbumin are clumped by antiovalbumin bodies, but oval chicken erythrocytes coated with bovine gamma globulin are dispersed; 2) when anti-*BGG *is used instead of antiovalbumin, the oval chicken cells become agglutinated while human cells remain dispersed; 3) next, a mix-*

stitutions occur with considerable frequency and other positions in which substitutions are rare or have not been observed. Interchanges of amino acids, when they do occur, can usually be accounted for by a single mutation in the gene (DNA) coding for these amino acids. There is evidence that certain regions having a high frequency of substitutions may be associated with the active site of the antibody molecule.

Substitutions of amino acids may also occur at one or a few specific positions in the "constant" part of the polypeptide chain. These are generally inherited variations and are the allelic variants referred to as allotypes.

Perhaps 100 or more human Bence-Jones proteins have been studied by sequence analysis or by less detailed comparative methods. It seems that no two of the L chains examined so far have been identical. There must be thousands of them, and thousands of different H chains as well. This would provide more than enough variability, or potential variability—more than enough different antibody specificities — to protect us.

One of the most important results of research to date is that it has served to sharpen our thinking about the biosynthesis of antibodies. In fact, our theories tend to become more precise, and more susceptible to experimental checking and modification, as our picture of the antibody molecule becomes clearer.

First of all, it seems that at least two kinds of cells, macrophages and lymphocytes, are necessary for production of antibodies to particulate antigens, such as bacteria or erythrocytes. The macrophage ingests the antigen and breaks it down enzymatically into smaller units. There is evidence that some antigen fragments form complexes with RNA, and that such complexes are highly potent in stimulating antibody synthesis when transferred to competent cells. It has not been proved, however, that this mechanism actually operates in vivo.

A provocative experiment has been described by Marvin Fishman and Frank Adler at the Public Health Research Institute in New York, and Sheldon Dray of the University of Illinois. They exposed macrophages from one rabbit to a bacteriophage virus; RNA (possibly complexed with antigen fragments) was then extracted from the macrophages and transferred in vitro to lymph node cells from a second rabbit. Synthesis of the antibody to the bacteriophage was seen to occur in these lymph node cells. And some of these antibody molecules were found to have genetic markers characteristic of the rabbit that had furnished the macrophages. The simplest interpretation of this experiment is that the genetic information, which is possibly related to antibody specificity, is transferred from macrophages to lymph node cells.

There is some evidence about the processes that produce antibodies within the lymphoid cells. The synthesis of antibodies, like the synthesis of other proteins, proceeds at the surface of the ribosome on the basis of information coded into the base sequence of RNA molecules. Recent studies suggest that L chains are liberated first and then combine with H chains, a process that may start even before the H chains come off ribosomal assembly lines. A probable final step is the union of two half-molecules, each consisting of a single H and a single L chain.

What about the elusive problem of specificity, the problem of explaining how the body achieves high-precision matching of antibody and antigen? One thing can be stated definitely on the negative side: The template theory cannot account for the facts. It no longer makes sense to think in terms of immunoglobulin molecules which are intrinsically nonspecific but which acquire specificity by folding themselves about antigens and taking on shapes complementary to those of the

wow

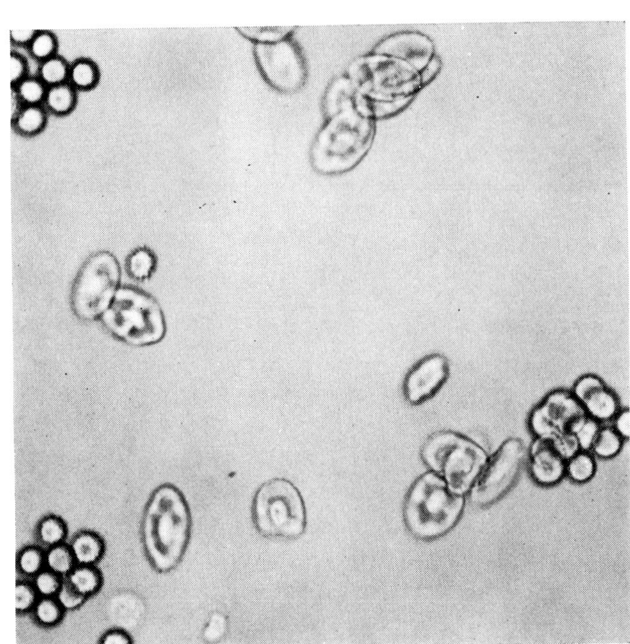

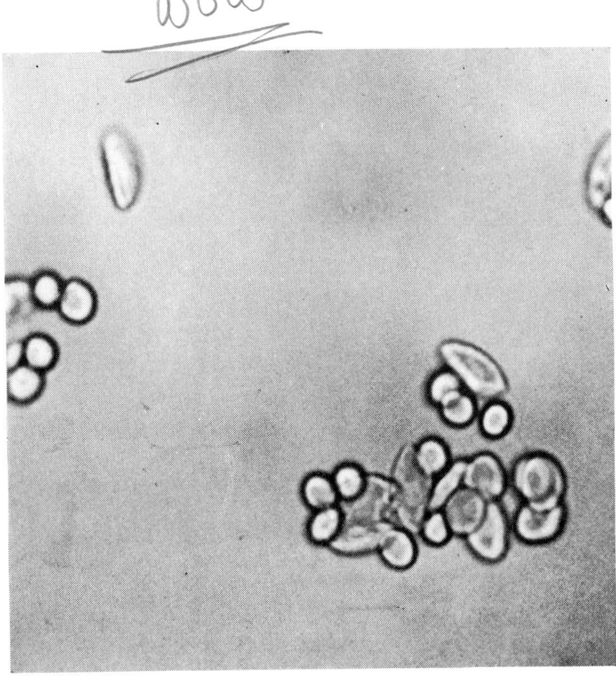

ture of antiovalbumin and antibovine gamma globulin causes discrete clumping of both round human and oval chicken cells; finally, when antibodies of dual specificity are used, agglutinates link together both the round human and oval chicken cells. These experiments were first described by Drs. H. H. Fudenberg and Genevieve Drews and the author.

enfolded structures. Evidence is quite conclusive that the folded structure of a protein is determined by its amino acid sequence.

This position has received strong support from experiments conducted by Charles Tanford at Duke University and Edgar Haber at Massachusetts General Hospital. Their work was done with antibody fragments, produced by the action of papain, containing single active sites. The fragments were thoroughly denatured by exposure to concentrated guanidine hydrochloride, which causes extensive protein unfolding. All the disulfide bonds and essentially all of the noncovalent bonds were broken. Yet upon removal of the reagent and reestablishment of disulfide bonds, the opened-up chains, made up of some 400 amino acids, spontaneously refolded and regained a substantial fraction of their initial antibody activity. It would be difficult to design a better demonstration of the validity of the theory that amino acid sequence determines protein structure.

If antigens play no role in the direct shaping of antibodies, the likely alternative is that in some sense the antibodies, or at least the potential for making them, must be ready and waiting. More concretely, this means that plasma cell precursors must differ genetically, that there must be a sufficient variety of genes to produce antibodies specific to whatever antigens might be encountered. In other words, there must be thousands of different strains of lymphoid cells to manufacture the variety of antibodies called for.

Broadly speaking, two theories have been formulated to account for this state of affairs. The first holds that all genes are inherited from preceding generations (implying the existence of a full complement of heavy- and light-chain genes in every cell, including the zygotes). This concept has been amplified by Dreyer and Bennett with the suggestion that one of the inherited genes for the variable portion of the molecule combines with the gene for the invariant part to give rise to a complete, functioning molecule. The alternate theory is that relatively few genes are inherited, but they are highly mutable and give rise to large numbers of different genes by somatic mutation or by crossing over and recombination.

There is now strong evidence that the heavy chain (and probably the light chain as well) is under the control of two separate genes, one coding for the variable segment and the other for the invariant segment of the chain. The best available data suggest that fusion of the two genes takes place, thus permitting synthesis of the single polypeptide chain. Although the number of inherited genes controlling the variable region is uncertain (see next page), there is strong evidence that the constant region of the chain is represented in the germ line by one (or a very small number) structural gene.

Notice that the time scales differ by an enormous factor. If the inheritance theory holds, most of the antibodies that protect us today appeared long ago (the general mutation rate for an ordinary protein is about one amino acid substitution in 10 million years). The alternative view implies that the great majority of antibodies arise during our lifetimes, with new genes appearing almost continuously. We do not yet know which theory is correct.

Theoretical questions also bear on the way in which the immune system evolved. One possibility is that the first antibody was a degenerate enzyme. After all, the architectures of antibodies and enzymes are similar in that both are proteins with highly specific active sites that occupy only a small fraction of the surface of the molecule. The difference is that enzymes perform a double duty, not only attaching to their substrates but also speeding up chemical reactions — whereas the job of the antibody is simply to complex with an antigen.

In any case, studies based on internal homologies or resemblances among amino acid sequences within the L and H chains suggest that the ancestor of present-day antibodies may have been a polypeptide made up of about 100 amino acid residues (half an L chain). The first L chain could have resulted from a duplication of the gene controlling the synthesis of this primitive protein. Half of this duplicated gene, corresponding to the variable portion of the L chain, may have been subject to mutation (and repeated replication if the germ-line theory is correct), whereas the other half, controlling the invariant half of the L chain, has remained highly resistant to mutation.

H chains may have arisen from the fusion of two L chains by a similar process of gene duplication. As previously noted, approximately three quarters of the H chain within any given class is essentially invariable. It is relevant here that amino acid sequence data, first obtained in the laboratories of R. L. Hill at Duke University and of S. J. Singer and R. Doolittle at the University of California, provided strong support for the common evolutionary origin of the light and heavy chains. A common origin for the immunoglobulins of widely divergent species has also been shown.

So far the order of amino acids has been determined in great detail for parts of the antibody molecule, and something is known about sequence in the rest of the molecule. Furthermore, there is a growing body of information that indicates how the four polypeptide chains may be arranged in space.

What remains to be done is fairly obvious and calls for a tremendous amount of work—nothing less than a final assault on the structural problem. Eventually we would like to have as complete a picture of the antibody molecule as John Kendrew and his associates at Cambridge University have of the myoglobin molecule—which means establishing the positions of all amino acid residues, finding out which residues are important in conferring specificity and which actually touch the antigenic determinants, and knowing how the H and L chains are folded upon themselves.

Such an analysis could be done by x-ray crystallography. This, of course, requires crystallized material and underscores the need for obtaining homogeneous antibody. So far only limited success has been achieved in this direction. One of Porter's fragments, derived from papain digestion, exists in a sufficiently pure state to crystallize spontaneously. But that represents only a fragment of the antibody molecule, one lacking a combining site and therefore lacking antibody activity. A complete and active antibody which also crystallizes was fortuitously produced for the first time in our laboratories. About a year ago we noted a rabbit producing an unusually large amount of antibody to a simple

Theories of Antibody Specificity (Variable Portion of Molecule)

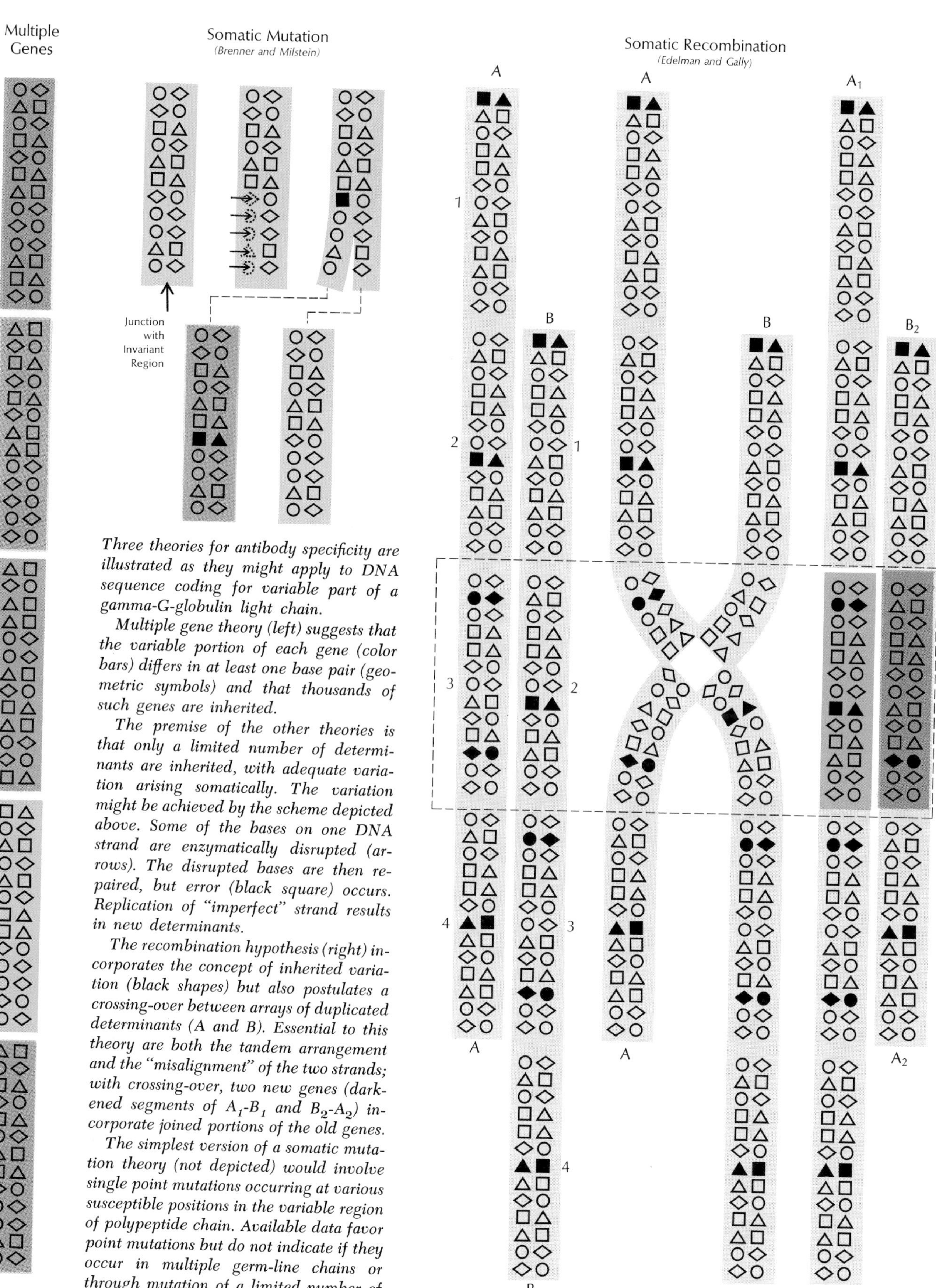

Three theories for antibody specificity are illustrated as they might apply to DNA sequence coding for variable part of a gamma-G-globulin light chain.

Multiple gene theory (left) suggests that the variable portion of each gene (color bars) differs in at least one base pair (geometric symbols) and that thousands of such genes are inherited.

The premise of the other theories is that only a limited number of determinants are inherited, with adequate variation arising somatically. The variation might be achieved by the scheme depicted above. Some of the bases on one DNA strand are enzymatically disrupted (arrows). The disrupted bases are then repaired, but error (black square) occurs. Replication of "imperfect" strand results in new determinants.

The recombination hypothesis (right) incorporates the concept of inherited variation (black shapes) but also postulates a crossing-over between arrays of duplicated determinants (A and B). Essential to this theory are both the tandem arrangement and the "misalignment" of the two strands; with crossing-over, two new genes (darkened segments of A_1-B_1 and B_2-A_2) incorporate joined portions of the old genes.

The simplest version of a somatic mutation theory (not depicted) would involve single point mutations occurring at various susceptible positions in the variable region of polypeptide chain. Available data favor point mutations but do not indicate if they occur in multiple germ-line chains or through mutation of a limited number of genes during life of animal.

hapten (the p-azobenzoate group). When the antibody was separated from all other serum proteins, it crystallized spontaneously under proper conditions. A number of physical measurements have indicated that this crystallization is attributable to the homogeneity of the antibody, possibly reflecting its synthesis by a single large clone of cells. The amounts available are not sufficient for x-ray crystallography, but the demonstration that an antibody can be crystallized indicates that complete structural analysis will eventually be feasible.

More recently, we have prepared crystals from the Fab fragments of several myeloma proteins, and one of these is being subjected to x-ray diffraction analysis by R. Poljak at the Johns Hopkins University School of Medicine. Similar analysis of a crystallized whole myeloma protein is proceeding in the laboratory of D. R. Davies at the National Institutes of Health. Since myeloma proteins are now considered to be typical immunoglobulins, and some have been shown to possess antibody activity, a knowledge of the three-dimensional structure of a myeloma protein may prove to be highly relevant to an understanding of antibody function.

At this stage it should be emphasized that fine-structure research has a value over and above its theoretical implications. In the process of taking immunoglobulin molecules apart and putting them back together, creating hybrid antibodies, and analyzing amino acid sequences, investigators are developing a battery of increasingly sophisticated techniques for handling proteins—techniques that will almost certainly bring about clinical advances as well as advances in fundamental knowledge. And, as already suggested, structural work on antibodies has had direct bearing on understanding of antibody synthesis.

One can logically anticipate that information about mechanisms of antibody production will be of great importance in providing the clinician with means of reinforcing natural immunologic processes or in substituting for them when they are absent or deficient; on the other hand, this information should have value in limiting host-versus-graft transplantation reactions, controlling allergies, and generally in dealing with pathological conditions stemming from immune reactions. To the extent that structural studies contribute to our understanding of biosynthetic mechanisms—and their contribution to date has been notable—it may be expected that they will suggest new approaches in many areas of medicine. After all, once you know how antibodies are formed, you can devise new ways for enhancing or inhibiting that formation.

Chapter 8

The Gamma A Globulins: First Line of Defense

THOMAS B. TOMASI
State University of New York at Buffalo

Why are some individuals particularly susceptible to repeated respiratory infections despite apparently normal circulating antibody responses? Why is it often impossible to correlate recovery from infection with serum antibody levels? Do antibodies help determine which viruses and bacteria will colonize the respiratory, gastrointestinal, and genitourinary tracts during the first hours or days of postnatal life? Can we augment our ability to predict which antibodies will cross the placental barrier? What role does antibody play in determining normal flora in the adult? Can "local" immunization be effective in certain respiratory diseases in which systemic vaccination has in general proved disappointing? Can autoimmune and/or hypersensitivity phenomena be related to local immunologic mechanisms?

These questions are obviously of prime relevance to clinical medicine. And while none yet lends itself to an unequivocal answer, investigations into the nature and behavior of the A class of immunoglobulins (IgA) give promise of leading to at least some of the answers. To be sure, our knowledge of the gamma A globulins is far less detailed at both structural and functional levels than is that for the gamma G globulins as described by Dr. Nisonoff [Chapter 7, "Molecules of Immunity"]. But we have already come far enough to be convinced that the IgA's – or at least one type of IgA – are important determinants of immunologic competence at most interfaces between the internal and external environments of the body.

The particular type of gamma A globulins which play this role have been designated as secretory gamma A globulins. Whereas the gamma G globulins form the dominant circulating antibodies in the serum and in other fluids that are completely confined within the body, the secretory gamma A antibodies are quantitatively and probably functionally dominant in all fluids bathing the organs and systems that are in continuity with the external environment — saliva, tears, breast milk and colostrum, gastrointestinal secretions, and probably the fluids elaborated by the mucoid tissues of the respiratory and genitourinary tracts. Thus these A globulins are uniquely situated to provide initial immunologic response to a host of bacterial and viral invaders and to affect the immunologic heritage of the new human.

Before detailing the evidence for and the significance of this last statement, it would be appropriate to place the gamma A immunoglobulins in the context of our understanding of all of the circulating immunoglobulins. Until recently, four major classes of human immunoglobulins had been defined; in the last few years, evidence for a fifth class has been presented. All are gamma globulins. The most thoroughly studied have been gamma G's (IgG), the dominant serum immunoglobulins. These IgG antibodies have a molecular weight of 160,000, a sedimentation coefficient of 7S, four polypeptide chains (two light and two heavy), and either a fast or slow electrophoretic mobility, depending on subclass; concentration in serum is normally about 12 mg/cc.

The gamma M globulins, in contrast, are large, complex molecules, with a molecular weight of 900,000 and a sedimentation coefficient of 19S. The molecules consist of 20 polypeptide chains (4 x 5), and have a fast electrophoretic mobility; normal concentration in serum is approximately 1.0 mg/cc. The IgA antibodies *in serum* — and this must be emphasized — are primarily 7S molecules, with a weight of 170,000 and four polypeptide chains; electrophoretic mobility is fast. Normal serum contains about 1.8 mg/cc of IgA. Gamma D globulins (IgD) are also 7S (150,000) globulins with a fast electrophoretic mobility. They are found in the serum in concentrations of only 0.03 mg/cc.

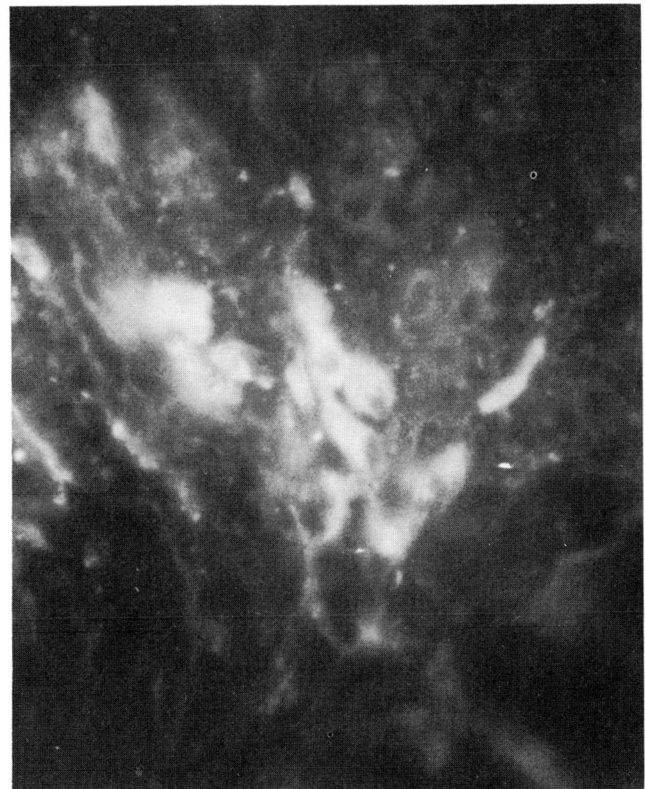

Fluorescent studies of human parotid document concentration and specificity of IgA. Tissue has been stained with fluorescein-conjugated antiserum to serum IgA. In area of gland near collecting ducts, cytoplasm of interstitial cells fluoresces.

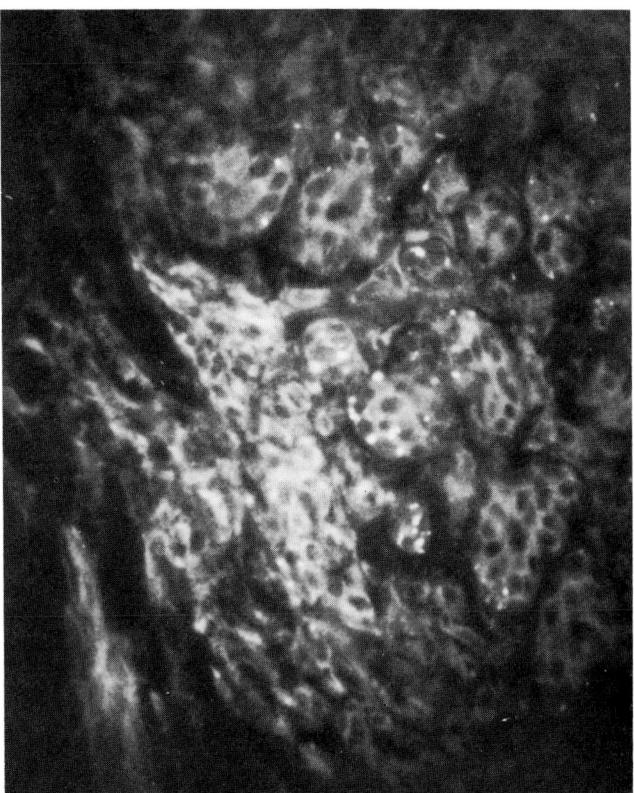

After absorption of the same antiserum with isolated serum gamma A immunoglobulin, an adjacent section of the parotid gland in the same area does not stain because the specific fluorescence of the interstitial cells has been abolished.

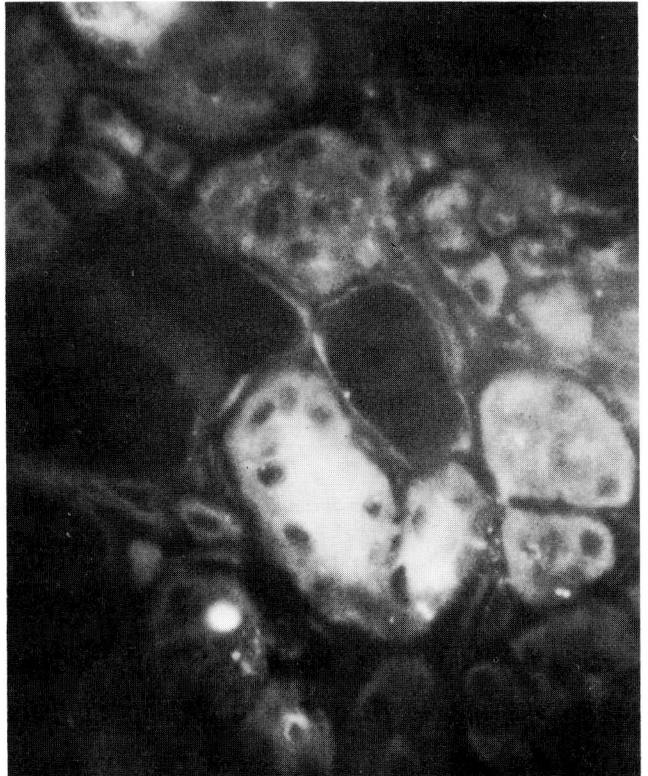

When gland is stained with fluorescein-conjugated antiserum to salivary IgA absorbed with isolated serum IgA, there is specific fluorescence of material in the cells of glandular acini, but there is no fluorescence of interstitial cells.

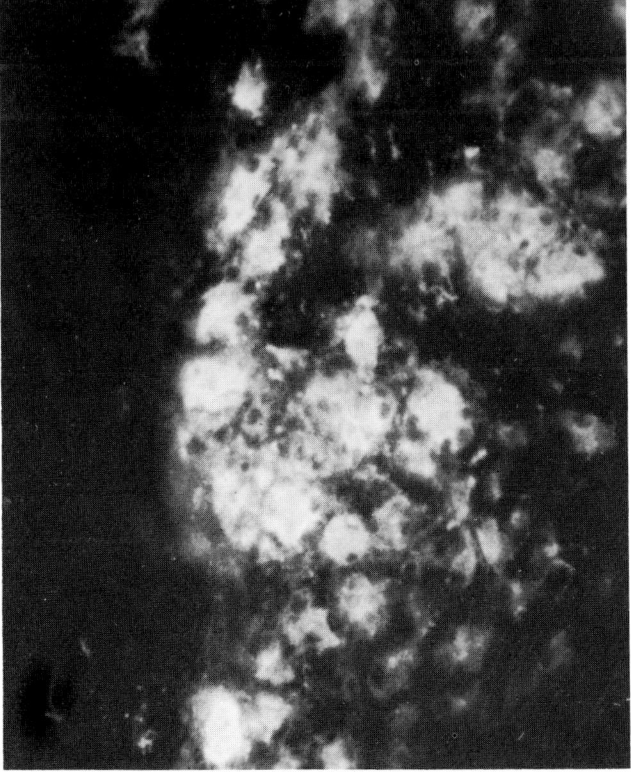

When the same salivary IgA antiserum absorbed with serum IgA is used to stain area of parotid near collecting ducts, there is widespread fluorescence of cytoplasm of the acinar cells. This is area where salivary IgA appears to be most abundant.

The most recently discovered class of immune globulins is the gamma E (IgE), described by Dr. K. Ishizaka and his colleagues at the University of Colorado. They appear to be present in normal serum in very small amounts and include the skin sensitizing or reagin antibodies in persons who are sensitive to ragweed and other allergens.

These characteristics by themselves do not serve to differentiate among the antibody classes. There are a number of other immunologic, genetic, and biologic properties that effect this differentiation. All immunoglobulins studied so far have class-specific antigenic determinants associated with their heavy (H) polypeptide chains. The binding of complement can be achieved by either IgG or IgM antibodies, but not by IgA. IgG antibodies cross the placenta, while the other classes do not. IgM appears to be associated with early response to antigens, while IgG is formed somewhat later.

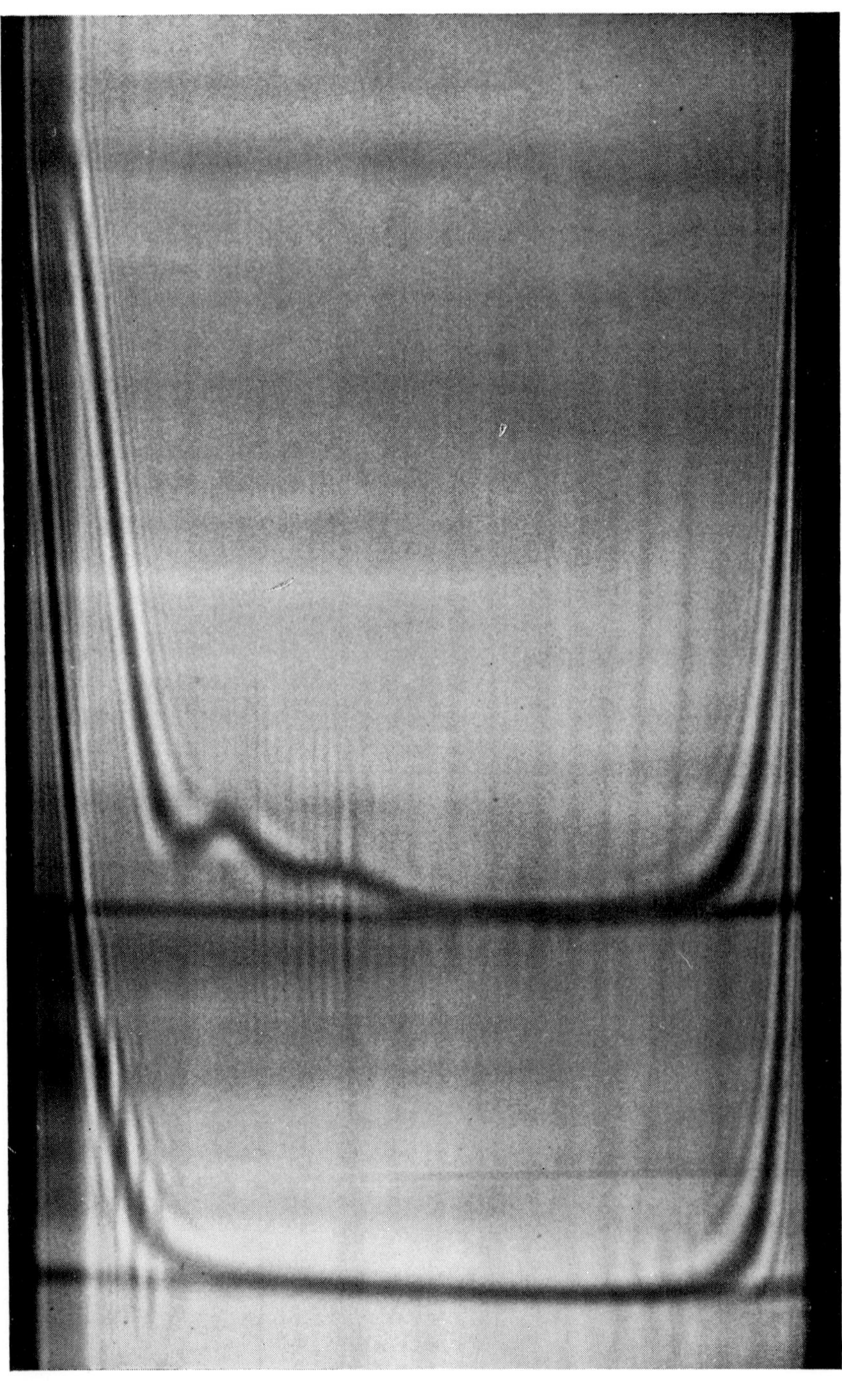

Evidence that salivary immunoglobulin is IgA is seen in ultracentrifuge patterns of normal individual (top) and patient known to lack serum IgA (bottom). Sedimentation is from left to right. Both 11S and 18S immunoglobulin components are present in the normal saliva, absent in that of the patient who is deficient in serum IgA.

Differences also exist in the antigens to which different antibody classes respond. Thus many gram-negative bacterial and blood-group antibodies are of the IgM type. For its part, the IgA class includes antibodies against a host of pathogens and other antigens — against diphtheria, brucella, escherichia, and many other bacteria, against blood-group and Rh antigens, against some of the nuclear factors involved in collagen diseases, and against many of the viruses associated with respiratory infections. I believe the importance of this last will emerge as this discussion continues.

It should be made clear that when it is said that the antibodies to any antigen belong to one class or another, this does not mean that other antibodies to the same antigen cannot belong to another class. If you look into the serum of a patient with brucellosis you will find brucella antibodies of gamma G, gamma M, and gamma A types. It is not yet known why the same antigen should elicit so many different types of antibody, nor is it known why there is wide individual variation in "typical" responses. However, the clinical significance of this variation is considerable even now, and its potential significance is much greater. For example, some anti-Rh antibodies are IgG, others are IgA. The former cross the placenta, the latter do not. Obviously, it would be highly useful to know whether the antibodies being produced in an Rh-incompatible pregnancy are IgG, with a potential for causing erythroblastosis fetalis, or IgA, without the ability to damage the fetus.

To sum up before returning to the discussion of the secretory gamma A globulins, it should be noted that immunoglobulins represent a tremendously heterogeneous population. No two are really alike. There are significant differences among classes — and even within each class — in amino acid composition. And they show exceptional specificity, which enables them to perform their immunobiologic function.

The gamma A globulins are found in serum, where there is about one IgA molecule for every five or six IgG

The Structure of Immunoglobulins

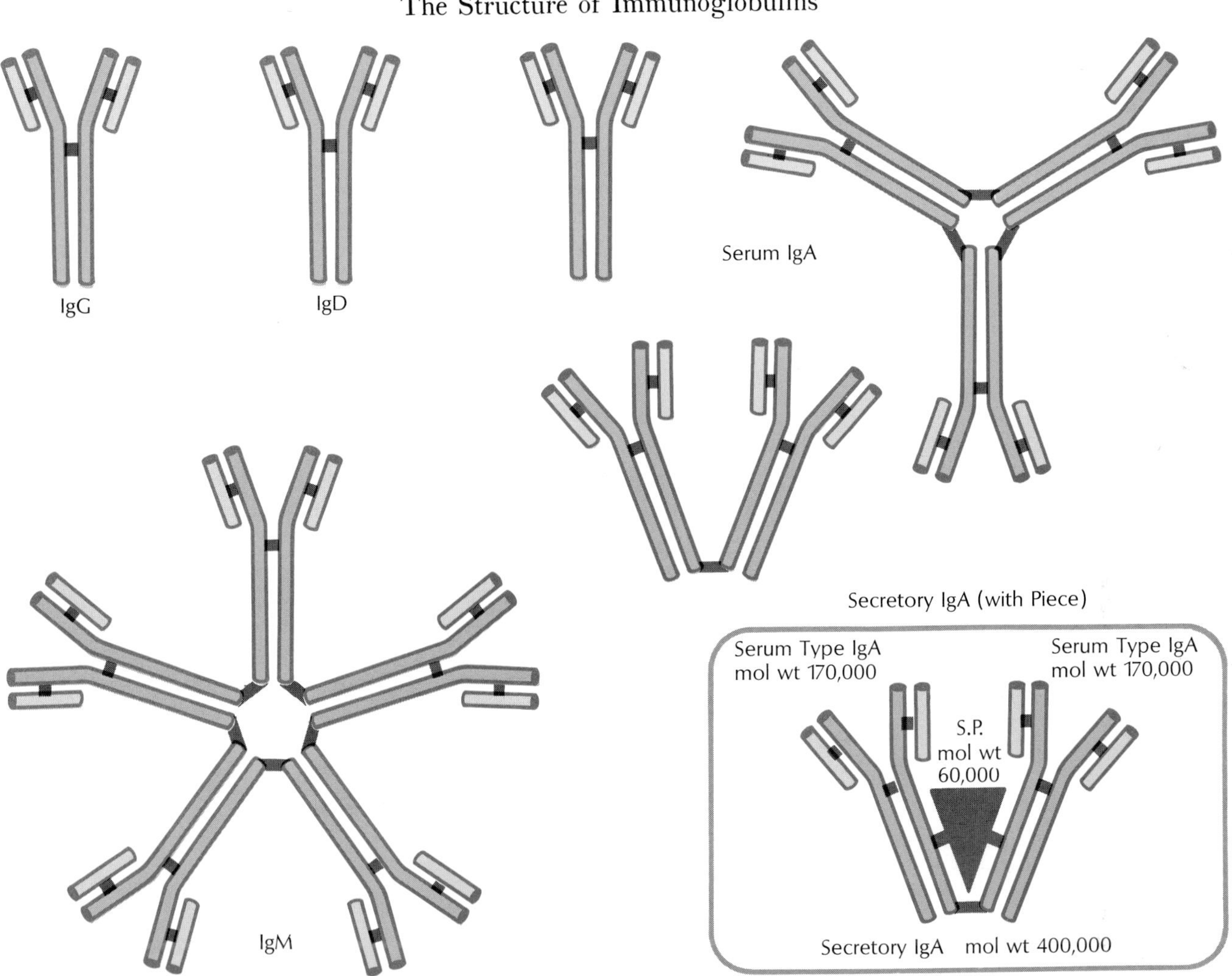

Comparative structures of the immunoglobulins are schematized. The IgG and IgD are seen as simple monomers, each with two light and two heavy polypeptide chains. Serum IgA is found in this form, but it frequently exists in the pictured dimer and trimer forms also, particularly in pathologic states. The large 19S IgM is visualized as a pentamer (as proposed by Miller and Metzger), while secretory IgA is seen as a dimer to which secretory piece has been added.

molecules. They are also found in almost every external secretion, with the ratio reversed and then some. In normal saliva, for example, the ratio of IgA to IgG is more than 20 to one. This relationship is essentially true for all the secretions previously mentioned that represent direct continuity with the external environment.

But much more than its ratio to other immunoglobulins is different about the secretory gamma A. Its molecule is much bigger than most IgA molecules found in serum, with a molecular weight of 390,000 (as compared with 170,000); it has a sedimentation coefficient of 11S rather than 7S and, unlike the polymers of IgA which are found in serum, particularly in pathologic states such as multiple myeloma, its disulfide bonds are not readily reduced by sulfhydryl reagents.

Work in several laboratories appears to have explained these differences. In one critical experiment, an antiserum was produced by injecting salivary A into an animal. This was absorbed with serum A, but even after absorption the antiserum retained specificity for the secretory globulin. This residual specificity is due to the presence of an additional nonimmunoglobulin component firmly attached to the IgA, probably by disulfide bonds. This nonglobulin component is called the secretory "piece." Work by Dr. Richard Hong in Dr. Robert Good's laboratory at the University of Minnesota, and by Dr. Mary Ann South, now at Baylor, as well as in our laboratory, has suggested that this piece is produced in epithelial cells rather than in the immunoglobulin-producing plasma cells that lie just below the basement membrane of the epithelium all along the GI and respiratory tracts.

The secretory piece has been partially characterized. It does not appear to contain any immunoglobulin antigenic determinants; it has a high carbohydrate content — about 9.5 percent — and contains sialic acid. Its amino acids are different from those in the gamma A polypeptide chains. Finally, there are four moles of disulfide bond per mole of secretory piece, which has a molecular weight of 50,000 to 60,000.

These data fit together very nicely.

If we keep in mind that the secretory gamma A has a molecular weight of around 390,000, then we can readily correlate this with the concept that it is a dimer of serum gamma A — with its molecular weight of 170,000 — plus secretory piece. In fact, our first realization that the secretory immunoglobulin was not simply a polymer of serum A came from our inability to dissociate it into 7S subunits by reduction, something accomplished readily with the serum polymers. Perhaps even more relevant has been the finding that the secretory gamma A globulins are highly resistant to proteolysis with enzymes such as trypsin, chymotrypsin, and pepsin, all of which will attack the serum immunoglobulins. Reasoning somewhat teleologically, you could say that if you set out to design a molecule capable of surviving and functioning in an environment rich in proteolytic enzymes and bacteria, you would rationally arrive at a structure like that of secretory A. It seems quite clear to us now that the piece conveys a great measure of stability to this antibody molecule.

But there is another possible function of secretory piece. It has been called by some investigators "transport piece," and it is certainly possible that it is related to the transport of the immunoglobulin from its site of production to the mucoid surface, although the evidence for this is far from conclusive. The hypothetical scheme for such transport (see pages 82 and 83) actually exemplifies the work now in progress in our laboratory, and in many others, through which efforts are being made to determine whether the secretory piece transports or facilitates the transport of immunoglobulin A across the mucous membrane. Such a demonstration would have great importance in biology. It should be noted here that we know very little about the transfer of proteins across biologic membranes. In contrast to the extensive and fruitful investigation of the mechanisms of electrolyte transfer, very little has been learned about the specific factors involved in protein passage. Clearly, then, one of the real interests in secretory piece is as a possible model for the biologic conveyance of proteins.

Even confirmation of the role of piece as a transport facility, however, would leave us with basic questions as to why the preference for gamma A along the mucous membranes, and why the plasma cells underneath these membranes are specific producers of IgA. There is considerable evidence that they are so specialized. If one takes fluorescent antigamma G and fluorescent antigamma A, one will find that in the lymph nodes and the spleen — the two major areas in which serum antibodies are produced — the plasma cells staining for G and those staining for A are in a ratio of about 4:1. On the other hand, using the same technique with plasma cells along the GI or respiratory tracts, or in the salivary gland or breast, one can pinpoint 20 or 30 IgA-producing cells for every IgG producer. This has been shown particularly well for the GI tract in studies by Drs. Crabbé, Heremans, and Carbonara of Belgium. These ratios of cells correspond very closely with the concentrations of the immunoglobulins found on the one hand in the serum and on the other in the external secretions. A few IgM cells and, interestingly, IgE cells are also seen in the gastrointestinal and respiratory tracts.

One cannot completely exclude the possibility that some sort of selection takes IgA antibodies from the serum and transports them to the secretory areas, but the weight of evidence certainly favors synthesis in local areas, followed by transport across the epithelial membranes directly into the secretions. In fact, we are inclined to the hypothesis that gamma A is elaborated in the "local" plasma cells and then transported in one direction into the serum, in another into the secretions, with the latter acquiring piece during its passage through the epithelial membranes. Thus local production in the GI and respiratory tracts could constitute significant synthesis of serum gamma A.

Possible Role of Secretory Piece

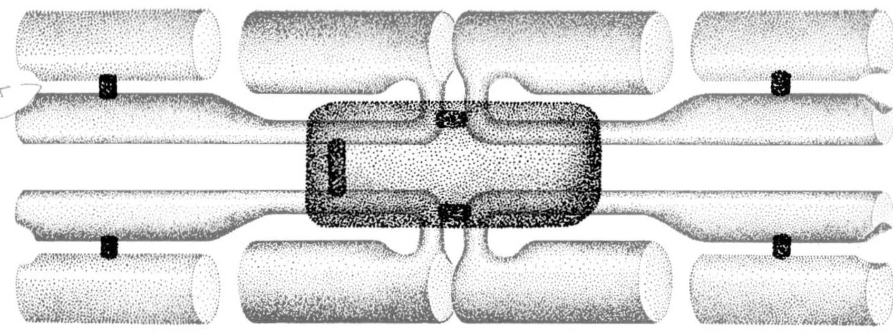

In this theoretic visualization of secretory IgA, the possible protective role of piece is seen. As projected here on dimer of antibody model [see Chapter 7, "Molecules of Immunity," by Alfred Nisonoff], piece straddles the bonds uniting the two components of the immunoglobulin, thus preventing its disruption by proteolytic enzymes.

Returning to the question of why plasma cells adjacent to the secretory areas are gamma A producers, we are still largely limited to speculation. Dr. Good [see Chapter 1, "Disorders of the Immune System"] and others have pointed out that immunocompetent organs such as the thymus and the bursa of Fabricius (in birds) are formed from epithelial cells, probably from endoderm. This would suggest a relationship among epithelial cells, the thymus, and the immunologically competent cells. Indeed, a number of groups, notably that of Dr. Aronson at the Pasteur Institute in Paris, have pointed out that thymectomized rats and mice appear to have specific defects in what he calls gamma A.

However, we are faced with a difficult problem here in determining what is gamma A in species other than the human. We are still hampered by inefficient means of isolating pure gamma A in good yields. Probably the best animal studies have been performed at the University of Florida by Drs. John Cebra, John Robbins, and Parker Small. They have isolated from rabbit colostrum a protein that has a molecular weight of 400,000; it is a

10.8S molecule that appears to be a dimer of serum IgA with an added component, which they call a T chain. In short, it seems quite analogous to the human secretory IgA. But in cows and sheep one finds a secretory gamma globulin with a distribution similar to that of human secretory A and having many other analogous characteristics – except that it is a fast gamma G globulin. Smaller amounts of an IgA-type protein may also be present.

What are the functions that can be assigned — speculatively at least — to the secretory IgA? Logically one can start with a possible role at birth. Within a matter of hours an essentially sterile gastrointestinal tract is colonized by many species and strains of bacteria. What determines which bacteria will colonize, what shall constitute normal flora thereafter? Undoubtedly multiple factors are at work, but the fluctuations in population may relate to the types of antibody present in the tract. Some of them may be ingested in mother's milk. These, the so-called coproantibodies, are predominantly secretory IgA; thus regulation of normal flora in both gastrointestinal and respiratory tracts may be included in any speculative list of functions of these immunoglobulins. Incidentally, in recent investigations, Dr. John Bienenstock and I have found that secretory gamma A is also contained in urine. Since it has been shown that IgA-type antibodies will react against organisms that are normal inhabitants of the bladder and other parts of the urinary system, this regulatory function may also be operative with this system.

As has been mentioned, colostrum has the same level of secretory IgA as do other external secretions. This predominance persists in breast milk, although the longer the mother nurses the more other immunoglobulins are found. We now know that colostrum contains a rich source of antibodies. Many, although not all, of these are of the secretory type and may well play a role in the resistance of the infant. Some animals, cows among others, are born agammaglobulinemic and receive no antibodies from their mothers. If colostrum is withheld, many of the calves will succumb to infection within a short period of time. Apparently they receive all their immunologic defenses postpartum. In the human, of course, the situation is more complex, not only because many gamma globulins are transmitted transplacentally, but because there is very little evidence of significant absorption of antibodies from the GI tract. Most people believe that the human GI tract is essentially impermeable to absorption of the whole antibody molecule. So if any significant role is to be postulated for the colostral and milk antibodies, it must be essentially at the local, gastrointestinal level.

Interestingly, GI tract permeability following birth is a species characteristic. In humans the GI tract is impermeable to intact proteins; in other animals it is permeable at birth but then shuts down — in two or three days in the cow and sheep, in 15 to 20 days in the rat. The mechanisms responsible for changing permeability are unknown, but I believe the phenomenon is a significant area for study, in terms of learning how a species acquires its immunologic competence.

Before we leave the perinatal aspects of secretory IgA research, an important observation should be reported. As noted previously, the human newborn receives gamma G from his mother, almost as the exclusive immunoglobulin. There is no gamma A, very little gamma M. If we look at the saliva of an infant in the first few days of life we find no immunoglobulin at all – but he does have secretory piece in a free state. Eventually, most of this piece material becomes attached to IgA. Thus the infant appears to be prepared with piece to develop a competent secretory immunologic system. This finding gains support from an observation by Dr. Good's group that the secretory A system develops earlier than the serum A. We have seen several infants 10 to 15 days old who had significant amounts of secretory IgA but no detectable serum IgA.

Another logical function for the secretory A globulins is, of course, as local defense against potentially pathogenic viruses and bacteria. Again the secretory gamma A has been shown to have antibody activity against a variety of different inhaled and ingested pathogens. Recent studies done at NIH in human volunteers have shown that recovery from upper respiratory infections of viral etiology is related more closely to the development of antibodies in the nasopharyngeal secretions than to serum antibodies. In fact, there is little consistent relationship to serum antibody at all. Moreover, it was found that the volunteers' resistance to challenge with respiratory viruses was related to secretory IgA antibodies measured in nasal discharge. Certainly, these studies would seem to have a bearing on the age-old

Comparison of Properties of IgA from Serum and Secretions

Property	Serum IgA	Secretory IgA
Sedimentation coefficient	6.9	11.4
Molecular weight	170,000	390,000
Percent hexose	5.0	6.2
Percent sialic acid	1.7	1.0
Moles disulfide per 170,000	15	16
Amino acid composition	Small but significant differences (greater than 10 percent) in eight amino acids: arginine, lysine, aspartic acid, glutamic acid, histidine, methionine, isoleucine, and glysine	
Gm (H-chain genetic factors)	—	—
InV (L-chain genetic factors)	+	+
3-Dimensional conformation	no helix ? cross beta structure	no helix ? cross beta structure

The sedimentation coefficient in this presentation is expressed at infinite dilution. As their absence here indicates, the Gm genetic determinants are specific for the H chains of the IgG molecule, while the InV genetic factors associated with the L chains are common to all classes of immunoglobulins. The three-dimensional conformation of IgA was determined by the technique of optical rotatory dispersion.

questions of why people get colds, why they recover from them, and why there seems to be little relationship between susceptibility, illness, and recovery on the one hand, serum antibody on the other. Indeed, the NIH studies showed that an individual with good serum antibody titers but no detectable local antibody would become ill when challenged with a respiratory virus, while the patient with good local antibody responses but little serum antibody would ward off the infection without manifesting any overt clinical signs or symptoms.

A related phenomenon is observable in the GI tract. There is suggestive evidence that susceptibility to reinfection with organisms such as cholera vibrios can be correlated with local antibodies — the coproantibodies. In experimental cholera in guinea pigs, for example, there is little relationship between serum antibody and susceptibility via the natural route of infection, the GI tract, but there is good correlation between resistance and coproantibody levels. When coproantibody levels disappear, the animals become susceptible again – even though serum vibrio antibodies may be rising and the animals can withstand systemic challenge. On a clinical note, it can be pointed out that cholera vaccines, heretofore administered parenterally, have not been optimally effective in preventing spread of the disease. Workers in Asia are most interested in the question of local immunity and the possibility of developing and testing vaccines that could be administered orally to act within the gastrointestinal tract.

Similarly, in relation to the respiratory tract, understanding of the secretory IgA raises questions about routes of administration and efficacy. One wonders if some of the older work suggesting that nebulization of antigens would provide an advantage in conferring immunity may not have more validity than has generally been accorded. Certainly these studies deserve review, repetition, and perhaps extension. Such studies on local immunization are presently under way in several laboratories.

Allergies are also conditions in which local factors play an important role. Work by Dr. Ishizaka, and investigations in our laboratories, have shown that in allergic persons ragweed antibodies are present in the external secretions. Especially important may be the IgE-type antibodies, and recent evidence suggests these may be produced locally. It is known that when a ragweed or pollen allergen is inhaled it is deposited on the mucous membrane surface of the respiratory tract. We believe it is a local antigen-antibody reaction, perhaps occurring on the surface of the mucous membrane, which elicits the release of such agents as histamine and serotonin, which actually cause the symptoms. Therefore the appearance of antiragweed antibodies in these secretions may well be important in determining allergic reactions. For this reason, along with Dr. Carl Arbesman here at the State University, we have been studying the desensitization regimens allergists have been employing for so many years. These procedures cannot be correlated with levels of serum antibody. Some individuals who are desensitized by small, repeated doses of the ragweed antigen may develop good levels of blocking antibodies in their serum — yet the clinical effect may be negligible. And the reverse is true. We are wondering if this apparent inconsistency might not be explicable on the basis of reactions in the local secretory system — that is, directly at the site of action.

In autoimmune disease, the role of secretory immunoglobulins is even more speculative, but it is receiving a good deal of investigative attention at this time. If we look at those diseases for which an autoimmune etiology has been postulated — pernicious anemia, ulcerative colitis, certain malabsorption syndromes, etc. — we can find very little good evidence that circulating antibody mechanisms are directly involved. Therefore, local immunologic mechanisms must be considered. We must seek to determine if locally produced, immunologically competent cells or antibodies may be producing the destruction characteristic of these diseases. Several groups are now looking at the secretions and the antibodies in the GI tract to see whether there are immunologic elements directed against intrinsic factor in patients with pernicious anemia, for example. Others are investigating the possibility of anticolon antibodies in individuals with ulcerative colitis. Some evidence for such locally produced antibodies has been obtained in these disorders, and in some cases the antibodies have been related to exogenous pathogens, but it is too early to draw conclusions as to the relevance of these findings.

Probably the area of clinical investigation in which knowledge of the secretory IgA system is being applied with the greatest intensity today is the study of that large group of patients, particularly in the pediatric age-group, who have repeated infections but who show no deficits in their circulating antibody systems. These patients are not agammaglobulinemic, dysgammaglobulinemic, or hypogammaglobulinemic. Yet they have one respiratory infection after another. The key question: Do these individuals represent a group in whom the local immune system is deficient? Such deficiency might be due to defects in local production — to absence of plasma cells or perhaps

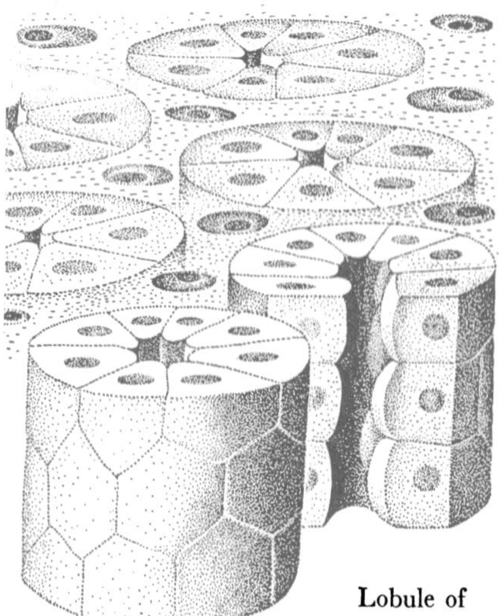

Lobule of Salivary Gland

Drawings suggest possible mechanisms of sy sis and transport of secretory IgA into the ex secretions. Above, the structure of a sal gland lobule is shown. The IgA is found u plasma-like cells in the interstitial spaces as as in the lumens of acini that feed int salivary duct. The rendering opposite corr structure with the general theory of form and transport of IgA. The theory holds th globulins are synthesized in the plasma cell then move in two directions – into the ge circulation and through the cells of the epit lining where secretory piece is acquired. On ing the epithelial cells and entering the secr tract, the globulin is now complete secretory even to a failure of the epithelial cells to produce piece.

Although the existence of such individuals has not been demonstrated in the population marked by susceptibility to respiratory infections, the suggestion of Drs. South and Good with regard to children with hereditary telangiectasia merits consideration. This disease is characterized by multiple infections superimposed on central nervous system pathology and by the lack of both serum and secretory gamma A globulins. It has been hypothesized that the lack of secretory A might explain the multiple respiratory infections from which these children often die.

From our studies we agree that secretory A is lacking in such patients, but we have found that it is replaced largely by gamma M. In itself this is an interesting finding; one would expect that gamma G would be a more likely replacement for A, but apparently there is some unknown relationship between A and M. The secretory gamma M in these children is active against some bacteria. It should also be stressed that the telangiectasia patient has many other immunologic abnormalities, including lack of IgE, defects in delayed hypersensitivity responsiveness and thymic abnormalities detectable on autopsy. Obviously, one cannot be sure that the multiple respiratory infections in these patients are a consequence of a deficiency in secretory IgA.

With Dr. Robert Schwartz of Tufts, we are studying another group of patients. These are individuals with disseminated lupus erythematosus, one of the so-called autoimmune diseases. A few of these patients have come to our attention because of frequent episodes of respiratory disease — as many as a dozen bouts of pneumonia in a single patient. All these patients have very highly elevated serum immunoglobulin levels, with the serum IgA particularly high. But in all cases the salivary gamma A is below the normal range, and there is no replacement by gamma M. These patients, then, may constitute a reasonable model for study of the relationship between secretory IgA deficiency and susceptibility to respiratory infections — certainly one of the most intriguing of the many intriguing and clinically promising aspects of the gamma A immunoglobulin system.

Synthesis and Transport of Secretory IgA

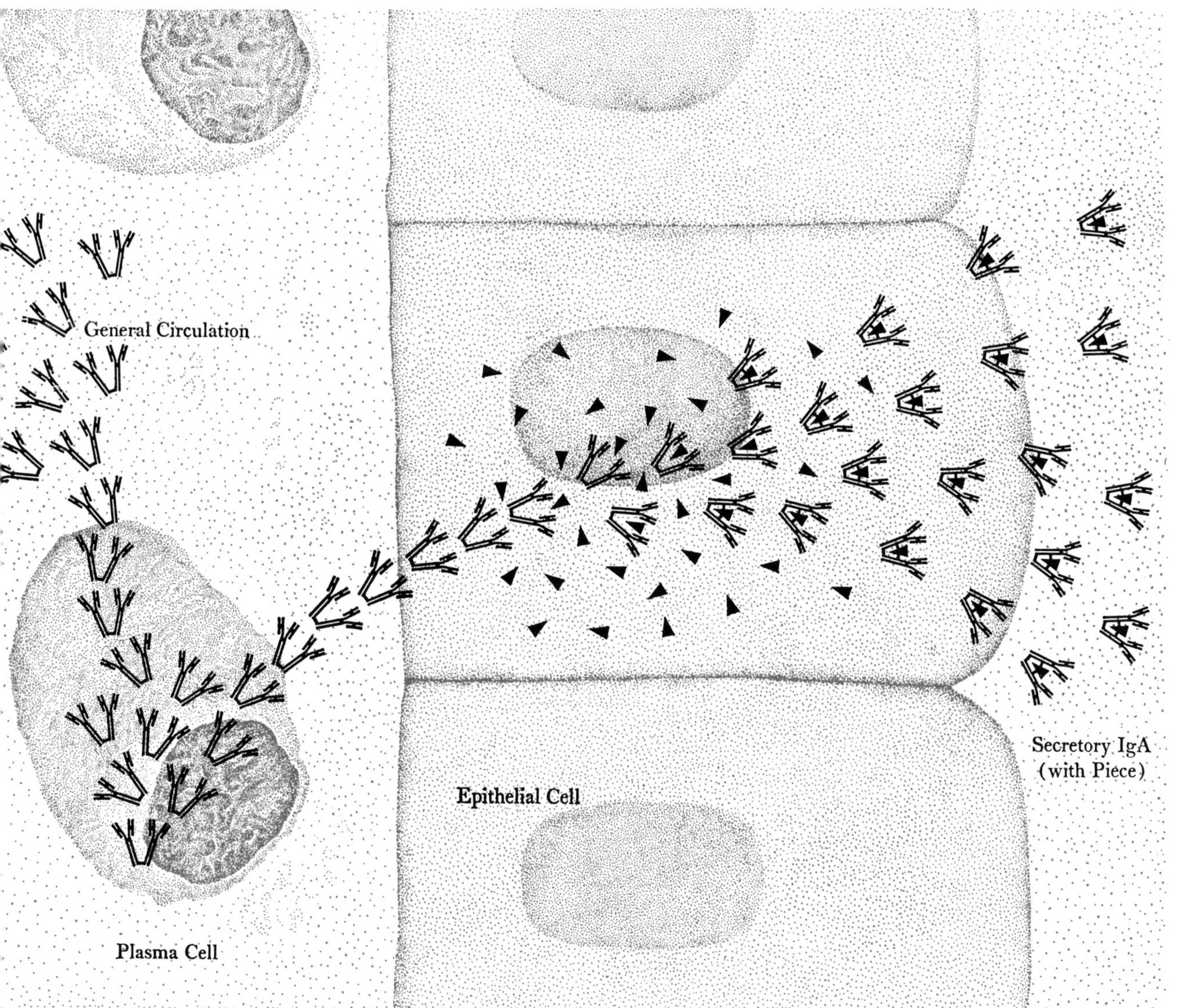

Chapter 9

The Identification and Significance of Gamma E

KIMISHIGE ISHIZAKA
Johns Hopkins University

IgE is a new class of immunoglobulin with a long history. Although only a few years have elapsed since work in our laboratory established IgE as a definable and distinct grouping among the gamma globulins, it is close to a half century since Prausnitz and Küstner first identified reaginic activity in human sera and began to correlate this activity with skin sensitivity in atopic allergic disease. The keystone of their classic experiments was the demonstration that skin-sensitizing activity could be transferred passively from individuals with allergy to normal individuals. This so-called PK phenomenon remains the hallmark of reagin as well as the first evidence that antibody is involved in this response.

In the intervening years concepts about the character of the reaginic antibody have undergone a series of revisions, interesting in themselves and in their import for the management of clinical allergy. They are perhaps even more interesting as a mirror of the sequential advances in immunologic concepts and techniques.

Early thinking was, of course, limited by existing boundaries of knowledge relevant to antibody and immunoglobulin classes. Effectively, this was restricted to gamma G (IgG) globulins. But as new techniques for fractionation and definition of proteins developed, the physicochemical properties that distinguished reaginic antibody from IgG emerged. Such facts as the electrophoretic distribution of reaginic antibody in the gamma 1 rather than gamma 2 region, the lack of reaginic antibody in the first globulin fraction by column chromatography (which contains the major component of IgG), and the slightly heavier sedimentation constant than IgG (7S) by ultracentrifugation brought reasonably general agreement that reaginic antibody at least does not belong to the major component of IgG. Next to be considered was gamma M immunoglobulin. Although the relationship between skin-sensitizing antibody and IgM was studied by a number of sophisticated investigators, the vastly different sedimentation constant (IgM is 19S) militated against such a relationship.

Then, about 10 years ago, Heremans first described IgA. Here, certainly, was a likely category for inclusion of reaginic antibody. Physicochemical properties were strikingly similar. The electrophoretic mobility of reagin is gamma 1; so is that of IgA. Both are pseudoglobulins rather than euglobulins, and by ethanol fractionation both belong to Cohn fraction III. With all of these common properties, the basis was laid for a hypothesis proposing that the reaginic or skin-sensitizing antibody is IgA.

Four apparently significant pieces of evidence were adduced in support of this hypothesis. The first was a result of the work of Heremans and Vaerman in 1962. They took IgA from the serum of a patient with atopic allergic dermatitis and were able to detect skin-sensitizing antibody in it. Subsequently, Fireman, Vannier, and Goodman added antiserum specific for IgA to reaginic sera, thus precipitating out the IgA. The remaining serum proved devoid of skin-sensitizing activity. Work in our own laboratory tended to add to the weight of evidence. We mixed IgA with reaginic serum, injected the mixture into normal individuals, and then tested to see if passive immunization had been achieved. We found that the path of passive sensitization had been blocked. Reasoning from knowledge that in guinea pigs IgG blocks the pathway of sensitization with IgG antibody, we suggested that IgA might have been the mediator of a similar blockade for reaginic antibody. Finally, Yagi and associates employed radioimmunoelectrophoresis to demonstrate IgA anti-ragweed antibody in a patient with atopic allergy. It was clear that IgA antibody could be found in the sera of patients with atopic allergic disease.

The first break in the chain of evidence, at least in our laboratory, came from what in a sense was a failed experiment. Our efforts to learn more about the skin-sensitizing antibodies had been somewhat impeded by the extremely small amounts of these antibodies that can be extracted from patients' sera. We therefore decided to see whether we could produce a more prolific antibody response by using blood group substances as antigens in a system that permits measurement of the actual quantity of antibody by radioimmunoassay. After we had done this with IgA, IgG, and IgM, we tested each of our purified antibody preparations by injecting them into the skin of normal individuals, in an effort to determine whether passive sensitization would be achieved. But the PK reactions were negative in all instances, including those in which IgA antibody had been injected.

Confronted with results that contradicted all prior work, including our own, that had pointed to IgA as the source of skin-sensitizing antibody, we undertook to repeat all the already described experiments. In analyzing the earlier experiments and comparing them with our most recent findings, we felt that we may have pinpointed the fallacy in the earlier experiments – the assumption that in so-called purified IgA preparations the only immunogenic proteins were IgA. We came to the conclusion that even when meticulously applied, the usual immunochemical methods might fail to detect contaminants or minor components. The problem seemed to us to be one of achieving true purity of the various fractions of the gamma globulin molecule.

The next step was to confirm the existence of what we now suspected to be a unique immunoglobulin class carrying the skin-sensitizing antibody. Our approach involved making antibodies against the immunoglobulin. We started with a reagin-rich fraction of sera drawn from patients with atopic disease; this we injected into rabbits to induce an antiserum. It took about six months before we could obtain a satisfactory reagent for our purposes, i.e., a hyperimmune serum containing antibodies against minor as well as major components of the immunoglobulin classes present in the

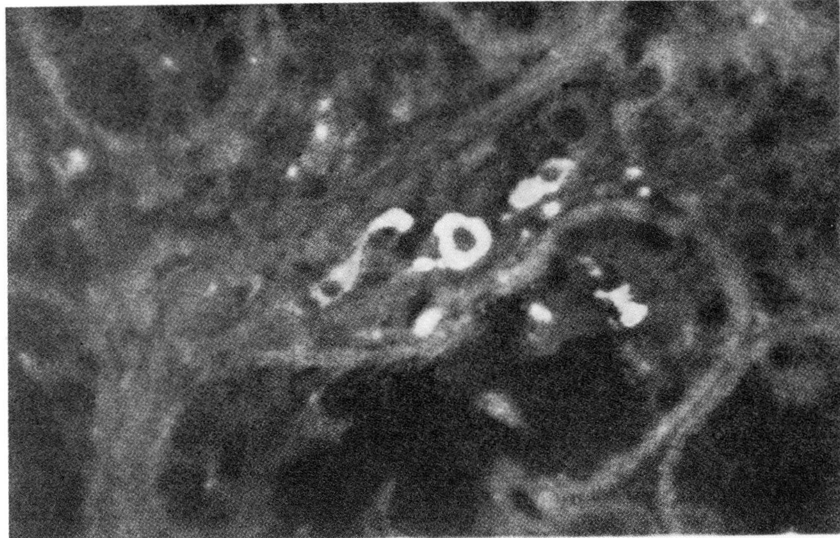

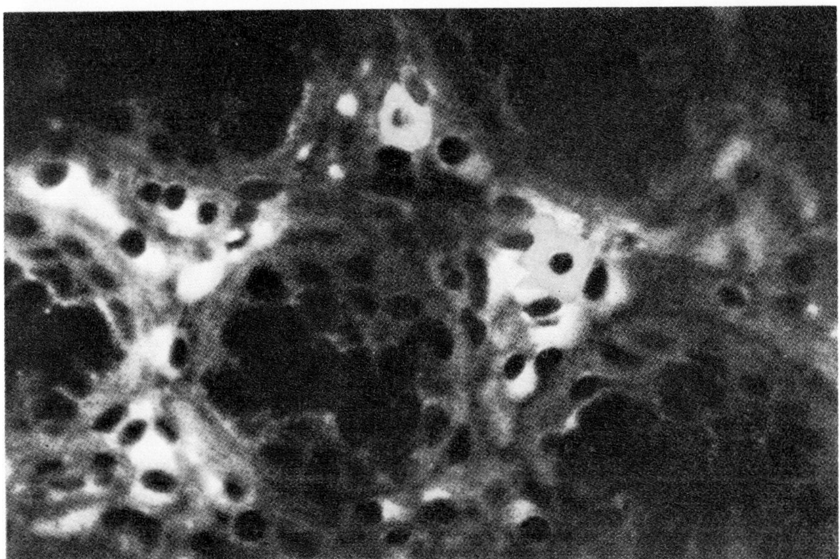

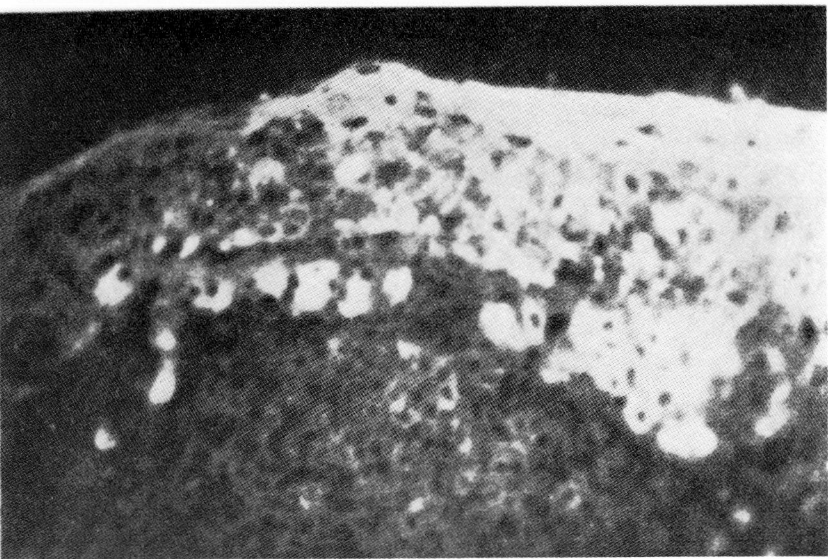

Localization of IgE-forming plasma cells is achieved through fluorescent antibody staining of bronchial mucosa (top), lamina propria of gastric mucosa (center), and tonsil (bottom). IgE-forming cells fluoresce green; the whitish areas, which were revealed by double staining, represent IgA-forming cells (center).

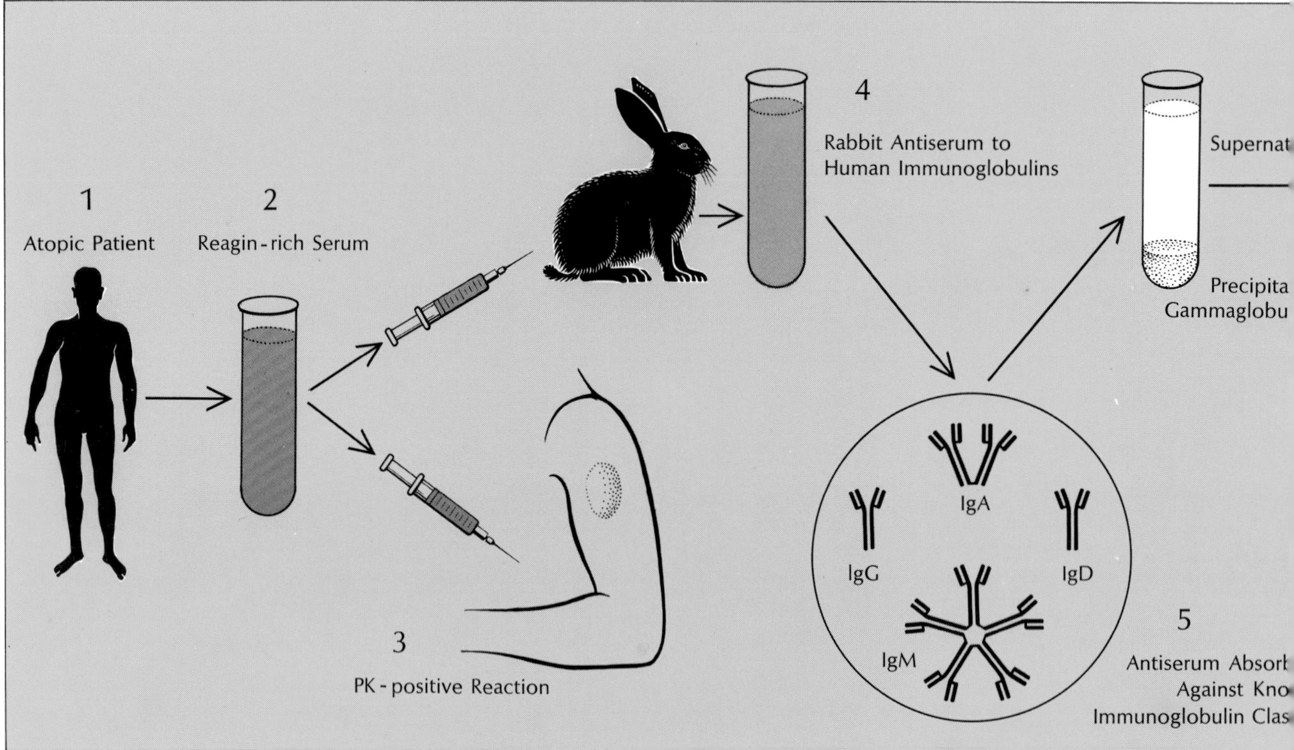

Scheme above outlines the critical experiments that led to conclusion that reaginic antibodies belong to a distinct immunoglobulin class—IgE. Patient with atopic allergy (1) acts as source of reagin-rich serum (2). Injected into arm of a nonatopic individual it gives positive PK (passive transfer) (3). The reagin-rich serum is infused into a rabbit to make an antiserum against human immunoglobulins (4). This antiserum is then absorbed against known immunoglobulin classes (5) so that the resulting supernatant is devoid of anti–gamma globulin antibodies, or "empty" (6). Next, a small quantity of reagin-rich serum is added

reagin-rich fraction. We then absorbed the antiserum against all known immunoglobulins – gamma A, G, M, and D – wherever possible using myeloma proteins to assure the purest possible forms of immunoglobulin. The resulting antiserum did not give precipitin bands for any of the known immunoglobulin classes. In effect, we produced what should have been an "empty" serum. We therefore incubated the "empty" serum with additional reagin-rich human serum and obtained a small amount of precipitate. The supernatant thus obtained was now devoid of skin-sensitizing activity on passive transfer. It appeared to us that we had evidence that reaginic antibodies belonged to a previously undiscovered antibody class.

Our next moves involved the setting up of immunodiffusion, radioimmunodiffusion, or radioimmunoelectrophoresis, using the "empty" rabbit antiserum to demonstrate the unknown immunoglobulin. And indeed, a gamma 1 precipitin band was demonstrated between the reagin-rich fraction and the rabbit antiserum. This precipitin band combined with radioactive allergen derived from ragweed extract. We now had satisfied two crucial criteria for an immunoglobulin class – a unique precipitin band and the ability to combine with antigen, indicative of antibody activity. We tentatively designated the precipitin band as a gamma E band and named the responsible immunoglobulin gamma E.

We then turned to the problem of correlating IgE with skin-sensitizing activity. Our studies showed that gamma E antibody could in fact be correlated with the presence of specific skin-sensitizing antibodies against particular antigens. For example, if one takes the serum of a patient who has antibodies against ragweed and reacts it in a radioimmunodiffusion system with radioactively labeled ragweed antigen, one can then detect a radioactive band corresponding to IgE. This, of course, is indicative of a reaction between the IgE antibody and the labeled specific antigen and of a qualitatively good correlation between the presence of IgE antibody and skin-sensitizing activity. Nor is this relationship limited to ragweed antigen. We have studied close to 24 patients with a variety of allergic sensitivities – grass pollen, house dust, horse dander, egg, and penicillin, in addition to ragweed. In all cases when anti-gamma E antibody was added to the serum to precipitate out the IgE, the supernatant was devoid of skin-sensitizing activity. It is clear that the IgE system is a multi-allergen reaginic system.

In addition to the qualitative correlation between IgE antibody and skin-sensitizing activity, a quantitative relationship has also been established. Again working with sera from patients with atopic disease, we tested the antigen-binding capacity in relationship to the skin-sensitizing activity of the sera. As might be expected, these patients had only negligible amounts of IgM antibody; their IgA and IgG antibody concentrations were uncorrelatable with their PK (skin sensitizing) titers; but there was a very close correlation between IgE antibody concentration, as measured

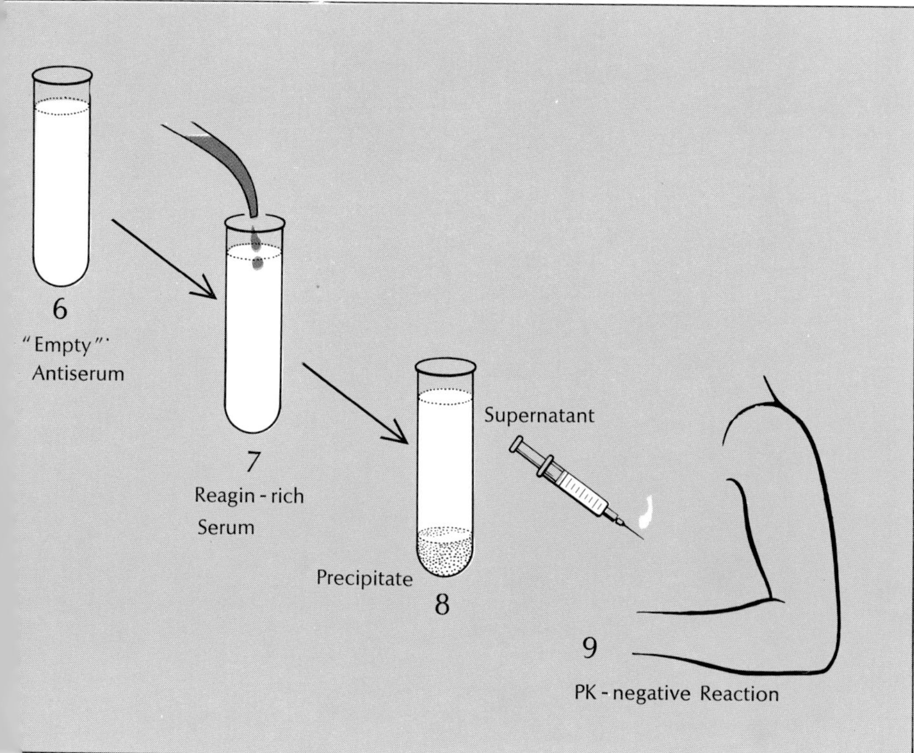

to the so-called empty antiserum (7) and another precipitate produced by ultracentrifugation (8). The supernatant is now injected into a nonatopic individual and there is no PK reaction, indicating that the antibodies possessing reaginic activity, introduced after other antibody classes had been removed, are now themselves precipitated out and the antiserum is truly empty in terms of immunoglobulin activity.

by antigen-binding capacity, and PK titers.

To the mounting evidence that IgE is a unique immunoglobulin class and that within it lies the skin-sensitizing activity of reaginic antibody, one can add physicochemical support. This can be summarized very simply. By any generally used fractionation process such as ion-exchange chromatography, gel filtration, sucrose density gradient ultracentrifugation, electrophoresis, etc., the IgE antibody against ragweed and the skin-sensitizing antibody to the same allergen will be distributed in the same fraction.

It was on the basis of these observations that we tried to isolate IgE from the sera of patients with atopic disease. Although we were not successful in completely separating the IgE from all other proteins, we did get out all molecules with known antibody activity – IgA, IgG, and IgM. The IgE preparation so purified had extremely high skin-sensitizing activity that was precipitated out by anti-IgE antibody. We felt that doubts about the identity between IgE antibody and skin-sensitizing activity were reasonably eliminated and that the evidence for IgE as a carrier of reaginic activity was irrefutable.

However, before one can classify IgE as a unique immunoglobulin class, there must be some data bearing upon the antigenic structure of the protein. To obtain such evidence we had to overcome the difficulties inherent in working with the extremely small amounts of IgE in the serum. (As far as we can estimate, IgE constitutes no more than 0.05% of the total immunoglobulins.) However, using the almost purified material described above and submitting it to radioimmunoelectrophoretic study, we were able to establish the following structural facts:

IgE has both kappa and lambda light-chain antigenic determinants. In addition, IgE has at least one unique antigenic determinant not shared by any other immunoglobulins. On the other hand, IgE does not have any of the major antigenic determinants of the other immunoglobulin classes. Taken together, these last two findings would seem to obviate the possibility that IgE is a subclass of any of the other immunoglobulin categories.

The uniqueness of IgE as an immunoglobulin class was further substantiated by the identification of an E myeloma protein by Johansson and Bennich in Sweden. The importance of this lies in the peculiar ability of myeloma patients to produce large quantities of immunoglobulin, which in all cases studied are virtually pure representatives of a single immunoglobulin class. The finding of E mye-

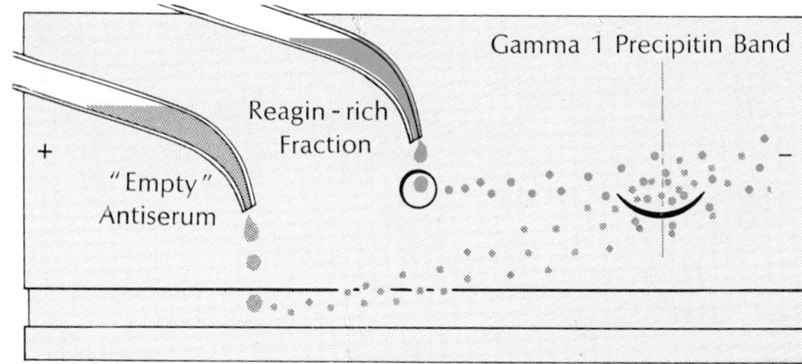

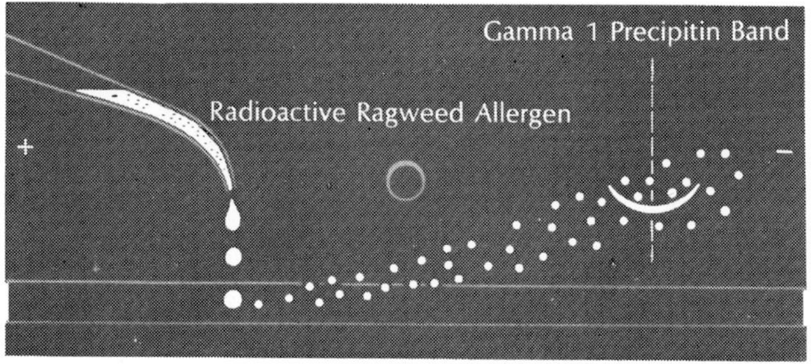

A unique electrophoretic precipitin band and an ability to combine with antigen – two crucial criteria for an immunoglobulin class – were demonstrated as schematized here. When reagin-rich serum was placed in well and "empty" antiserum in trough, the two combined, as proved by precipitin band in gamma 1 position. Tagged ragweed allergen was then added to system and this too, as autoradiography showed, proved capable of combining with reaginic antibody and localizing at the gamma 1 position.

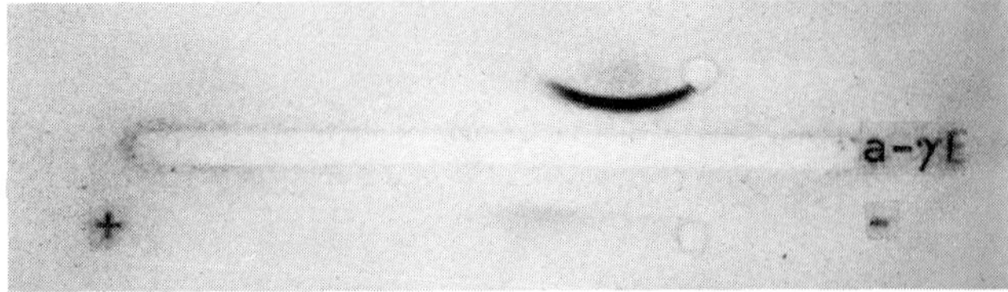

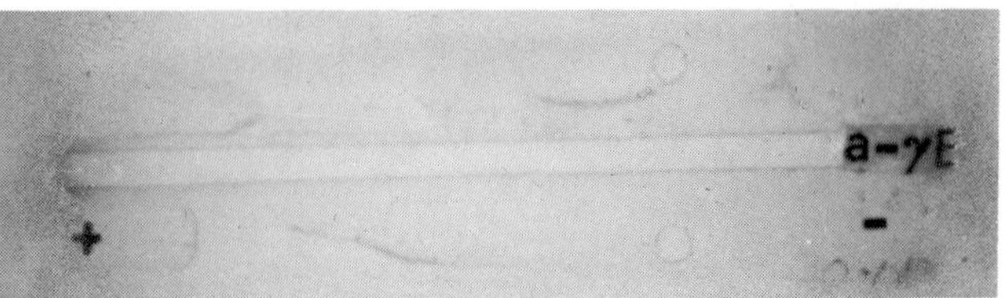

The radioimmunoelectrophoresis schematized on previous page is shown in actuality above. Photo at left is stained slide with IgE precipitin band at gamma 1 position. Autoradiogram on right reveals the radioactive ragweed allergen combining at same place.

loma protein facilitated confirmation of some of our physicochemical findings and several important extensions of knowledge about the IgE molecule. We had placed the sedimentation coefficient at around 8S; Johansson and Bennich reported it as 7.9S. Electrophoretically and chromatographically, they found the IgE in the same position as we had. In addition, they reported the molecular weight at about 200,000 and carbohydrate content at a rather high 11%. By all of these parameters, IgE could be distinguished from other immunoglobulins.

Bennich and Johansson also pursued structural studies with their E myeloma protein and identified an antigenic determinant on the Fc portion of the heavy chain, which is designated as the epsilon chain. In all, they were able to describe the IgE molecule as one containing two heavy and two light chains.

Ragweed antigen–IgE antibody complexes induce erythema-wheal reaction (E), while complexes with IgG (G) and IgA (A) and IgE antibody alone (C) do not.

After identification of reaginic antibodies as IgE and quantitation of IgE antibodies, we turned to studies of their immunochemical properties. Some salient facts: IgE antibodies are capable of sensitizing not only human skin but also monkey skin; in in vitro reactions, the antibodies agglutinated red cells coated with antigen and this hemagglutinating activity of the antibodies was comparable on a weight basis to that of gamma G antibodies. This evidence and structural studies both strongly suggest that gamma E antibodies are divalent.

Participation of complement in reaginic hypersensitivity has been a matter of discussion for a long time. When leukocytes from atopic patients are incubated with ragweed allergen (or other antigens capable of stimulating atopic allergic responses), histamine is released. It was Lichtenstein and Osler who first demonstrated that this release leaves the cell intact, that it is not a response to a lytic system but rather a cell surface phenomenon. However, because of the minimal amounts of reaginic antibody involved, we were not completely satisfied that reaginic antibodies are incapable of complement fixation. Perhaps, we thought, the amounts of complement activated and fixed were too small to be detected by conventional means. In the first stages of this investigation, we simply sought to get the highest possible concentration of skin-sensitizing IgE antibody, but no matter how high the concentrations we were unable to detect any evidence of complement-fixing activity.

We then decided to work with nonspecifically aggregated IgE. Our rationale for this approach was the knowledge that such aggregates of IgG will fix complement through the same mechanisms as IgG antibody-antigen complexes. The same parallelism exists for aggregated IgM and IgM antibody-antigen complexes, while IgA aggregates and IgA antibody-antigen complexes will not fix complement. In fact, the IgE aggregates would not fix complement even when we used large amounts – as much as 800 μg – of nitrogen. The failure to fix complement applies also to the various C′ components. We tried using C′3 and even C′1a, which, of course, is the complement component directly involved in interaction with antibody. The evidence at this time is strong that complement is not involved in reaginic hypersensitivity reactions.

If complement is not involved, one can hypothesize that another enzyme system must be. Possibly the system or systems are complement-like, even if they differ from the complement in hemolytic reactions. Whatever this system is, it appears to participate in histamine release; identification of this could have primary importance in understanding the mechanism of allergic reactions in the atopic patient.

The heat lability of IgE also suggests an area for investigation that could be clinically important. If purified IgE is heated at 56°C for four hours, IgE antibody will lose its ability to sensitize. Similarly, nonantibody IgE will lose its capacity to block sensitization. However, the antibody will still combine with antigen, so we can assume that the antibody combining site remains intact. We have postulated that some structure, other than the combining site, which is present in the Fc portion of the molecule and is actually involved in passive sensitization, is destroyed by heat treatment. It would be a significant advance if we could identify this structure, since it might suggest a means of inhibiting the sensitization mechanisms without the need to suppress the entire immune system involved in IgE elaboration.

Direct evidence for the attachment of IgE to its target cells can be elicited by injecting specific anti-IgE antibody intradermally, inducing an erythematous wheal. This is apparently a reverse type of allergic reaction resulting not from antigen combining with IgE antibody but by the complexing of IgE with anti-IgE antibody. This is not only a skin reaction; we can also induce histamine release by the addition of anti-IgE antibody to isolated leukocytes – support for the idea that IgE antibody is directly involved in the histamine release that occurs as a part of an allergic reaction. Furthermore, the sensitivity of leukocytes to anti-IgE is increased by pretreating the cells with IgE, followed by washing. This suggests that IgE sensitizes the leukocytes by actually combining with them.

More recent experiments actually showed that IgE is present on basophil leukocytes. If one incubates radioactively labeled anti-IgE with leukocytes, the radioactive protein is demonstrated on basophils by autoradiography but not on the other leukocytes. We have also demonstrated that E myeloma protein incubated with leukocytes bound to basophils but not to the other cells. On the other hand, IgG combined with neutrophils and monocytes but not with basophils. Preferential binding of IgE with basophils has biologic significance because basophils have the major portion of histamine in human blood. One can visualize that the combination of either allergen or anti-IgE with basophil-bound IgE may result in the release of histamine from the cells.

A system employing the reverse type of allergic reaction and monkey lung tissue has apparently served to identify a second chemical mediator of IgE activity – the so-called slow-reacting substance of anaphylaxis (SRS-A). The monkey lung tissue, sensitized with either reaginic serum or E myeloma protein released both SRS-A and histamine upon exposure to anti-IgE.

What are the mechanisms of histamine and SRS-A release? In an attempt to answer this question, we fragmented the anti-IgE antibody by pepsin digestion and by subsequent reduction of the pepsin fragment to obtain a 5S Fab dimer and a 3.5S Fab monomer of the antibody. The dimer proved capable of inducing both histamine and SRS-A release in passively sensitized human leukocytes and in passively sensitized monkey lung tissue. But the monomer fragment did not stimulate such release, suggesting that the bridging of cell-bound IgE molecules might be the initial step in the mechanism of releasing chemical mediators.

This idea was supported by experiments with antigen-antibody complexes. When IgE antibodies against ragweed allergen were incubated with the allergen and the mixture was injected intracutaneously into normal individuals, erythema-wheal reactions were induced. Mixtures of the same

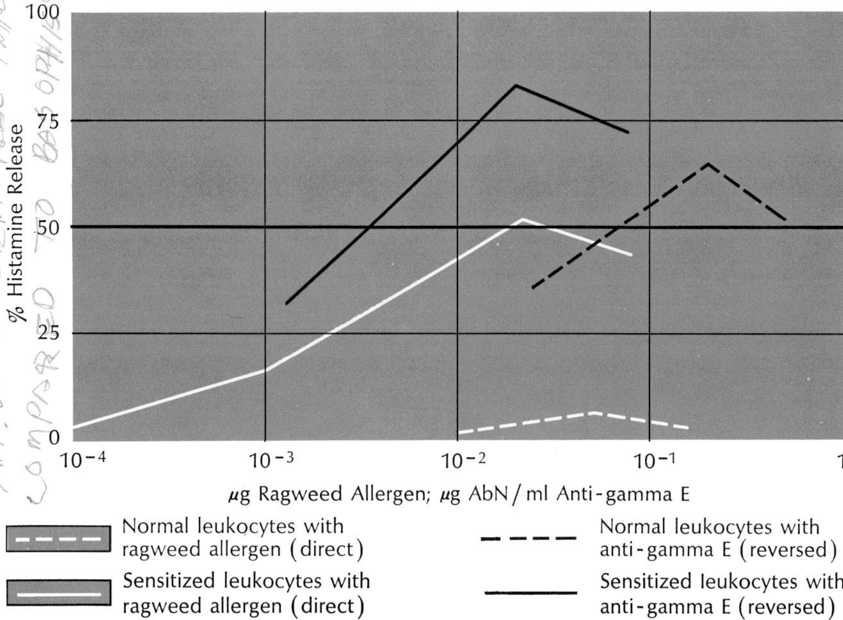

Some relationships between histamine release and reaginic antibody activity have been clarified in vitro. Normal human leukocytes manifest no significant histamine release when incubated with ragweed allergen but do with anti-gamma E antibody. After sensitization with reaginic serum, release is seen with either allergen or antibody.

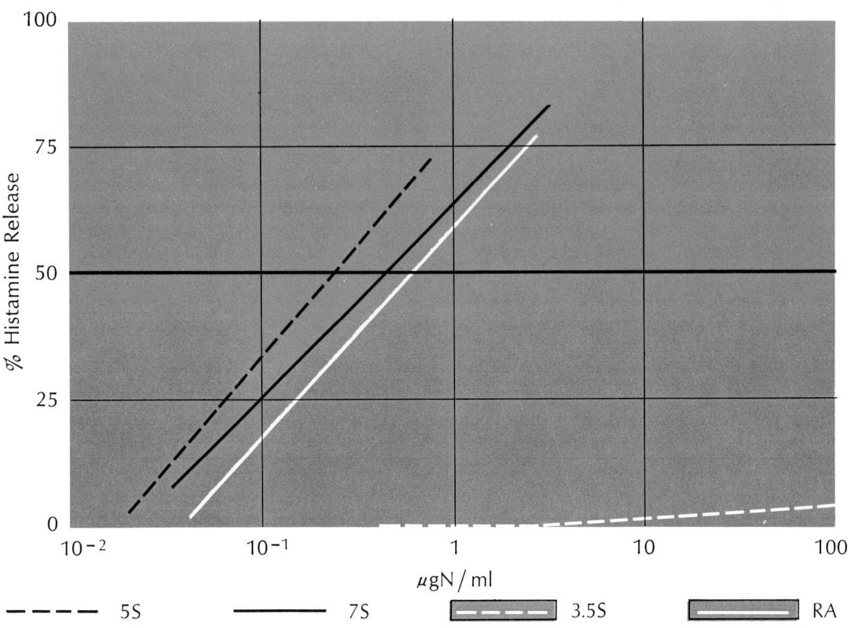

Dose response curves quantify histamine release by whole anti-gamma E molecule (8S), Fab dimer (5S) and reduced alkylated antibody (RA), and by Fab monomer (3.5S).

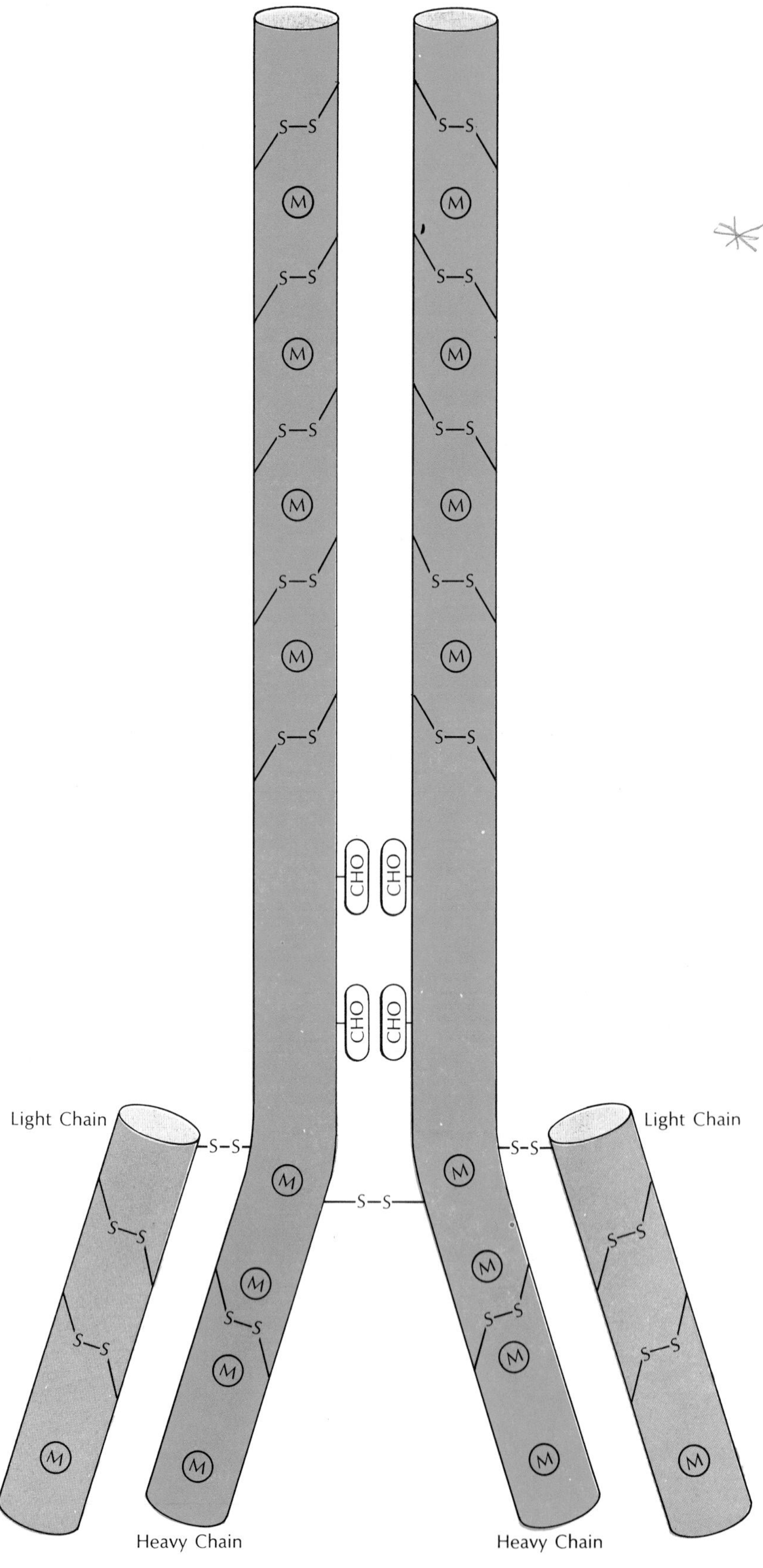

Working with an E myeloma protein, Johansson and Bennich in Sweden have elucidated a number of the structural characteristics of the IgE molecule. Among them: molecular weight 196,000; sedimentation constant 7.9S; two heavy chains (mol wt 75,500); two light chains, each with 214 amino acid residues (mol wt 22,500); abundance of carbohydrate (about 11%), methionine (M), and disulfide bonds (S-S).

allergen with either IgG or IgA antibodies did not have the activity. Sucrose density gradient ultracentrifugation analysis of the allergen–IgE antibody mixtures showed that preformed allergen–IgE antibody complexes were responsible for the induction of the skin reaction and that at least two IgE antibody molecules are necessary to form a biologically active complex.

We also employed nonspecifically aggregated E myeloma protein, which it will be recalled mimics the antigen-antibody complex, and found that extremely minute quantities of the aggregated gamma E provoked erythema-wheal reactions. When the monomer form of IgE was injected no such reaction occurred even at concentrations 100 times greater than that of the aggregates giving a positive skin reaction. We believe that allergic reactions occur when IgE molecules interact or when such interaction leads to structural changes in the molecules. Participation of allergen apparently is not essential for the induction of the reactions.

Since the second case of E myeloma was found in this country, further studies were carried out with the myeloma protein. The protein was digested with papain or pepsin to obtain its fragments. It was demonstrated that the Fc fragments, which represent the carboxyl terminal half of epsilon chains, bind to leukocytes and passively sensitize the cells. This finding indicates that structures essential for sensitization are present in the Fc portion of gamma E molecules. We have also found that nonspecifically aggregated Fc fragments induce erythema-wheal reactions in normal human skin, but monomer Fc fragment does not. Furthermore, incubation of the aggregated Fc with leukocytes in vitro resulted in the release of histamine, and the incubation of the material with monkey lung tissues resulted in the release of both histamine and SRS-A.

Based on these findings, we can speculate about the molecular mechanisms of reaginic hypersensitivity reactions. In the sensitized state, IgE antibody molecules are fixed on certain tissue cells, probably mast cells, by a region of the antibody surface corresponding to Fc. As the result of the combination of allergen and the cell-bound IgE antibody, antigen-antibody complexes will be formed and antibody molecules combining with the same antigen may interact with each other. A structural alteration in the Fc portion of the IgE molecules may occur as the result of the antibody-antibody (IgE-IgE) interaction. The final structure will stimulate enzymatic sequences in the cells, leading to the release of histamine and/or SRS-A, depending on the cells involved.

Our most recent studies with IgE have been designed to map the distribution of IgE-forming cells in the body of both man and monkey. Using fluorescent antibody techniques we have sought both IgE-forming cells and germinal centers that would stain with anti-IgE. We have found these in tonsils, adenoid tissues, bronchial and peritoneal lymph nodes, and in the Peyer's patches of monkeys. In contrast, very few have been located in spleen or subcutaneous lymph nodes. Apparently, the distribution is quite different from that of IgG. The appendix, incidentally, remains a question since we have not been able to obtain human appendices for study as yet, and the *Macaca irus* monkeys we work with lack appendices. We have also located IgE-forming cells in mucosal tissues of the nose, respiratory system, stomach, small intestine, and rectum (see photos on page 85).

It would seem to be plausible that this distribution is related to allergic disease or at least to such disease in the respiratory tract. The possibility that locally formed IgE may be involved in respiratory allergy is raised.

IgE distribution is particularly intriguing if one notes its striking similarity to the distribution of IgA. In fact, IgE was demonstrated in nasal washings and sputa from some asthmatic patients. If one recalls that until recently the reagin was thought to be IgA and that the two immunoglobulin classes are similar in many respects, then the possibility arises that the protective role that has been assigned to secretory IgA at the interfaces between our internal and external environments may be played in part by IgE. Indeed, Ammann et al. recently obtained suggestive data that deficiency in IgE may be related to recurrent respiratory tract infection.

For the investigator primarily interested in understanding the IgE system, the concept that it has some role in protection against infections is a tempting one. The detrimental role of IgE in mediating allergic reactions has been established. Logically, one must ask what is the positive evolutionary motivation for the development of the IgE system. In a sense this is analogous to the situation we were confronted with when transplantation made us aware of the body's ability to produce antibodies directed against histocompatibility antigens. If we reason that this ability does not exist merely to frustrate the surgeon, then we must also reason that IgE was not "put there" just to produce wheezes and rashes.

Section Three

Mediators and Effectors of Immunity

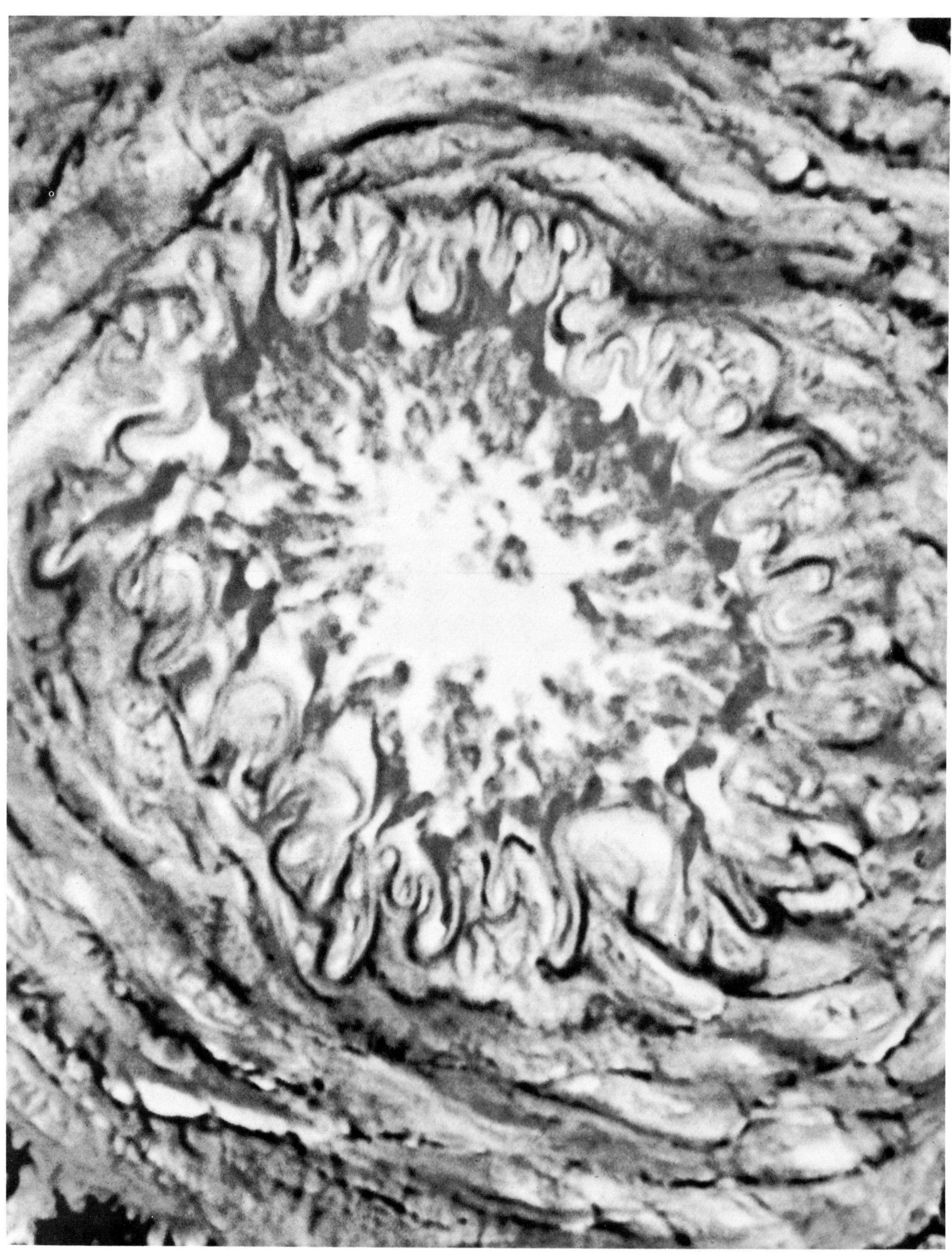

The role of complement is critical in accelerated transplantation rejections. The photograph shows spasm in a medium-sized artery of rabbit kidney that had been transferred to a dog. Deposition of eosinophilic material on the endothelium is notable. Studies by Dr. D. S. Clark at the University of Minnesota showed this material to be predominantly degranulating platelets, the enzymes of which probably contributed to immunopathology. Such xenografts are, of course, rejected in minutes. If complement activity is suppressed, appearance of the endothelial lesion is delayed and graft life may be extended up to 30-fold.

Chapter 10

The Immunologic Role of Complement

HENRY GEWURZ
Rush Medical College

In a recent series of experiments in our laboratories, a gram-negative endotoxic lipopolysaccharide was obtained from *Veillonella alcalescens* and reacted with fresh guinea pig serum. Extensive lesions — "holes" approximately 90 angstroms in diameter — were formed on the lipopolysaccharide membrane. Drs. Howard A. Bladen, Stephan E. Mergenhagen, and I did further studies with this system and demonstrated conclusively that the lesions were produced by the action of the serum complement, thus providing new evidence that endotoxin is a substrate for complement.

These experiments and similar ones in other laboratories are significant in themselves and provide support for a suggestion first made about five years ago by Dr. Wesley Spink of the University of Minnesota. He hypothesized that the clinical effects of endotoxin shock may actually be due not to the endotoxin itself but to a serum factor (complement) acting on the endotoxin and on vascular and cell surfaces coated with endotoxin. This suggestion is eminently logical, since the biologic effects of endotoxin are strikingly similar to the phenomena mediated by complement (see illustration on pages 98 and 99). The logic becomes even more forceful if one views under the microscope the dramatic lesions produced as the complement sequence goes to completion on the endotoxin.

Beyond this specific significance, these experiments serve to exemplify the expanding horizons of complement research. Since the turn of the century, complement has been an important but limited immunologic tool, its action being observable almost exclusively at the end point of cytolysis either in the erythrocyte or in the bacterial cell. But in the past few years the field of complement research has expanded into diverse clinical and experimental directions, with results that are at once fruitful and frustrating.

More and more, investigators are looking into the particular relationship between complement and renal disease, a relationship expressed in the form of lowered complement titers in acute nephritis, in some forms of chronic nephritis and congenital nephrosis, in systemic lupus erythematosus, in plasma cell hepatitis associated with kidney damage, and in rapid rejection of renal homografts. The role of complement in inflammatory reactions, even when they are not related to classical antibody, is also coming in for increasing investigative attention. So too is the possibility of inhibiting complement activity as a modality of suppressing the immune response and of manipulating inflammation.

Before launching a fuller discussion of these lines of research and their clinical implications, it is appropriate to review the underlying work that has made it possible for us to deal with complement not simply as a mediator of cell lysis but as an effector of immune response, one with a wide range of activities and of activity inhibitions. These actions add up to a most remarkable control system for some of the most basic functions in physiology. Essentially this has led to recognition of the complement system as consisting of at least nine discrete protein substances. All seem to be globulins of either the alpha or beta class, with one intriguing exception — a gamma globulin. Obviously the unraveling of such a complex system has involved work by many different research groups, but it should be noted that the chemistry has been defined largely in five laboratories, those of Manfred M. Meyer at the Johns Hopkins University, H. J. Müller-Eberhard of the Scripps Clinic and Research Foundation, R. A. Nelson at the University of Miami, Irwin H. Lepow at Western Reserve, and Herbert J. Rapp and Tibor Borsos at the National Institutes of Health.

The triggering event which, of course, must precede complement activity is the steric modification of antibody by antigen. In a sense, once antibody has combined with antigen, its basic immunologic function has been served. This is recognition. After antibody has recognized foreign protein, it takes on a form that permits it to activate any of several enzyme systems present in serum. These enzyme systems, the most important of which appears to be complement, serve as the "muscles" to effect the secondary immunologic actions — phagocytosis, chemotaxis, cytolysis, etc.

The first of the complement components to act (C′1) reacts directly with the antigen–modified antibody. C′1 is much heavier than the other eight proteins, with a molecular weight of around one million and a sedimentation coefficient of 19S. All the other components lie between 4S and 10S. C′1 has, in turn, been subdivided into three components (C′1q, C′1r, C′1s), and it is interesting to note that the first of these subunits to act — C′1q — is the only gamma globulin thus far identified in the complement system. It is certainly provocative to consider that the first complement component that reacts with antibody is itself a gamma globulin. Moreover, as first shown at Rockefeller University by Drs. Müller-Eberhard and Henry Kunkel, C′1q is deficient in certain individuals with agammaglobulinemia.

After C′1, the next component involved is C′4 (the numbers here reflect the historic sequence of discovery, rather than the order of action). The first component acts upon the fourth, modifying the latter so that it combines with the first component, with the antibody, or with the cell surface. The fourth component is therefore the first one capable of direct interaction with the cell. As C′2 comes along, it is also acted upon by C′1. The second component is modified by the cleaving out of inactive substance, as shown by Drs. Robert Stroud and Mayer at Hopkins. A complex of activated second component and modified fourth component is created. This complex has been found to have actual enzyme activity, designated by Müller-Eberhard as C′3 convertase.

It is the third component, C′3, which seems to have the greatest biologic role within the complement system. It must come along during the very brief time when the enzyme site created by the second and fourth components is active. If it does, many C′3 molecules may be brought to the cell surface (as shown by Müller-Eberhard and colleagues), and the way will be prepared for phagocytosis and subsequent functions. This is a key function of C′3. Equally important is that the amplification produced by the action of C′2 on C′3 provides for a tremendous enhancement of the efficiency of the immune system. One antibody molecule may bring hundreds of complement molecules onto the cell surface, with consequent intensification of phagocytosis. In short, C′3 greatly potentiates antibody-mediated phagocytosis, and C′3 is activated most effectively after antibody, C′1, C′4, and C′2 interact as has already been described.

Clearly, then, there is a major need for complement in the immune system long before the cytolytic action occurs, which is at the end of the reactivity chain. We now have the beginning of an answer to why nature has been so sophisticated in creating the complement system. If cytolysis were the sole function, then a single enzyme should have served as well, even as it does in the bacterial hemolysis system. A fantastic degree of control is implied in the nine-component system. It now seems that the first three components act as a check, so that nothing gets into the area of action of the last six components unless conditions and events are just right.

Much of what can be concluded from this is extremely speculative, which is why complement research was described earlier as both fruitful and frustrating. The frustration comes because so much of what we suspect cannot be demonstrated —

The Complement Components

In the schematic presentation on the facing page, the complement sequence is traced from the combination of antibody with antigen to the point where the criteria for much of the biologic activity of complement have been fulfilled. It is based largely on presentations made by Müller-Eberhard, Mayer, and Lepow. To facilitate following the sequence, a graphic glossary of the symbols used is given below.

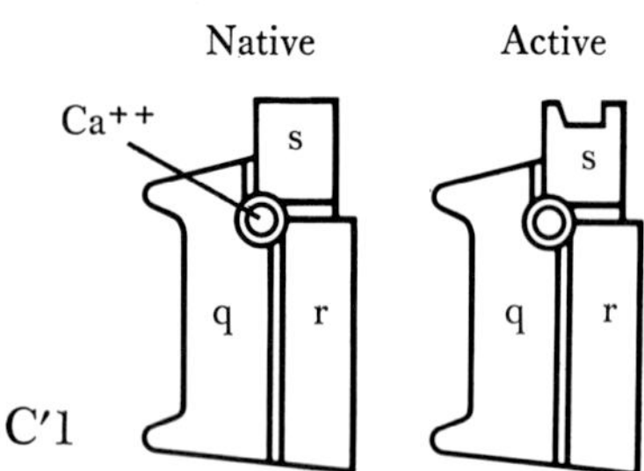

The first component (C′1) is made up of three subunits — C′1q, C′1r, and C′1s — held together by calcium ion.

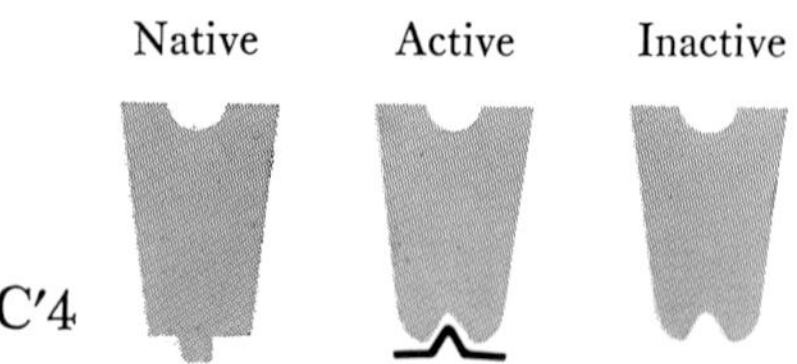

Next in order of activity is C′4. Interaction with C′1 enables the native molecule to combine with a nearby receptor.

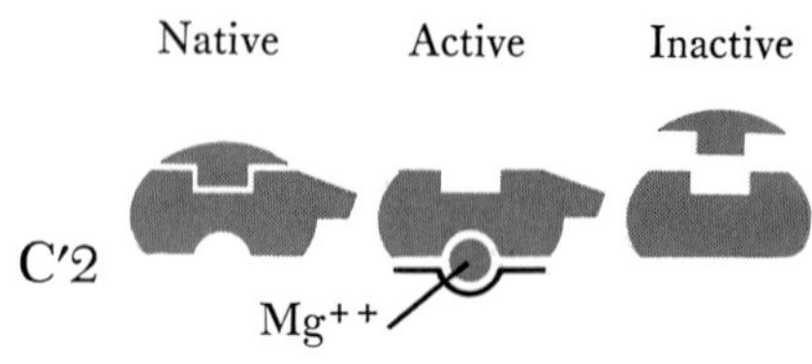

C′2 also interacts with C′1 and is split into active and inactive fragments.

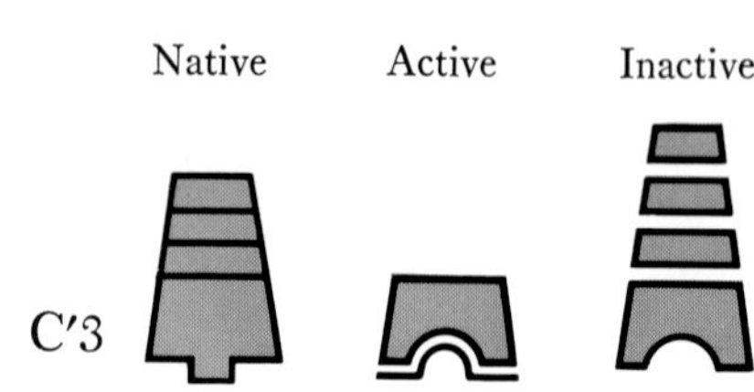

C′3 is quantitatively dominant in the complement group. One of the fragments into which it is cleaved may be active in the hemolytic sequence.

The Complement Sequence Leading to Biologic Activity

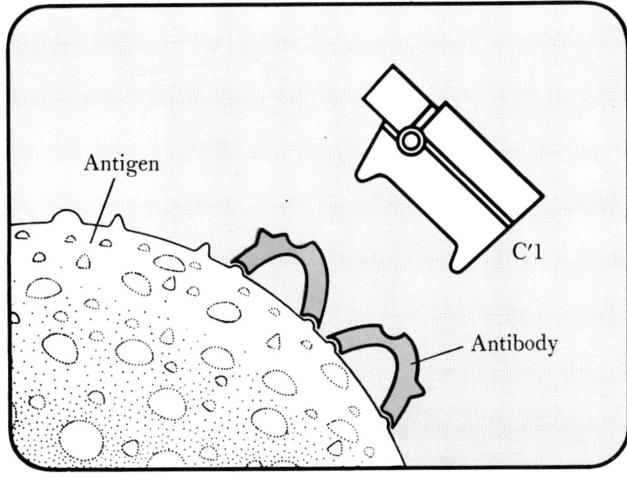

Initiating the sequence is the combination of antigen and complement-fixing antibody. It is hypothesized that under certain conditions, complement binding sites are then exposed.

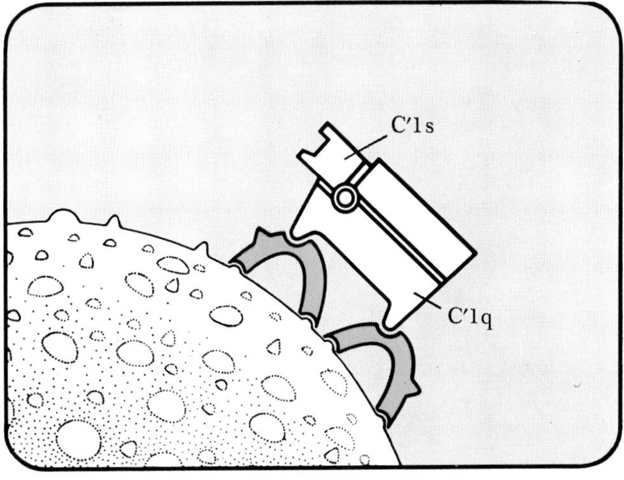

C'1 combines with these sites, with C'1q (a gamma globulin) attaching to the antibody. Enzymatic site (at C'1s) capable of acting with next component is converted to its active form.

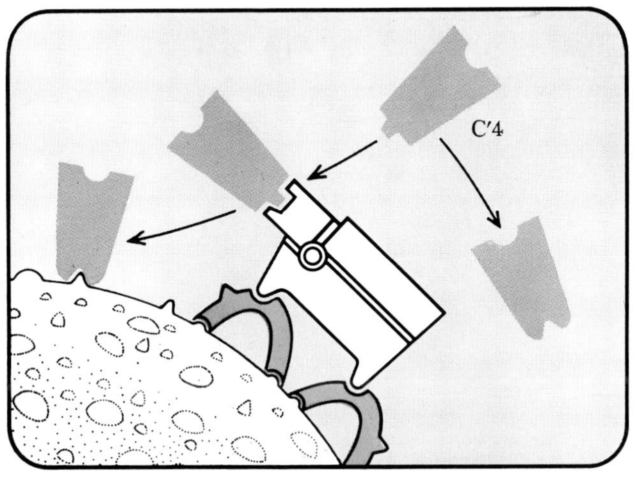

Next in order of appearance is C'4, which is acted upon by C'1s, exposing site for binding C'4 to the surface of the antigen or to the antibody. If unbound, C'4 cannot function in hemolysis.

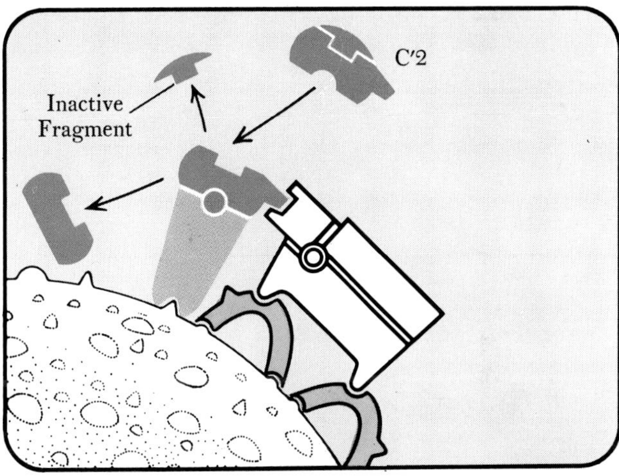

C'2 also interacts with C'1. An inactive fragment is cleaved out, preparing activated C'4-C'2 complex to act on next component. Magnesium is needed for integrity of this complex.

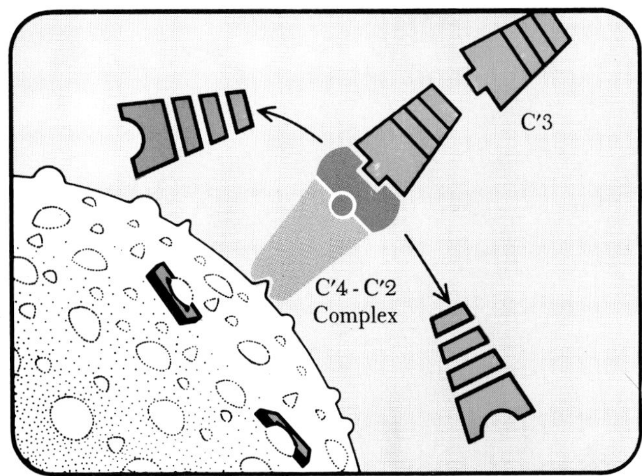

If C'3 appears during the few minutes the C'4-C'2 complex is active, it may be cleaved into at least four parts, one of which may become bound to the surface of the cell.

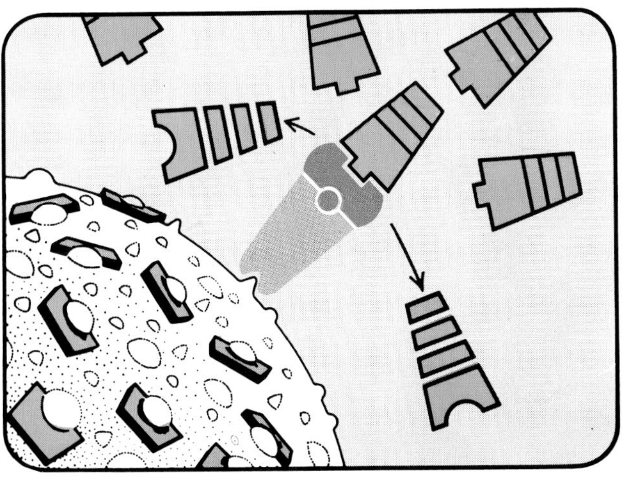

Each C'4-C'2 complex can apparently mobilize hundreds of C'3 molecules, thus providing tremendous amplification of immunologic functions served by C'3 and perhaps later C' components.

Some Biologic Functions of Complement Components

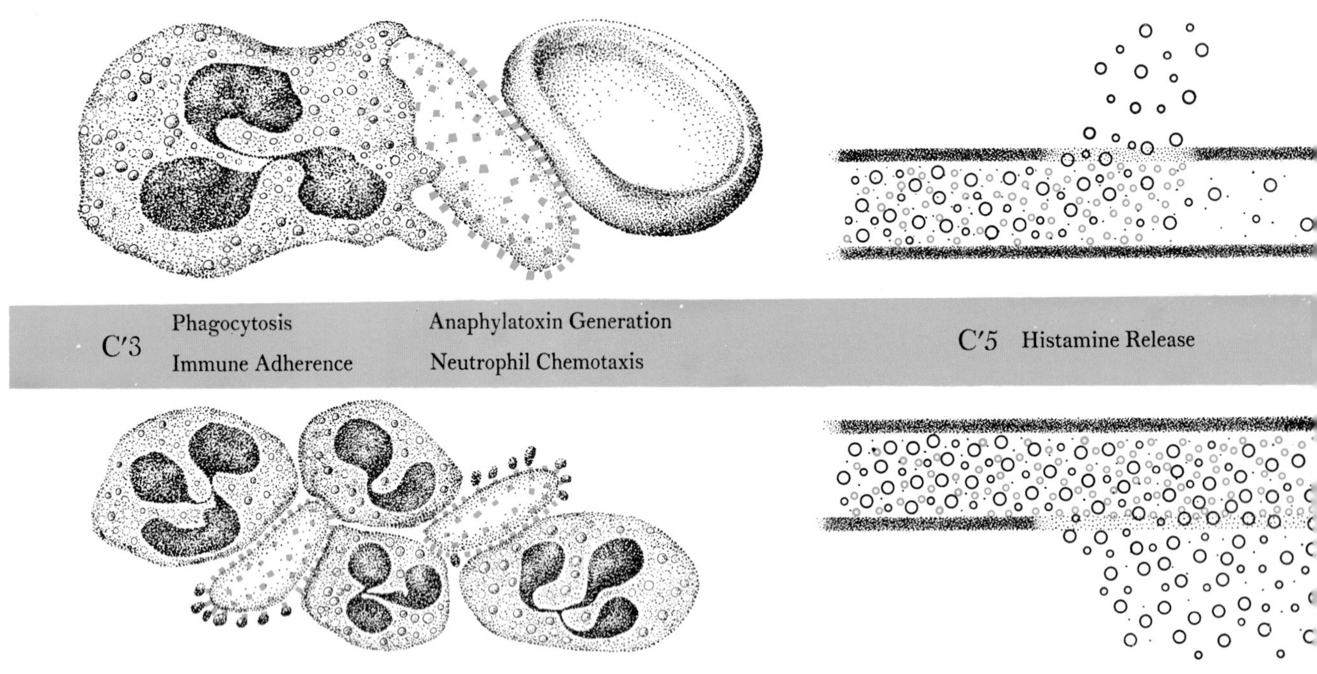

A biologic function served by C'3, the coating of organisms, which leads to imbibition and reticuloendothelial clearance, may be particularly critical in facilitating phagocytosis of pathogens (a beneficial effect of complement illustrated above the color band). Immune adherence may contribute to this process by fixing an organism to a cell surface. Anaphylatoxin leads to vasodilation, thus expediting delivery of cellular elements to bolster immune and inflammatory responses. A plasmin-mediated chemotactic factor may further enhance cellular defenses. On the negative side (illustrated below the color band), these functions in excess may lead to platelet and leukocytic thrombi, while enzymes released by degranulating cells may contribute to systemic and local necrosis.

The activities attributable to C'5 are in a sense continuous with those of C'3. Frank histamine release, triggered by anaphylatoxin, may be mediated by this component, leading to increased vascular permeability and resultant access of cellular and humoral elements to site of inflammation or infectious process (above band). If carried to excess, vascular integrity may be compromised (below band) to the point where shock intervenes.

but then our tools are still very new.

At any rate, the complexity of the complement system is all the more valuable in terms of permitting biologic control, because each component seems to be subject to the activity of inhibitors. These inhibitors may come into play at any time to stop the sequence in its tracks. This is one of the most exciting areas for investigation, since it suggests that we may eventually be successful in one of our prime goals — the manipulation of the complement system in the laboratory and at the bedside. There is reason to believe that such manipulation may occur naturally in rheumatoid arthritis, for example.

Rheumatoid factor can be considered as an inhibitor of complement. Like C'1, it combines with aggregated gamma globulin. By competing for the same binding site, it will impede the initiation of the complement sequence. In this way, instead of acting as an autoantibody and producing immune destruction, rheumatoid factor may act as a bar to progressive complement destruction at sites where there are aggregated gamma globulins. This speculation is provocative in several respects. If, for example, rheumatoid arthritis is triggered by a virus, and that virus induces an antibody response, you might have a pathogenic antigen-antibody complex as a result. The body's control of this might be the manufacture of a large globulin molecule that can blanket or douse the complement-combining sites and prevent complementary lysis, a concept advanced by Drs. Frank R. Schmid at Northwestern, I. M. Roitt of London, and John S. Davis at the University of Virginia.

Returning now to the functions subserved by C'3, in addition to phagocytosis, it has been shown that this component cleaves into at least four parts after the C'4-C'2 complex acts upon it. Each of these four parts was identified by Drs. H. S. Shin and Mayer. One of these may participate in the hemolytic sequence while another may be a plasmin-mediated chemotactic factor which brings neutrophilic white cells into the area of an inflammatory reaction. Another activity of C'3 may be responsible for anaphylatoxin, which has the potential of inducing smooth muscle contraction and which increases vascular permeability. However, it is also possible that anaphylatoxin release may be a result of the action of C'5.

In fact, the sequence between C'3 and C'7 is quite cloudy in the present state of knowledge. This is not surprising, since it is only in the last few years that complement research has dealt with more than four components, and it is largely from classical C'3 that the activities of the remaining factors have been dissected. In this connection Müller-Eberhard has postulated that factors five, six, and seven form a trimolecular complex and act in concert after the action of C'3 to prepare the cell for the final cytolytic event. It should be noted that some investigators who have worked with

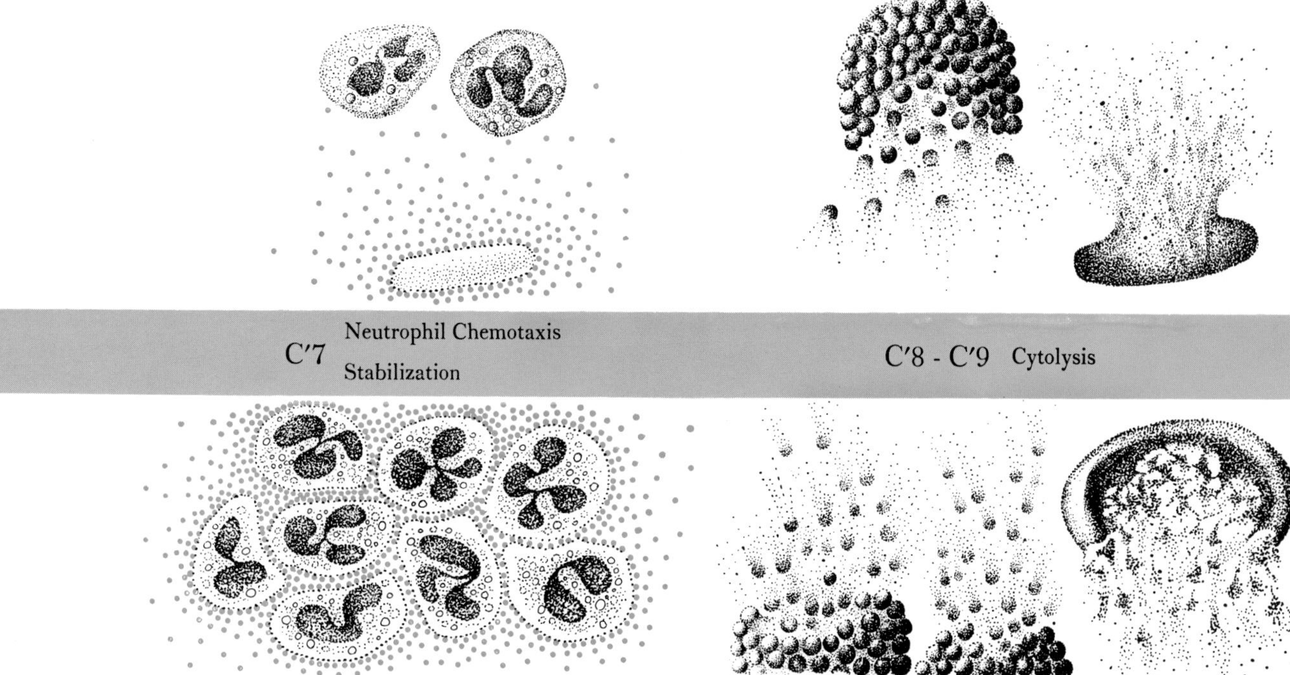

While specific activities related to C′6 are still not identifiable, with the involvement of C′7 a chemotactic stimulus to neutrophils occurs that may greatly augment the population of these cells in areas invaded by pathogens or in sites of inflammation. It is also believed that C′7 stabilizes the complement sequence, paving the way for cytolytic action at its conclusion. In terms of host benefit (above the color band), C′7 may reinforce phagocytic processes previously initiated. On the debit side (below color band), it may produce vessel-clogging agglomerations of cellular elements.

The final components, C′8 and C′9, are responsible for lysis of bacteria, red cells, etc. On the positive side, the process appears to be the last step in the destruction of bacteria and, possibly, tumor cells. On the negative side are the hemolytic effects and, perhaps, destruction of transplant cells. A corollary function is the opening up of mast cells, with resultant histamine release. Cell lysis and enzyme release may not only be involved in the effects of C′8 and C′9 but may feed back into other steps of the sequence. Additional biologic functions have been suggested for the complement system, but it is not yet possible to relate them to specific components.

guinea pigs are inclined to oppose this view; they suggest that C′5, C′6, and C′7 have sequential functions. Either way, in this part of the C′ sequence histamine release may take place, and here the stage is set for the activities of C′8 and C′9 — destruction of the bacterial cell or erythrocyte by lysis. It is generally believed that at least one, and perhaps both, of these components are enzymes.

In addition to the biologic functions shown schematically above and on page 98, several other effects of the C′ system have been suggested, though their relationship to specific components is not yet defined. These include viral neutralization, bactericidal action in the serum, mediation of graft rejection, destruction of normal and neoplastic cells, and participation in some types of immediate and delayed hypersensitivity, suggesting some of the clinical implications now envisioned by those investigating complement. The traditional role for complement has been in the detection of antibody. (Those antibodies which can utilize complement can be detected in vitro because complement is subsequently unavailable for hemolysis.) However, it is obvious that complement did not evolve for this specific purpose.

Rather, in reviewing research conducted at the University of Minnesota with Drs. Joann Finstad and Robert A. Good, on the phylogenetic development of the complement system, one finds that an antibody-complement system exists in all vertebrates studied which are phylogenetically distal to the lamprey. Apparently, then, the humoral C′ system dates back to the lower vertebrates, and its continued presence strongly suggests that it has provided a survival advantage to all species which appeared later than the primitive fishes.

Complement appears early in the ontogenic sequence too. In cows, for example, we have detected C′ titers early in the second trimester, long before circulating immunoglobulins are detectable. In humans, although complement is believed not to cross the placenta, neonatal titers are between 50 and 80 percent of adult levels. Therefore the C′ system seems to develop early and independently of the immunoglobulins, again suggesting a potential importance to the developing organism.

What, then, is the purpose of complement fixation?

The question can be answered only speculatively by noting that the existence of antigen-antibody complexes that are either effective or ineffective in complement fixation would seem to provide a remarkable control mechanism, one which would prevent complement activity just anywhere in the body. Non–complement-fixing complexes — such as the rheumatoid factor — could serve to prevent autoimmune injury resulting from antibodies not otherwise controllable by the body. Study of nature's own experiments — for example, the changes in complement concentrations that occur

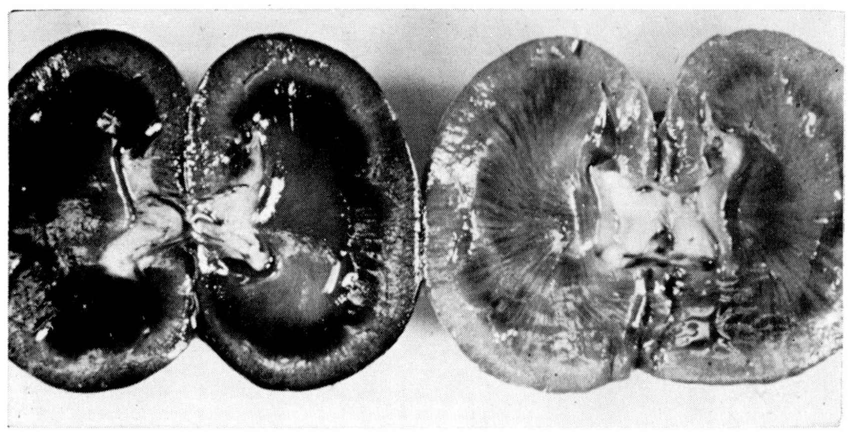

Rabbit kidney (right) rejected by dog in xenografting experiment is compared with normal rabbit kidney. Graft shows zone of vascular congestion at the corticomedullary junction. There is strong evidence of occlusions on the venocapillary side of the circulation.

in disease — may, when correlated with experimental findings, help us find a less speculative answer.

The complement system may also be utilized to unravel etiologies of immune-mediated disease. Certain of the system's components may be altered in ways characteristic for a given disease state or immunopathologic mechanism. Indeed "profiles" of serum concentrations of selected C′-dependent functions can be composed which, when compared with appropriate experimental models, may aid in elucidating the pathogenesis of certain diseases, much as determining the serum electrolyte composition aids in understanding the etiology or pathogenesis of disorders of metabolism. Drs. Richard J. Pickering and Good and the author have utilized this approach in studying several diseases associated with either known immune damage or repeated infections, including those shown in the graphs on page 55.

Perhaps of more immediate practical importance have been the experiments seeking to relate complement activity to graft rejection. While at the University of Minnesota I participated in a series of such experiments along with Drs. D. Scott Clark, Richard L. Varco, Pickering, and Good.

We began with the fact that a number of diseases that are known to precipitate an immunologic attack on the kidney are associated with low complement levels. However, early studies of renal homografts done without immunosuppression had failed to reveal any diminution of complement activity. If anything, C′ had been found to be elevated in the serum during rejection. We felt that such findings could stem from a number of phenomena that did not really relate to the possible status of complement during graft rejection. We therefore sought a system which would make the aspects of rejection that might be attributable to complement stand out in bold relief. For this reason we resorted to a physiologically extreme measure — the xenografting into dogs of kidneys from sheep, rabbits, pigs, and cows.

Following such transplantation, rejection is extremely rapid. Blood flow ceases in four to 12 minutes in the sheep or rabbit grafts. Microscopically, the typical lesions in the dissected kidney are made up of depositions of platelets and polymorphonuclear neutrophils on almost every blood vessel in the kidney. These platelets and polymorphs show pronounced degranulation; in short, one sees a fulminant example of endothelial damage, a clear example of the immunopathology associated with humoral factors. And in association with these lesions we found marked reductions in serum complement levels, and in the measurable levels of all C′ components assayed (C′1, C′4, C′2, and classical C′3). At the same time, there was a dramatic uptake of complement-fixing antibody in the system, suggesting the possibility that there was excessive complement utilization underlying the hypocomplementemia.

We were then confronted with the question of whether the role of complement was causative of or coincidental with the rapid xenograft rejections. In an effort to answer this question, we employed the cobra venom C′3 inhibitor isolated and described by Nelson. We found that when complement activity was thus suppressed, there was a remarkable prolongation of graft survival in the rabbit-dog transplants, with survivals of up to 150 minutes recorded. Parallel results were achieved with other inhibitors.

Turning to human transplantation, we measured complement levels during rejection processes occurring after human renal homografts. Of 20 patients selected for this study, seven showed well-defined rejection reactions within their first postoperative week. Five of these, including three whose grafts crossed the ABO barrier, showed unusual falls in both complete C′ titers and in C′2 titers. Another 10 patients showed rejection reactions only after good initial organ function that lasted a week or more after transplantation. Seven of these patients then had what can be defined as "accelerated" rejections, and all showed drops in C′ and C′2 titers. On the other hand, the three patients who had "indolent" rejections showed no abnormal diminution of complement, nor did the three who did not reject their grafts during observation.

To sum up, it appears the complement system can both mediate certain graft rejections and serve as an indicator of an ongoing graft rejection, particularly of the accelerated type. Available morphologic data suggest that the accelerated rejections are associated with more profound endothelial damage, reminiscent of that observed in the xenograft rejections by dogs. Therefore, one can clearly state that in addition to the more prominent cellular rejection mechanisms, there are humoral rejection mechanisms which become readily detectable when reactions are so rapid that serum pools are measurably depleted. But even in slower reactions, the humoral factors are probably participating. Indeed there is some preliminary evidence that close scrutiny of the vascular walls in such situations may reveal C′ deposition.

Be that as it may, it seems clear that complement, activated and directed by complement-fixing antibodies, can cause or participate in transplant rejection. And perhaps one can also infer that present efforts to create more effective techniques for immunosuppression as an adjunct of transplantation surgery should not ignore the need for suppression of the complement and other humoral systems, as well as for suppression of cellular immune mechanisms.

That such complement inhibition can be achieved has already been demonstrated by the cobra venom extract mentioned in the description of the xenograft experiments. Using the venom factor we have been able to selectively reduce C′ in dogs and keep it reduced for periods of five to seven days. The venom factor appears to be directed against C′3. This means that for the first time we have at our disposal a method for depleting C′ without using it. This is important because in the process of utilizing complement it is possible to induce toxicities. Even more significant, we now can foresee the possibility that venom — or, more likely, some other inhibitor, since the venom works only transiently — may be applied in human disease and, of course, in transplantation problems. It stands to reason that since anticomplementary factors can be isolated in cobra venom, such factors most likely exist elsewhere in nature, so we have taken a long step toward the ability to manage serum complement levels when necessary. Finally, we have another important tool for manipulating and studying complement in vivo. Since most of the studies with complement to date have been in vitro, this could be extremely helpful.

Having mentioned the possibility of using complement inhibitors to manipulate human disease, it is probably wise to state quickly that to date we have not been able to definitely assign to complement an etiologic or pathogenetic role in any disease. The evidence for the existence of such a role is largely inferential. We know, to cite an obvious instance, that the effects seen in hemolytic anemias parallel the effects that can be attained with complement in vitro. We also know that complement components can be detected on red cells in various anemias, and they can be involved in both erythrophagocytosis and hemoly-

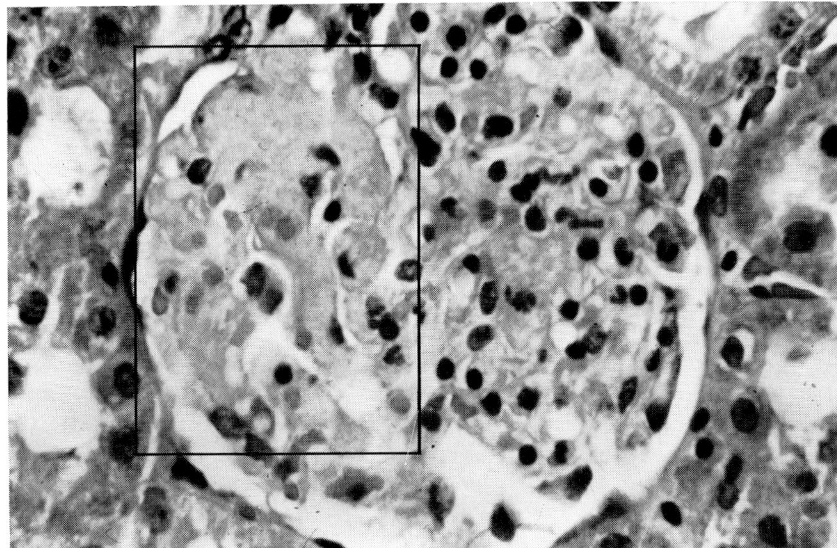

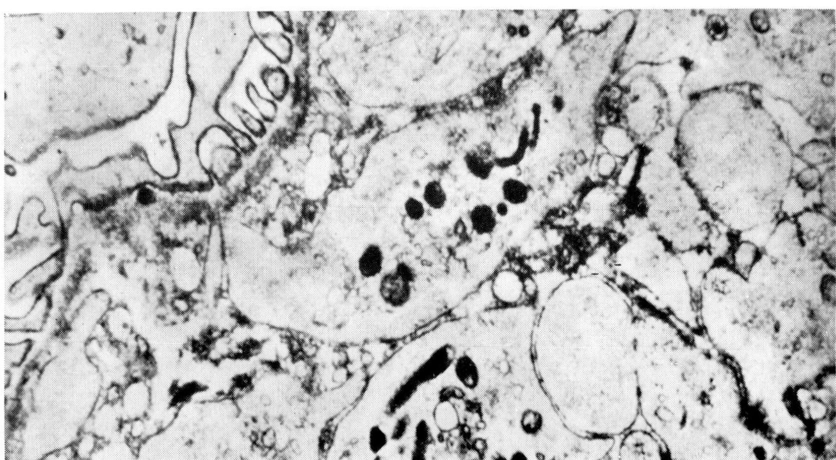

After rabbit kidney was transplanted to dog, eosinophilic material (boxed area) was deposited along glomerular endothelium. The result nine minutes later was clogging of blood vessels and cessation of blood flow. Electronmicrograph close-up (below) of glomerulus from rejected rabbit kidney identifies the eosinophilic deposits as being composed predominantly of platelets.

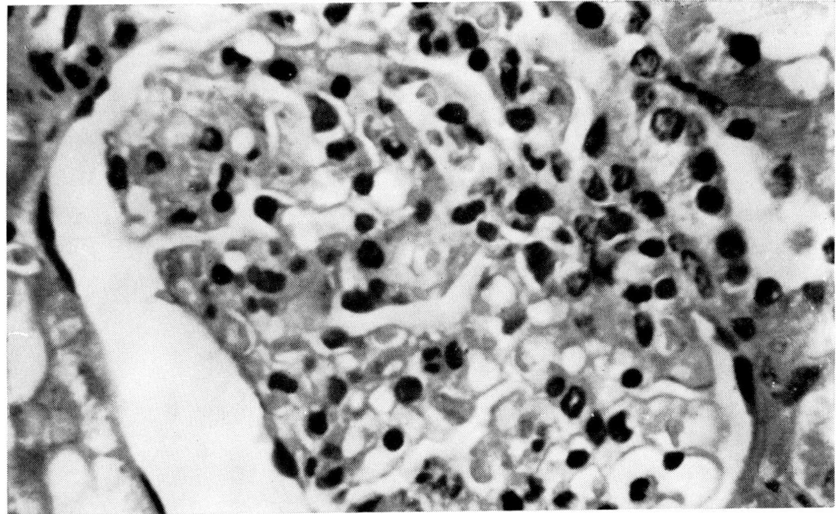

When cobra venom extract was used to inhibit complement activity, xenograft was still functioning at 17 minutes, and marked retardation of morphologic changes associated with rejection was apparent in the glomerulus.

Complement Profiles in Human Disease

The possibility that complement measurements may one day serve as diagnostic aids to the clinician, even as electrolyte measurements are employed today, is raised by the finding that various diseases marked by serum complement abnormalities appear to have "complement profiles" in which alterations can be traced from component to component. Such clinical applications would be greatly aided by the development of laboratory models mimicking the human syndromes. The profiles of typical patients are presented below, along with an incomplete profile for experimental serum sickness. The last, of course, has always been considered a model for acute glomerular nephritis, but it will be noted that its pattern actually is closer to that of systemic lupus erythematosus. This pattern may be suggestive of circulating immune complexes and indeed may be seen in the early stages of acute glomerular nephritis.

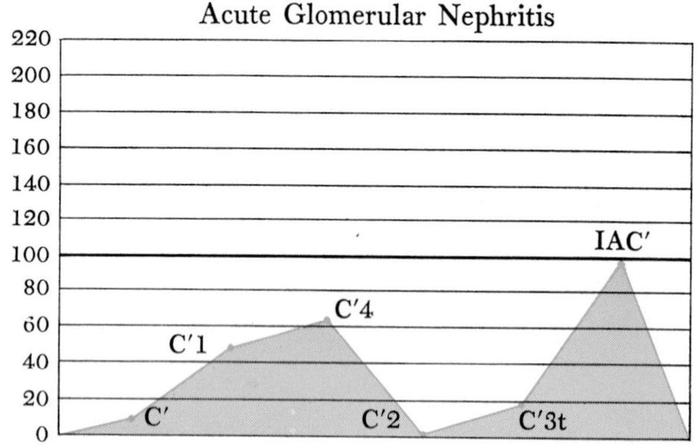

Total complement is very low, but the C′1 and C′4 components are only moderately depressed and immune adherence activity (IAC′) remains normal.

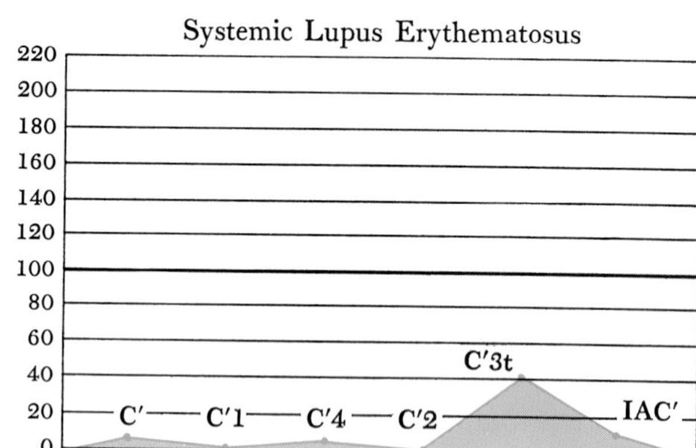

Total complement is extremely low, as are most of the complement components. In these profiles, C′3t designates the cumulative activities of C′3, 5, 6, 7, 8, and 9.

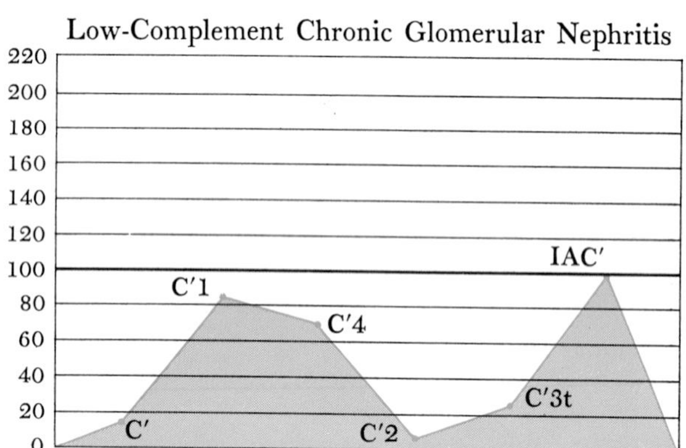

Although total complement is quite low, the first two components in the sequence and the immune adherence activity are near normal.

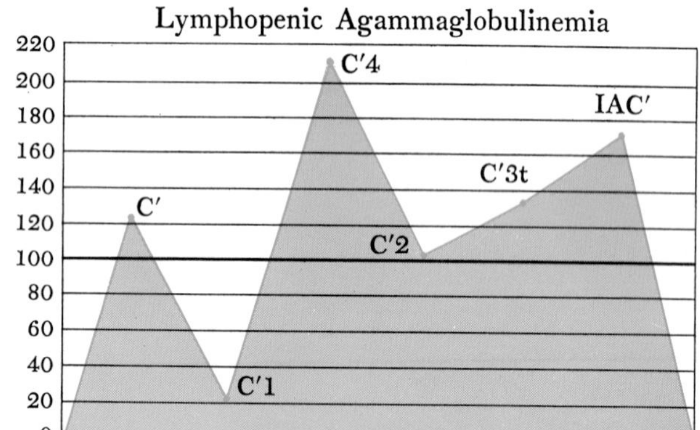

Total complement is elevated, as are all components except C′1 (which includes a gamma globulin). C′1 is also depressed in patients with nonlymphopenic agammaglobulinemia.

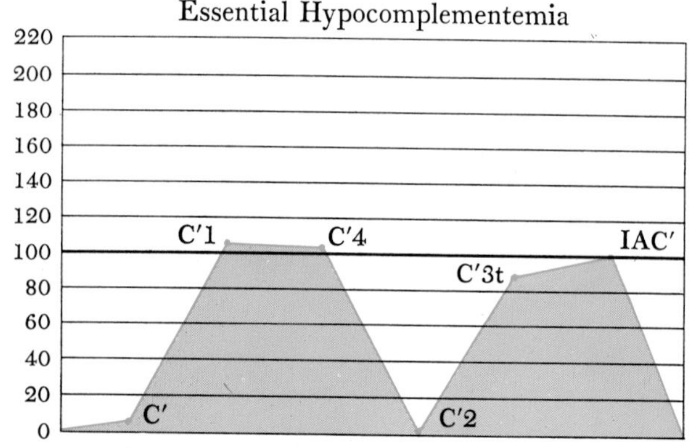

Despite the great depression of total complement and C′2 hemolytic activity, the other components and immune adherence C′ activity are at normal or slightly elevated levels.

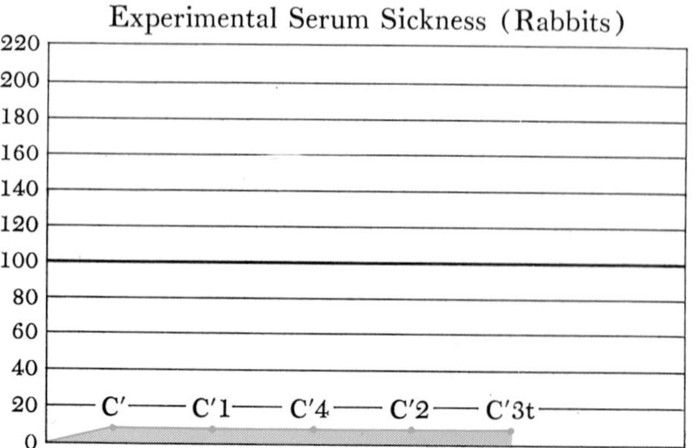

The level of total complement and that of all complement components are equally depressed. The pattern is suggestive of systemic lupus erythematosus.

sis. As a matter of fact, an almost more pressing question is why complement-induced hemolysis is not a universal in vivo fact. The answer, we feel, may lie in the control mechanism built into the complement system, or possibly in our endowment of non–complement-fixing antibodies or other functional C′ inhibitors.

What value, then, would there be in suppressing complement activity? Hypothetically, at least, those diseases that are marked by low complement titers — systemic lupus erythematosus and the nephrotic and nephritic syndromes, among others — might in fact be diseases of excessive complement utilization. In fact, in these diseases histochemical microscopy has revealed complement deposition on the basement membrane in patterns characteristic for the disease. Such patterns can be reproduced after passive deposition of antigen-antibody complexes in animal models. At any rate, the findings suggest that complement may be essential to the destructive processes characteristic of the disease, in which case there would be a logical reason for employing therapy to reduce the amount of C′ available.

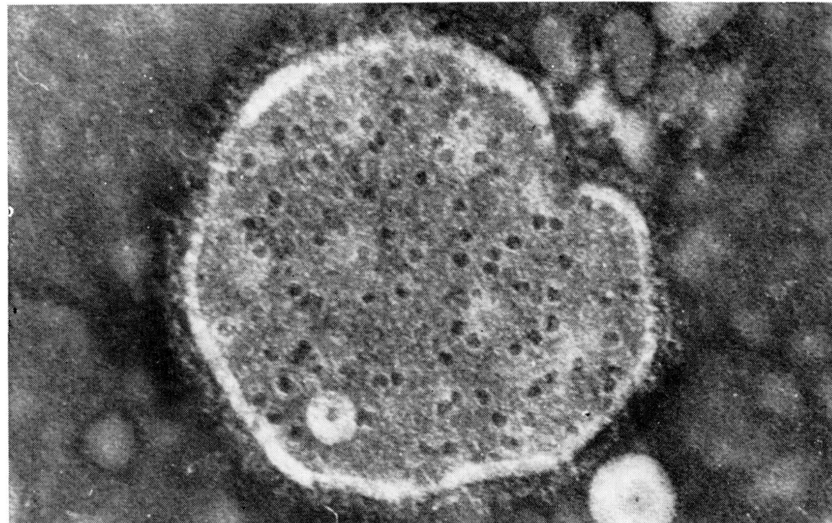

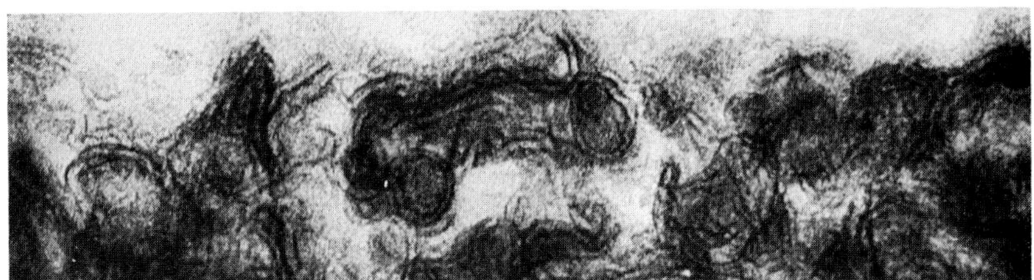

Lesions on Veillonella alcalescens *endotoxin (top) suggest the complement sequence has been carried through to completion on endotoxin substrate. "Cross-sectional" view below shows that endotoxin is itself a membrane, with two 30 Å layers separated by one of 25 Å. These experiments were performed by Dr. Bladen.*

Another clinical area of particular interest is inflammation. Here complement may be able to play a central role. Studies done with Rebuck skin windows provide a convenient indication of this role. These investigations were carried out in Minnesota in cooperation with Drs. Arthur R. Page, Pickering, and Good, and involved patients who had chronic and acute glomerulonephritis. There was a suggestive correlation between the finding of lowered serum C′ in these patients and a depressed neutrophil exudation in response to the inflammatory stimulation created by the skin window. And in vitro studies with sera from these same patients revealed the presence of a heat-labile substance that interfered with the expression of the complement-dependent neutrophil chemotactic factor. It was with this inhibitor that a near-perfect association with the neutrophil response could be made. Further, depressed chemotaxis was seen in an individual with congenital deficiency of complement; it was rarely seen in the general population. Chemotaxis was normal in patients with Bruton-type agammaglobulinemia. (In addition, Pickering found a heat-labile inhibitor of hemolytic C′ in some of these patients.) All these observations suggested that neutrophil exudation in response to a mechanical stimulus is mediated or increased by complement.

Obviously, inflammatory processes subject to bacterial and viral stimuli may also be mediated by complement. Is it not possible, then, that complement components are involved in most of the major parameters of inflammatory response — potentiation of phagocytosis, opsonification, immune adherence, increased vascular permeability due to anaphylatoxin and histamine release, and white-cell chemotaxis? One also wonders if anti-inflammatory agents such as steroids might not act in part through complement.

At the start of this article, experiments demonstrating the ability of complement to "punch holes" in endotoxin were touched upon. The fact that endotoxin is a substrate for C′ is very exciting from an investigational standpoint and even more intriguing in its clinical implications. The latter, of course, are inherent in the possibility that the shock syndromes may be attributable to complement's ability to lyse cells and destroy cell membranes, to induce histamine and anaphylatoxin release, etc. It has been found that the endotoxin molecule is the most efficient complement fixer we have seen; microgram quantities will fix complement far more effectively than will antigen-antibody complexes. One is tempted to postulate that endotoxin has a unique ability to interact with complement by virtue of its strong antigenicity and its richness in substrates for C′ components.

From the investigational point of view, the endotoxic lipopolysaccharide represents a relatively "pure" model of the cellular target of complement. It is membranous, and its surface is susceptible to the hole-punching effects of complement. Thus it represents a biologically reactive prototype of a cell surface—bacterial or mammalian. With such a prototype we may soon be able to answer many of the questions we now have about the complement system. We may be able to change some of our frustrating speculations into fruitful facts.

Chapter 11

Transfer Factor and Cellular Immunity

H. SHERWOOD LAWRENCE
New York University

The discovery by Landsteiner and Chase that delayed hypersensitivity could be transferred by cells from sensitive to nonsensitive guinea pigs proved a milestone in progress toward an understanding of cellular immunity, as this class of reactions is now termed. Cellular transfer thus separated the immunologic responses mediated by cells from those resulting from circulating antibody and at the same time provided a sorely needed immunologic end point for analysis of underlying mechanisms.

In the years that followed, and as the Landsteiner and Chase findings were extensively confirmed, the importance of delayed hypersensitivity as a distinctive category of altered tissue reactivity became increasingly appreciated. Its biologic ramifications have proved to be widespread indeed. Notably, it has been found that the select population of delayed-type hypersensitive cells (DTH cells, i.e., circulating, thymus-dependent small lymphocytes) are centrally involved in apparently diverse functions that encompass immunologic surveillance of neoplastic cells, rejection of homografts, mediation of certain autoimmune diseases, and recovery from intracellular microbial and viral infections in man.

It is the purpose of this article to touch upon selective aspects of the work on transfer factor (TF), the active moiety residing in such DTH cells that converts normal lymphocytes in vivo and in vitro to a specific antigen-responsive state, thereby resulting in the transfer of long-lived systemic delayed hypersensitivity. The importance of TF in analysis of the particular deficit in cellular immune deficiency syndromes as well as its potential usefulness as a therapeutic agent in such deficiency diseases will also be considered. Although emphasis will be placed on work emanating from our laboratory, many other groups have contributed substantially to the elucidation of the nature and function of transfer factor.

Our studies began with the adaptation of the Landsteiner and Chase principle and resulted in the finding in humans that viable blood leukocytes are effective in the transfer of delayed cutaneous sensitivity to tuberculin and to streptococcal antigens. As in the guinea pig, we also found that successful transfer in humans depended on critical quantitative variables such as the degree of sensitivity possessed by the donor and the dosage of leukocytes required. However, it soon became apparent that the cellular transfer system in humans exhibited different properties from that studied in the guinea pig. The differences related chiefly to the smaller dosage of cells found effective in humans and the prolonged duration of transferred sensitivity observed.

These species differences led to observations which showed that in humans extracts of leukocytes prepared by freezing and thawing or by osmotic lysis are as effective as intact viable cells in the transfer of enduring systemic states of delayed hypersensitivity. This finding permitted initiation of attempts to isolate and characterize the active material (TF) in blood leukocytes. The experimental approaches taken were conditioned by the biologic activity of the material, i.e., the fact that a minute quantity of leukocyte extract could confer upon recipients the precise immunologic memories of the donor promptly (as early as four to six hours and usually by 18 to 24 hours) as well as for prolonged periods (one to two years). This event in the face of the dilutional factors encountered in the recipient (e.g., an intra- and extracellular fluid compartment of 35 liters) suggested the possibility of replication of TF. This notion was reinforced by our finding that nonviable leukocyte extracts were capable of transferring either tuberculin or streptococcal sensitivity from natively sensitive donor A to recipient B and thence from recipient B to

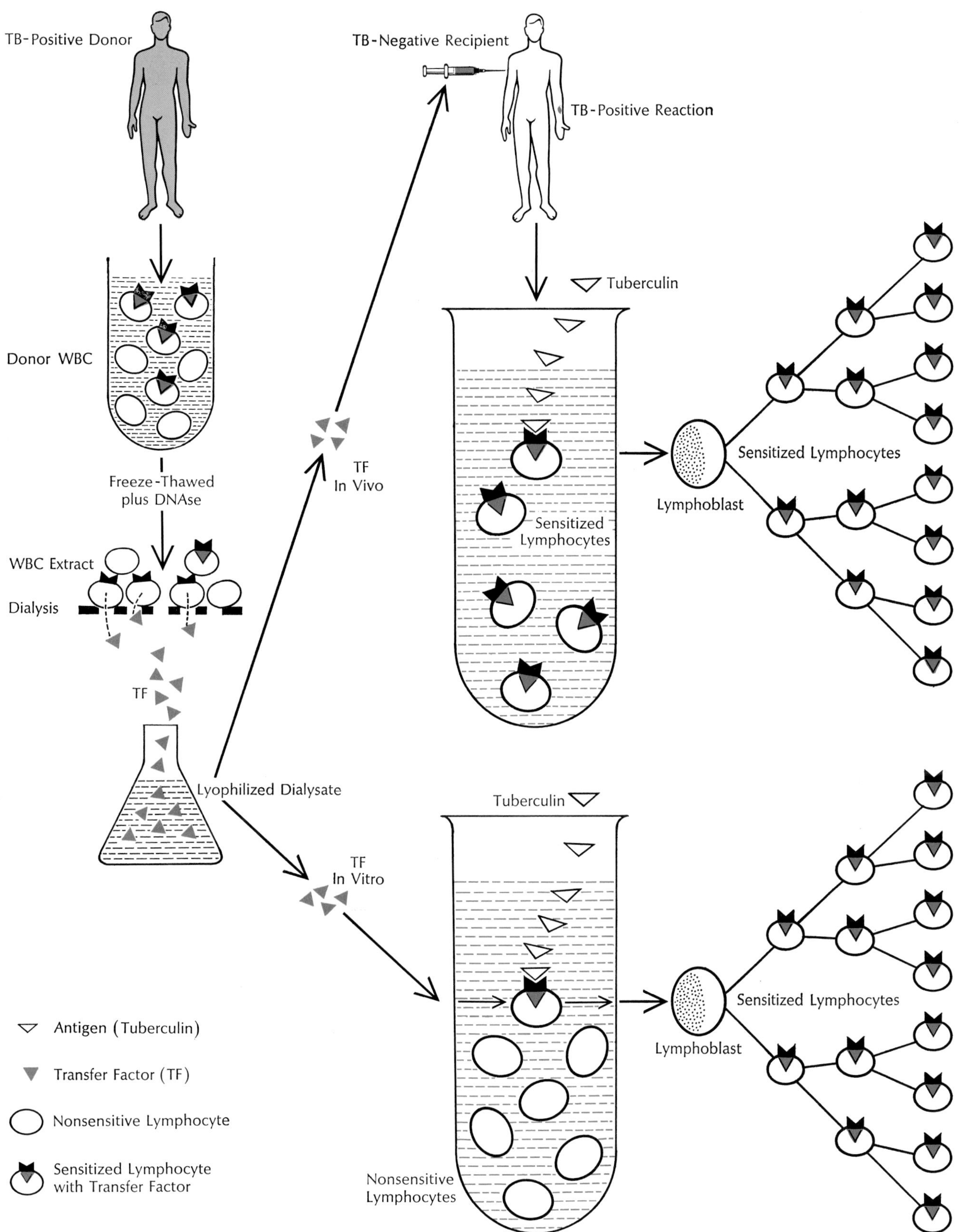

The ability of dialyzable transfer factor to confer sensitivity to a specific antigen either in vivo or in vitro is demonstrated in experiments schematized above. Preparation of TF from leukocytes of tuberculin-sensitive individual is shown at left. When injected into TB-negative recipient (top center), the dialyzable TF converts subject to tuberculin-positive state. Lymphocytes from such a TF-sensitized person, when incubated with antigen, can undergo lymphoblast transformation and produce clone of specifically sensitized lymphocytes (top right). Similarly, when TF is added to preparation of nonsensitized lymphocytes in vitro (bottom center) it induces lymphoblast transformation that leads to production of clone of tuberculin-sensitive cells.

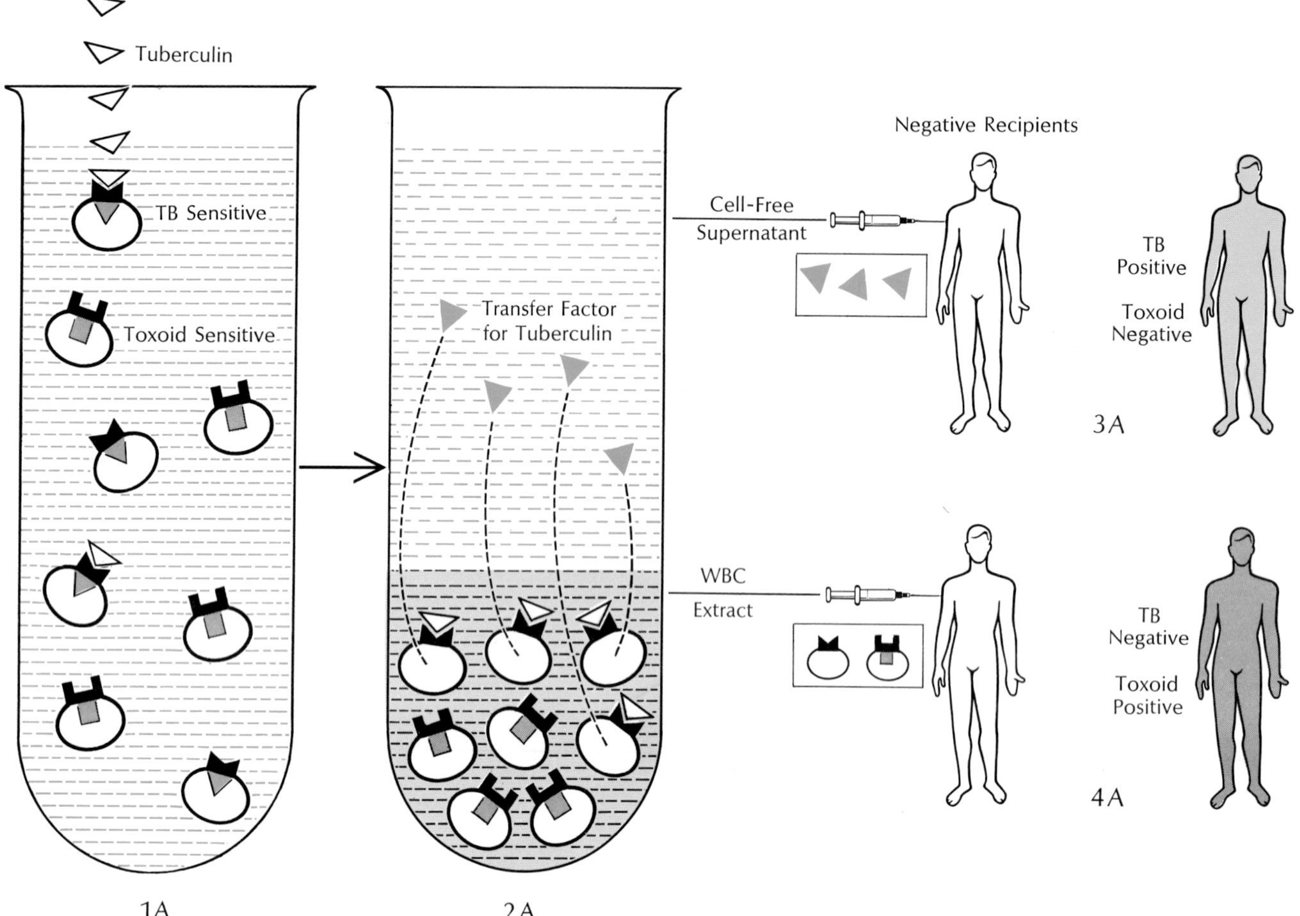

Role of antigen in releasing specific transfer factor from sensitive lymphocytes is illustrated above. In the first series, TB antigen is incubated with mixed population of TB-sensitive and diphtheria toxoid-sensitive lymphocytes (1A). After centrifugation the cell-free supernatant is separated from lymphocytes by sedimentation (2A). Supernatant, containing the TF released through WBC interaction with tuberculin, is able to transfer sensitivity for TB but not for diphtheria toxoid (3A). WBC extract is exactly

recipient C. The application of a skin test to recipient B in each instance, however, could have contributed to this result.

In any event, to test the assumption that either DNA or RNA or protein contributed to this unusual biologic activity, leukocyte extracts containing TF were treated with DNAse, RNAse, or DNAse plus trypsin. This exogenous enzymatic treatment had no effect on the capacity of such extracts to transfer sensitivity, nor did the endogenous nucleases or lysosomal hydrolases activated by leukocyte lysis. Transfer factor is stable in leukocyte extracts, and its activity is not impaired after 8 to 10 hours storage at 25° C or 37° C, or when storage-frozen at −20° C for two to three years, or stored as lyophilized dialysate at 4° C for five years.

A. M. Pappenheimer Jr. and I turned to the diphtheria toxin-antitoxin system to explore the relationship between TF and serum antibody synthesis and the transfer of a secondary immune response. We used tuberculin sensitivity as a marker and were able to transfer tuberculin and toxoid sensitivity to the same recipient. Nevertheless, using a sensitive biologic test, we were unable to detect antibody (diphtheria antitoxin) in either the leukocyte extracts used to transfer delayed sensitivity to toxoid or in the sera or skin of the recipient at the time he expressed delayed cutaneous reactivity. Thus the state of delayed sensitivity in the recipient of TF is expressed in the absence of detectable specific immunoglobulins, a finding subsequently confirmed by Good and his associates in agammaglobulinemic patients.

Studies with coccidioidin as antigen attempted to assess the possibility that TF produced its effects by enhancing latent sensitivity. Coccidioides infection is restricted to the western United States, and recipients were selected who had remained on the eastern seaboard. Coccidioidin sensitivity was transferred with leukocyte extracts, and the sensitivity persisted for one to one and a half years without known exposure to antigen.

The subsequent demonstration of the transfer of homograft sensitivity (accelerated rejection of skin homografts), with my colleagues Rapaport, Converse, and Tillett, established clearly that TF does indeed confer de novo sensitivity. Thus the host exposed to the histocompatibility antigens of another individual is stimulated to produce a cell population containing a *new* transfer factor with specificity directed against those particular antigens. We therefore also found that the action of TF is immunologically specific in initiating rejection only of the

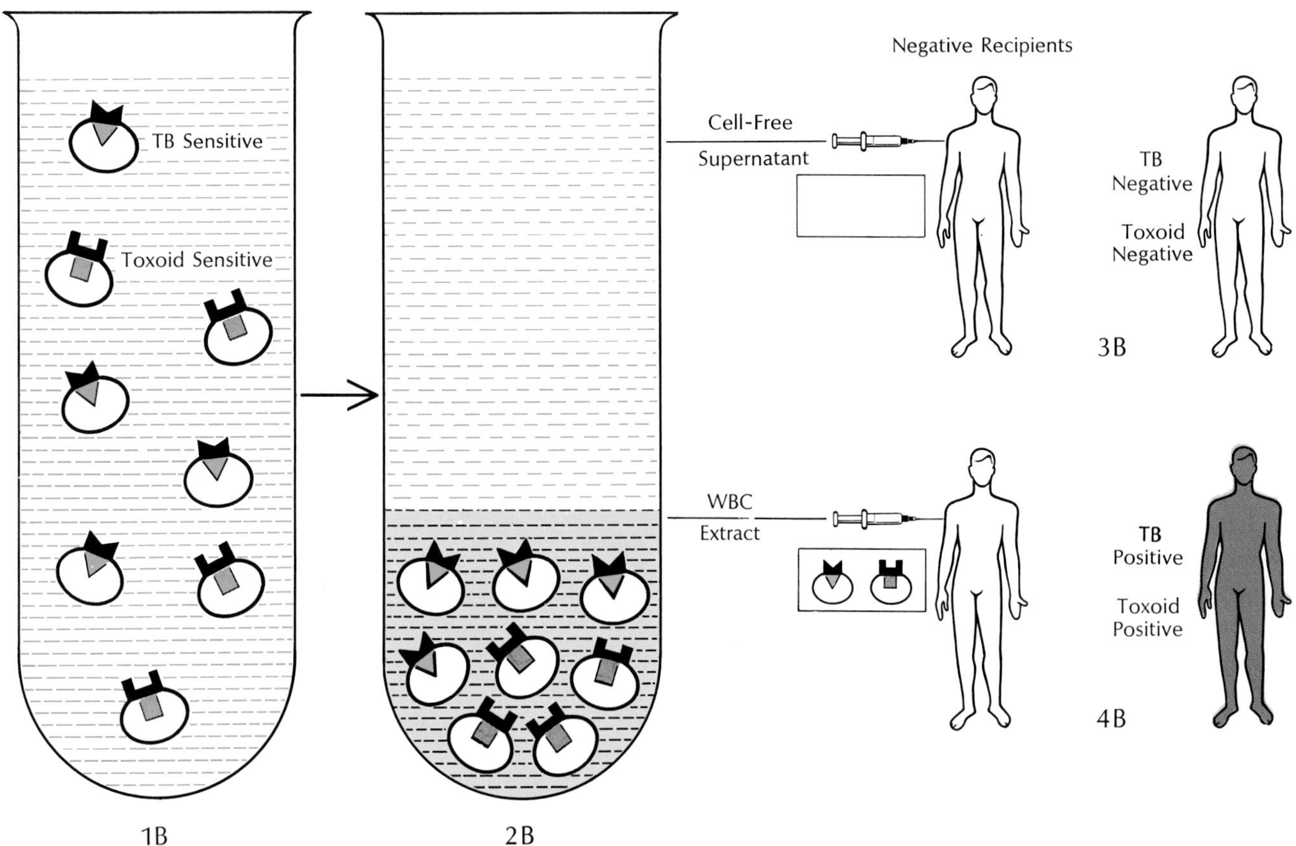

opposite in its specificity, retaining transfer capacity for toxoid sensitivity but lacking ability to transfer TB sensitivity (4A). However, when a mixed lymphocyte population with antigen is used (1B), supernatant is free of transfer activity, while cells retain such activity for both sensitivities (2B). This is demonstrated when supernatant fails to convert negative recipient (3B), while cell extract makes the negative recipient positive in reactions to both tuberculin and diphtheria toxoid (4B).

related graft and not of unrelated grafts placed on the same recipients. Thus TF alone without the intervention of serum antibody can initiate a series of events that bring about the downfall of the homograft.

Taken together, these data suggest that the immunosuppressive effects achieved with drugs, and more particularly with antilymphocyte serum, in recipients of organ transplants could be due in part to the deflection or engagement of those few circulating small lymphocytes that bear the specific transfer factor elaborated against the histocompatibility antigens of the transplant donor.

Subsequent findings obtained with Rapaport and Dausset have clearly established that human histocompatibility antigens of leukocyte extracts are nondialyzable and therefore are readily separated from TF, which is dialyzable. Thus, in this system at least, the antigenic materials that actively induce sensitization are distinct from the material that cannot actively induce but can only transfer a state of sensitivity to homografts. This finding also suggests an explanation for the long duration of transferred sensitivity in man, even when viable cells are used. It appears that although the cellular vehicle of TF is rejected via a homograft response, TF itself is not.

The long-term goal of identification and purification of transfer factor was greatly facilitated by our subsequent finding that it is a dialyzable moiety of <10,000 mol wt and that it is not an immunoglobulin. Its exact biochemical nature remains to be established. However, the main candidates in the dialysate for this type of biologic activity are polynucleotides and polypeptides. In these studies it was again established that dialyzable TF is insensitive to pancreatic RNAse, despite evidence of RNAse activity on known substrate added to the dialysate. Further, studies with dialyzable TF in patients with sarcoidosis reconfirmed this insensitivity to pancreatic RNAse. We also showed that TF could be inactivated by heating at 56° C or 100° C for 30 minutes. Additionally, we have found that dialyzable TF is not immunogenic in rabbits or in man.

The finding in humans that leukocyte extracts are as effective as viable cells was confirmed and extended by several groups of investigators, notably Maurer, Jensen et al., and Baram and Mosko. The further purification and separation of TF from other cell constituents as a dialyzable moiety of <10,000 mol wt was subsequently also confirmed and extended by Baram et al., Arala-Chaves, Fireman et al., Brandriss, and Good and David and their colleagues. The consensus ar-

Some Properties of Dialyzable Transfer Factor

BIOLOGICAL	BIOCHEMICAL	IMMUNOLOGICAL
Properties of whole extract: Prompt onset (hrs) Long duration (> 1 yr) Equal intensity	Soluble, dialyzable, lyophilizable	Not immunoglobulin
Dissociable from transplantation antigens	< 10,000 mol wt	Not immunogenic
Small quantities → magnified effects	No protein, albumin, α or γ globulin	Immunologically specific
	Orcinol positive	Converts normal lymphocytes in vitro and in vivo to antigen-responsive state
	Polypeptide/polynucleotide composition	Transformation and clonal proliferation of converted lymphocytes exposed to antigen
	Inactivated 56°C–30 min.	Informational molecule/derepressor/receptor site
	Resists pancreatic RNAse	
	Retains potency (5 yr)	

rived at through these investigations has firmly established TF as a dialyzable moiety of low molecular weight occurring in dialysates comprised mainly of polynucleotides and polypeptides. There has also emerged the suggestion, particularly from Baram's studies, that some residual activity may be nondialyzable. In any event, the path leading to the precise biochemical identification of TF is clear.

Not clear, however, is the exact mechanism by which transfer factor so promptly confers on the recipient's lymphocytes the precise immunologic memories possessed by the donor and thereby initiates a state of enduring specific sensitivity. Recently, clues to this mechanism have arisen from an extension of in vitro studies initiated with Pappenheimer some years ago. Pappenheimer and I found that incubation of sensitive leukocytes with antigen liberated TF into the cell-free supernatant and thereby desensitized the cells. When cell populations sensitive to tuberculin and to diphtheria toxoid were incubated with tuberculin, the TF for tuberculin was liberated into the supernatant, while that for toxoid remained in the cell pellet, as shown by in vivo transfer of sensitivity. The supernatant of control tubes incubated without tuberculin contained no TF, whereas the cell pellet transferred both tuberculin and toxoid sensitivity.

Our subsequent discovery that transfer factor is a dialyzable moiety that is not immunogenic in vivo and that it is free of histocompatibility antigens has led us to employ it for studies on in vitro lymphocyte transformation response. This assay system for TF has been studied by Fireman et al. and by Valentine and the author. The basic finding is that incubation of dialyzable TF prepared from tuberculin-sensitive cells with nonsensitive human blood lymphocytes in culture causes no discernible effect. However, addition of tuberculin to such cultures causes a very small proportion of lymphocytes to undergo transformation to lymphoblasts (i.e., they behave as if obtained from a tuberculin-sensitive donor).

In one series of experiments, Valentine and I were able to show that tuberculin-positive, diphtheria toxoid–negative dialysate caused in vitro transformation of lymphocytes from individual A, who was not sensitive to either antigen, in the presence of tuberculin but not in the presence of toxoid (i.e., the effect is immunologically specific). Of further interest, the in vivo injection of an aliquot of the same positive dialysate into that same negative individual A transferred delayed cutaneous reactivity to tuberculin but not to toxoid. Lymphocytes obtained from individual A after transfer in vivo now responded in culture to tuberculin alone but not to toxoid.

This type of result suggests that dialyzable transfer factor confers on a select population of nonsensitive lymphocytes the capacity to respond specifically to antigen by transformation and clonal proliferation in vitro and that this same event occurs in vivo. The consequence of this conversion of normal lymphocytes to the sensitive state is the expression of delayed cutaneous reactivity or homograft rejection by the recipient upon exposure to the specific antigen. The recent work of David and Good and their colleagues has also shown that dialyzable TF injected in vivo not only induces cutaneous reactivity but also confers on the recipient's circulating lymphocytes the capacity to make migration inhibitory factor (MIF) in the presence of specific antigen in vitro. One may conclude from these cumulative observations that once the nonsensitive lymphocyte is converted to a sensitive state by dialyzable TF it is then capable of all the in vitro and in vivo activities heretofore detected only in sensitive lymphocyte populations. It should also be emphasized that what has been revealed in recipients of TF occurs in the natively sensitive host whenever he is exposed to the appropriate antigen. This exposure may take the form of an intradermal tuberculin test, a growing population of tubercle bacilli in the lung, or transplantation of a renal homograft.

In additional studies of this type, Valentine and I have found that culturing sensitive human blood lymphocytes with antigen (tuberculin) results in the production of a material with similar activity in the cell-free supernatant. Addition of such active supernatants to nonsensitive lymphocytes in culture causes their conversion to the sensitive state. In the presence of antigen the result is the transformation of such activated cells to lymphoblasts. This supernatant material is inactivated by heating at 56° C for 30 minutes and is not sedimented at 100,000 x G. It differs from dialyzable TF in being unable to pass through a Visking cellulose dialysis bag.

The preparations of dialyzable transfer factor resulted, as noted, in the transformation of only a very few nonsensitive lymphocytes (around 3% at seven days culture). The question then arose: How is this effect amplified? Does antigen liberate TF from a few sensitive cells to recruit a large population of nonsensitive cells, as originally postulated by Pappenheimer, or is TF a vehicle for immunologic information passed from cell to cell?

Marshall, Valentine, and I approached this question by continuous time-lapse cinematography of lymphocytes in culture, held captive in a plastic ring under one microscopic field for seven days. From these observations we estimated that $<2\%$ of the total circulating lymphocyte population in natively sensitive humans was antigen responsive, and we observed that these few cells undergo blast transformation, repeated cell division, and clonal proliferation. Thus, at least after 48 to 72 hours in tube culture, we found no evidence for recruitment, and the large numbers of transformed lymphocytes (20% to 30%) observed at the end of seven days arose by a process of repeated cell division from the very few antigen-responsive cells present at the start. That recruitment may occur in the first 48 to 72 hours of culture is likely, but this cannot be established by these experiments.

Using this cinematographic technique, we next examined the behavior of nonsensitive lymphocytes cultured with supernatant material produced by tuberculin-stimulated sensitive cells. Here, also, an equally small population of nonsensitive cells (about 2%) were initially "converted" or "recruited" to an antigen-responsive state by the active supernatant. In the presence of tuberculin these few cells undergo transformation, repeated cell division, and clonal proliferation, and become amplified into 15% to 20% transformed cells by the seventh day of culture (see photographs, page 113).

This type of observation, particularly those obtained using dialyzable TF, provides direct visual evidence in favor of Burnet's clonal selection theory – especially the finding of an immunologically specific engagement of a highly restricted number of cells in the total circulating lymphocyte population. The implication is that those nonsensitive cells engaged may be a clone held in reserve that is predestined to become amplified to a much larger population of sensitive cells should the tuberculin-negative individual meet the tubercle bacillus.

What then of transfer factor and its mechanism of action? The experiments on serial transfer of delayed sensitivity from individual A to B to C diminished the possibility of an antibody or superantigen effect. Dialyzable TF excluded immunoglobulins and was found not to be immunogenic. The polynucleotides present in the dialysate appear too small to code for the amount of information required, and thus the informational aspects of TF are difficult to explain. From the in vitro studies and the direct visual evidence secured by cinematography, our results suggest that TF may act as a "derepressor" of a select few circulating lymphocytes, allowing them to respond to specific antigen by transformation and clonal proliferation. Thus the data that suggested replication of transfer factor by the host appear to result from the repeated cell division and clonal proliferation of the few antigen-stimulated lymphocytes following their conversion to an antigen-responsive state by TF. That additional TF is synthesized by such cells and passed to each new generation is suggested by in vivo data but is not yet established.

A recent upsurge of interest in the field of cell-mediated immunity has been occasioned by the perfection and versatility of in vitro correlates of in vivo phenomena. Such studies have resulted in an appreciation of the wide spectrum of latent responsiveness detected in sensitive lymphocyte populations following interaction with antigen. The activities liberated from or produced by the few antigen-responsive cells of the total circulating human lymphocyte population are shown in the illustration at the left.

It may be seen that in addition to the prompt liberation of transfer factor, interaction with antigen triggers the sensitive lymphocyte into production of a heat-labile, nondialyzable material that converts nonsensitive

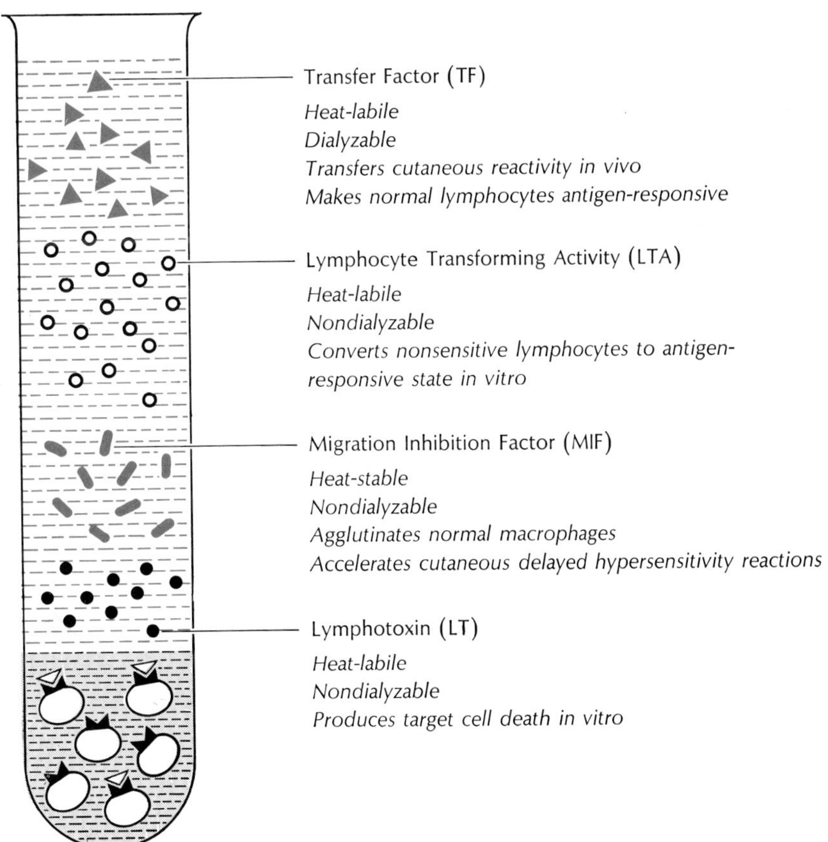

When the sensitive lymphocyte is cultured in the presence of antigen, at least four mediators of cellular immunity, including TF, are known to be produced, and there may be others. Those thus far established, with their properties, are schematized above.

lymphocytes into the antigen-responsive state. Also produced are a heat-labile, nondialyzable lymphotoxin that results in damage and death of indifferent mammalian cells in tissue culture and a heat-stable MIF that causes normal macrophages to adhere to each other and agglutinate. The importance of this family of molecules in specific and nonspecific recruitment of other lymphocytes to the antigen-responsive state and the subsequent escalation of the capacity for further production of similar mediators is readily apparent. The secondary involvement of other cell populations in the inflammatory response by such soluble mediators, expressed as delayed reactivity in the skin, rejection of homografts, and perhaps caseation necrosis in the lung, for example, is also implied.

The points to be emphasized are:

1) The catalogue of mediators of cellular immunity is far from complete.

2) The effector activities detailed may be a function of one molecule in varying concentration or of a family of molecules simultaneously present in the same supernatant – a critical point to be resolved.

3) As yet, only dialyzable transfer factor is sharply delineated from the other moieties present by virtue of its low molecular weight and distinctive properties. Transfer factor also differs significantly in its specificity and in its function as an "initiator" or "derepressor" molecule, unlike the other materials that function as effector molecules and lack specificity.

4) Demonstration of in vivo activities for these in vitro products is in progress. TF initiates the chain of events that results in cutaneous reactivity or homograft rejection in vivo as well as conferring antigen responsiveness on nonsensitive recipient lymphocytes in vivo and in vitro. MIF in its function as an effector molecule results in an accelerated delayed cutaneous reactivity upon intradermal injection. An in vivo function of the lymphocyte-transforming activity and of lymphotoxin should also be defined in the near future.

It should be noted that leukocyte donors selected for in vivo transfers are normal individuals who have donated blood for clinical use and have not transmitted hepatitis.

TF and Cellular Immune Deficit

With the extension of the principle of cellular transfer to man, a technique became available that elucidated mechanisms of delayed hypersensitivity in normal individuals and thus allowed its adaptation to the analysis of specific derangements in congenital or acquired immunologic deficiency disease syndromes. Although most of the studies on cellular transfer in such diseases have utilized viable leukocytes, the transfer of delayed sensitivity can occur only by virtue of the specific TF liberated from the cellular vehicle that is employed.

Good and his associates showed that patients with congenital agammaglobulinemia are anergic yet are capable of acquiring delayed sensitivity via transfer factor, and thus the mechanisms of cellular immunity are functional although dormant in such patients. Urbach et al., using viable cells and the technique of local transfer, observed that although patients with sarcoidosis could acquire local tuberculin sensitivity, they were incapable of expressing the systemic sensitivity so characteristic of the normal individual's response. We have recently confirmed and extended these observations, using dialyzable transfer factor. Our studies revealed that sarcoidosis patients can respond to TF with the development of local sensitivity, and only two of seven patients studied were capable of developing even low-grade systemic sensitivity.

These results point to an impaired production or function of the patient's own specific transfer factor for the usual delayed sensitivities as the basis for the anergy characteristic of this disease. The systemic unresponsiveness to TF also suggests that the impairment lies in host cells that are ordinarily converted to an antigen-responsive state, presumably circulating, thymus-dependent small lymphocytes. However, the occasional transfer of systemic sensitivity and, indeed, the regular transfer of local sensitivity suggest the deficit is only partial.

Clues to the origin of the anergy detected are suggested by recent reports from Belgium and Germany of the transfer of delayed reactivity to Kveim antigen by means of leukocytes of Kveim-positive patients with sarcoidosis. These results taken together suggest that the cellular immune mechanisms of the sarcoidosis patient are so taken up with their response to the Kveim antigen (i.e., producing TF to it) that they are somehow deflected from producing the transfer factors stimulated by earlier exposures to delayed allergens. The Kveim antigen may thus preempt the production or function of the "memory cells" for delayed hypersensitivity. This immunologic amnesia can be only partially restored locally and transiently by someone else's TF engaging a few, presumably uncommitted, immunocompetent lymphocytes.

The situation in Hodgkin's disease, as elucidated by Good and his associates and others, appears even more extreme in that the cellular immune deficiency seems total. The Hodgkin's patients not only appear uniformly unable to accept systemic transfer but they also differ from the sarcoidosis patients in failing to respond to local transfer as well. This defect suggests that the impairment results in the lack of enough immunocompetent cells capable of engagement by TF to initiate a local reaction.

The response to transfer factor of patients with other types of neoplastic disease, chiefly carcinomatous states, varies with the presence, extent, and duration of metastases. Amos and Hattler, using lymphocyte suspensions, were able to transfer only local but not systemic sensitivity to 18 patients with advanced malignancy. With Solowey and Rapaport, we have evaluated a comparable group of such patients, using dialyzable TF, and have also transferred local sensitivity. Each of these 10 patients also developed systemic sensitivity; however, it was weak in intensity and short in duration. These results suggest a variable involvement of immunocompetent host cells in tumor-bearing individuals. Whether this cellular immune deficiency reflects a faulty immunologic surveillance mechanism that permitted neoplasia to develop or is a consequence of the neoplastic process itself cannot be decided at this time.

Considerable evidence has been accumulated to highlight the central role of cellular immunity in resistance to or recovery from infectious diseases caused by intracellular microbes. This beneficial role of cell-mediated immunity has been repeatedly emphasized by studies of congenital and acquired cellular immune deficiency diseases, as well as from observations on the consequences of immunosuppressive therapy now commonplace in transplant recipients. In each instance such patients may succumb to infection with indigenous bacterial, fungal, or viral parasitism of the intracellular type, usually in the presence of an adequate serum antibody response and despite appropriate antibiotic therapy.

Recognition of this reality has led to attempts at immunologic reconstitution of such cellular immune deficiency states. Effectiveness of such attempts is based on knowledge of the precise locus of the cellular deficiency. For example, children with the Di George syndrome suffer a complete absence of cellular immunity that stems from the congenital absence of a thymus. This deficiency can be overcome only by the transplantation of a thymus, which confers on thymus-dependent peripheral lymphocytes the capacity to initiate and sustain cellular immune responses. Intermediate in degree are those children with the lymphopenic form of congenital agammaglobulinemia who have been immunologically reconstituted with histotreatment pioneered by Good and by Bach [Chapter 23, "Immunologic Reconstitution: The Achievement and Its Meaning"]. This remarkable treatment appears to result in proliferation of the thymus-dependent lymphocyte population among other hematopoietic stem cell lines in the transplant.

At the other end of this spectrum there exists the great bulk of "acquired" cellular immune deficiency states. These become manifest in individuals originally endowed with a full complement of normal thymic and marrow components that are selectively deranged in association with certain diseases such as sarcoidosis or Hodgkin's disease; disseminated, indolent, intracellular infections such as leprosy and moniliasis; or with immunosuppressive therapy (drugs or ALS). It is in these states, where the locus of the deficiency appears to reside at the peripheral or effector level (i.e., the circulating, thymus-dependent lymphocytes), that the therapeutic use of transfer factor for immunologic reconstitution appears to hold promise.

In this regard, administration of transfer factor has been shown effective in several specific instances. The first example studied is that of Kempe's report of a child with progressive generalized vaccinia following smallpox inoculation, despite the production of high-titer circulating antivaccinial antibody. The continued dissemination of vaccinial lesions was not inhibited either by amputation of the inoculation site or by passive administration of high-titer antivaccinial gamma globulin. Nevertheless, the disease was halted promptly following cellular transfer with viable blood leukocytes from sensitive adult donors. Recovery was coincident with the acquisition of delayed sensitivity to vaccinia virus.

This successful use of TF is impressive in the light of the usual fatal outcome of such infections, the long control period of observation, and the ineffectiveness of both natural antibody and passively administered gamma globulin in halting the progress of the disease. This accomplishment has since been duplicated in other patients, including one adult. The results achieved in the adult with generalized vaccinia are of interest in that cellular transfer was associated with spontaneous delayed reactions around the vaccinia sites, and in this case also the prior administration of antivaccinial gamma globulin had been without effect. Of further interest is the observation of a relapse following the first cellular transfer. A second cellular transfer done by O'Connell et al. from the same sensitive donor brought a prompt and effective response, with eradication of the disease.

This type of immunologic reconstitution via transfer factor was also achieved in a child with disseminated cutaneous moniliasis of many years duration, reported by Buckley et al. The circumstances were similar in that both high-titer natural antibody and passive administration of specific antimonilial antibody had been without effect despite concurrent courses of amphotericin therapy. Yet the disease was terminated by cellular transfer from a sensitive donor, in the form of a parental marrow graft.

We have suggested elsewhere that transfer factor may be adapted to convert lepromatous leprosy to the tuberculoid type. Lepromatous leprosy, like disseminated vaccinia or disseminated coccidioidomycosis, is a disease process that goes virtually unchecked in the host despite the presence of a high titer of serum antibody. There is no inflammatory reaction in the patient's skin or tissues to the lepra bacilli or their products. Moreover, there is a loss of established delayed type responses as well as a diminished capacity for active delayed sensitization. The tuberculoid type of leprosy is characterized by a benign, self-limited course. There are few lepra bacilli detectable in tissues, little or no serum antibody response, and a positive delayed cutaneous reactivity to lepromin. Coincident with the above suggestion, it was demonstrated by de Bonaparte et al. that lepromin sensitivity can indeed be transferred into anergic lepromatous patients by means of leukocytes from sensitive donors. It is too early to assess the effect of this reconstitution of delayed reactivity on the course of the disease.

The use of viable immunocompetent cells as a source of transfer factor can be hazardous when administered to a host with markedly deficient cellular immunity, who is rendered incapable of rejecting the transferred cells via a homograft response. Such cells may initiate a graft-versus-host reaction against the recipient and may result in an equivalent of runt disease in proportion to the genetic (i.e., antigenic) disparity between cell donor and recipient. We have suggested elsewhere that this hazard may be avoided by using dialyzable TF prepared from donor cell populations. Dialyzable TF is a safer, more effective preparation for immunologic reconstitution of the peripheral type since it is not antigenic in animals or man; it is free of all macromolecular cell constituents, including histocompatibility antigens; it retains potency in the lyophilized state for at least five years; and it can be administered repeatedly without immunologic or other reactions. Using dialyzable TF, David and Good and their colleagues have transferred delayed cutaneous reactivity to candida antigen to one of two children with disseminated candidiasis. Moreover, the lymphocytes of the recipient also acquired the capacity to produce MIF in vitro when exposed to candida antigen following transfer. It is too early to detect any beneficial effect on the course of the disease in this patient.

When dialyzable transfer factor is given repeatedly, from the same or from pooled donors, to the same recipient over a prolonged period, the only detectable result is a boost in the intensity and duration of the transferred sensitivity. Tuberculin sensitivity is an example. We have also pointed out that the dosages of TF that we or others have used to date are deliberately minute and scaled down to study mechanisms of cellular immunity. For immunologic reconstitution therapy, however, a much higher dosage given repeatedly over a prolonged period may prove desirable. The means for increasing the dose of TF (dialysis, concentration, lyophilization) have been described. The potential value of transfer factor in such disseminated infections will depend on the precise locus and nature of the particular underlying cellular immune deficiency among a host of other variables. However, the judicious use of dialyzable TF in otherwise fatal infections caused by intracellular microbes may be worth serious consideration and evaluation. In this connection, it has been demonstrated that whole blood transfusion, by virtue of leukocytes bearing TF, will transfer tuberculin sensitivity to recipients.

Immunologic Surveillance

This is all fascinating in its own right and has yielded potentially useful, practical information for assessment of disease and perhaps for the design of rational treatment. Yet what is the real function of cellular immunity and what evolutionary pressures were exerted to develop such potent and diversified activities of a particular stem cell line? Thomas was the first to suggest that for survival of multicellular organisms, cell-mediated immunity had to evolve if mutant cells were to be recognized as foreign and rejected as if a homograft. In his view, suspension of this function results in neoplasia, and its efficient operation protects against this hazard. Thomas' postulate has been termed "immunological surveillance" by Burnet and has been in large measure substantiated by an increasing body of clinical and experimental evidence. Two examples will suffice: 1) the increased incidence of "spontaneous" malignant growth in "totally" immunosuppressed animals treated with thymectomy plus antilymphocyte serum; 2) the fact that upon cessation of immunosuppressive therapy, recipients of renal transplants who have acquired donor tumor cells and developed metastases will reject the kidney, tumor, and metastases as well.

These considerations, among others, have led to a revival of interest in the immunologic approaches to treatment of neoplastic disease. Early attempts at cellular transfer for immunologic reconstitution of the cancer-bearing human host have been either suggestive or equivocal. However, the underlying principle is a sound one but difficult to demonstrate as unequivocally in patients as in experimental animals. Much depends on whether, as seems likely, the tumor bears specific histocompatibility antigens distinct for it and distinct from those of the host. In that case, the degree of specificity for individual histocompatibility antigens revealed by transfer factor in respect to homograft rejection becomes critical. The latter experience would suggest that a specific TF would also have to be produced to reject the tumor. Since sensitization of one individual to another's tumor is neither a desirable nor practical undertaking in vivo, it is possible that techniques may be adapted to sensitize a normal individual's lymphocytes to tumor antigens in vitro. The recent availability of normal lymphocytes maintained as continuous cell lines in culture may provide the machinery for such an undertaking.

We are thus approaching, at a quickened pace, the point where the judicious clinical evaluation of transfer factor may be feasible in otherwise potentially fatal illnesses associated with cellular immune deficiency syndromes. Transfer factor is a new immunologic principle that may prove of benefit in such clinical situations where antimicrobial therapy alone has proved ineffective and the prognosis for recovery is exceedingly grave.

TF and Immunologic Homeostasis

We have seen that transfer factor exhibits a predilection and exquisite specificity for foreign histocompatibility antigens, which are the chief targets of transfer factor. Thus, the diverse functions of TF subserve a single role – policing unwanted foreign cells.

Such alien cells may arise from within or without the host. Examples of the former occur when the host's cells undergo alterations in the configuration of their histocompatibility antigens. Two mechanisms that may lead to this change are 1) mutation and neoplastic transformation and 2) amicable intracellular residence of virions, microbes, and fungi. We originally suggested the latter in the "self + x" hypothesis, an idea that has since received experimental confirmation and that virtually identifies all delayed hypersensitivity response as homograft reactions. Examples of overtly foreign cells introduced from without are supplied by cellular or organ transplants. This concept is more fully developed in two specialized reviews, "Transfer Factor and Cellular Immune Deficiency Disease" by H. S. Lawrence and "Transfer Factor and Other Mediators of Cellular Immunity" by Lawrence and F. T. Valentine [see Selected Readings]. Thus it is the specific TF induced in the respective circulating lymphocyte population that in my view equips this cell to seek out and attempt to destroy all other cells that present the appropriate antigenic configuration.

It is understood that once such cellular interaction occurs, the initially small stimulated lymphocyte population undergoes transformation and becomes amplified by clonal proliferation. The elaboration of effector molecules, such as lymphocyte transforming factor (LTF), migration inhibitor factor (MIF), and lymphotoxin (LT), will probably be shown to further amplify this triggering event and its consequent tissue damage in vivo as well as in vitro.

Frames from time-lapse cinematography show lymphoblastic proliferation in an individual microchamber following culture of lymphocytes stimulated with tuberculin. Sequence 1 through 4 on opposite page begins on day 3 of culture and continues through day 6; sequence 5 and 6, not followed with time-lapse, illustrate magnitude clones may reach by day 7 or 8. Experiment suggests that clonal formation (at least after day 3) results from repeated cell division of a few antigen-sensitive cells rather than from recruitment (Marshall, Valentine, and Lawrence. J. Exp. Med. *130:2:327).*

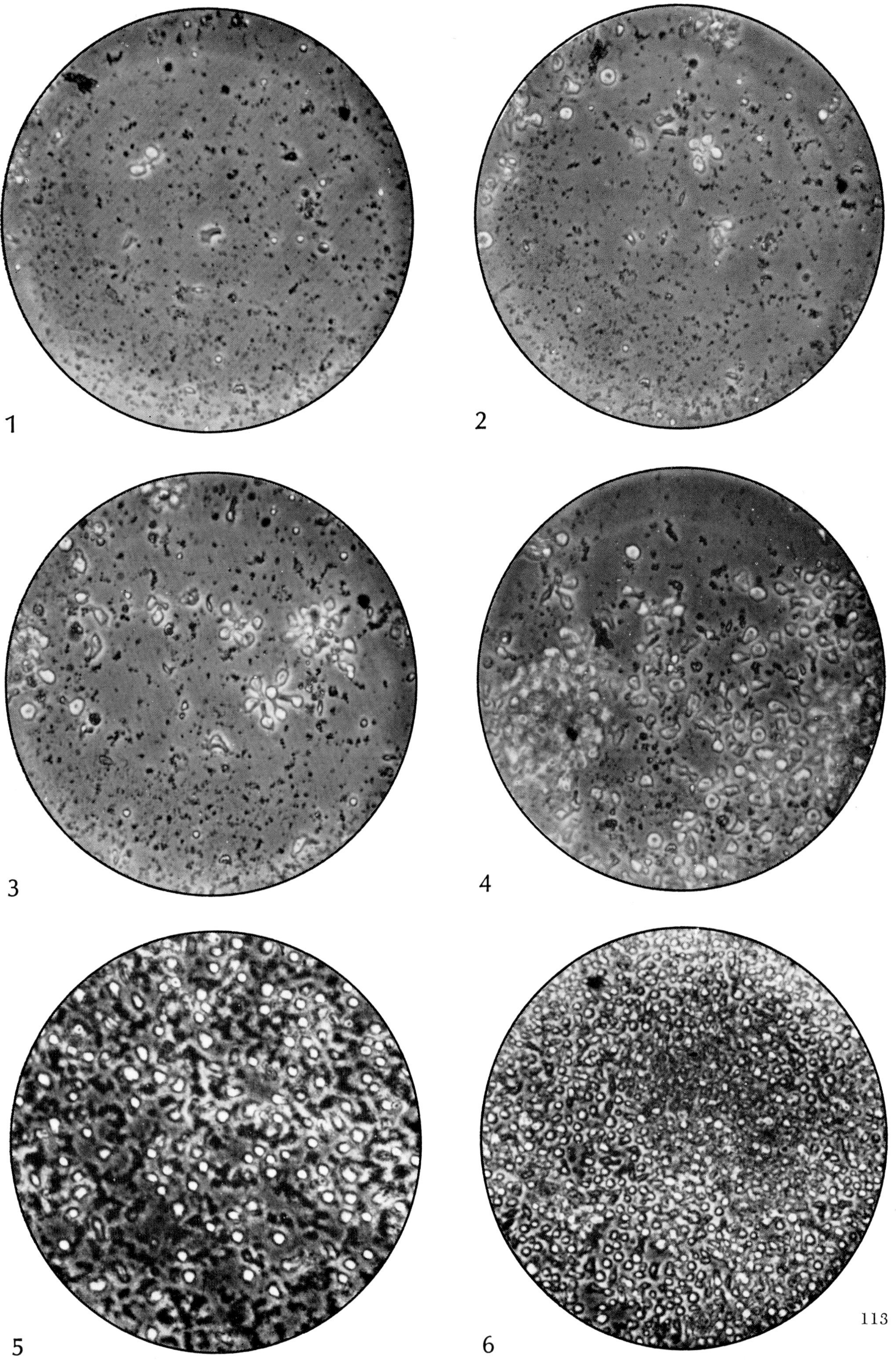
1
2
3
4
5
6

Chapter 12

Chemical Mediators of Immediate Hypersensitivity

ROBERT P. ORANGE *and* K. FRANK AUSTEN
Harvard Medical School

Sir Henry Dale demonstrated in the early 1900's that the anaphylactic reaction of the actively sensitized guinea pig could be substantially duplicated by the intravenous injection of histamine into a normal animal. Sir Thomas Lewis then demonstrated that the "triple response" was associated with the endogenous release of a histamine-like substance. Sometime later, Best and his coworkers, using a simple chemical extraction procedure, recovered significant concentrations of histamine from lung and liver tissue. These three observations led to the hypothesis, prevailing for many years, that histamine was the single mediator of immediate-type hypersensitivity reactions in man.

Evidence suggesting more than one chemical mediator of anaphylaxis first appeared in 1940 when C. H. Kellaway and E. R. Trethewie demonstrated that antigenic challenge of sensitized guinea pig lung tissue in vitro resulted in the release not only of histamine but also of a second substance that could slowly contract the guinea pig ileum; it was then termed "slow-reacting substance." Proof that this second material was not histamine was subsequently furnished by W. E. Brocklehurst when he showed that it contracted the isolated guinea pig ileum even in the presence of a potent antihistamine. He named it "slow-reacting substance of anaphylaxis" (SRS-A) to distinguish it from other materials that also could produce such contraction in the presence of antihistamines but that were not formed or released as a result of an immunologic event.

When similar studies were conducted with species such as the rat or mouse, whose mast cells contain serotonin as well as histamine, serotonin was also detected as a result of the immunologic reaction. In 1950, in South America, Beraldo demonstrated that the plasma of a dog undergoing active systemic anaphylaxis contained a hypotensive, smooth-muscle-contracting principle termed "bradykinin."

Thus, present evidence suggests that antigen-antibody reactions involve the release from mammalian tissue of at least four distinct chemical materials – histamine, serotonin, bradykinin, and SRS-A – each with the potential for mediating responses of immediate hypersensitivity, such as smooth-muscle contraction or local increase of vascular permeability. This would account for the failure of antihistamines to relieve in man all the clinical symptoms of allergic reactions. Antihistamines are also relatively ineffective inhibitors of certain experimental models of the allergic reaction, i.e., the Schultz-Dale response.

Of the four potential chemical mediators, histamine has been the most intensively studied. In mammals, it is found primarily in the granules of mast cells located in the perivascular connective tissue, where it is stored by electrostatic binding to a heparin-protein complex. It may be released from this bond by interaction of human reaginic antibody with its specific antigen at cell surfaces. This form of immunologic release of histamine from either the human polymorphonuclear leukocyte or the rat mast cell is a process unaccompanied by the discharge of other intracellular molecules. It is probably a secretory event, not destructive of the target cell. Collaborative work with E. L. Becker has demonstrated that this type of histamine release seems to involve activation of a cell-bound esterase.

As for serotonin, there is as yet no compelling evidence that it contributes to immediate hypersensitivity in man. It is present in the mast cells of the rat and mouse but not in those of most other species. It is particularly prominent in the platelets of some species and in the enterochromaffin cells of the gastrointestinal tract. Like histamine, serotonin in its final form exists in the primary target cell and is released as a result of a relevant immunologic event.

The kinins are peptides formed by the enzymatic action of kallikrein on the alpha-globulin plasma substrate kininogen. Plasma kallikrein elaborates the nonapeptide bradykinin; tissue kallikrein yields the decapeptide kallidin, which is rapidly degraded to bradykinin by a plasma aminopeptidase. Thus, these enzymes must be activated before the kinin system is implicated. The system is set off by any change in surface because the first protein triggering the pathway is Hageman factor of plasma, which also initiates the clotting sequence. Thus, whenever the kinin cascade is activated it is essential to determine whether such activation is primary, as a result of an immunologic event, or secondary to nonspecific tissue injury. In either case, it may aggravate the response and contribute to further tissue injury. O. Jonasson and E. L. Becker showed that the antigen challenge of sensitized guinea pig lung tissue in vitro is associated with the appearance of a kinin-forming enzyme in the perfusate. New methods for more refined assays of kallikrein, bradykinin, and kininogen may at last permit us to determine whether the presence of kinins in anaphylactic reactions is due to a specific immunoglobulin or is secondary.

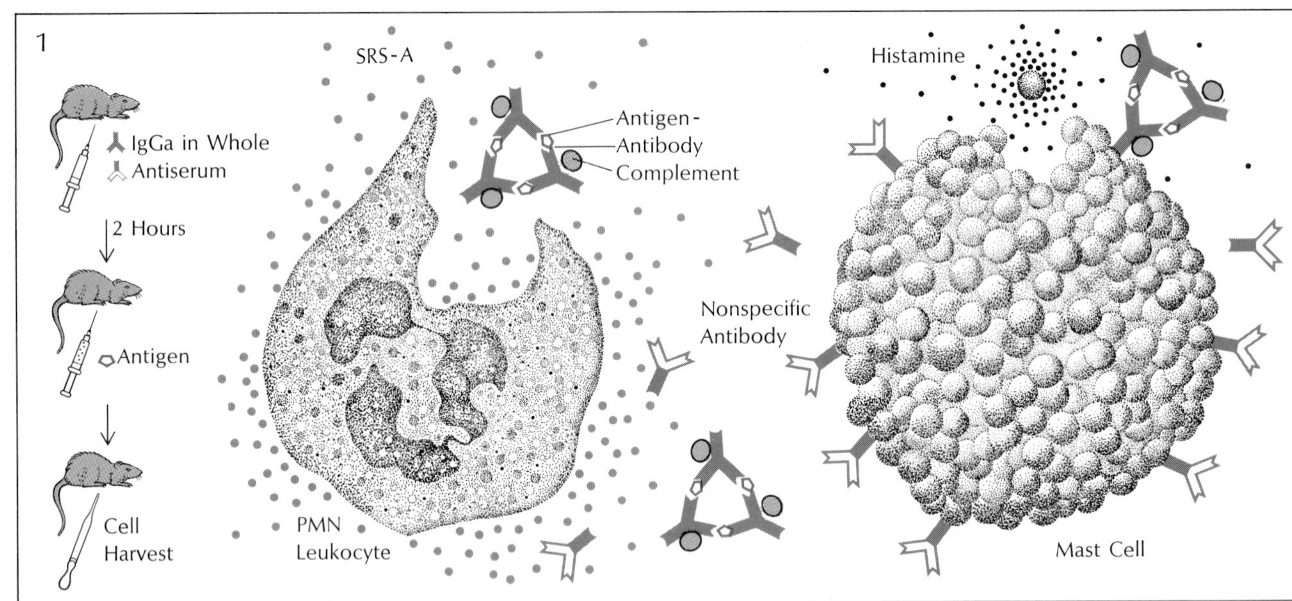

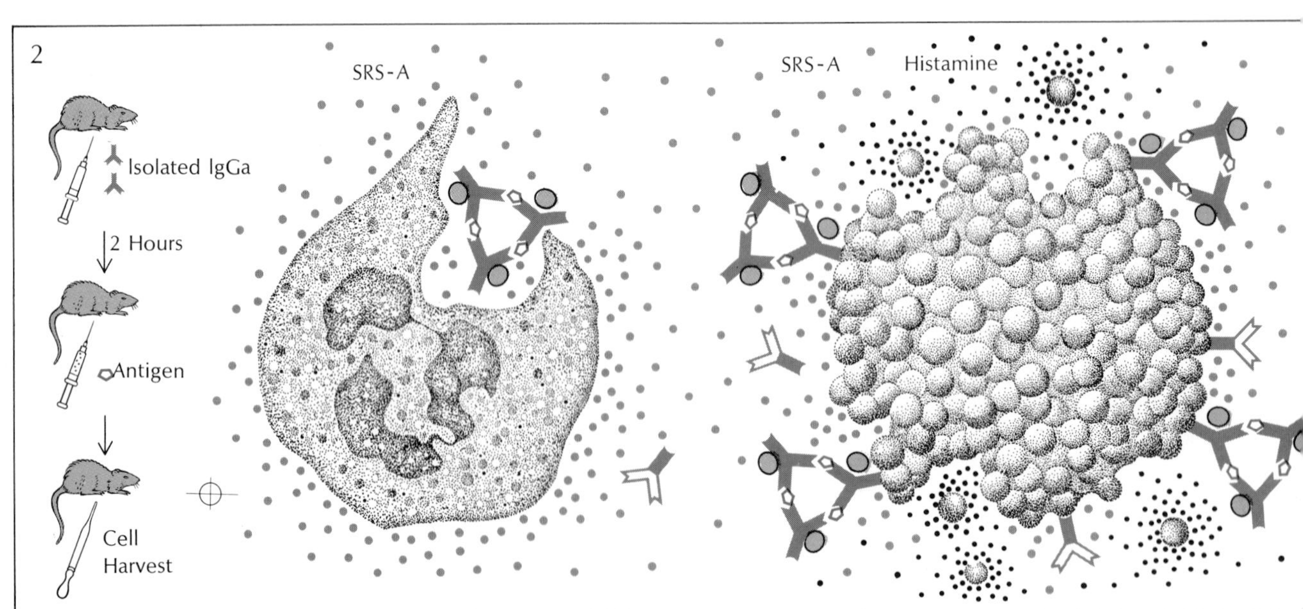

Although two different immunoglobulins, IgGa and IgE, are able to mediate histamine and SRS-A release in the rat peritoneal cavity, the cellular and humoral events involved differ. When whole antiserum is used as a source of IgGa (1), polymorphonuclear leukocytes and an intact serum complement system are required for SRS-A release. Mast cells contribute little to release of histamine or SRS-A, apparently because nonspecific immunoglobulins preempt their receptor sites. However, when the IgGa globulins are isolated by ion exchange chromatography (2), SRS-A release is derived from reactions involving both PMN leukocytes and mast cells, while histamine is mast cell–derived. This pathway appears to be operative only when competition

The precise chemical structure of the acidic lipid SRS-A is unknown. It is distinguished from histamine by its ability to contract the guinea pig ileum in the presence of antihistamines; it is distinguished from bradykinin and serotonin in having no effect on the estrous rat uterus. It is further distinguished from serotonin because its biologic activity is not antagonized by specific serotonin antagonists and because it fails to produce tachyphylaxis when it contracts a smooth-muscle preparation. Further distinction from bradykinin is demonstrated by the failure of SRS-A to be affected by a number of proteolytic enzymes, including chymotrypsin and pronase, which are known to inactivate bradykinin. In having no effect on isolated gerbil colon or estrous rat uterus, SRS-A differs from the available prostaglandins, which are active on such tissues. In addition to differing from all other chemical mediators in terms of its effects on smooth muscle, SRS-A is further differentiated by its permeability-producing activity in the skin of guinea pigs treated with antihistamine and antiserotonin agents.

The potential biologic significance of SRS-A in man derives from three observations: 1) it is released from the lungs of allergic humans on challenge with specific pollen antigen, 2) human bronchiolar smooth muscle is exquisitely sensitive to the contracting activities of SRS-A preparations, and 3) the clinical finding that antihistamines are of rather limited benefit in controlling allergic bronchospasm. The isolation and identification of SRS-A have been facilitated by the recent development of methods for its large-scale production and by the discovery of a simple scheme for maintaining its biologic activity during storage. These two procedures have permitted the further purification of SRS-A by chemical fractionation and thin-layer chromatography, which reveal a mobility distinctly different from that of the available prostaglandins. While SRS-A has been found to be a unique acidic lipid chemical mediator obtainable from a variety of mammalian species as a result of an immunologic event, it has not yet been possible to differentiate among SRS-A obtained from the rat, guinea pig, monkey, and man.

Study of the immunologic mechanisms involved in releasing these chemical mediators is not feasible with actively sensitized animals because the clinical syndrome resulting from antigenic challenge represents a complex response involving a variety of immunoglobulins and sensitized cells. Passive sensitization, however, permits the use of isolated immunoglobulin fractions and allows precise definition of the contribution of the various immunoglobulins. Some years ago B. Benacerraf, Z. Ovary, and associates at New York University demonstrated in vivo that physicochemically different homologous immunoglobulins had distinctly different biologic functions in the guinea pig. They showed that a guinea pig immunoglobulin termed gamma 1 could mediate cutaneous or systemic anaphylactic reactions, but this electrophoretically rapid immunoglobulin did not react with antigen to activate

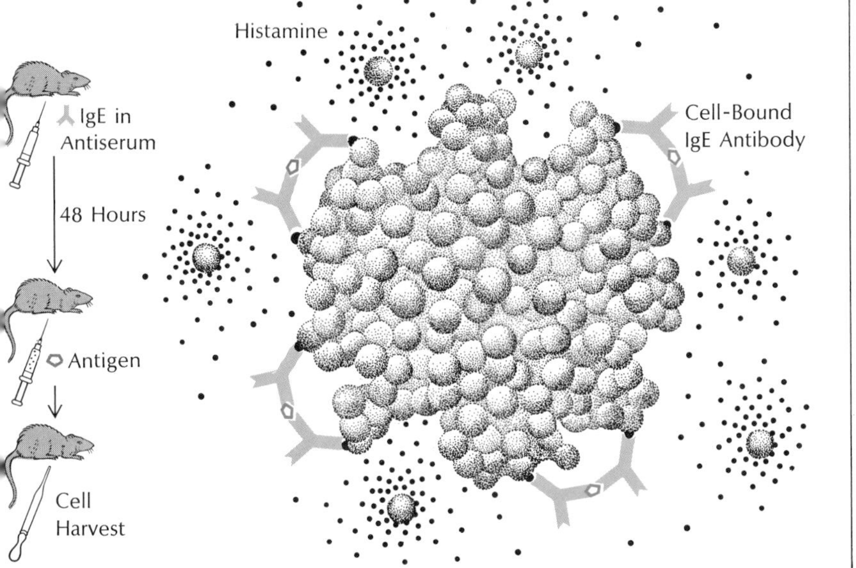

with nonspecific gamma globulin is minimal. Rat IgE antibodies mediate the antigen-induced release of both histamine and SRS-A by mast cells (3) without involvement of complement system, probably by acting as fluid phase antigen-antibody complexes when time between antibody administration and challenge is short. However, when challenge is delayed (4), some IgE molecules become firmly attached to mast cell receptor sites and mediate release of histamine without SRS-A upon exposure to antigen.

the complement system. A second immunoglobulin, gamma 2, with essentially the same molecular weight but slower electrophoretic mobility, did react with antigen to activate complement and mediate the passive Arthus reaction; however, it did not mediate cutaneous or systemic anaphylaxis.

With K. Bloch, who had participated in the early in vivo studies, we confirmed those observations by demonstrating that only gamma 1 antibody and not gamma 2 of the same specificity mediated the release of histamine from guinea pig lung tissue passively sensitized in vitro. Conversely, gamma 2 antibody sensitized an antigen-coated red cell for lysis by complement in vitro while gamma 1 antibody did not. Shortly thereafter, we demonstrated that the gamma 1 antibody of the guinea pig prepared the lung tissue not only for the subsequent antigen-induced release of histamine but also for release of SRS-A. Inasmuch as immediate hypersensitivity appeared to involve a number of distinctly different chemical mediators, it seemed possible that the formation and release of these mediators might also involve distinctly different immunoglobulins or target cells or both. Thus, we directed our efforts toward developing a model system that would allow us to determine the biologic activity of homologous immunoglobulins in terms of capacity to release the various chemical mediators.

Previous in vivo studies of immediate hypersensitivity had been based largely on the lesion of passive cutaneous anaphylaxis (PCA). In an assay extensively employed by Ovary, an antibody is placed in the skin of an animal and the animal is then challenged intravenously with specific antigen. The resulting intracutaneous antigen-antibody reaction results in the discharge of some unknown material that produces a local increase in vascular permeability. A blue dye, injected at the time of antigen challenge, diffuses out of the damaged vasculature and produces a blue spot, the extent and intensity of which permits some quantification of the PCA lesion. While this phenomenon was used to make a number of important observations, it offered no insight into the nature of the mediators involved.

Accordingly, we used a system in which the peritoneal cavity of the rat functions as a sort of in vivo test tube, thus assuring that none of the essential ingredients are absent from the system. In this simple model, the animal receives an intraperitoneal injection of whole antiserum or an immunoglobulin fraction derived therefrom. After an appropriate latent period to permit sensitization, the animal is challenged with specific antigen either intraperitoneally or intravenously. The resulting antigen-antibody reaction in the peritoneal cavity releases the chemical mediators of immediate hypersensitivity. Five minutes after antigen challenge, the peritoneal contents are harvested, the cells sedimented by centrifugation, and the supernatant fluid analyzed for its contents of histamine, serotonin, SRS-A, and bradykinin by bioassay. Histamine is assayed on the isolated guinea pig ileum in the presence of atropine. Serotonin, which is released from rat mast cells in association with histamine, is assayed on the estrous rat uterus as is bradykinin, but the concentration of bradykinin in the peritoneal fluid is low, perhaps because of its rapid degradation in vivo. SRS-A is assayed on guinea pig ileum in the presence of a potent antihistamine.

Studies in our laboratory suggested that such release of SRS-A in rat peritoneum was mediated by a subpopulation, IgGa, of precipitating antibodies present in whole homologous antiserum. Isolated IgGa fractions were also capable of mediating histamine

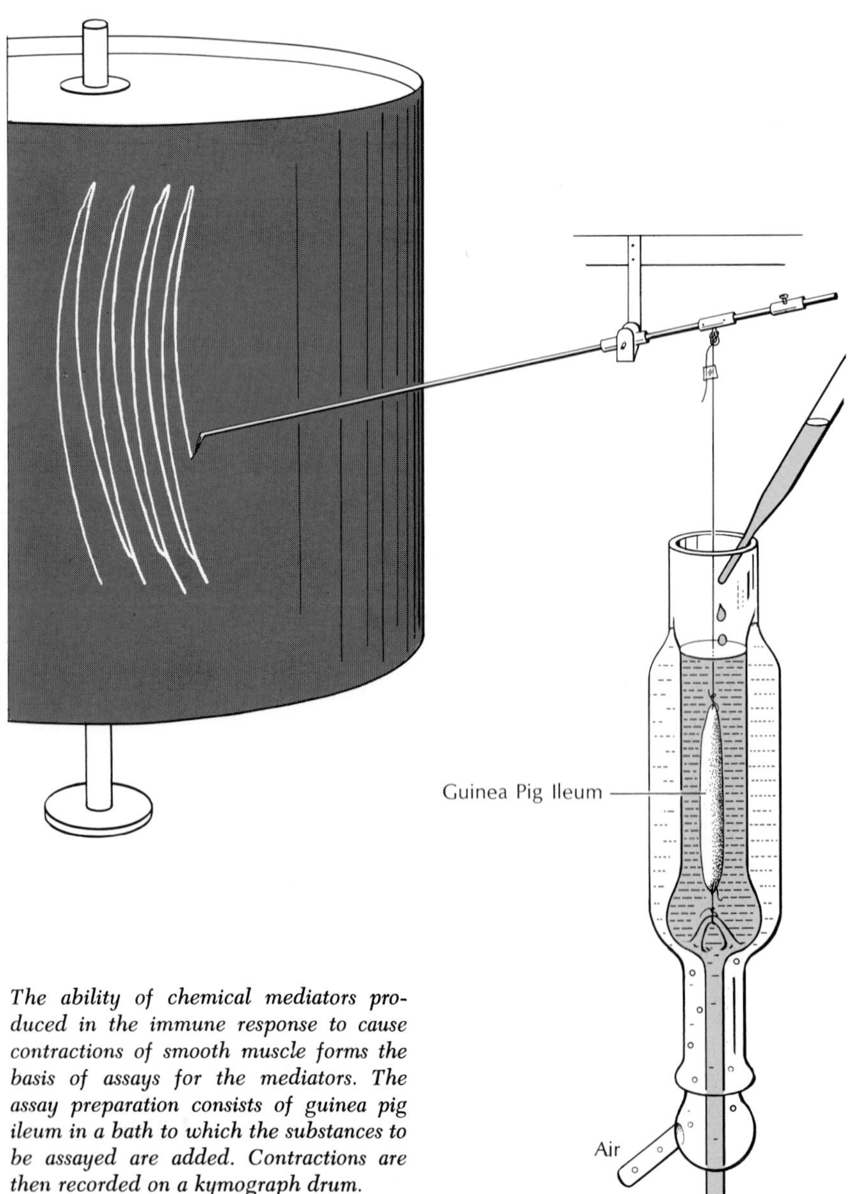

The ability of chemical mediators produced in the immune response to cause contractions of smooth muscle forms the basis of assays for the mediators. The assay preparation consists of guinea pig ileum in a bath to which the substances to be assayed are added. Contractions are then recorded on a kymograph drum.

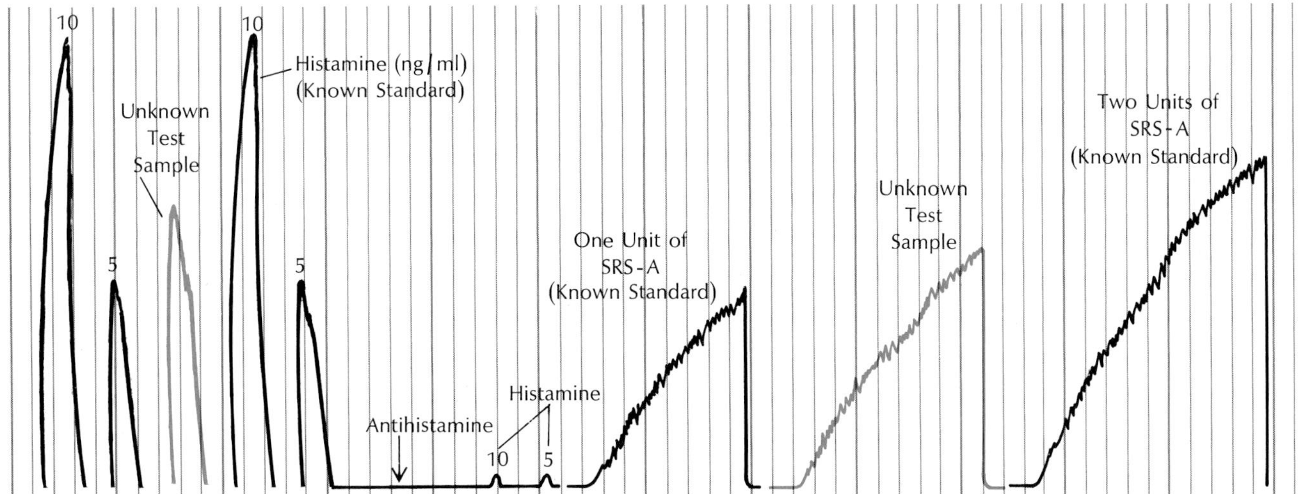

In assaying for SRS-A, contractile activity of an unknown test sample is compared with that of known standards. Antihistamine blocks histamine response; methysergide may be added to block serotonin, chymotrypsin to abolish kinin-like activity. SRS-A-mediated contraction ensues after brief latent period. In this illustration, the unknown is bracketed between known amounts of histamine and SRS-A. Value obtained times reciprocal of dilution yields concentrations of mediators per ml in the unknown.

release. IgGa was characterized as a 7S immunoglobulin of slow electrophoretic mobility, insensitive to treatment with mercaptoethanol or heat, and capable of fixing complement. A second homologous but heat labile immunoglobulin, IgE, analogous to human reagin, also mediated the antigen-induced release of SRS-A and histamine. It is differentiated from rat IgGa not only by its heat lability but also by mercaptoethanol sensitivity, inability to fix complement, fast electrophoretic mobility and an approximate molecular size of 8S. The immunologic release of SRS-A mediated by the IgGa antibodies in whole serum requires the presence of the polymorphonuclear leukocyte and an intact serum complement system (see illustrations on pages 116-117). However, when the IgGa antibodies are isolated by ion exchange chromatography they may mediate the release of SRS-A and also histamine through an immunologic pathway involving the mast cell. This latter pathway occurs only when competition by nonspecific gamma globulin of the same class is minimal. Rat IgE antibodies interact with rat peritoneal mast cells to mediate the antigen-induced release of histamine, a reaction that does not require serum complement. With short sensitization periods, rat IgE also prepares the peritoneal cavity for the complement-independent, mast cell-dependent release of SRS-A. Thus, two physicochemically distinct homologous immunoglobulins are capable of mediating the intraperitoneal release of histamine and SRS-A in the rat, but the cellular and humoral prerequisites for these reactions are quite distinct.

Our model, permitting quantification of the in vivo immunologic release of the chemical mediators, also made possible a study of agents that might selectively block these reactions. Attention was directed to the antifilarial agent diethylcarbamazine by M. S. Mallen, who observed a reduction in severity of concomitant asthma in some of his patients when filariasis was treated with that drug. When he administered the antifilarial to patients who had asthma but not filariasis, he again observed some clinical improvement. In our laboratory, the drug proved to be an active inhibitor of immunologic release of SRS-A in the rat, without being an end-organ antagonist of SRS-A. Its action was unique in that it occurred after antigen-antibody interaction and prior to formation and release of SRS-A, thereby permitting desensitization of tissues without inflammatory response. Studies of the essential structures required for inhibition established that the carboxamide side chain was essential for optimal inhibitory activity. The piperazine-ring structure could be modified by employing either a pyridine or piperidine ring without loss of inhibitory activity provided the carboxamide side chain was intact. Diethylcarbamazine is metabolized by the rat at a rate of 100 mg/kg/hr and its LD_{50} is 150 mg/kg. The dose that reliably gave 50% inhibition of SRS-A release was 20 mg/kg administered five seconds to five minutes before antigenic challenge. An inhibitory concentration was no longer present after five minutes because of the rapid metabolism of the drug. Therefore, structural modification of the molecule permitting a longer half-life must be accomplished before this agent can be used in other model systems or clinically.

A second agent receiving much clinical attention at the present time is disodium cromoglycate. An allergen-sensitive British clinical pharmacologist, Roger A. Altounyan, troubled by the lack of a useful pharmacologic agent for treating bronchial asthma, decided to test in himself various materials that might block histamine or SRS-A release by mechanisms other than the specific end-organ antagonism of histamine. Challenging himself with methacholine, histamine, and antigen, he observed that khellin protected him against antigen challenge but not against histamine or methacholine. He then persuaded his colleagues in chemistry to synthesize structurally related compounds. As a result, disodium cromoglycate was developed and shown to be effective against aerosol challenge tests in man. In vitro studies have been difficult to interpret because the dose response for inhibition is not lin-

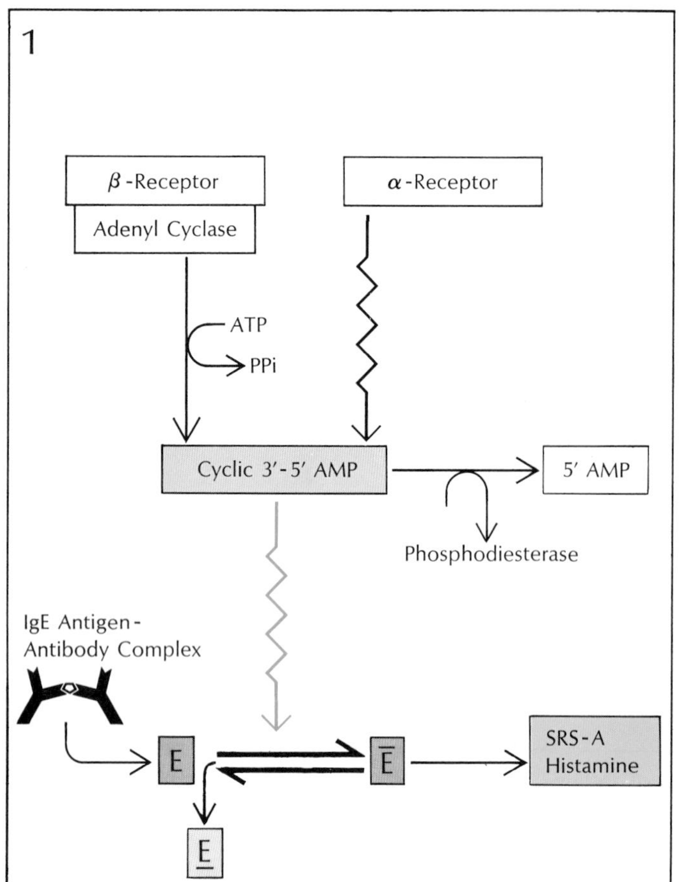

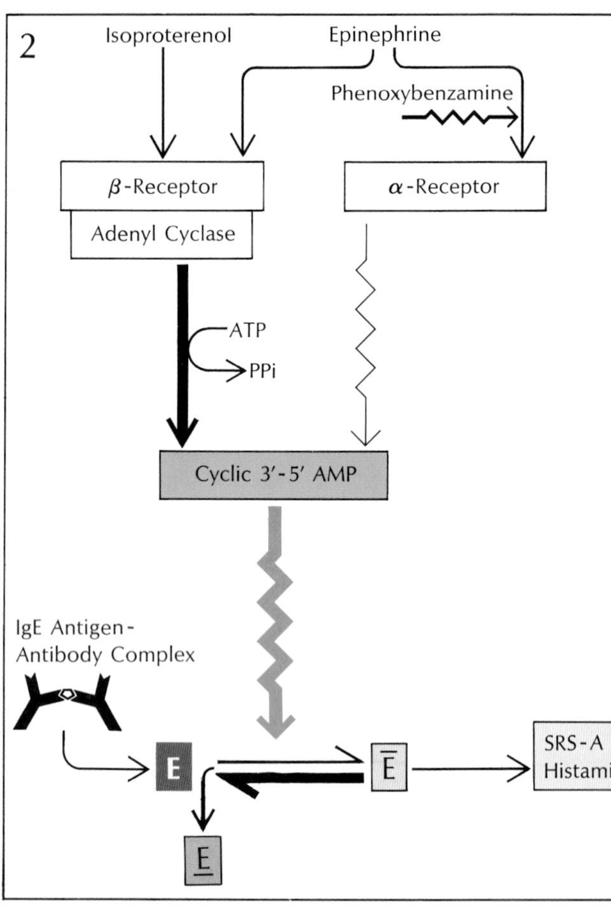

IgE antibody interacts with specific antigen (1) to activate a reaction sequence, presumably enzymatic, represented as $E \rightleftharpoons \bar{E}$, leading to the release of histamine and formation and release of SRS-A. Certain steps in this reaction sequence may also decay to nonactivatable products, $\underline{E}$. The reaction sequence appears to be modulated by the cellular level of cyclic-AMP. Beta-adrenergic stimulation (2) by agents such as isoproterenol or epinephrine, which interact with the β receptor in tissues to activate membrane-bound adenyl cyclase and increase the synthesis of cyclic-AMP, results in an increase in cellular cyclic-AMP and

ear. When the rat intraperitoneal test system was used, disodium cromoglycate was found to block the immunologic release of histamine mediated either by heat-labile homocytotropic antibody or by heat-stable IgGa, but against SRS-A release it was effective only when the IgE antibody was used. The concentration of disodium cromoglycate required to inhibit the PCA lesion was much greater than that effective against histamine release from peritoneal cells, an observation consistent with current clinical use of the drug as an aerosol preparation for prophylaxis and treatment of allergic asthma. The point should not be missed that these two simple chemical agents act after antigen-antibody interaction and before release of mediators, thereby permitting tissue desensitization without inflammation.

In collaboration with K. and T. Ishizaka, we have shown that monkey lung fragments sensitized with IgE-rich human serum from ragweed-sensitive individuals and challenged with specific ragweed antigen release histamine and SRS-A. The antibody mediating the direct release of both substances was identified as IgE by showing that specific removal of IgE with an immunosorbent prevented release of both mediators. Furthermore, in a reverse release experiment, monkey lung sensitized with IgE-rich human serum or the Fc fragment of an IgE myeloma released histamine and SRS-A with anti-IgE but not anti-IgG, anti-IgA, anti-IgD, or anti-IgM. The collaboration is continuing and has revealed that diethylcarbamazine will block the pathways to the release of histamine and SRS-A. The system is also being used to search for a heat-stable human antibody that might be the counterpart of gamma 1 in the guinea pig and IgGa in the rat.

The studies of E. S. K. Assem and H. O. Schild and of L. M. Lichtenstein have suggested that β-adrenergic agents inhibit the IgE-mediated release of histamine from human lung and peripheral leukocytes, respectively. In collaboration with K. and T. Ishizaka, we have extended these studies using monkey lung fragments sensitized in vitro with human atopic serum and challenged with the ragweed extract, antigen E. Four lines of evidence indicate that agents capable of increasing the intracellular level of cyclic adenosine-3′5′-monophosphate (cyclic-AMP) also inhibit the release of histamine and SRS-A from primate lung. β-adrenergic agents such as isoproterenol capable of activating membrane-bound adenyl cyclase inhibit the release of histamine and SRS-A. Methylxanthine derivatives such as theophylline, which block the phosphodiesterase-mediated catabolism of cyclic-AMP, are inhibitory. A marked synergism between β-adrenergic agents and the methylxanthines is ob-

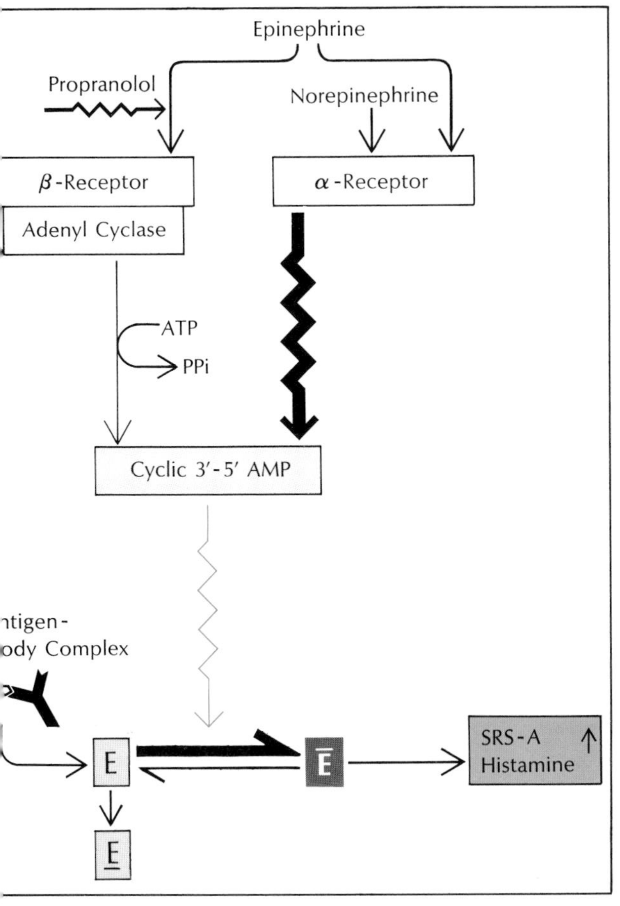

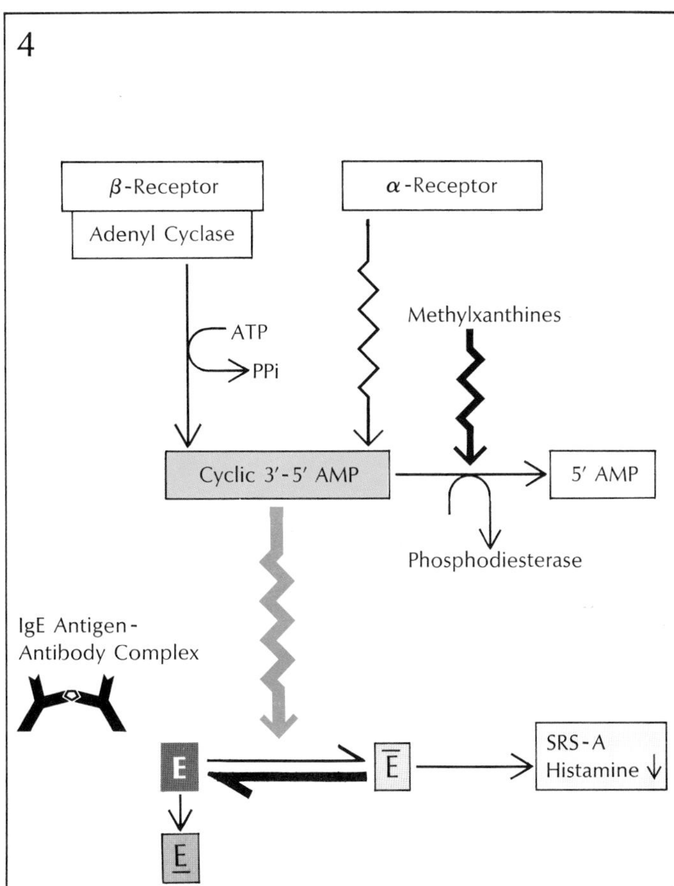

inhibition of the release of histamine and SRS-A. The β-adrenergic activity of epinephrine is enhanced by blockade of its α-adrenergic activity with phenoxybenzamine. Alpha-adrenergic stimulation (3) with norepinephrine, or epinephrine in the presence of the β-adrenergic blocking agent propranolol, results in a decrease in tissue cyclic-AMP levels and an increased release of the mediators. Cyclic-AMP is normally broken down to 5′-AMP by a cytoplasmic phosphodiesterase. When the phosphodiesterase is inhibited by a methylxanthine (4), the level of cyclic-AMP increases and inhibition of the immunologic pathway is observed.

served. Finally, an alkylated derivative of cyclic-AMP itself (dibutyryl cyclic-AMP) inhibits the IgE-mediated release of histamine and SRS-A from primate lung. Our laboratory, too, has observed the modulating effect of cyclic-AMP on the IgE- and IgGa-mediated release of SRS-A but not histamine in the rat.

The enormous complexity of immediate-type hypersensitivity may be explained by its origin in an immunologic event, involving many or all of the mediators of acute inflammatory response – amines, peptides, and acidic lipids. Local change in vascular permeability due to release of factors from cells may also result in the accumulation of non-tissue-fixing immunoglobulins that in turn may react with antigens to activate entirely humoral mediator systems such as serum complement. Such complexity need not be discouraging. If immediate hypersensitivity does indeed involve various immunoglobulin classes, different cell types, and a diverse group of chemical mediators, then we must look to effective management of the phenomenon through the development of selective blocking agents. Diethylcarbamazine and disodium cromoglycate are early examples of such agents. The systems now exist that permit the selection of other and perhaps more effective agents, acting alone or in combination, for the drug control of immediate hypersensitive clinical conditions in man.

Chapter 13

Immunologic Unresponsiveness

WILLIAM O. WEIGLE
Scripps Clinic and Research Foundation

Discussion of immunologic unresponsiveness, or tolerance, may conveniently be initiated by the introduction and definition of the word "tolerogen."

A tolerogen is an antigen existing in a form or under conditions that induce the immune mechanisms of an organism to be unresponsive to itself. It is the counterpart of the term immunogen, the form of antigen that stimulates the immune mechanisms to produce antibody or to commit leukocytes against itself.

By starting from these definitions, we focus on two key facts about immunologic unresponsiveness: 1) it is a distinct phenomenon, and not simply an absence of response; 2) it is specific to the antigen (tolerogen) that induces it, even as immunologic responsiveness is specific to the antigen (immunogen) evoking it.

In this context, understanding of immunologic unresponsiveness demands knowledge of those factors that cause antigen to turn off, rather than turn on, immunoresponsive mechanisms. We know that these factors must operate in order to provide for the organism's recognition of its own antigenic determinants as "self," and that they must break down to precipitate autoimmune disease and, quite possibly, malignant disease. And we have learned that certain maneuvers can be employed to induce immunologic unresponsiveness in both newborn and adult animals. Before pinpointing the conditions leading to tolerance, however, it is important to define as far as possible the elements participating in the immune response to an antigen, particularly the cellular populations involved.

At least two different cell populations are actively involved in responding to antigen. One, derived from bone marrow, consists of the actual antibody-producing cells and their precursors; the other consists of thymus-derived cells. These cells migrate from the thymus and bone marrow to lymphoid tissues. In addition, macrophages seem to play an important part, in at least some immunologic reactions, as nonspecific "handlers" of antigen. It should be stressed that in specifying the two cell populations involved in immunologic reactions, we are not differentiating between the humoral antibody response mechanisms and the cellular immune response mechanisms. Rather, we are talking about a synergistic activity of the two cell populations required for the production of antibody.

There is abundant evidence that such synergism takes place in the spleen and other lymphoid tissues. There is evidence also that both types of cell have specific receptor sites for antigen so that both must react with antigen in some way before the bone marrow cells are stimulated to proliferate, differentiate, and produce antibody. Why the bone marrow cell must interact with the thymus-derived cell is not known.

Numerous experiments have documented this need for two cellular populations to interact. For example, experiments undertaken by Claman and his collaborators and by Miller et al. have shown that when mice were rendered immunologically unresponsive by whole-body irradiation, restoration of the responsiveness to a specific antigen – sheep red blood cells – could be achieved only by injecting them with both bone marrow and thymus cells from animals able to respond to the antigen.

In our own laboratory, a similar collaborative effect between bone marrow and thymus cells has been shown to be involved in the immunologic responses to aggregated human gamma globulin (HGG). Inbred mice were made unresponsive to this antigen by its injection in a tolerogenic (deaggregated) form. Such specifically tolerant animals were then used as donors of bone marrow and thymus cells in combinations with normal syngeneic animals. The recipients were all irradiated to eliminate their own immunoresponsive cell populations. They were found able to make antibody responses to aggregated HGG only when bone marrow and thymus cell injections consisted of cells derived from normal animals. When the attempt to reconstitute specific response involved either cell type from tolerant donors, no immune response to the HGG was elicited.

Dr. Weigle is in the department of experimental pathology, Scripps Clinic and Research Foundation, La Jolla, Calif.

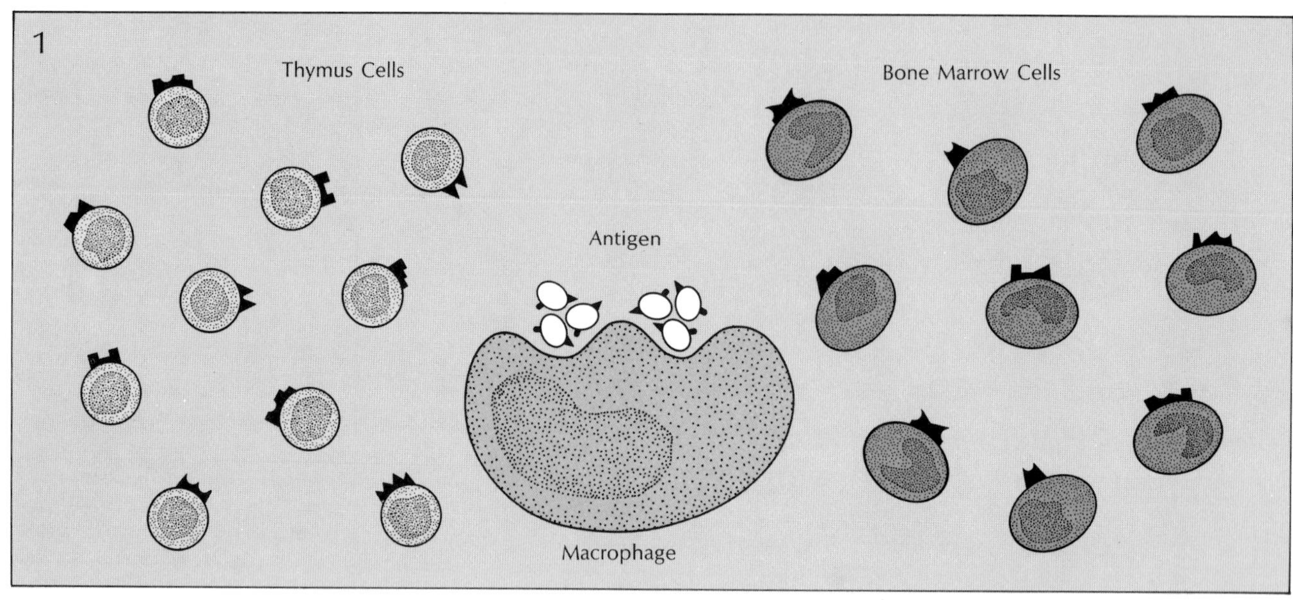

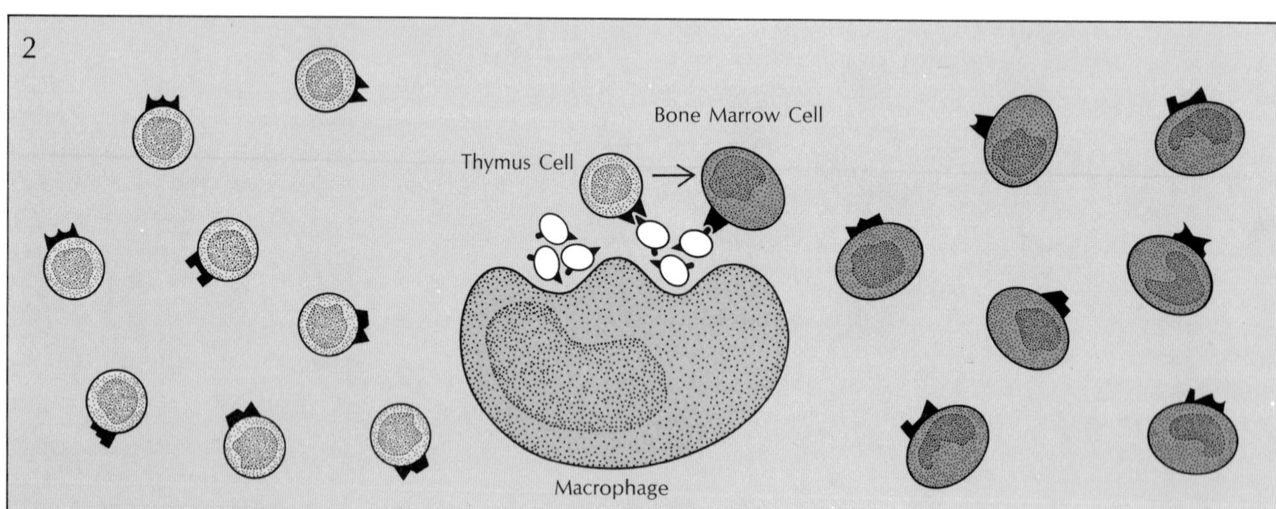

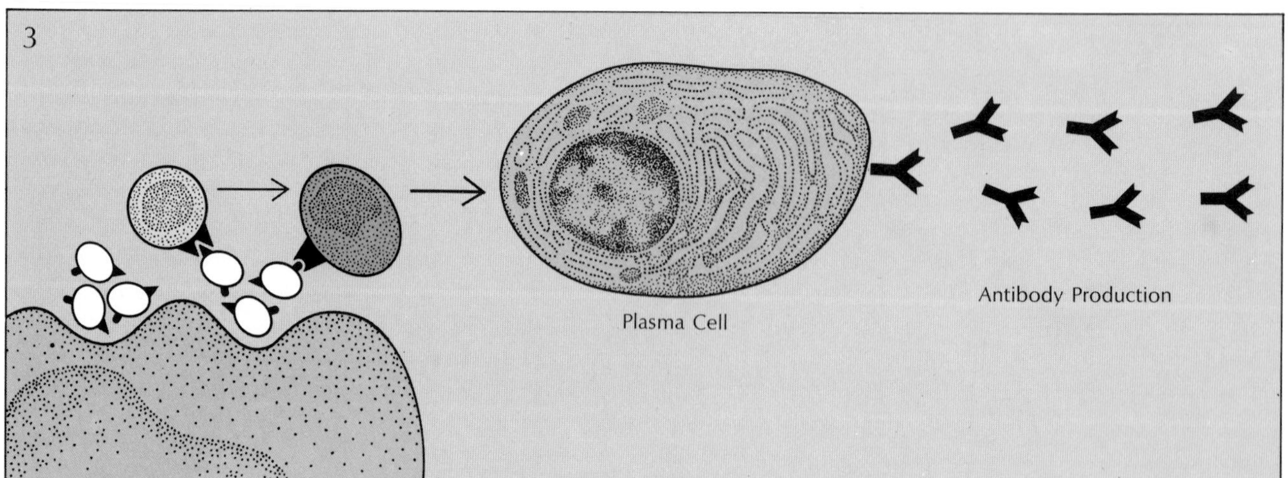

Thymus-derived and bone marrow cells interact synergistically in the development of an antibody response. As schematized above, the macrophages first fix antigen on their surface membranes (1). Specifically committed cells of both lymphoid populations then attach to different determinants of the aggregated antigen. As a result of this interaction with antigen, the bone marrow and thymic cells are brought into close proximity for a sufficient period of time to permit passage of information from the thymic to the bone marrow cell (2). This interaction provides a signal to the bone marrow cell, probably in the form of a change in surface membrane configuration. In response to this signal, the synthetic mechanisms of the marrow cell are activated, and the cell differentiates and proliferates into plasma cells that elaborate the specific antibodies (3).

The obvious implication of these and similar experiments is that immunologic unresponsiveness is created by unresponsiveness in either of the two cell types required to mount an antibody response. However, it should be noted that in most situations in which unresponsiveness pertains, most notably our normal unresponsiveness to self antigens, all evidence shows that both cell types are unresponsive. But this is not always so. We now believe that the occurrence of certain autoimmune diseases is limited to situations in which the individual has been living with only one cell type unresponsive. Thus, when this tolerance breaks down, that individual becomes immunologically responsive to a self antigen.

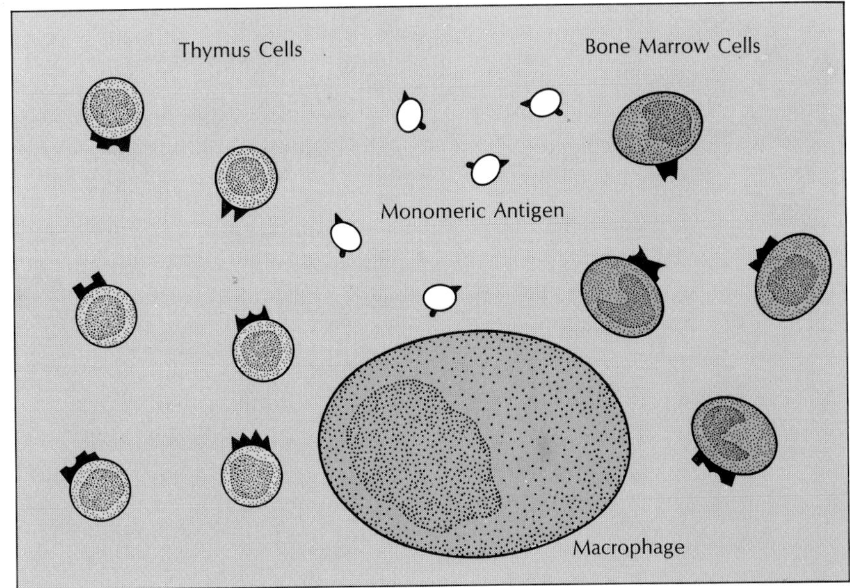

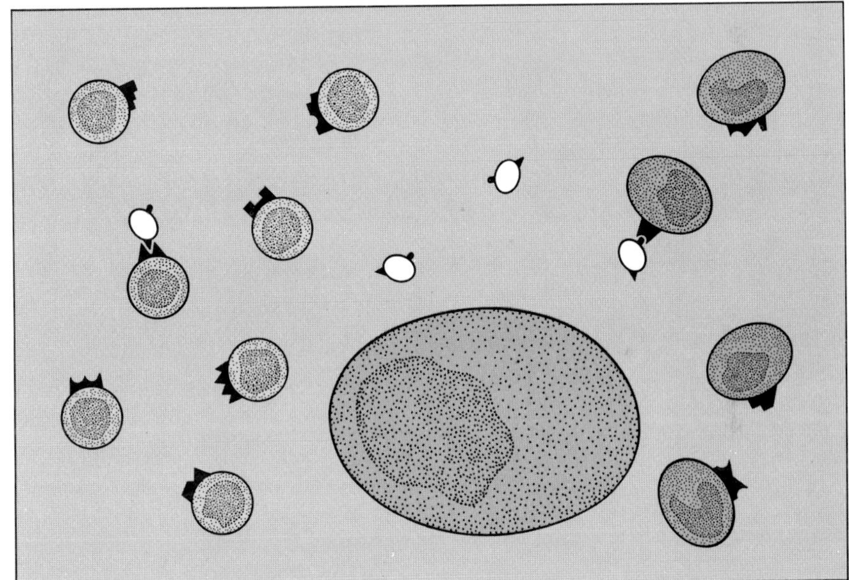

Monomeric or deaggregated forms of antigen have been shown to be tolerogenic. An important clue to the mechanisms involved has been derived from studies showing that monomers are not fixed by macrophages (top). For this reason, although both bone marrow and thymus-derived cells can complex with monomeric antigen, the two cell types are not brought into the proximity required for synergistic interaction. Not only does this preclude the production of antibody but those cells capable of reacting to a specific antigen, having reacted to the tolerogen, will not subsequently react upon exposure to aggregated or other immunogenic forms of the antigen.

Recent experiments with Chiller and Habicht tend to support this hypothesis and to elucidate certain cellular kinetic patterns that appear relevant to understanding the pathogenesis of autoimmunity. Groups of mice were made tolerant to HGG by the injection of deaggregated antigen. Suspensions of thymus cells and of bone marrow cells were then transferred from these tolerant animals to previously irradiated syngeneic recipients. The irradiated mice were challenged with immunogenic (aggregated) HGG on days 0 and 9. On day 14, the spleens of the recipient animals were assayed for plaque-forming (immunoresponsive) cells to HGG. It was found that the thymus cells from the tolerogen-treated animals were essentially nonresponsive from day 2 after challenge and remained unresponsive for the duration of the experiment, 100 days. Bone marrow cells, on the other hand, remained responsive for 11 days, then began to lose their responsivity, becoming completely tolerant by day 21. Thereafter, there was a progressive resumption of responsivity so that by day 100, the bone marrow cells had regained full responsivity to HGG.

Thus, a clear dichotomy in the kinetic behavior of the two immunocompetent cell populations was demonstrated, with thymus-derived cells becoming unresponsive sooner and remaining so much longer than bone marrow cells. Additional experiments showed that the tolerogenic dose response curves of the two cell populations also varied. When three different dose levels of deaggregated HGG were employed – 0.1, 0.5, 2.5 mg – there was no difference in that all induced total unresponsivity in thymus cells. But there was a direct relationship between dose and degree of unresponsivity in the bone marrow cells, with only 9% becoming unresponsive with the small dose, 56% with the intermediate, 70% with the large dose.

The results of these experiments are consistent with the possibility that, while in most cases tolerance to self antigens involves both thymus and bone marrow cells, there could be situations in which tolerance is actually induced to only one type, most likely the thymic cells; or if induced to both types, it may be maintained to only one type, again the thymic. It is known that autoimmune disease most often involves the type of semisequestered antigen that circulates in the body in extremely small quantities, so that the dose-tolerance relationships observed in the experiments just described may well be pertinent to the question of why tolerance is only partial and therefore breakable. We leave a fuller discussion of this until later in this presentation when we shall attempt to put the clinical problems of autoimmunity into the context of our experimental knowledge of immunologic unresponsiveness.

The involvement of both the bone marrow and thymus-derived cells in immune response is a specific one. That is to say, only a limited number of either type of cells are capable of reacting with a specific antigen. The role of the macrophage, on the other hand, is nonspecific. Nor, as a matter of fact, is this role as firmly documented as that of the other cell types, and it is probable that macrophages participate in some but not all immunologic reactions. The most plausible hypothesis for its role is that the macrophage either alters the antigen in a particular way to make it available for the specifically reactive cells or that it fixes the antigen on its surface for the same purpose. Perhaps it provides a surface to which antigen is attached and on which the bone marrow and thymus-derived cells are held in close proximity for a long enough time to permit whatever interaction is required between the two specific cell types. This interaction would be a signal for the bone marrow cell to initiate the proliferation and differentiation needed for the production of antibody.

From a chronologic standpoint, the sequence may start with the macrophage interacting with and fixing the antigen upon its surface. In this process, certain of the antigenic determinants effectively become sites upon the macrophage membrane. The thymus-derived and bone marrow cells, which are biologically precommitted to react with these antigenic determinants, can then get to them. The result is a fixed cellular aggregation that permits the cells to interact for the time required to initiate the biosynthetic mechanisms needed for antibody production, a situation that would not pertain if the antigens were moving freely through the circulation. Although the nature of the synergistic action among the cells is not fully understood, it seems likely that it involves a change in surface membranes and a consequent perception of a signal for DNA synthesis.

With this sequence, two different directions might be followed. If the contact with antigen is sufficient, i.e., if the concentration of antigen is great enough and maintained for a sufficiently long period, then the precursor cells could differentiate into antibody-forming cells and actually produce antibody. With shorter periods of contact or lesser concentrations of antigen, the process might be less complete but nevertheless sufficient for the antibody-cell precursors to be

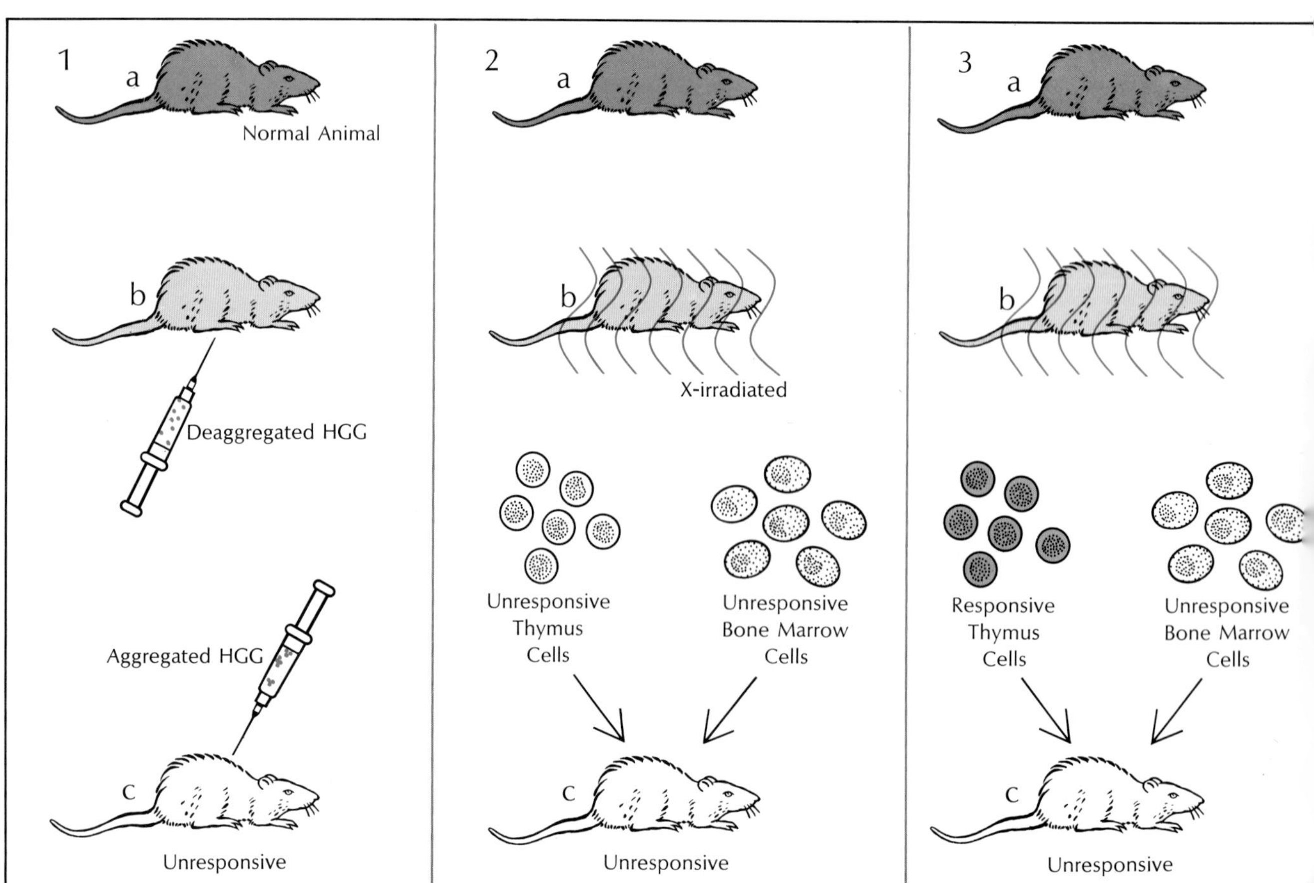

To demonstrate experimentally that specific immunologic unresponsiveness is maintained unless both responsive bone marrow and thymic cells are present, inbred mice are injected with tolerogenic (deaggregated) human gamma globulin and are then unresponsive to aggregated HGG (1). When mice are irradiated to destroy their own lymphoid cell populations, they remain unre-

committed as memory cells for the involved antigen. And, of course, subsequent contact with the antigen would once again turn on the committed cells, this time to complete antibody production via the anamnestic response.

This construction of events therefore suggests an explanation for both the primary immunologic response as mediated by humoral antibodies and for secondary or memory responses. It also, when viewed from a different perspective, serves to indicate a possible point of confluence and departure for humoral antibody and cellular hypersensitivity responses. It should be remembered that any antigenic molecule has multiple, differing antigenic determinants. Thus, a simple serum protein may have as many as 30 determinants, each totally different from all others. We believe that in any particular reaction, the determinant or determinants that react with the bone marrow cell are different from those that react with the thymus-derived cell. If humoral antibody is to be elicited, then it will have to be in response to the determinant(s) that react with the bone marrow cell. On the other hand, for the immunologic response to be directed toward delayed hypersensitivity, the determinants would have to interact with the thymus-derived cell. Nor is it excluded that both reactions could take place either simultaneously or sequentially. Indeed, there are many bacterial and other antigens known to be capable of inciting both humoral antibody and delayed hypersensitivity or cellular antibody responses.

It may appear that the discussion has digressed considerably from the subject of this paper, immunologic unresponsiveness. It is not a true digression, however, since the mechanisms of immune response are essentially variations of the mechanisms of immunologic nonresponse. The basic factors that separate immunocompetence from tolerance reside for the most part in the inciting antigen.

Historically, the study of immunologic unresponsiveness can be dated from Burnet's prediction that specific unresponsiveness would result from the injection of antigenic material early in life. This prediction was then given reality by Billingham, Brent, and Medawar with their demonstration that mice could be made tolerant to histocompatibility antigens by injection of replicating allogeneic cells during neonatal life. Those classic experiments, of course, opened the broad highway leading to clinical transplantation. They also had the effect of defining the first set of conditions under which exposure to antigen would lead to immunologic nonresponse rather than to immunologic response. The governing condition, in this case, was the immunologic immaturity of the recipient animals. Subsequent work has demonstrated that this is but one of several sets of circumstances fulfilling the generalization that an unresponsive state to subsequent injections of an antigen will usually ensue when the initial exposure occurs under conditions that obviate the development of an immune response. Irradiation, administration of immunosuppressive drugs, administration of antilymphocytic sera, and manipulation of the antigen have all been employed to provide temporary failure of immune responsivity so that the administered antigen acts as a tolerogen rather than as an immunogen.

Of these approaches, the one that is in many ways the most intriguing and from which the most has been learned about the mechanisms of unresponsivity is manipulation of the antigen. Many of the experiments in this regard have been performed with heterologous serum proteins, which have a number of attributes making them particularly suitable for the induction of immunologic unresponsiveness. These properties include a relatively simple molecular structure and a diminished immunogenicity in comparison with other antigens. They can be obtained relatively pure in large quantities. Significantly, the serum proteins are soluble, they rapidly equilibrate between intra- and extravascular spaces, and they persist in the circulation.

Enumeration of these properties here is not intended to document the

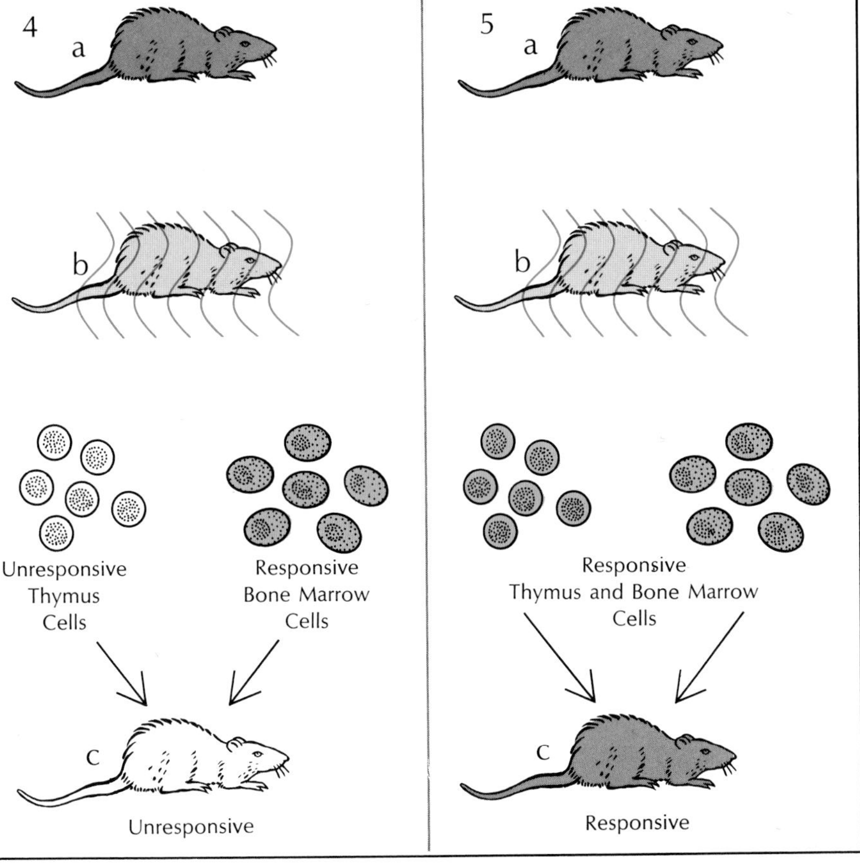

sponsive to aggregated HGG after injection of two unresponsive cell populations (2) or of one responsive and one unresponsive cell population (3, 4). Only with both bone marrow and thymic cells from responsive donors will the animal respond (5).

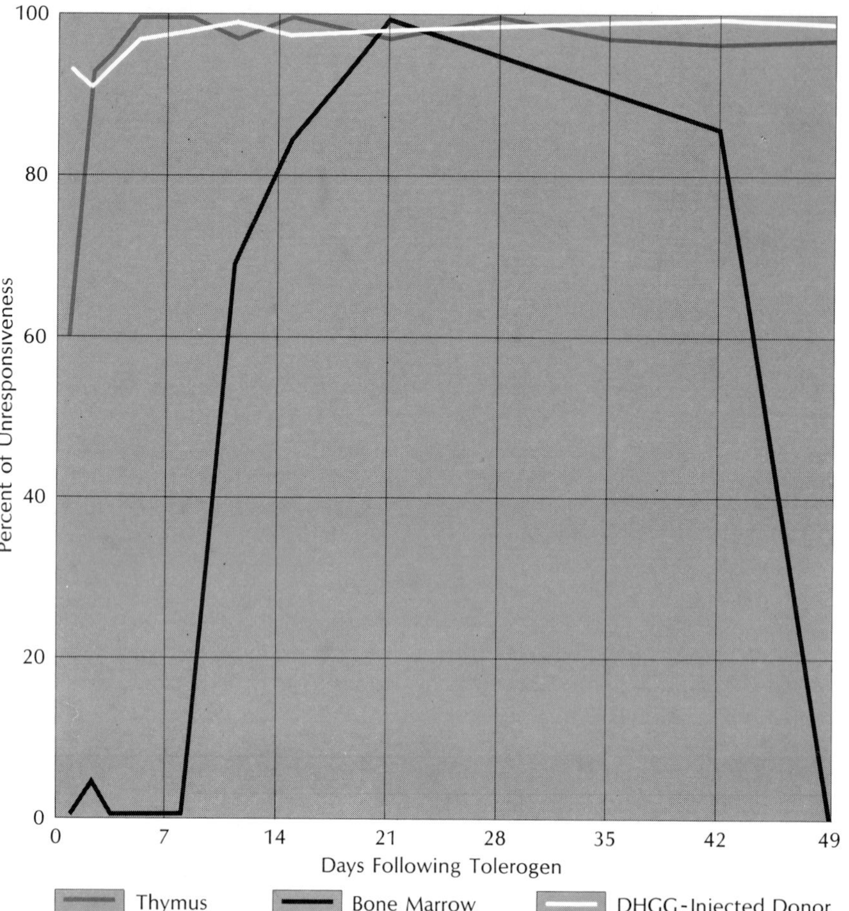

Mice injected with deaggregated HGG (white line) remain unresponsive to aggregated HGG with respect to their marrow and thymic cells. When such cells are injected into irradiated animals in combination with normal cells, it is found that marrow cells become unresponsive later and return to responsiveness sooner than thymic cells.

validity of the choice of investigators in using these antigens to study immunologic unresponsiveness. Actually, the characteristics that make them suitable are also clues to many of the mechanisms involved in tolerance. Thus their solubility, the ability to reach both intra- and extravascular sites and to persist all add up to an ability to reach all antigen-reactive cells in effective concentrations; all relate to the previously stated generalization that unresponsiveness is achieved when exposure to the antigen initially occurs under conditions in which antibody response is inhibited.

One cannot achieve unresponsiveness if only a part of the cell populations capable of making antibody encounters antigen under conditions of tolerogenesis. This explains why, for the most part, it is much more difficult to achieve immunologic unresponsiveness with microbial and viral antigens or with heterologous erythrocytes, which neither persist in the circulation nor readily equilibrate into the extravascular spaces. Such antigens probably do not come into contact with all of the antigen-reactive cells in effective concentrations. In addition, these antigens are usually quite complex, containing many different antigenic determinants so that unresponsiveness may be induced to some but not all determinants present.

Tolerance to Small and Large Doses of Antigen

Just as the distribution pattern of the antigen affects its ability to create an unresponsive state, so does the dose of antigen used. The concept that a massive antigen dose can cause "immune paralysis" has been widely discussed, particularly in relationship to organ homografts and second grafts transplanted after the rejection of initial grafts. The original experiments related to this phenomenon were performed here at the Scripps Clinic by Dixon. He employed extremely large doses of serum protein (1 gm/day), which, as has been noted, persisted in the circulation for long periods of time. And the recipient animals did indeed become unresponsive to these antigens. However, these experiments raised a key question: Were these animals really becoming tolerant or was the amount of antigen given so large that it was continually neutralizing the antibody being produced before it could be detected?

Recent experiments in our laboratory, in which we directly observed antibody production by cells, rather than depending on detection of the antibody in serum, have shown that when these animals are first given very large doses of antigen they make an extremely good antibody response. This response first rises very sharply and then disappears. Additional injections of antigen will not result in antibody production, and one now sees a prolonged state of immunologic unresponsiveness.

These results can be interpreted in the light of the previously noted relationship between antigen concentration and the development of antibody-producing and memory cells. What appears to be happening is an exhaustive differentiation of cells. At very high levels of antigen concentration, all of the antibody-producing cells are being activated to produce antibody. None of the exposures are in the intermediate range calculated to direct a portion of the immunocompetent cells toward becoming memory cells. No precursor cells capable of responding to the specific antigen remain, and a true unresponsiveness is induced.

It may be noted, almost parenthetically, that some investigators have suggested that in addition to this clearly established high-dose tolerance there is also a phenomenon of low-dose tolerance. This would be unresponsiveness induced in some way by extremely low doses of antigen. We have not been able to demonstrate such a phenomenon in the systems we employ and, on theoretical grounds, tend to doubt its importance in induction of tolerance. Rather, we believe that so-called low-dose tolerance occurs because the inciting antigenic stimulus is provided by a combination of immunogenic and tolerogenic materials and, under certain conditions, the tolerogenic forms may successfully compete with the immunogens.

From the previous discussion, it is obvious that under certain circumstances the induction of unresponsiveness is dependent upon the status of the host. Thus, the newborn animal becomes unresponsive to an antigen because his potential antibody-producing cells are exposed to and interact with that antigen before they have matured to a state of competence to make antibody. Similarly, when irradiation or immunosuppression is employed to induce specific unresponsiveness, one is taking advantage of a temporary inability of the immunocompetent cells to respond to interaction with antigen by producing antibody. There is, however, another means of inducing tolerance in adults, one dependent entirely on manipulating the antigen. This technique involves the centrifuging of the antigen so that it is presented to the recipient entirely in monomeric or deaggregated forms.

Monomeric Antigen

Monomeric antigen is as fully able to interact with bone marrow and thymus-derived cells as is the usual aggregated or polymeric antigen. However, the interaction will be tolerogenic rather than immunogenic and no antibody production will result. The explanation for this is still somewhat hypothetical, but there is evidence that permits the presentation of this hypothesis with some degree of confidence. A major clue is the demonstrated inability of macrophages to fix monomeric antigen. It seems likely that for essentially steric reasons, the monomer is unable to "bridge" the gaps among bone marrow cells, thymus-derived cells, and macrophages. The configuration necessary for exchange of the information directing antibody synthesis is thereby prevented from developing. In the absence of the clustering of cells required for initiating antibody production, the antigen removes or inhibits those cells able to react with it from the pool of immunoresponsive cell populations. The result is that subsequent exposures to immunogenic forms of that antigen will not be met with any response.

Although, for the most part, this approach to the induction of immunologic unresponsiveness – using monomeric forms of the antigen – has been employed as an experimental tool, the technique has some obvious clinical possibilities. One such would be the development of an antilymphocytic serum (ALS) or antilymphocytic globulin (ALG) that is itself nonimmunogenic. In using ALS or ALG to depress immune response to histocompatibility antigens, as is being done in organ transplantation, one of the major problems is that the ALS or ALG is itself antigenic. Therefore, efforts to induce and maintain tolerance to histocompatibility antigens and to prolong graft survival have been seriously hampered by the immunologic reaction to the substance itself. With each additional dose, the ALG is rendered less effective by the immunologic response to it.

It has now been shown experimentally that this problem can be circumvented by preparing the initial dose of normal globulin in a deaggregated form. As could be predicted, a subsequent injection of ALG is just as potent against the lymphocytes mediating the histocompatibility reaction but is not itself immunogenic. ALG can then be administered at will, under the cloak of tolerance that is provided by the initial tolerogenic preparation of normal globulin.

This approach works extremely well in animals. We have been able to make mice unresponsive to rabbit gamma globulin, then inject them with rabbit ALG and obtain complete and prolonged immunologic unresponsiveness. In humans, the approach has not been as successful, but I believe this is simply because we still lack precise information on the specific gamma globulin fractions involved in lymphocytotoxicity. In the horse ALG now being used clinically, there are both gamma 1 and gamma 2 globulins. We do not know which is the effector of antilymphocytic action. Once this has been learned, the problems of purification and manipulation should prove manageable.

Before leaving the subject of the induction of immunologic unresponsiveness, let us turn briefly to the other approaches that have been used to accomplish this in adult subjects, specifically the use of irradiation or immunosuppressant drugs. In a sense, creation of such tolerance is analogous to returning the subjects immunologically to their prenatal or neonatal state in which the bone marrow and thymus-derived cells are incapable of participating in the production of antibody. When this is done, antigenic exposure is tolerogenic, and, as in the immature animal, induction of unresponsiveness is dependent upon the administration of antigen following immunosuppression.

It is also worthy of note that in some cases the route of injection of the antigen will determine whether immunogenicity or tolerogenicity will result. For example, Battisto and Miller have shown that when bovine gamma

Tolerance Induction: Dose/Cell-Type Relationships

Dose of Tolerogen Injected (mg)	*Percent Unresponsiveness* in* Thymus	Bone Marrow
0.1	96	9
0.5	99	56
2.5	99	70

** 11 days after injection*

The greater sensitivity of thymic cells to induction of tolerance is reflected in the above table showing that a dose of tolerogen that affected only a small portion of the bone marrow cell population made almost all thymic cells unresponsive.

globulin (BGG) is injected into the jugular vein of a guinea pig, an antibody response is elicited. But BGG injected into the mesenteric vein will produce tolerance. The key here apparently is the direct pathway between the mesenteric vein and the liver. It is probable that the liver deaggregates the BGG so that the form of antigen presented to the antibody-forming cells is analogous to the monomeric forms produced in the laboratory. It has been shown also that certain haptenic chemical allergens injected into guinea pigs intradermally will couple to tissue proteins and invoke both humoral antibodies and delayed hypersensitivity. The same haptens given orally will invoke neither, and the animals will subsequently be unresponsive to intradermal administrations.

From Sensitivity to Tolerance

Up to now, we have been talking about the induction of unresponsiveness in subjects immunologically virgin with respect to the antigens employed. Unresponsiveness can also be induced in previously sensitized animals. To do this, the experimentalist must seek to eliminate specific memory cells by exhaustive differentiation into antibody-producing cells, much as is done in the induction of immune paralysis with massive doses of antigen.

Paul, Siskind, and Benacerraf approached this problem by first immunizing rabbits with pneumococci and subsequently injecting them with booster doses of a pneumococcal polysaccharide, the latter being a tolerogen. The resulting progressive decrease in immune response was compatible with the concept of exhaustion of memory cells. Among numerous other studies along these lines was one in which Mitchison found that mice injected periodically with 100 mg doses of bovine serum albumin first made antibody responses, then became unresponsive. And Humphrey has been able first to terminate a previously induced unresponsive state, then reinduce it. In our laboratory, Dr. Von Felton has been able to induce an unresponsive state to HGG in animals previously immunized with this antigen. Clearly, these and other studies provide a strong suggestion that the induction of tolerance in a previously sensitized subject is a feasible concept and one that deserves priority in our thinking because of its obvious implications in the management of autoimmune diseases and chronic transplant rejection reactions.

Maintenance of Tolerance

For many years, it was generally believed that the maintenance of tolerance depended upon persistence of antigen in the circulation or elsewhere in the animal. This proposition depended upon the concept that the antigen plays an active role in immunologic unresponsiveness through residence on the surface of antibody-producing cells and physical blockade of antibody synthesis. It has been suggested that once the antigen falls below a critical level, the cell would be permitted to resume its responsive state and tolerance would spontaneously remit. However, in the past half dozen years or so, I believe that more than enough evidence has been accumulated to refute this construction and to suggest a more passive role for antigen, one in which it is responsible for deleting or inactivating some step necessary for antibody production. If such is the case, animals could become unresponsive and remain so for at least a limited period of time without any persistence of antigen. The need for persistent antigen as a maintainer of tolerance would be limited to the suppression of responses by new antibody-producing cells arising out of spontaneous mutations or migrating from a primitive lymphoid organ such as the thymus. This latter possibility is strengthened by experiments showing that thymectomized animals are not as likely to show spontaneous loss of unresponsiveness as intact ones.

If the role of antigen is passive, what are the mechanisms involved in the fulfillment of this role?

It has been previously noted that the cells involved in antibody production – both bone marrow and thymus-derived – have receptor sites on their surfaces. It is possible that these receptor sites have very much the same configuration as the antibodies (or sensitized lymphocytes) that these cells are predestined to produce. Thus, they are capable of complexing with the antigen and initiating the membrane changes that signal antibody synthesis. It may be that the change in membrane signalled by a tolerogenic antigen is different from that triggered by an immunogen; or perhaps it is the absence of change in a surface membrane that leads to loss of responsiveness, mediated by some event such as the stripping off of the antigenic receptor sites from the cell. This is a plausible although, it must be stressed, not a demonstrated recapitulation of events that could lead to a "lesion of unresponsiveness." What has been demonstrated, to the extent that one can demonstrate a negative, is that there is no detectable antigen present in animals during a period of immunologic unresponsivity. These observations do not rule out the possibility that some tolerogen may be tightly bound to the receptors on the lymphocyte.

Within the concept of a passive role for antigen, one can suggest three possibilities to explain the persistence of immunologic unresponsiveness: 1) the complexing of antigen and the immunocompetent cell would result in cell death, with subsequent phagocytosis of the cell-antigen complex; 2) the antibody-producing cells and their precursors could be irreversibly inhibited and forced to differentiate in a direction away from antibody production; 3) the antigen could eventually be eluted from the receptor site, leaving a cell free of antigen but unresponsive.

Termination of Tolerance

The immunologically unresponsive state may be terminated either specifically or nonspecifically. The former implies that the events that cause the individual to regain ability to respond are specific for the antigen or antigenic determinant to which he has previously become unresponsive. Nonspecific termination implies some overall change in the immunologic status of the subject, causing him to lose unresponsiveness in a manner not solely directed against a single antigen or antigenic determinant.

Perhaps the best example of nonspecific termination is the spontaneous revival of immunocompetence. Even with rabbits made unresponsive at birth – and this is probably the most stable form of induced tolerance – there is after six months or so a loss

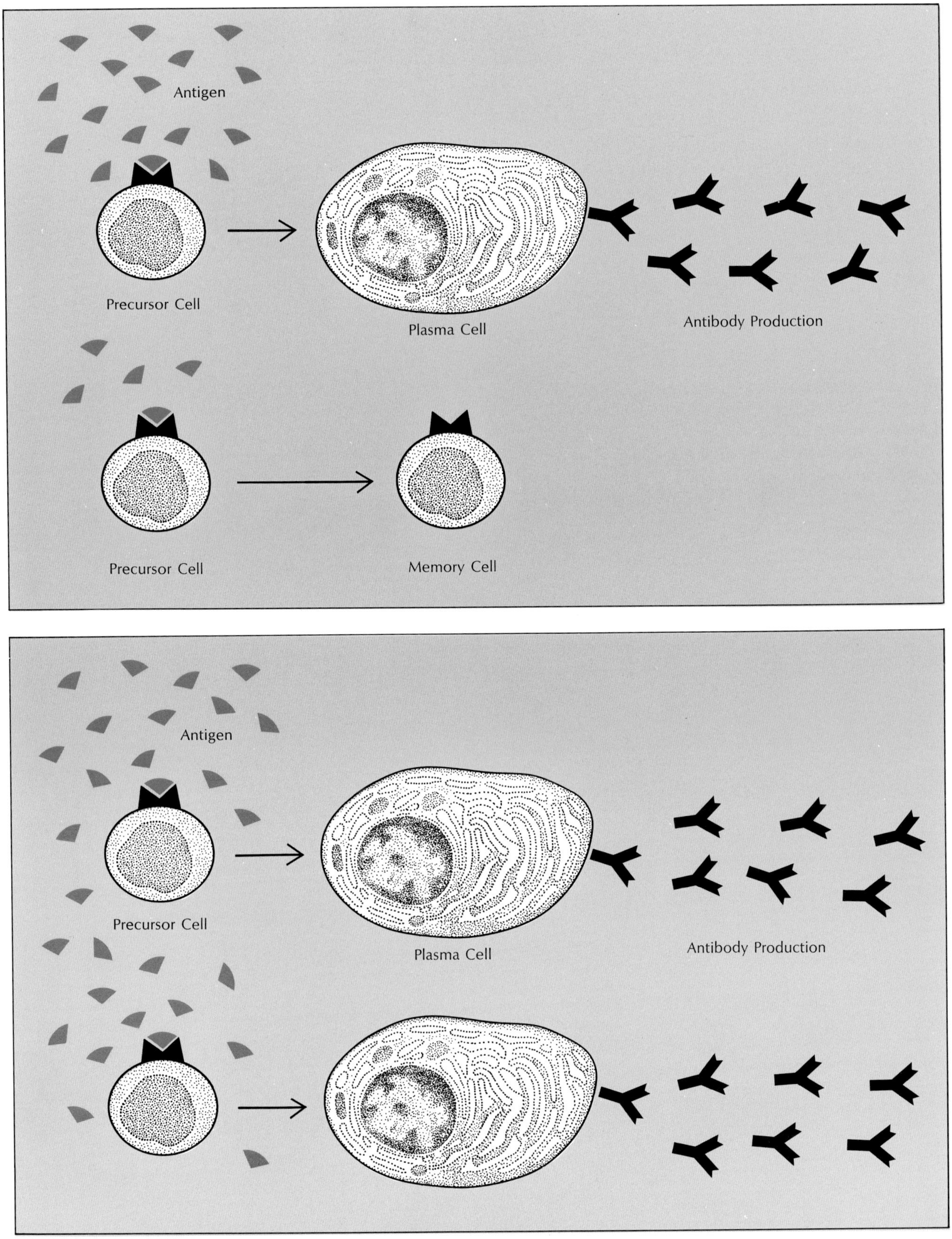

Antigen

Precursor Cell

Plasma Cell

Antibody Production

Precursor Cell

Memory Cell

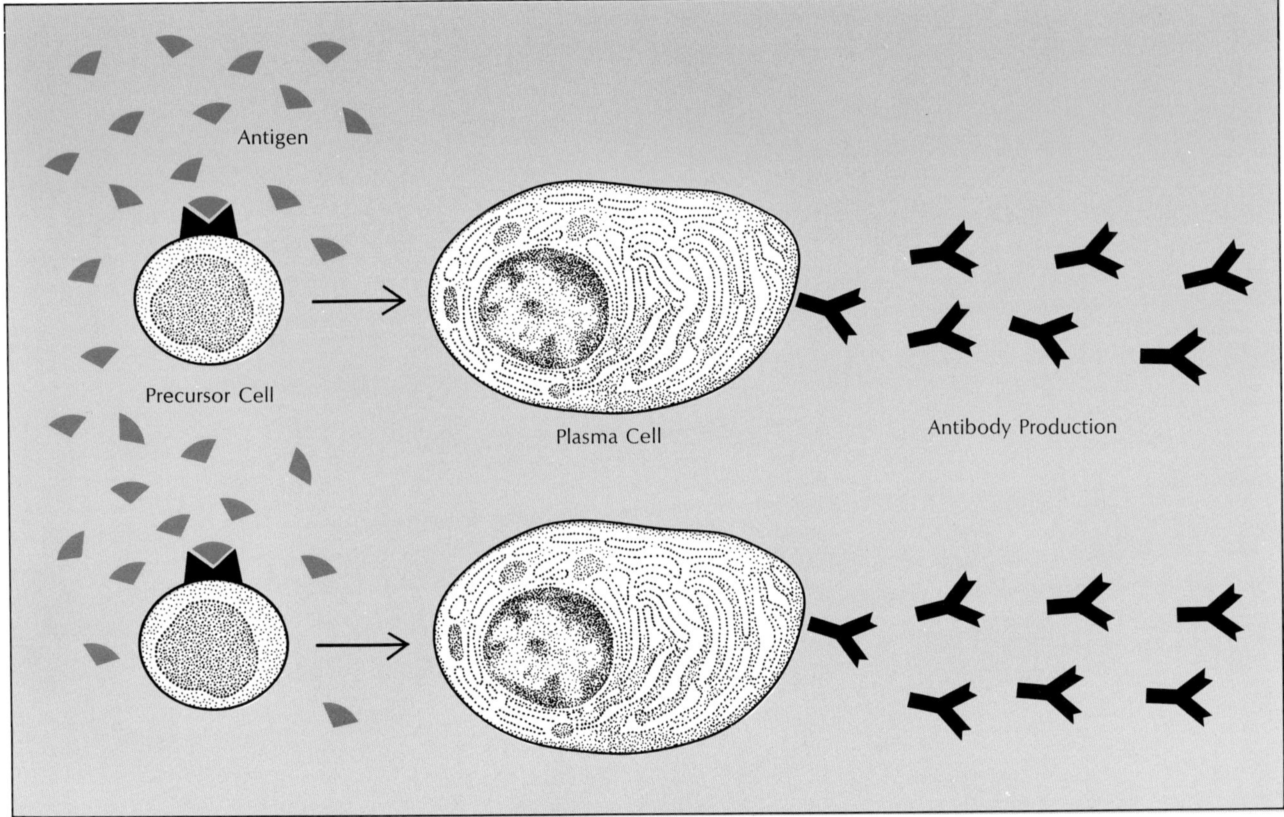

The concept of "immune paralysis" induced by very high antigen doses probably relates to antigen concentration around the immunocompetent precursor cells. When concentration is high enough the precursor cell will be fully activated and produce antibody. With lower concentrations of antigen, activation will be incomplete and memory cells, capable of anamnestic response, will result (top). If the total antigen dose is high enough to provide all precursor cells with the stimulation to produce antibody, no committed memory cells will be left behind to respond to subsequent antigenic exposure (bottom).

of unresponsiveness, regardless of which antigens they have been tolerant to. Thus, if these animals had been made unresponsive by exposure to human gamma globulin and bovine serum albumin (BSA), they now begin to make antibody to both of these antigens. It will be recalled from discussion of maintenance of tolerance that spontaneous mutations arise and that persistent antigen may play a "surveillance" role in maintaining unresponsiveness. However, when the antigen has disappeared, mutations might lead to a return of immunocompetence. Alternatively, stem cells in the bone marrow might make new immunocompetent cells that could express themselves in the absence of tolerogenic antigen.

Interestingly, some investigators have suggested that whole-body irradiation might have the same effect through its mutagenic capacity. However, critical examination of these experiments makes it seem much more likely that, rather than itself terminating tolerance, irradiation only enhances the spontaneous termination phenomena. Experiments in our laboratory showed that whole-body irradiation of rabbits made unresponsive to BSA neonatally failed to alter the unresponsive state, while similar irradiation of rabbits made hyporesponsive but not completely unresponsive to BSA resulted in the animals having a more enhanced antibody response than nonirradiated normal controls.

Specific termination of tolerance can be achieved by using a protein with a number of antigenic determinants similar to those on the tolerated protein and also with a number of determinants that are different. In other words, what is needed is a cross-reacting antigen but not one so closely related to the tolerated antigen that it would share its fate. This has been shown in a number of experiments, such as those using adult rabbits made unresponsive to bovine serum albumin neonatally. Pig, human, equine, and guinea pig serum albumins, which cross-react with BSA 30%, 15%, 15%, and 6% respectively, all will terminate the specific unresponsive state, but sheep serum albumin, which is 75% cross-reactive with the BSA, usually will not do so. Similar results can be obtained with altered preparations of the tolerated antigen; that is, those too close to the tolergen will not terminate tolerance, those that are cross-reactive, but more remote, will.

This relationship can be expressed in terms of a verbal model. Imagine two serum proteins. The first has a set of determinants that can be labeled A, B, C, D, E, and F (using six to represent a sample of the 30 or more determinants found on serum proteins). This protein is the antigen to which the subject is unresponsive. A second protein is injected with determinants H, J, K, L, F, and D. The animal will make antibody to the second protein, including the 33% (F and D) of the antigenic determinants that are shared. This antibody response will terminate tolerance only to the determinants shared with the second antigen.

In this context of termination, quotation marks should probably be used around the word tolerance. One has not directly interfered with the specific unresponsive state in this situation, but rather has presented the antigen in a way that permits normal non-

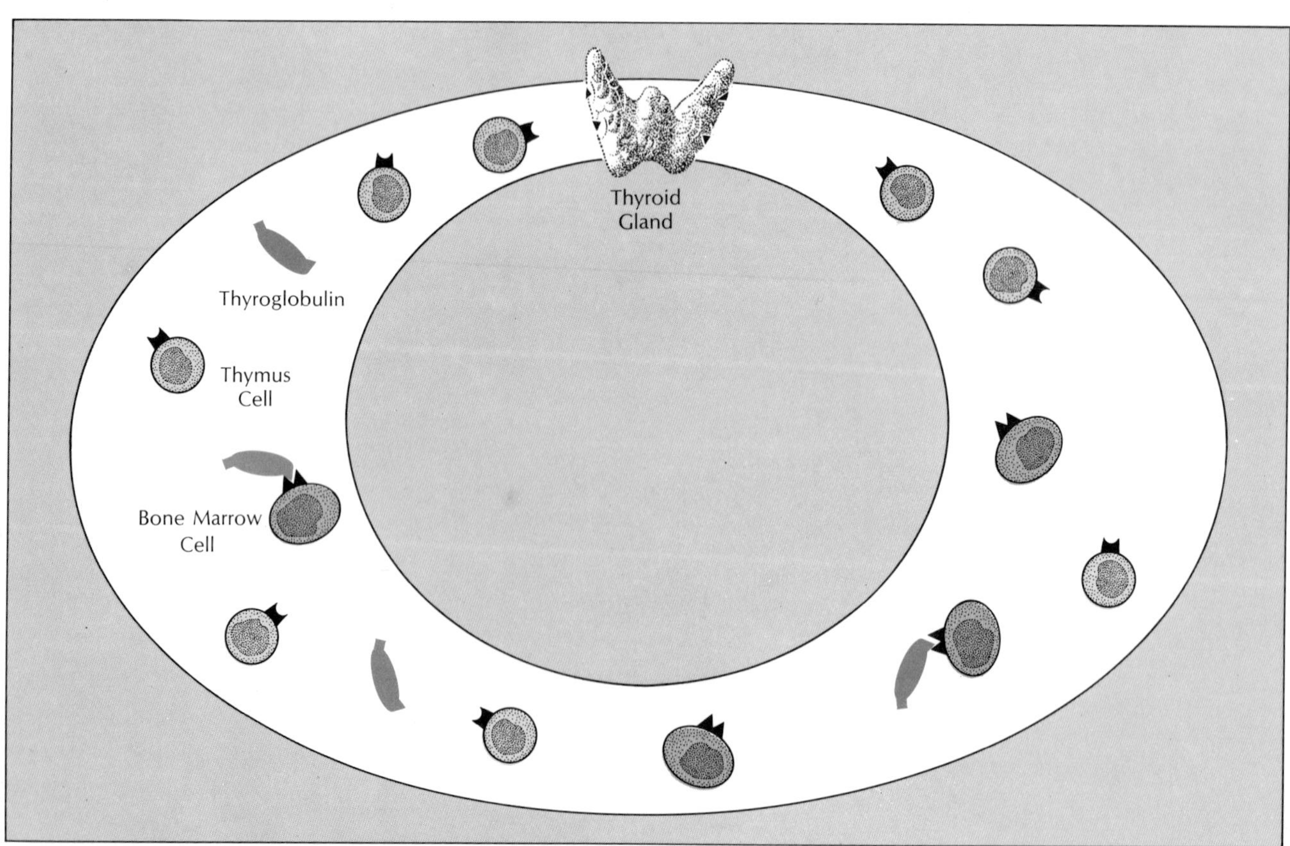

In this scheme for the pathogenesis of autoimmune disease, exemplified by thyroiditis, small amounts of thyroglobulin are in the circulation. While only the thymic cells are tolerant to the antigen, the interaction that takes place with the marrow cells will

tolerant cells, probably precursor cells in the bone marrow, to mount an antibody response. Obviously, the second antigen did not create these cells; they were there all the time. Perhaps the animal was unresponsive only at the level of the thymus-derived cells and not with respect to the bone marrow cells. By providing sufficiently different antigenic stimulation (sufficient cross-reactivity), one permitted the recruitment of responsive thymus cells capable of interacting with the bone marrow cells and producing an antibody response. Conceptualizing experiments of this type in parallel to the actual experiments, such as those with the various serum albumins, not only demonstrates a method for terminating tolerance but also provides indirect evidence for the synergistic participation of two cell types in the antibody response. Recent experiments, discussed previously, strongly suggest that at the time of injecting the second antigen a tolerant state exists in the thymus but that the bone marrow cells are responsive.

What happens now when the animal is challenged with the previously tolerated antigen?

With the first challenge, a response to D and F is elicited, mediated by the memory cells to those two determinants. An antibody response occurs, but it is not directed to A, B, C, and E because there are still no thymus-derived cells recruited to interact with the bone marrow cells. Therefore, with only a few additional injections of antigen, the limited pool of specific memory cells is exhausted and unresponsiveness is restored.

We have come to think that this sequence of events is particularly important because we believe that it closely parallels the sequence of events occurring spontaneously and resulting in certain autoimmune disease.

Autoimmunity

It is our working hypothesis that the pathogenesis of some experimental autoimmune disorders can be traced back to extremely low concentrations of self-antigens–thyroglobulin, sperm antigens, brain antigens, etc. – in the circulation. These concentrations could be sufficient to maintain tolerance to the thymus-derived cells but not to the bone marrow cells. This is a completely normal condition, since the unresponsiveness at the thymus level is adequate to inhibit any antibody response. However, if one now superimposes upon this situation a viral transformation or, more probably, a genetic mutation that permits the thymus cells to react with the altered portion of the self antigen, interaction takes place with the already immunocompetent bone marrow cells and immunopathology ensues.

I believe that experiments in our laboratory have adduced significant evidence in support of this hypothesis. We have been working with thyroglobulin in rabbits to create a model for autoimmune thyroiditis resembling Hashimoto's disease in humans. Although the evidence is that in some species of animals the effector cell population is of thymus and in others of bone marrow origin – that is to say, in some the disease is one of delayed hypersensitivity, while in others it is mediated by humoral antibodies – all the experiments previously described for termination of tolerance can be

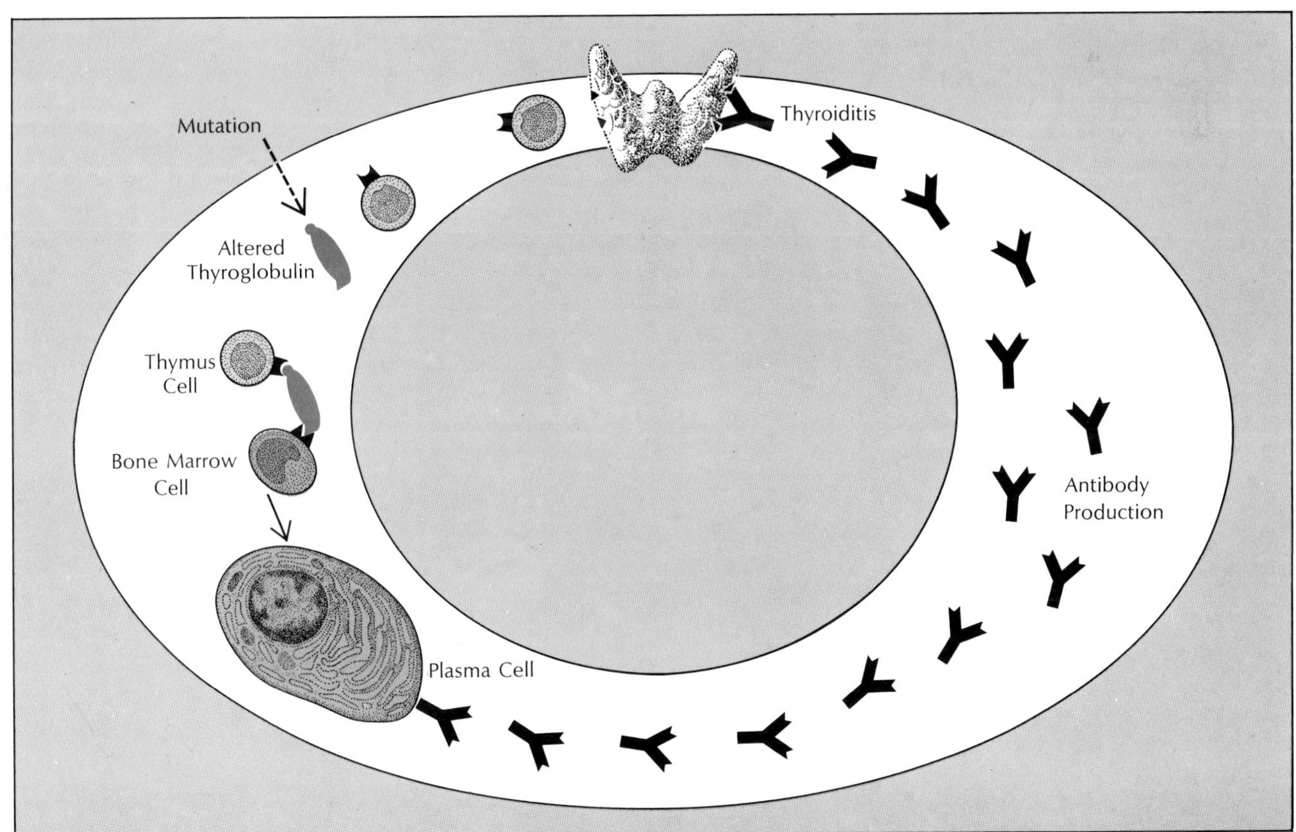

not result in antibody (left). With a genetic (or other) alteration of the thyroglobulin, the thymus cells lose their unresponsivity. Now both cell types respond to antigen and interact with each other to produce autoimmune antibodies against the thyroid.

reproduced with the thyroglobulin antigen. It appears that experimental thyroiditis in the rabbit is the result of circulating antibody.

Thyroglobulin is a semisequestered antigen present in the circulation in very small amounts and able to equilibrate between intravascular and extravascular spaces. In the rabbit, immunologic unresponsiveness can be induced to heterologous thyroglobulin by injecting it in amounts just sufficient to get a concentration equal to that found in the normal human. It has been known for years that if one takes thyroglobulin and injects it in complete Freund's adjuvant, this form of grossly altered protein will elicit an antibody response and thyroiditis in rabbits. However, we have found that in rabbits made unresponsive to heterologous thyroglobulin, tolerance can be terminated by using aqeous solutions without adjuvant, provided one makes specific antigenic alterations on the protein by adding certain chemical groups. The result is a circulating antibody to thyroglobulin and immune thyroiditis. We believe it is directly due to the antigenic alterations that permit the altered antigen to react with the thymus-derived cells, which in turn will interact with the bone marrow cells not tolerant to all of the native determinants on the thyroglobulin. Experiments in mice demonstrated that large amounts of tolerogen are required to induce tolerance in the bone marrow cells, while only small amounts are required for the thymus cells. Since thyroglobulin is present in such low levels in body fluids it is most likely that only the thymus cells are tolerant to autologous thyroglobulin.

Additional experiments have shown that native thyroglobulin injected along with the altered thyroglobulin will prevent the development of lesions. Even after repeated injections of altered thyroglobulin, which produce progressive disease marked by severe lesions and high antibody titers, an injection of native thyroglobulin will reestablish tolerance.

In some animals, we have been able to reverse immune thyroiditis by accompanying injections of native thyroglobulin with the antimetabolite cyclophosphamide. The results are variable, however, and I would be very cautious about interpreting them as a forerunner of an approach to the treatment of human disease. Unresponsiveness to self components at the thymus but not the bone-marrow-derived cells may be involved in rheumatic fever and rheumatoid arthritis, where there appears to be tolerance at the level of thymus-derived cells.

Equal caution is indicated in regard to one of the major goals of transplantation immunologists, the development of techniques to induce tolerance to the homograft. There are many who are optimistic that such tolerance might be induced with preparations containing small doses of tolerogenic transplantation antigens. Our own experiences with the so-called low-dose tolerance concept, discussed earlier in this presentation, tend to minimize this possibility. It is our best estimate that larger doses of antigen will be needed and, for that, the histocompatibility antigen or antigens will have to be purified. Much work is being done in this direction now, and when it is successful the outlook for making recipients truly immunologically unresponsive to organ transplants will improve immeasurably. This development, however, still appears to be rather far off.

If the problem of therapy for autoimmune disease is one of reestablishing unresponsiveness that has been spontaneously terminated, then that of treating cancer may be one of terminating an unresponsiveness that has spontaneously developed. Many investigators have suggested recently that tumors may arise as the result of the immune mechanism's failure to recognize new antigenic determinants on neoplastic cells. In this context, the failure may be analogous to that of the rabbits made unresponsive to BSA and thereby unable to recognize unrelated determinants on the closely cross-reacting sheep serum albumin. If this assumption proves valid, it might be possible to terminate this unresponsive state by immunizing patients with appropriately altered membranes or membrane fractions from the tumor cells. However, this would not be likely to work with metastases since the presence of tumor antigens in the circulation, even in trace amounts, would probably inhibit the termination of an unresponsive state. The termination of unresponsiveness to tumor antigens may have limited application if the observations of the Hellströms, suggesting that the failure of tumor rejection is caused by enhancing antibody-blocking rejection by cellular sensitivity, prove true.

Again, this is a development for some time in the future. But goals such as the treatment of autoimmune and malignant disorders and the facilitation of transplantation serve to assure continued interest in and investigation of the mechanisms of immune unresponsiveness. Such persistent research seems certain to provide us with both biologic and clinical insights of abiding importance.

Chapter 14

The Interrelationship of Clotting and Immunologic Mechanisms

OSCAR D. RATNOFF
Case Western Reserve University

The scientific investigator tends to narrow his sights and to simplify his experiments so that the questions asked pertain to or at least give the appearance of pertaining to a single variable. Pragmatically, this has value in making scientific investigation more manageable. But such simplification tends to produce an isolation or compartmentalization of various aspects of physiology. We create separate systems into which we fit all the phenomena that relate to the ability of the blood to clot, or of a clot to lyse, or those actions and reactions through which the body defends itself against infectious agents or other foreign proteins. And, of course, having created these systems, we promptly forget that they are man-made, that in nature many of the processes that we think of as discrete are really need-determined variations of similar or closely related biochemical events. In other words, the body probably has a finite number of responses to the stresses it encounters; in order to mobilize these responses appropriately, there must be an intermeshing of "systems."

From an evolutionary viewpoint, "need determination" is obviously closely related to natural selection. The enzymes involved in clotting, for example, must have evolved from functionally more simple substances by mutation and genetic reduplication, with the mutant gene coding for an enzyme with specificities slightly different from its ancestor. Logically, one must assume that enzymes evolving in this manner would have multiple substrates. In fact, from considerations of physiologic economy one is tempted to speculate that only those mechanisms with such versatility would be retained.

Several early investigators had the insight required to connect the blood clotting process with immunologic defenses even before the experimental techniques required to provide evidence for these insights were available. During World War I, Ludwig Herzfeld in Poland published a series of papers in which he proposed a relationship between the blood clotting enzymes and the complement system. The main pillar upon which this concept rested was fractionation experiments in which Herzfeld found that prothrombin and what was then called complement midpiece (C′1) were found together in a single fraction.

At about the same time, Jobling and Petersen were reporting experiments that appeared to link immunologic responses to the release into the blood of proteolytic enzymes that we would today identify with plasmin. They were, for example, able to demonstrate the release of such proteolytic substances upon exposure of plasma to kaolin, an experiment that has echoes in recent work.

Much more recently, just after World War II, Rocha e Silva in Brazil advanced the concept that blood clotting liberates a biologically active polypeptide, bradykinin. In essence Rocha e Silva, by demonstrating that the precursor of bradykinin was present in much greater quantities in plasma than in serum, was able to suggest the utilization of this precursor in clotting processes. This linking of bradykinin to blood clotting, as will be seen later in this discussion, identifies one of the significant points at which the immunologic and clotting systems touch.

These are only three of many possible examples of the early work that groped toward the relationship between clotting and immunologic processes. As we approach this relationship in a more organized manner, a pivotal point is the role of what I, as a coagulationist, think of as factor XII, or Hageman factor.

As blood circulates in the intact organism, it is essentially inert with regard to clotting. This lack of activity is, of course, absolutely necessary; one would otherwise be confronted with the constant development of thrombi. However, when blood is drawn from the vasculature into

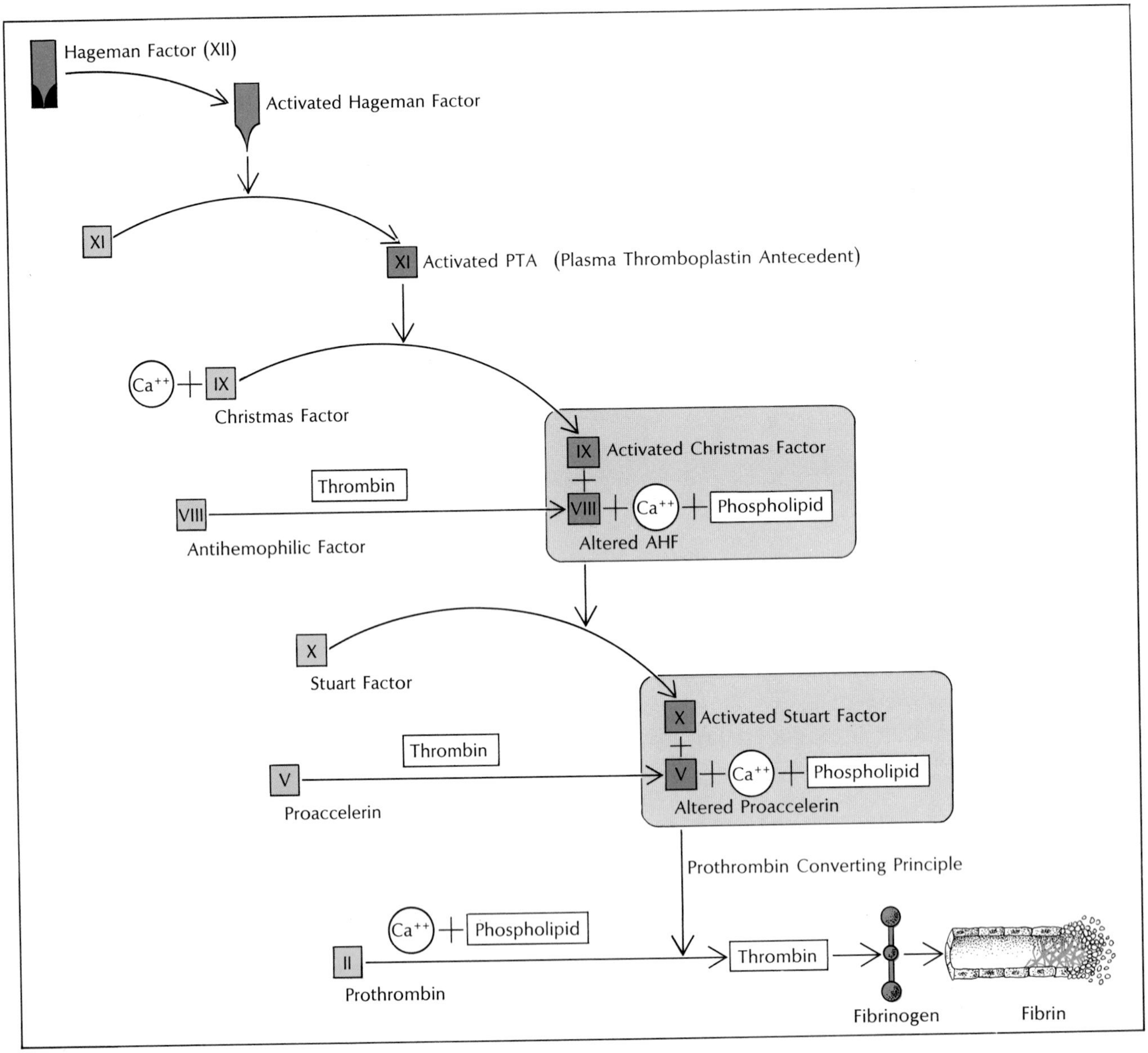

Hageman Factor (XII)
Activated Hageman Factor
XI
XI Activated PTA (Plasma Thromboplastin Antecedent)
Ca^{++} + IX
Christmas Factor
IX Activated Christmas Factor
+
Thrombin
VIII
VIII + Ca^{++} + Phospholipid
Antihemophilic Factor
Altered AHF
X
Stuart Factor
X Activated Stuart Factor
+
Thrombin
V
V + Ca^{++} + Phospholipid
Proaccelerin
Altered Proaccelerin
Prothrombin Converting Principle
Ca^{++} + Phospholipid
II
Thrombin
Prothrombin
Fibrinogen
Fibrin

The clotting sequence is initiated when factor XII (Hageman factor) is activated and then interacts with plasma thromboplastic antecedent (PTA, or factor XI). Two explanations have been suggested for this event. The most widely held is that Hageman factor's interaction with PTA causes the latter to change from its inert form into an active proteolytic enzyme. Alternatively, some believe Hageman factor and PTA combine into a complex that triggers subsequent steps in the clotting cascade. By whichever route, it is now established that Hageman factor's use of PTA as a substrate leads to clot formation.

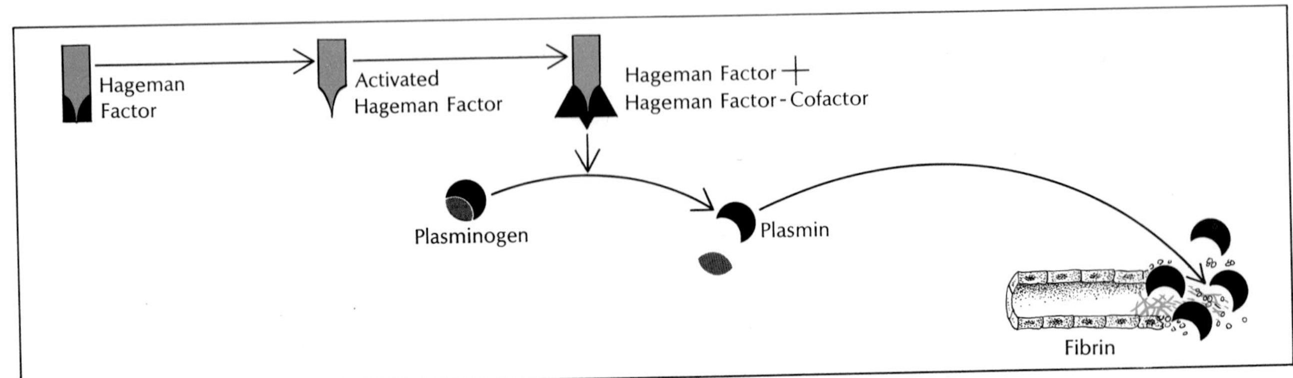

Simultaneously with initiating clotting, Hageman factor sets in motion the events that result in dissolution of clots through fibrinolysis. In this sequence Hageman factor acts in association with a cofactor to convert inert plasminogen to proteolytically active plasmin. It is the plasmin that directly attacks the fibrin clot and disrupts it enzymatically, as depicted above.

a glass container, a change from an inert to a biologically active form takes place. The exact nature of the change is poorly understood. The two most likely possibilities are either the formation of a giant macromolecule or a change to a hydrophobic state that causes the molecules to be thrown out of solution, giving much the same effect as the formation of a macromolecule.

By whatever mechanism, the phenomenon is now known to result from contact between factor XII and glass. Factor XII – Hageman factor – is activated and then participates in a variety of different reactions, all mediated in a number of sequential steps. In the clotting sequence, factor XII interacts with plasma thromboplastic antecedent (PTA), or factor XI. It is generally believed that the interaction is enzymatic and factor XI changes from its inert form to an active proteolytic enzyme. Some investigators have suggested alternatively that the Hageman factor and PTA form a complex and that this complex is responsible for subsequent events leading to the formation of thrombin and to clotting. At any rate, PTA, activated by Hageman factor, does lead to clotting. But Hageman factor does a good deal more than that.

At the same time that it initiates the sequence eventuating in clotting, specifically in fibrin formation, Hageman factor acts in association with a cofactor to activate the fibrinolytic mechanism by converting plasminogen to its active proteolytic form, plasmin. Thus, the substance that starts the clotting process in its active form also initiates the steps leading to the destruction of the clot.

A third role of Hageman factor is to induce the formation of agents that bring about some of the events observed in inflammatory states. Thus, Hageman factor participates in the elaboration of an agent, apparently a proteolytic enzyme, that experimentally enhances vascular permeability in guinea pig skin. This agent, named PF/Dil (for permeability factor evolving in plasma upon dilution), in turn activates another plasma proteolytic enzyme, kallikrein, from its inert precursor. Plasma kallikrein has the property of splitting off biologically active polypeptide fragments from an alpha globulin in plasma. These frag-

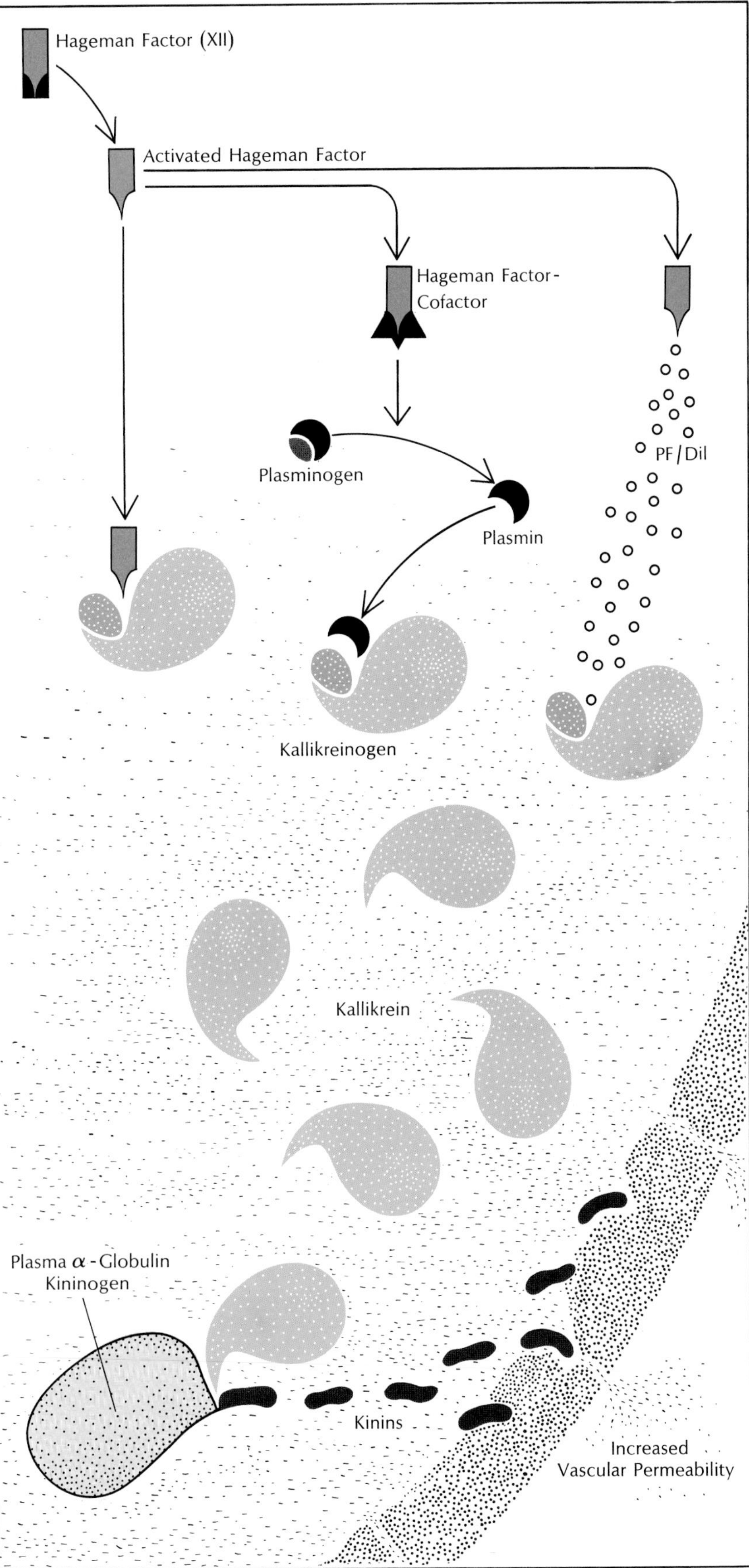

Kallikrein activation, leading to increased vascular permeability, is initiated by Hageman factor via three pathways: direct effect on kallikreinogen, via plasmin, through PF/Dil elaboration. Kallikrein splits off kinins from kininogen, a plasma alpha globulin.

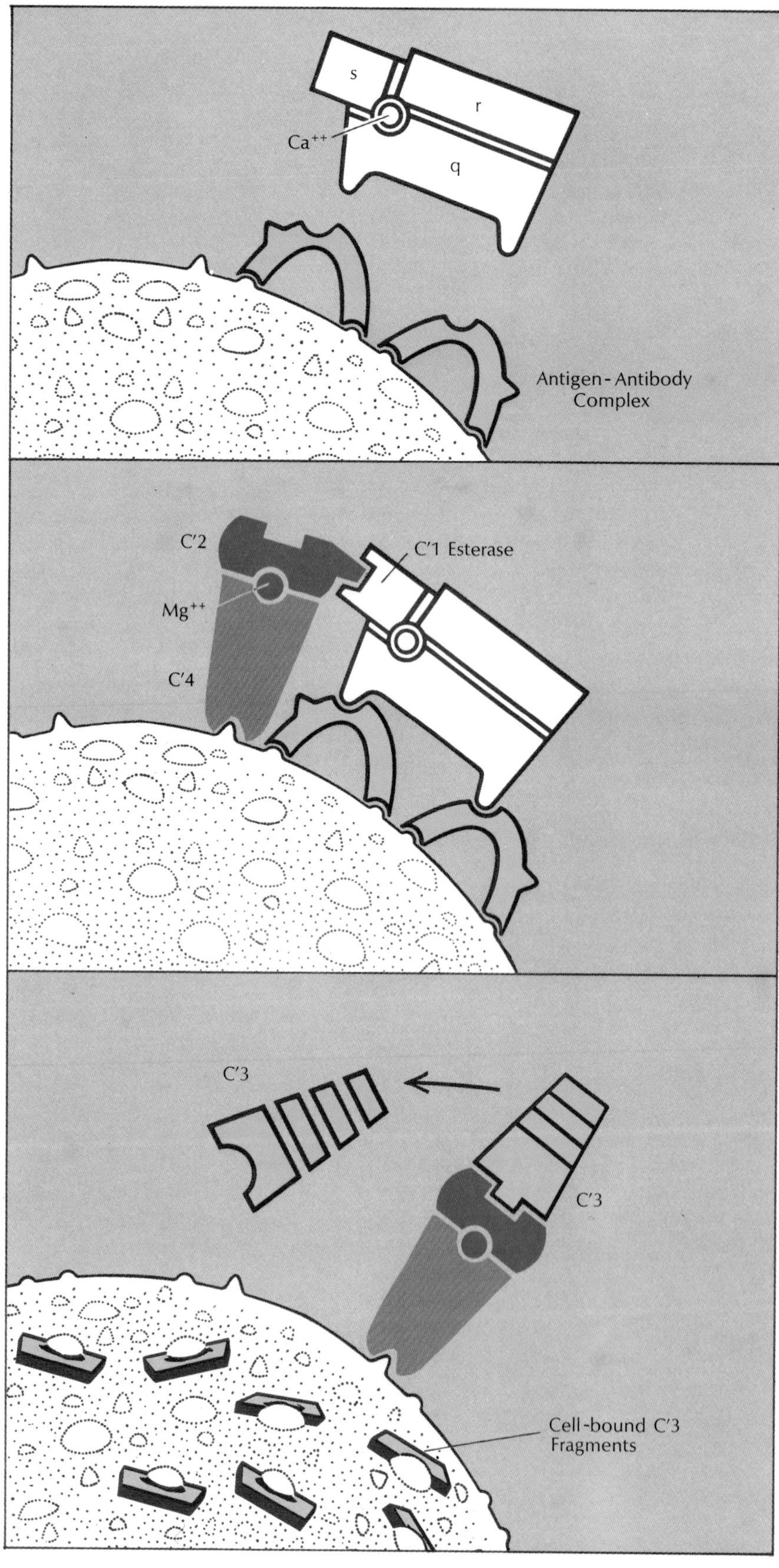

The immunologic events involved in complement activation begin with adherence of the antigen-antibody complex to the cell surface. The first component (C'1) is a complex molecule having three components, q, r, and s. C'1 esterase, derived from the s component, catalyzes subsequent reactions. The ability of Hageman factor to initiate the complement sequence, without immune complexes, is depicted on next page.

ments, known generically as kinins – and including bradykinin, lysyl-bradykinin (or kallidin) among others – enhance vascular permeability; dilate small blood vessels, leading to hypotension; contract certain smooth muscles; and perhaps bring about the migration of leukocytes into extravascular tissues. Effectively, then, a fourth role of Hageman factor involves the activation of plasma kallikrein. An alternative view, for which some evidence has been provided, suggests that Hageman factor may activate kallikrein directly.

Among the first demonstrations of this activity of Hageman factor, a series of experiments undertaken by Keele and coworkers in England points to yet another function of the kinins. This group was interested in the mechanisms of pain and discovered that an individual's own plasma, applied to the exposed base of a blister, produced excruciating pain. Moreover, the induction of pain with plasma could be obviated by protecting the plasma from contact with glass. Keele's group also showed that the actual induction of pain was attributable to a polypeptide of the kinin class. At this juncture, J. Margolis, who had worked out the methodology that led to the discovery that glass activated Hageman factor, came to work with Keele. Margolis provided the missing link in the sequence of events that led to the induction of pain. That link, of course, was Hageman factor, which now could be shown to be involved in the release of kinin polypeptides. More specifically, Margolis was able to show that Hageman factor was initiating events that activated kallikrein from its precursor, kallikreinogen. This activation, as I have noted, is achieved either directly or through the mediation of PF/Dil.

We have now considered four different substrates with which Hageman factor can act – with PTA in the clotting sequence, with a cofactor to initiate fibrinolysis, with PF/Dil, and with the precursor of plasma kallikrein – to bring about some of the phenomena associated with inflammation. A new complication should be noted: Plasmin, the proteolytic enzyme responsible for fibrinolysis, has the capacity to liberate kinins from their precursors and probably to activate kallikrein. Thus, Hageman factor can participate in kinin formation in separate ways: through direct action upon PF/Dil and plasma kallikreinogen and, indirectly, by bringing about the formation of plasmin.

Certainly the evidence described so far gives substance to some of the evolutionary speculations at the outset of this discussion, specifically those that suggested the likelihood that enzymes have multiple substrates and that what we think of as discrete systems are really parts of an integrated physiologic continuum. However, we have not yet broached the question of how clotting mechanisms might be linked with immunologic defenses. For this, we turn to the complement system.

It will be recalled that complement achieves its classic effect, exemplified by the hemolysis of a sensitized red cell, via a cascade of at least nine separate components working in a specific sequence. En route, various effects – chemotaxis of neutrophils, phagocytosis, elaboration of anaphylatoxin, histamine release, etc. – are mediated.

The first component in the series, C′1 is in fact a complex molecule in which three subcomponents – C′1q, C′1r, and C′1s – are held together, possibly by calcium bonds. When antigen-antibody complexes interact with C′1, a proteolytic enzyme, C′1 esterase, is elaborated and catalyzes the subsequent reactions with C′4 and C′2. The esterase is specifically derived from the C′1s subcomponent. With these facts in mind one can now review the experimentation linking clotting and other hemostatic mechanisms with the complement system and other immunologically involved reactions.

A logical starting point for such a review is experiments performed with Lewis Thomas more than two decades ago. We found that complement could not be measured in the presence of plasmin. We were unable to explain this anticomplementary action of plasmin until further experiments with Pillemer and Lepow showed that plasmin in some way led to the destruction of the fourth and second components of complement. At this point Lepow and I hypothesized that what we were really doing was causing the formation of C′1 esterase with the plasmin, and the esterase was affecting C′4 and C′2.

To test this hypothesis, experiments were undertaken with Naff in which, instead of using the whole C′1 complex, we used the isolated subcomponents. We were able to demonstrate that plasmin directly converted C′1s to C′1 esterase without the participation of the C′1q and C′1r subcomponents and, therefore, without the need for participation of antigen-antibody complexes. Once again, the trail led back to Hageman factor. Hageman factor activates plasmin; plasmin activates C′1s, triggering the elaboration of C′1 esterase; and C′1 esterase reacts with C′4 and C′2. Now, normally, the participation of C′4 and C′2 is subsequent to antigen-antibody-complex interaction with C′1 and represents a key event in the development of the entire complement sequence. We now have, in vitro at least, a system for the activation of complement that starts with Hageman factor and bypasses the key immunologic event.

Studies with C′1 esterase also led in another immunologically related direction. Among the well-established consequences of antigen-antibody-complex activity are inflammatory reactions, and critical to inflammation is increased vascular permeability. The possibility that C′1 esterase might be a permeability factor therefore seemed worthy of investigation. Studies with Lepow showed that not only did C′1 esterase increase vascular permeability in guinea pig skin but that it did so through the release of histamine from mast cells. Further studies (with Smink and Abernathy) showed that the effects of C′1 esterase on vascular permeability could be enhanced by preincubation of the esterase with guinea pig serum.

This finding struck a responsive chord historically, with investigative lines going at least as far back as the work of Friedberger and Friedemann around 1910. These investigators had found that incubation of antigen-antibody complexes with serum resulted in the elaboration of substances that, when injected into an animal, evoked signs and symptoms resembling those of anaphylaxis. The agent produced by the incubation of antigen-antibody complexes with serum (or by incubation with serum of such materials as kaolin or agar) had been

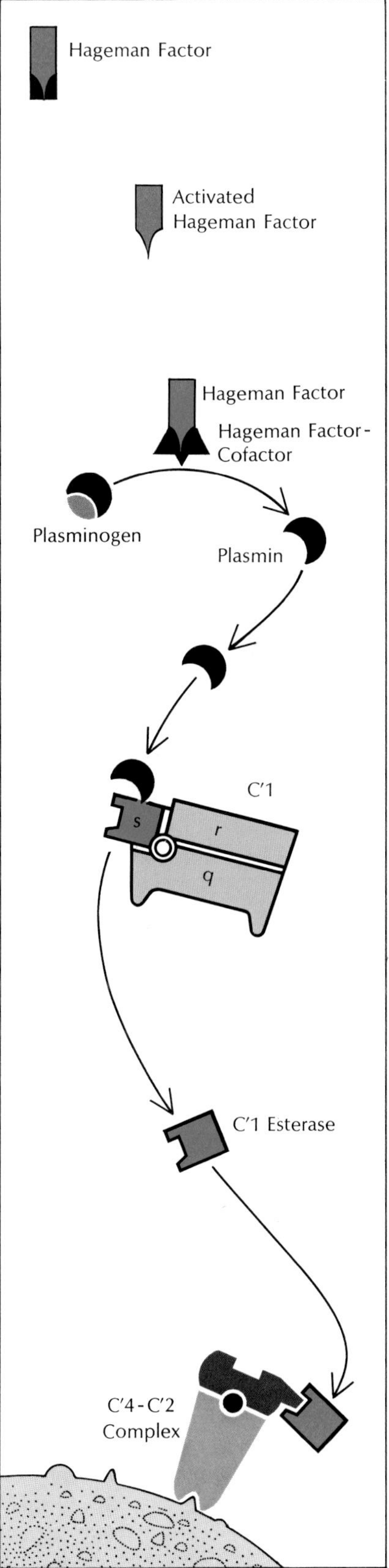

The complement sequence can be initiated by Hageman factor via activation of plasmin. Plasmin actually serves to stimulate the release of C′1 esterase from the C′1s component in a fashion paralleling that observed in antigen-antibody reactions.

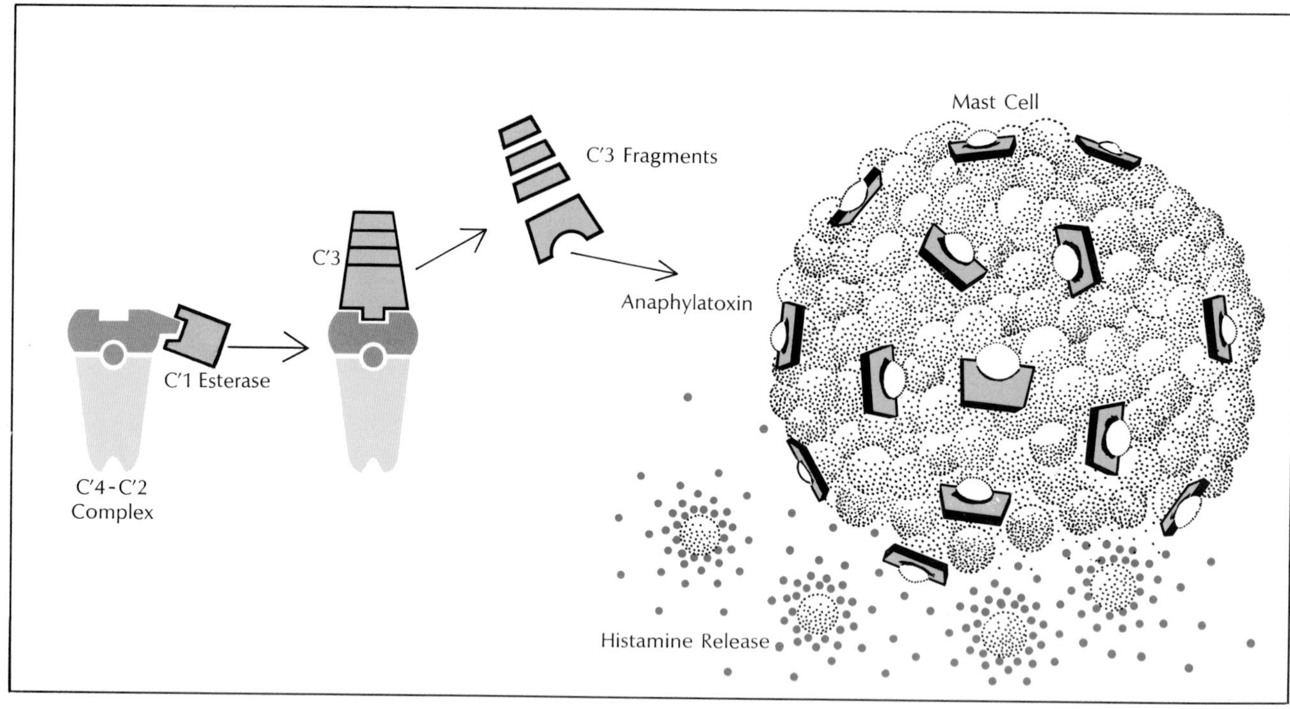

Studies have shown that C′1 esterase release following either antigen-antibody complexing or plasmin activation leads to increased vascular permeability. This phenomenon has been traced to action by the C′1 esterase on C′3 fragments. The result is the elaboration of anaphylatoxin, which in turn triggers the release of histamine from mast cells.

named anaphylatoxin. As research in this field progressed, it became clear that the action of anaphylatoxin was mediated either in vivo or in vitro by histamine-like substances.

With this background, Dias da Silva and Lepow at Case Western Reserve University set out to integrate into the picture the observations concerning the ability of C′1 esterase to increase vascular permeability via histamine release. They proceeded to show that the mechanisms first described nearly 60 years before were actually mediated by C′1 esterase. Under the conditions of their experiments, C′1 esterase incubated with C′4 and C′2 split off a fragment from C′3 that had the properties of an anaphylatoxin. Moreover, other experiments, by Ward, showed that another biologically active fragment of C′3, released through the action of plasmin, is chemotactic for leukocytes. In the context of this discussion, it is important to keep in mind that the activation of C′1 esterase and all of the activities subsequent to this event can be initiated not only by antigen-antibody complexes but by the Hageman factor–induced activation of plasmin. Clearly, separation of the clotting, fibrinolytic, and immunologic processes can no longer be sustained.

The projection of some of these findings into the clinical area was first accomplished by Dr. Virginia Donaldson, then in Cleveland and now at the University of Cincinnati. Lepow and I had observed that plasma contains a potent inhibitor of C′1 esterase. Dr. Donaldson reasoned that alterations in concentration of this inhibitor might be expected in inflammatory and immunologic disorders in which complement might participate. She chose as one of the syndromes to study, along with inflammatory states, the noninflammatory disorder hereditary angioneurotic edema. This familial disease, inherited as an autosomal dominant trait, is characterized by the episodic appearance of sharply localized noninflammatory edema. The site at which edema appears during any particular episode determines whether it is harmless or severely distressing or lethal. A commonplace terminal event is complete and sudden airway obstruction.

Dr. Donaldson discovered that the plasma of patients with hereditary angioneurotic edema was devoid of C′1 esterase inhibitory activity. Simultaneously, Landerman and his associates in Washington showed that in patients with hereditary angioneurotic edema the normal capacity of plasma to inhibit plasma kallikrein was diminished, although never wholly absent. The observations made by Landerman and Donaldson were quickly reconciled. Pensky in Cleveland had purified C′1 esterase inhibitor separated from human plasma. This agent was found by Kagan and Becker to inhibit not only C′1 esterase but PF/Dil and plasma kallikrein as well. Indeed, C′1 esterase inhibitor has turned out to be an agent blocking many different enzymes participating in the defenses of the body, including plasmin, activated Hageman factor, activated PTA, and the C′1r component of C′1.

From the experiments in our laboratory showing the relationship between C′1 esterase activity and histamine release, Dr. Donaldson hypothesized that the mechanisms of the maintenance, if not the initiation, of edema in hereditary angioneurotic edema were dependent on the release of histamine. She reasoned that in some way C′1 esterase became active at the site of an edematous lesion and, because of the lack of C′1 esterase inhibitory activity, this activation resulted in large-scale elaboration of histamine from mast cells. To her surprise, when the plasma of patients with hereditary angioneurotic edema was incubated under suitable conditions polypeptide kinins were released instead of histamine or anaphylatoxin. Although similar to bradykinin and kallidin in their biologic activities, the polypeptide kinins generated in hereditary angioneurotic edema differed in their chemical properties from these two substances. It should be stressed that Dr. Donaldson's original hypothesis that histamine was being released and her later finding that a biologically active kinin was generated are not mutually exclusive. In patients with this disease both mechanisms could be operative.

Be that as it may, we still do not have any hard evidence with respect to the processes by which edema formation in the syndrome is initiated. Dr. Donaldson's work provided two intriguing clues: 1) in test tubes, plasma from patients with hereditary angioneurotic edema will produce permeability-enhancing substances when treated with plasmin, and 2) ellagic acid added to the plasma of patients with this disease will lead directly to the elaboration of C′1 esterase.

Some years ago, Crum and I found that ellagic acid, a product of tannic acid, had powerful clotting effects on the blood, which could be related to its ability to activate Hageman factor. Thus either of Dr. Donaldson's clues could lead to a solution to the problem of how edema is caused in the hereditary syndrome, that is, either by activation of plasmin or by activation of clotting. One fact favors the former explanation. It has been observed that individuals with the disease are likely to have episodes of edema in response to emotional stress. And it has been demonstrated that plasmin is more readily evolved in blood from a patient under stress than in blood from a "calm" individual.

From the clinical point of view, among the most intriguing and most pertinent interactions between hemostatic and immunologic processes are those relating to platelet aggregation. It is this interrelationship, for example, that accounts for a number of the most common idiosyncratic reactions to drugs.

It has been shown that when immune complexes come into contact with platelets in solution, aggregation of platelets results, and a number of biologically active constituents – phospholipids, ADP, and serotonin, among others – are liberated from these cells. In the presence of complement, such platelet aggregation can take place even though the amounts of antigen-antibody complex are small; without complement, the phenomenon is observable only with larger concentrations of immune complex. Platelets have another important relationship to immune complexes. Although these are, of course, nonnucleated cells, they have been shown to phagocytize small quantities of antigen-antibody complex. Large quantities of complex are believed able to disrupt platelets without involving phagocytosis.

These facts can be related to drug sensitivity reactions, as demonstrated by the work of Ackroyd in Great Britain and of N. R. Shulman at the National Institutes of Health. In classic drug hypersensitivity, e.g., to quinidine or quinine, the patient is sensitized by initial exposure to the agent. Subsequent exposure results in the rapid development of petechiae over the entire body, including the head and the extremities. These hemorrhages are manifestations of thrombocytopenic purpura.

Shulman has shown that the initial exposure of the patient resulted in the development of circulating antibodies to the drug. When a second dose provides a challenge, the drug, probably in haptenic combination with a carrier protein, reacts with the circulating antibody to form immune complexes. In the presence of complement these adhere to the platelets and facilitate premature removal of the platelets from the circulation, presumably by the spleen and other reticuloendothelial organs. The life span of the platelets is thereby shortened. With their disruption, the platelets release phospholipids, serotonin, and ADP, all of which have biologic activities.

Movat in Toronto has proposed an alternate explanation for the thrombogenic effects subsequent to the interaction between immune aggregates

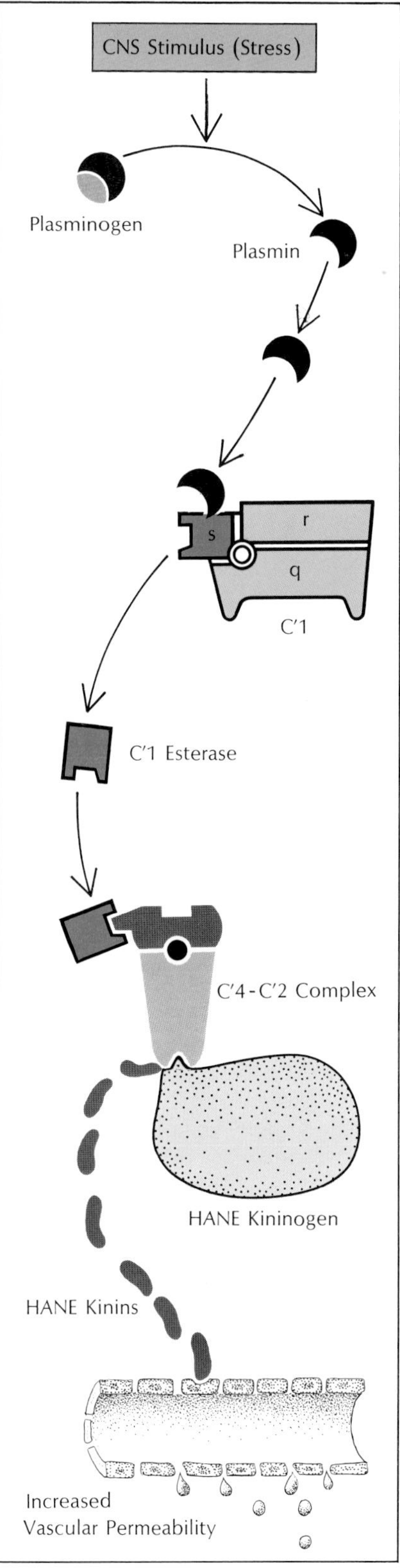

In this suggested scheme for the pathogenesis of hereditary angioneurotic edema, a CNS stress initiates the activation of plasmin, a phenomenon that appears to correlate with clinical findings. Plasmin activates C′1 esterase, leading to elaboration of specialized (HANE) kinins and increased vascular permeability and edema.

and blood, one suggesting the involvement of Hageman factor. In his experiments antigen-antibody complexes accelerated clotting if they were first brought into contact with normal human serum. But with serum devoid of Hageman factor, that is, prevented from contact with glass, clotting was not accelerated. These experiments also suggested a liberation of kinins in the process.

Investigations into the relationship between immune complexes and clotting have also been directed toward understanding the mechanisms of endotoxic shock. This involves a concept in which endotoxin plays a role analogous to antigen. The evolution of this concept, and it remains largely hypothetical, can be traced in the work of Thomas, Stetson, Rapaport, Horowitz, and others, which has led to the view that endotoxin may induce diffuse intravascular coagulation. After the injection of endotoxin, a slow formation of fibrin ensues. Monomeric units of fibrin, induced by the elaboration of thrombin, may polymerize with fibrinogen or may form microscopic fibrin thrombi that are phagocytized by the reticuloendothelial system and thus removed from the circulation.

Experimentally, if a second intravenous injection of endotoxin is made a day after the first, the generalized Shwartzman reaction may ensue, in which fibrin is laid down in vulnerable sites such as the physiologic filters in the glomeruli, the small vessels of the lung and liver, and so forth, an event often lethal to the experimental animal. The failure of the animal to resist the second injection of endotoxin can be traced to the paralysis of the reticuloendothelial system (RES) that follows the initial injection.

Essentially, this hypothesis has just been expressed in mechanical terms. However, one can also interpret the same sequence in immunologic terms as, indeed, Stetson has done. This interpretation is built on two premises: 1) that antigen-antibody complexes initiate clotting in the presence of whole blood; 2) that most individuals have antibodies against endotoxin. The endotoxin reaction may then be described as an antigen-antibody reaction leading to intravascular coagulation. On first challenge, the complexes that are formed are handled by the RES and removed from the circulation so that the intravascular clotting sequence does not develop. Subsequent endotoxin forms circulating complexes and the immunologic reaction causes clot formation.

A number of experimental findings and observations lend credence to this thesis. For example, Shwartzman showed that the two-step induction of experimental endotoxic shock could be achieved if antigen-antibody complexes were used for the initial injection in place of endotoxin. It has also been shown that pregnant animals require only one injection of

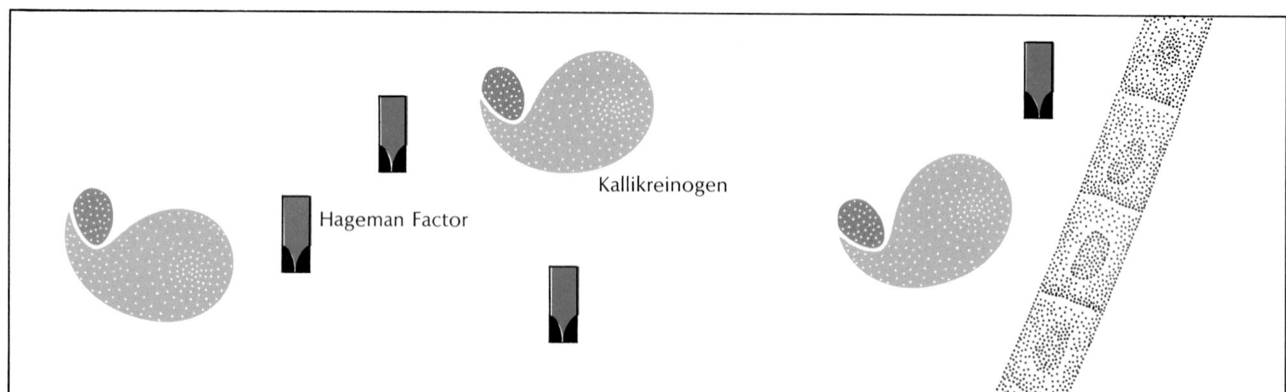

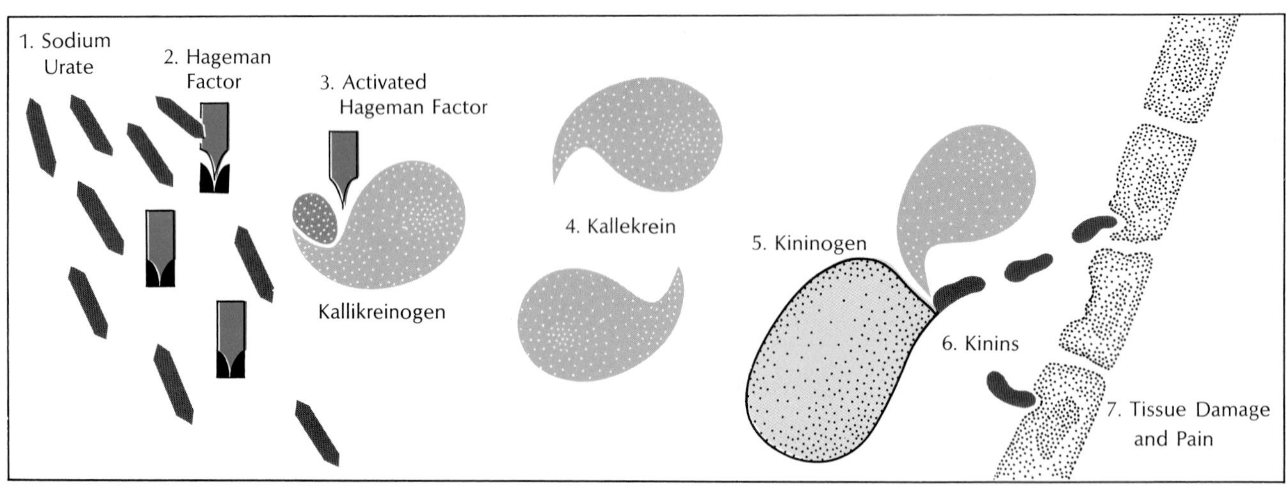

Work by Kellermeyer and Breckenridge has suggested a possible role for Hageman factor in the development of the symptoms in acute gout attacks. The basic findings are that sodium urate crystals activate Hageman factor and that normal joint fluid contains Hageman factor and precursors of PF/Dil, kallikrein, and kinins. On this basis, one can hypothesize the scheme in the lower panel, starting with sodium-urate-crystal activation of Hageman factor and eventuating in tissue damage and pain.

endotoxin for shock to supervene, and it is known that the pregnant animal frequently has a hypofunctional RES. It has been shown, too, that large doses of anticoagulants can inhibit the Shwartzman reaction under appropriate experimental conditions.

There is also considerable evidence for an effect of endotoxin on clotting time, although the direction of the effect is somewhat controversial and, in fact, seems to depend on how one sets up the experiment with regard to various complex phenomena involved in intravascular clotting. In a technique that, in many respects, seems to recapitulate much of what has been learned of the immunologic induction of clotting, McKay in San Francisco has produced the Shwartzman phenomenon with a combination of ellagic acid, to activate Hageman factor; phospholipid (analogous to that liberated from disrupted platelets), to enhance clot promotion; epsilon-aminocaproic acid (an inhibitor of plasmin), to prevent clot dissolution; and norepinephrine, to stimulate alpha-adrenergic receptor sites. With this mixture the events usually associated with the injection of endotoxin are reproduced by a nonimmunologic procedure and without use of endotoxin.

The combination of antigen-antibody complexes and whole blood, leading to acute tissue damage mediated by thrombotic events, has taken on an additional clinical context in recent years with the advent of organ transplant surgery. I believe that the so-called hyperacute rejection, in which a graft will be violently reacted against within hours of transplantation, may be an expression of the pathologic phenomena we have been discussing. For example, when a kidney is so rejected, one sees thrombi composed of fibrin and platelet clumps occluding its small vessels. Certainly, consideration of antigen-antibody complexes as the initiator of thrombogenesis is entirely plausible. In this context, Mustard in Toronto has suggested that prolongation of graft survival might be achieved by use of drugs that might inhibit platelet breakdown.

This proposal is based on certain assumptions that are not yet solidly grounded experimentally. Thus one cannot say that the clot-promoting effects of phospholipids from disrupted platelets are major factors. It is alternatively, or perhaps additively, possible that the antigen-antibody complexes damage vascular endothelium and that the debris from such damage is as clot-promoting as platelet debris. Possibly platelet damage is actually a sequel of vascular endothelial damage. If so, this might explain why immune complexes do not always damage platelets. If such damage were secondary to vascular endothelial damage, it might not occur at all if the particular antigen-antibody aggregate did not injure the vascular endothelium.

As must be apparent by now, it is difficult to discuss any aspect of the relationship between the clotting and immunologic mechanisms without returning with almost monotonous regularity to Hageman factor and its activators. Consideration of foreign body reactions – both exogenous and endogenous – is not exceptional in this respect. In the current epidemic of drug abuse, a number of bizarre clinical observations have been made. Among these have been the response seen in the lungs of "blue velvet" addicts. These individuals inject themselves intravenously with mixtures of concentrated paregoric and crushed tripelennamine tablets. After repeated injections, pulmonary hypertension may develop, with diffuse arterial and arteriolar thrombosis, followed by formation of foreign-body granulomas in vascular walls. Both clinical and laboratory investigators have established the offending agent as talc derived from the tablets containing tripelennamine. We have a reasonable basis for suggesting that the major role of talc is activation of Hageman factor.

When Hageman factor activation was first studied, the agents found capable of doing this were insoluble, starting, of course, with glass but also including such compounds as barium carbonate, talc, asbestos, and even spider webs. Subsequently, a number of soluble materials, including ellagic acid, cellulose sulfate, and carrageenin, were identified as Hageman factor activators. Finally, certain naturally occurring constituents of the body, including sebum and some types of collagen, have been shown to activate this factor.

From this very incomplete list of Hageman factor activators, one can project certain clinical situations involving foreign-body reactions. The possibility exists that such Hageman factor–mediated responses may be involved in some of the reactions to talc seen after accidental introduction of this agent during surgery. Even more intriguing is the work done by Kellermeyer and Breckenridge. They discovered that the sodium urate crystals found in the joints of individuals with gouty arthritis are a Hageman factor activator and that joint fluid normally contains Hageman factor as well as the precursor forms of PF/Dil, kallikrein, and the kinins.

While it would be extrapolating too far to suggest that these findings suggest an etiology for gouty acute arthritis, it seems quite reasonable to hypothesize that some of the symptoms of this syndrome might start with the precipitation of sodium urate crystals within the joint, activation of the Hageman factor, and elaboration of pain-inducing kinins. Indeed, there is evidence that just this sequence is unfolded when one puts sodium urate into a joint. This course of events does not deny that other mechanisms are operative to bring about acute gouty arthritis. Thus, sodium urate crystals are known to be ingested by leukocytes, resulting in the release of lysosomal enzymes that may induce acute arthritis. Complement, too, may be involved in the pathogenesis of acute gouty arthritis, for Naff has shown that sodium urate crystals deplete serum of C′2, C′3, C′4, and C′5. Thus, whatever its role in the induction of acute gouty arthritis, Hageman factor cannot account for all the known events.

Moskowitz took cartilage mucopolysaccharides, ground them up, and added them to plasma. With normal plasma, kinins are produced; with plasma lacking Hageman factor, there is no kinin production. Moreover, when rheumatoid joints, presumably containing degenerated cartilage, are aspirated, kinins are found in the fluid. Clearly one must entertain the possibility that rheumatoid arthritis involves the sequences we have been discussing, initiated by activated Hageman factor.

Another set of experiments conducted here in Cleveland by Warren and Kellermeyer have focused on the ability to incite inflammatory reactions with "inert" plastic beads. Once again, the ability to achieve the reaction is dependent upon the presence in plasma of Hageman factor. What is most interesting about these experiments is the suggestion that they provide an animal model for such diseases as pneumoconiosis, in which inhalation of silica crystals leads to pulmonary fibrosis. In studying lungs from patients with pneumoconiosis, one finds the silica crystals at the center of the inflammatory areas. In view of what has already been described it would not be surprising to learn that between the inspiration of silica-rich dusts and the development of lesions, activation of the Hageman factor and evolution of kinin activity has taken place.

In investigating the interrelationships of the clotting processes and host defense responses, a great temptation arises to follow the many clinical roads that are opened up. As physicians, it is entirely appropriate that we yield to this temptation. At the same time, as physiologists and biologists, we would be remiss in not recognizing the opportunity afforded to gain a deeper understanding of the interrelated nature of biologic reactions and in this way to grope toward a more holistic and more realistic concept of the design of life.

Chapter 15

Lymphocytic Factors in Cellular Hypersensitivity

JOHN R. DAVID
Harvard Medical School

The participation of two different cell types in reactions of cellular hypersensitivity is well established, as is the importance of these mechanisms in a wide array of immunologic events, including delayed hypersensitivity, certain allergic manifestations, autoimmunity, homograft rejection, immunologic responses to cancer cells, and defense against intracellular bacteria, viruses, fungi, and parasites. The cells involved are primarily lymphocytes that through contact with antigen become sensitized to the antigen, and macrophages that employ their phagocytic capacities to attack, to destroy, and to sequester autologous or foreign materials.

With the recognition of the importance of both lymphocytes and macrophages in these events, it became central to establish the means by which these cell types communicate with each other. The evidence is now accumulating that cell-free factors elaborated by the sensitized lymphocytes subsequent to stimulation by specific antigen can involve macrophages as well as other cell types. Perhaps a dozen or more such factors have now been identified. However, it should be stressed that for the most part what has really been shown is a dozen or more different *activities*. Since for the most part these activities have been assayed by different investigators using different techniques and test systems, often in search of different functions, it is highly unlikely that each of the activities separately identified is actually a function of a distinct substance. Rather, it is probable that several of the factors have multiple activities and that, for example, one man's lymphotoxin may be another's inhibitor.

Before the various factors are described, it should be reiterated that in investigating any of them one generally starts with lymphocytes derived from an individual having cellular hypersensitivity to a particular antigen. The lymphocytes are stimulated in vitro by incubating the cells with that antigen for a given time, most often 24 hours.

The culture medium is then made cell free and the activity assayed in the supernatant. With certain exceptions to be noted below, the production of the various factors is highly specific in that the lymphocytes will produce them in vitro only against the antigen with which sensitization of the lymphocytes was accomplished in vivo. In fact, it has been shown that when hapten protein conjugates are used for sensitization, subsequent production of active factor by the sensitive lymphocytes is dependent on incubation with the same hapten carrier protein conjugate. Thus, when sensitization is achieved with dinitrophenol (DNP) conjugated to guinea pig albumin, lymphocytes will not respond when incubated with DNP conjugated to ovalbumin or with no antigen.

The exceptions noted in the preceding paragraph involve the ability of certain mitogenic agents such as phytohemagglutinin (PHA) or conconavalin A to stimulate lymphocytes nonspecifically. Such lymphocytes will produce active factors, but it is still not certain whether or not these are identical with the factors resulting from antigen-stimulated lymphocytes. Another possible exception relates to experiments that have shown normal lymphocytes can be made sensitive in vitro by using RNA from specifically sensitized lymphocytes. These RNA-treated lymphocytes can then be stimulated by the parent antigen to produce lymphocytic factors. The whole question of transfer of sensitivity with RNA remains somewhat controversial and will not be explored here.

The best known of the lymphocytic mediators is the migration inhibitory factor (MIF), so named because of its ability to inhibit the migration of macrophages out of capillary tubes. Closely related are the macrophage activating factor and, probably, macrophage aggregation factor.

Another mediator to which we will devote discussion is the chemotactic factor for macrophages; there is also a chemotactic factor for neutrophils. Then there is a group of factors having as their prime characteristic the ability to kill cells in culture – the cytotoxic or lymphotoxic factors. Other mediators have been found that do not kill cells but will prevent their growth. This group includes the cloning inhibition factor of Lebowitz and Lawrence, the proliferation inhibition factor of Green et al., and the factor described by Adler and Smith, which can inhibit DNA synthesis. In all cases, when these factors are removed from the culture, the cells will resume growth.

Bloom and Bennett and subsequently other investigators have also demonstrated a skin-reactive factor, one that when placed in the skin of a guinea pig causes an erythematous reaction, with induration and a histologic picture (mobilization of large numbers of mononuclear cells and some polymorphonuclear leukocytes) closely akin to that seen in a classic delayed hypersensitivity reaction. The difference between the reaction obtained with this factor and a naturally occurring delayed hypersensitivity reaction is one of time. The supernatant-mediated reaction occurs in 4 to 12 hours, rather than the 24 required for delayed hypersensitivity. One would expect that a supernatant containing preformed factors would elicit a reaction in less time than lymphocytes would require to reach the reaction site by normal vascular routes and produce the factors at the site.

The skin-reactive factor serves to illustrate that the study of the lymphocytic factors not only produces insights into the mechanisms of cellular hypersensitivity but also reinforces the need to differentiate between the phenomena subserved by activated supernatants and the existence of discrete factors. While the skin-reactive factor is at this time considered operationally to be a definite entity, it would seem much more likely that it represents the combined activities of several other factors, most likely a combination of a chemotactic factor and MIF and perhaps also of a toxic factor. Having said this, rather

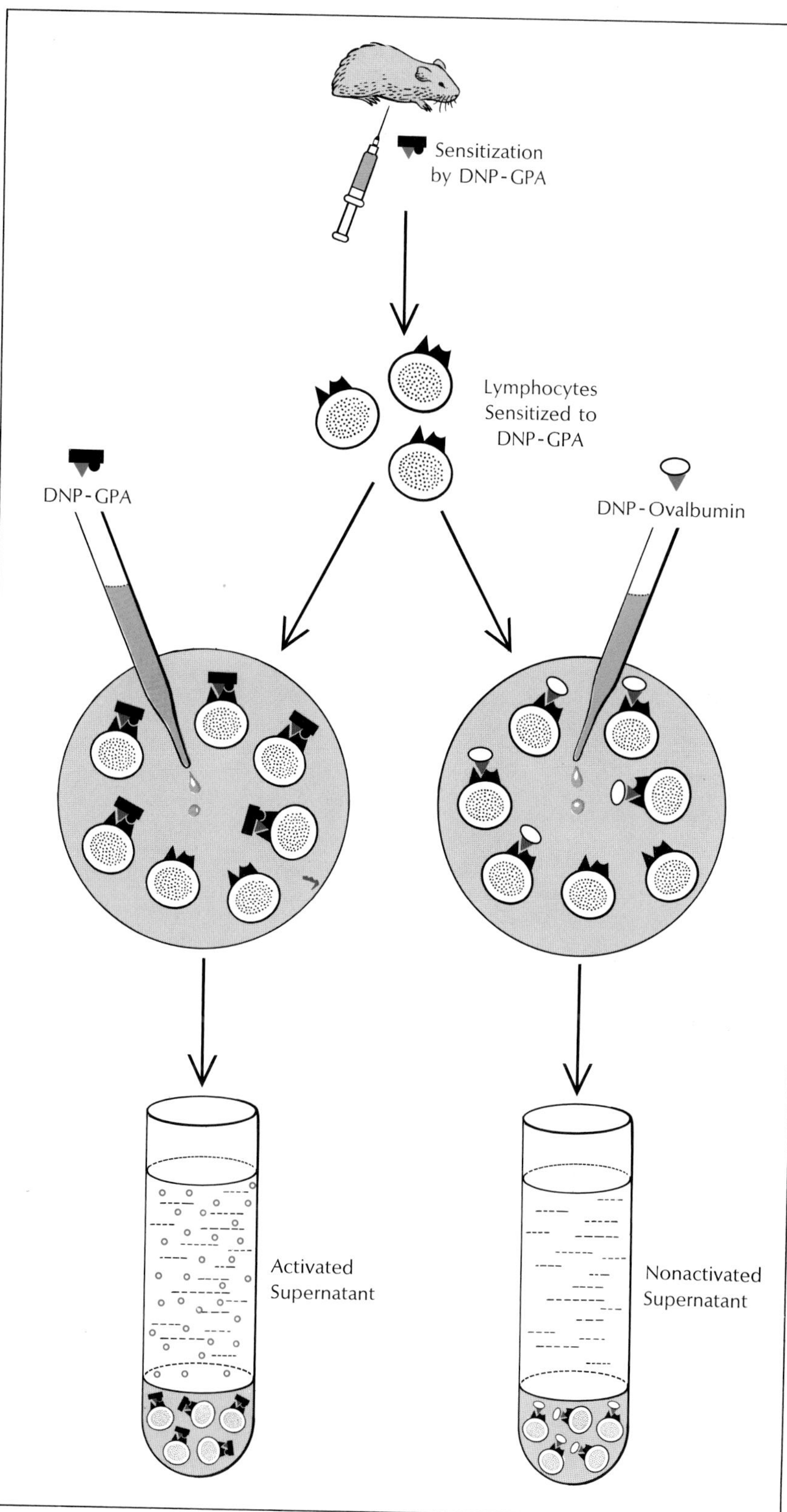

One demonstration of the specificity required for the production of lymphocytic mediators is provided by this experiment in which two different antigens, each with DNP but with different carrier proteins, are employed. The animal is sensitized with DNP conjugated with guinea pig albumin, and its lymphocytes are harvested and placed on two different cultures. On one, the sensitizing antigen is placed; on the other, DNP conjugated with ovalbumin. After incubation, lymphocytes from each culture are suspended and centrifuged; those incubated with DNP-GPA produce a mediator-containing (activated) supernatant; those incubated with DNP-OVA conjugate or without any antigen result in a supernatant without mediator activity.

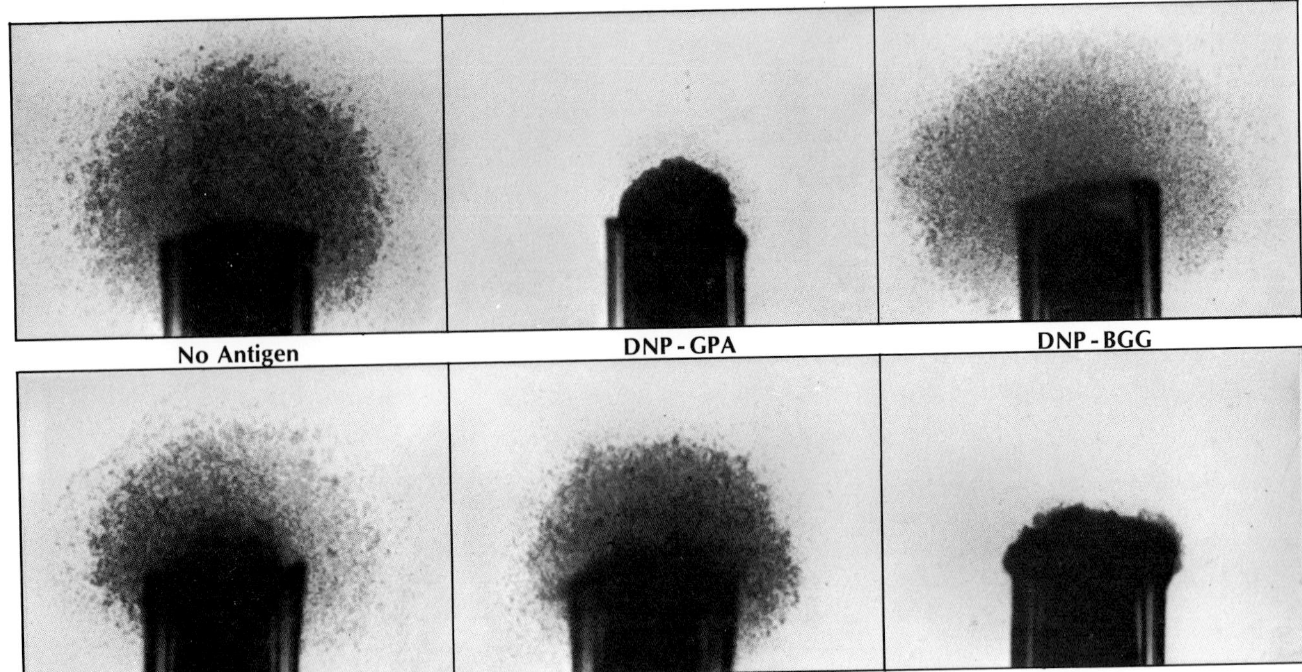

Quantitative assays of migratory inhibition of macrophages by MIF show the high degree of specificity of activity. The migration of cells from an animal sensitized to DNP-GPA (top) is inhibited only by the DNP-GPA antigen and not by DNP conjugated with another carrier protein (DNP-BGG). With animals sensitized to DNP-BGG (lower panel), MIF activity is similarly specific; in this case DNP-GPA produces a "control" result. Method is capillary tube technique of George and Vaughan.

than extend the discussion of how many factors there are, let us proceed to more detailed description of those factors whose properties have been most completely defined. I will pause only to note the existence of two other lymphocytic factors: interferon, produced in response to antigenic stimulation and being studied most extensively because of its possible role in defense against viral infections [see Chapter 26, "Interferon and Interferon Inducers: The Clinical Outlook," by Thomas C. Merigan Jr.], and the transfer factor of H. S. Lawrence [Chapter 11, "Transfer Factor and Cellular Immunity"].

Migration Inhibitory Factor

To begin with MIF, the in vitro study of cellular hypersensitivity had its origins in the work of Rich and Lewis nearly 40 years ago. They showed that if explants of spleen or lymph node cells from sensitized animals were placed in vitro with specific antigen, cell migration from these lymphoid explants was inhibited. More recently, eight years ago, George and Vaughan developed a more quantitative system for studying this phenomenon. They placed sensitive peritoneal exudate cells in small capillary tubes that were cut at the cell-fluid interface after the cells had been spun down and allowed to migrate on glass. With this system it was possible to measure precisely the cells' migration after 24 hours. Not only is this a more quantitative procedure than is possible with lymphoid cell explants but it also permits the manipulation and purification of the exudate cells before they are placed in the capillary tubes.

Through this system it was found that the migration of the entire cell population – consisting of lymphocytes, macrophages, and a few polymorphonuclear leukocytes – appeared to be inhibited by specific antigen. Early in this research, the participation of two cell types in the hypersensitivity reaction was suggested by the observation that if peritoneal exudate cells from a sensitized guinea pig were added to normal exudate cells, migration inhibition of the entire cell population could be achieved if only 2% of the cells in the culture came from the animal sensitized with specific antigen.

Further experiments showed that if one purified lymphocytes derived from lymph nodes of sensitized animals and placed them in capillary tubes, no inhibition was demonstrable. Yet only a few of these same cells, added to normal macrophages, were enough to inhibit migration. Further, Bloom and Bennett took peritoneal exudate cells from sensitized animals, separated the lymphocytes from the macrophages, and added antigen to the macrophage fraction. These cells were no longer inhibited by antigen unless the lymphocytes were returned to the preparation. Clearly, one could now delineate a picture of cellular hypersensitivity involving both a sensitive lymphocyte population and a normal macrophage population.

Defining the relationship mathematically produced an estimate that one lymphocyte was sufficient to affect the migration of about 1,000 macrophages. In terms of designing an in vitro model for cellular hypersensitivity, this relationship suggested a far more efficient system operating through mediators than would be possible if cell-to-cell interaction were required. Moreover, it suggested a huge amplification of the hypersensitivity reaction having significant biologic advantages. Thus, a huge cellular reaction can be mobilized by a few sensitive lymphocytes against, for example, an invading microorganism.

The identification of migration inhibitory factor, the soluble mediator produced by lymphocytes that is capable of inhibiting the in vitro migration of macrophages, was followed by extensive research in several laboratories to determine both the properties of the lymphocytes producing the mediator and the properties of MIF itself. The lymphocytes must, of course, be capable of being sensitized by and, subsequently, of reacting with antigen. They also must be living metabolizing cells, for if one either kills the lymphocytes or inhibits their protein synthesis by such agents as puromycin they will cease to produce MIF.

The first physical properties of MIF to be demonstrated were its heat stability at 56° C for 30 minutes and its nondialyzability, the latter suggesting that it is a macromolecule. Thereafter a variety of fractionation and other techniques were used to further define MIF properties. The results of these experiments by Remold using Sephadex fractionation, acrylamide disc gel electrophoresis, degradation by chymotrypsin and neuraminidase, and cesium chloride ultracentrifugation indicate that MIF from guinea pigs sensitized to a hapten BGG conjugate is an acidic glycoprotein with a molecular weight between 35,000 and 55,000 and that it is not an immunoglobulin.

By taking the Sephadex fraction containing MIF and applying it to monolayer cultures of macrophages, one can also study in vitro the effects of the mediator on these cells. Recently, Nathan in our laboratory showed that after 72 hours of incubation many more macrophages stick to the bottom of the culture dish in the MIF-treated cultures than in control cultures, so that the mediator clearly affects the stickiness of the macrophages (without increasing their rate of multiplication). If radioactive starch is then added to these monolayers, the amount of starch phagocytized by the macrophages is increased three- to fourfold in the MIF-treated cultures. While most of this enhancement can be accounted for by the increased number of macrophages, one also finds that phagocytosis per cell is increased by about

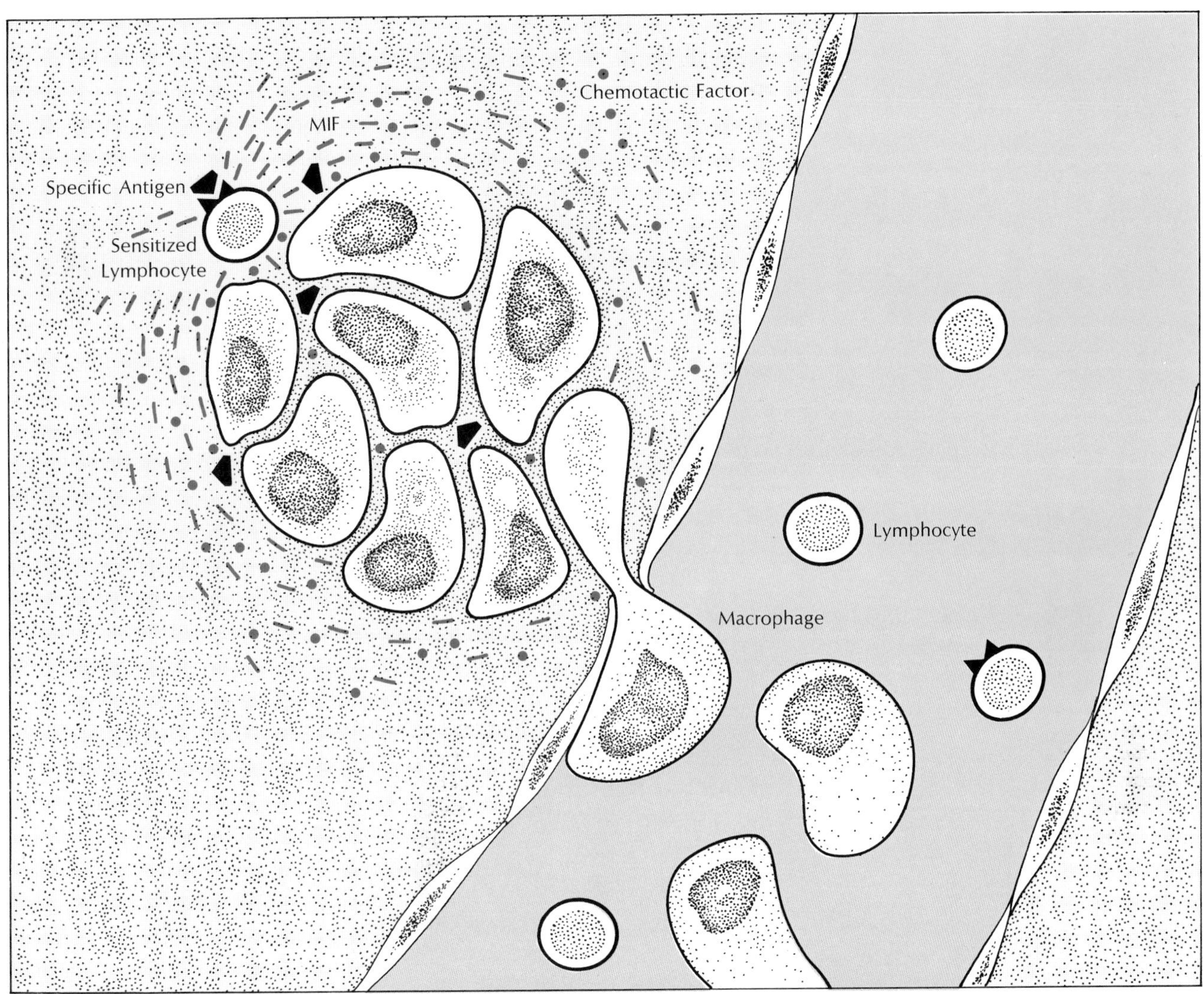

The role of chemotactic factor and MIF in the cellular hypersensitivity reaction is suggested schematically. If an animal is challenged with an antigen to which it has been sensitized, a small number of specifically sensitized lymphocytes make contact with antigen at the challenge site, and chemotactic factor and MIF are elaborated. Chemotactic factor attracts macrophages to this area; MIF keeps them there and activates them. Macrophages are the major component of cell population at the reaction site.

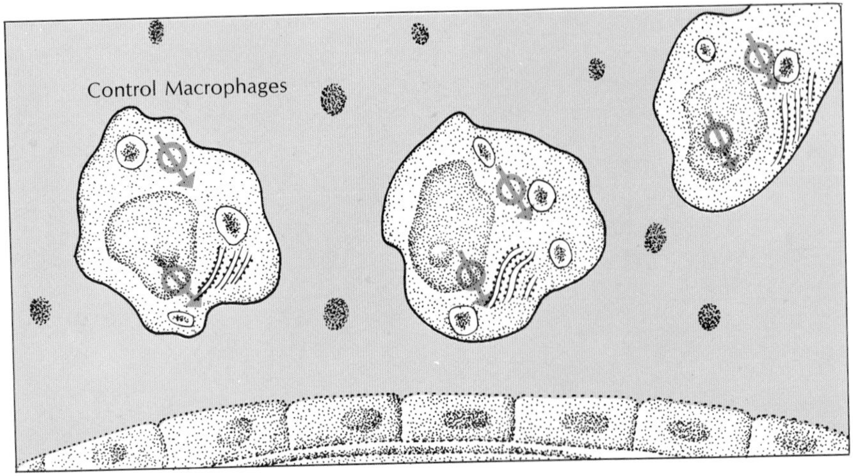

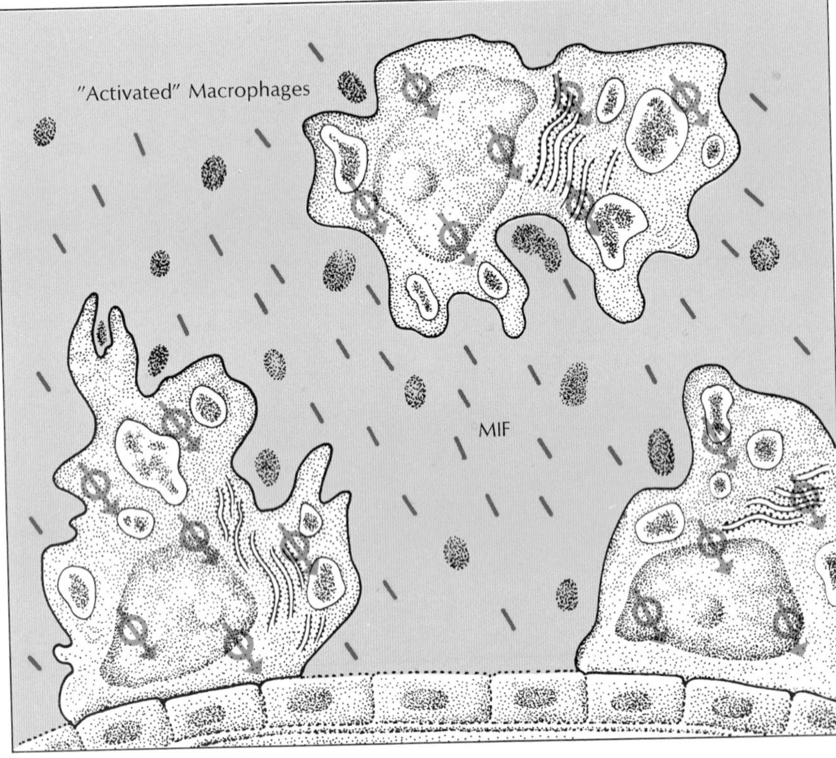

The influence of MIF-rich supernatants is much broader than simple inhibition of migration. When control macrophages (top) are compared with MIF-treated cells, one sees that the latter are spread out and have greatly enhanced ruffled membrane activity. They are more active in phagocytosis and have greatly enhanced glucose oxidation through the hexose monophosphate shunt. It seems likely that MIF and the factor activating the macrophages are the same substance assayed for different activities.

20%. If dead tubercle bacilli are substituted for starch, the increased phagocytosis per cell is even more marked.

Most recently, Nathan compared glucose carbon-1 oxidation in macrophages treated with MIF-rich fractions with glucose oxidation in control macrophage cultures. He found that under the influence of MIF, the treated macrophages increase their glucose oxidation from four- to eightfold. This is probably the most dramatic change observed in MIF-treated macrophages.

The elevated glucose oxidation was found to represent increased metabolism through the hexose monophosphate shunt, which may well be related to a potential heightening of bactericidal capability. It was especially interesting that a latent period of two days was required before the stimulation to increased glucose oxidation could be observed.

If the MIF-treated macrophages are incubated for 72 hours and time lapse cinematography is done, the cells appear far more spread out than control macrophages and there is more extensive ruffled membrane activity. These pictures appear to resemble closely the activated macrophages described by Mackaness [Chapter 5, "Cell-Mediated Immunity to Infection"]. The scheme is almost complete. Influenced by MIF-rich fractions, the macrophages increase their phagocytic capacity, are metabolically more active, and exhibit more membrane activity. What is still to be demonstrated is the ability of these macrophages to kill bacteria more effectively than unstimulated macrophages and whether MIF and the substance that activates the macrophages are the same. It will be recalled that in listing lymphocytic factors, we included the macrophage aggregating factor described by Lolekha and his coworkers. On the basis of the evidence now available, it seems likely that this factor is MIF being assayed on the basis of a property other than the ability to inhibit migration in vitro, that is, the clumping of macrophages in a test tube.

Chemotactic Factors

In work with Ward on chemotactic factors, our starting point was the knowledge that in delayed hypersensitivity reactions, notably in skin reactions to tuberculin or other antigens, accumulation of macrophages occurs at the reaction site. If this phenomenon is considered in the context of chemical mediators, it becomes reasonable to ask whether a lymphocytic factor is responsible for attracting the macrophages. To test for this possibility, Ward assayed chemotaxis in vitro using a Boyden chamber – a double chamber in which the two parts are separated by a Millipore filter. By placing cells above the filter and activated supernatant below, one can determine chemotactic activity by counting the number of cells that pass through the filter. With this system, it was found that the MIF-rich supernatant (compared with control supernatant) was indeed chemotactic for macrophages and, to a lesser extent, for neutrophils.

Was this chemotactic factor actually MIF being assayed for different properties? Like MIF, the chemotactic factor was nondialyzable and heat stable at 56° C. Also, both activities were found in the same fractions after Sephadex gel chromatography, with the peak activity eluting just after albumin. However, when electrophoresis on acrylamide gels was used, chemotactic factor was found in a different gel fraction than MIF. Further procedures were employed to show that the difference was not simply a matter of concentration, of dilution, of binding to albumin, or of assay sensitivity. Macrophage chemotactic factor was indeed a separate factor from MIF. Another piece of evidence for the difference between the two factors was the effects that each has on cells from different species. MIF made by guinea pig lymphocytes does not inhibit migration of rabbit macrophages, while chemotactic factor made by guinea pig lymphocytes is as chemotactic for rabbit macrophages as it is for cells from its own species.

Although the molecular weight of macrophage chemotactic factor is similar to that of MIF – in the range between 35,000 and 55,000 – Ward also demonstrated some chemotactic activity in heavier fractions, those corresponding to the gamma globulins. The data suggest that this could be accounted for by aggregation of the chemotactic factor molecules.

It was noted above that some attraction for neutrophils was also present in the Boyden chamber assays for macrophage chemotaxis. Subsequent disc gel electrophoresis experiments have shown that the neutrophil chemotactic factor can be separated from MIF and chemotactic factor and has a molecular weight somewhat less than that of the macrophage factors.

Lymphotoxic Factors

The lymphotoxic factors have emerged against a background of many years of research on the specific cytotoxicity of lymphocytes for target cells where cell-to-cell contact has apparently been essential for lymphocyte killing. It has not been simple to demonstrate an effect by soluble mediators in some of the long-established systems and, consequently, the lymphotoxic factors are somewhat more controversial than the lymphocyte mediators discussed so far. The initial experiments in this field were done by Ruddle and Waksman using tuberculin-sensitized rat lymphocytes to which PPD was added in vitro. The supernatant from this preparation was then applied to rat fibroblasts and cell killing was demonstrated. These experiments appeared to show that a soluble mediator could produce an effect previously considered the result of a direct lymphocyte–target cell interaction.

Granger and his colleagues, using lymphocytes nonspecifically stimulated with PHA, found either mouse or human lymphocytes so stimulated would produce in one to three days a factor capable of killing mouse L cells. This cytotoxicity could be quantified by measuring amino acid incorporation. Interestingly, the lymphotoxin obtained by Granger's method can also be prepared with human lymphocytes from either tonsils or spleen. The lymphotoxin derived from PHA-stimulated cells, as described by these workers, seems to affect almost all types of tissue culture cells, including macrophages. However, there is a variation in the susceptibility of different target cell types. In our own work with a guinea pig antigen-stimulated lymphotoxic factor, macrophages are not killed by the factor. Rather, more of the macrophages actually remain viable and more of them are present in the cultures after three days. Before discussing the work with guinea pig lymphotoxin, one should note some of the properties of the factor elaborated in Granger's studies.

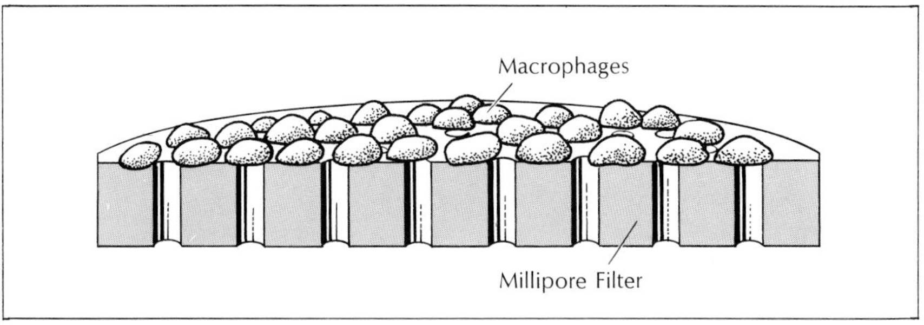

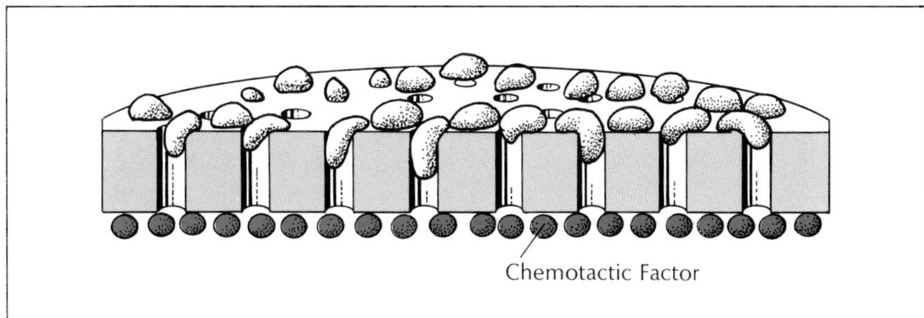

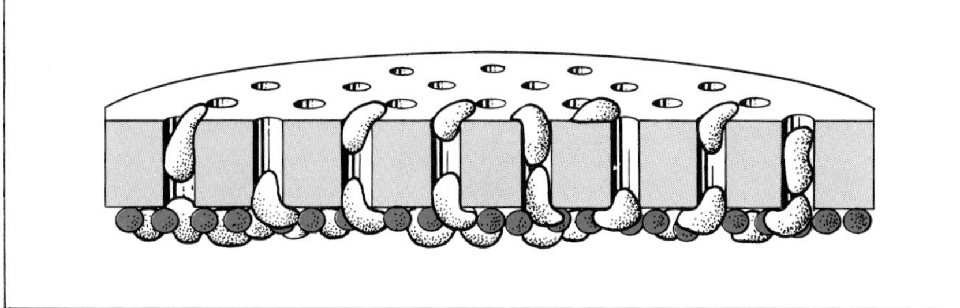

The presence of guinea pig chemotactic factor can be detected in vitro by using a Boyden chamber in which the two compartments are separated by a Millipore filter. Macrophages are placed on the upper side of the filter and supernatant from specifically sensitized lymphocytes on the underside. Movement of macrophages through the filter indicates that chemotactic activity is present in the supernatant.

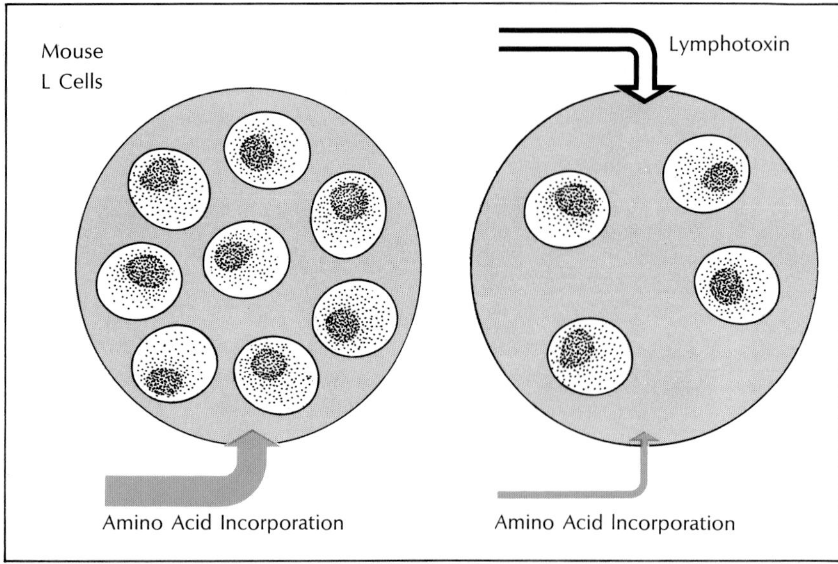

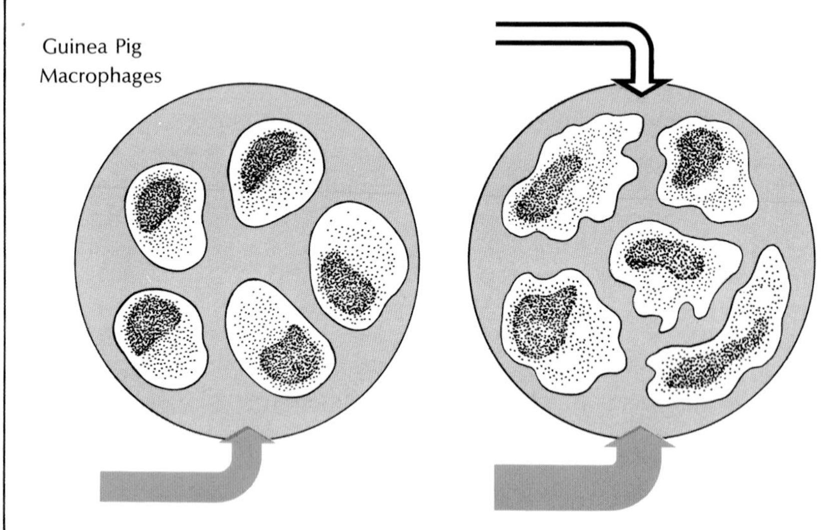

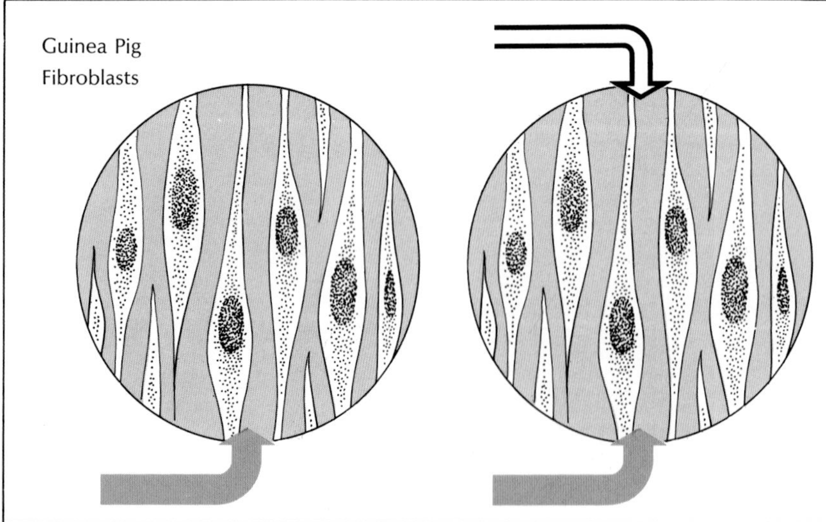

The differential cell susceptibility to lymphotoxin is measured in terms of amino acid incorporation of different cell lines. Mouse L cells appear highly susceptible and treatment with lymphotoxin results in marked depression of amino acid incorporation. Amino acid incorporation is increased in guinea pig macrophage cultures containing supernatants with lymphotoxin, while incorporation of amino acids by cultures of guinea pig fibroblasts remain essentially unaffected by lymphocytic activity.

It has been found to be a protein with a molecular weight in the human material of 80,000 to 90,000. When applied to cell cultures, its action appears to be reversible during the first 24 hours, i.e., the cells will resume growth if the factor is removed during this period. Thereafter, toxicity is irreversible.

Mention of molecular weight brings us to one of the major areas in which observations on lymphotoxins by different groups of investigators appear to be contradictory. Heise and Weiser, working with guinea pig lymphocytes and PPD antigen, found their cytotoxic factor had a molecular weight of 150,000; Dumonde et al., using the guinea pig and bovine gamma globulin as antigen, reported a 68,000 molecular weight; in our own work with guinea pig lymphocytes and BGG-hapten conjugate antigens, we find peak activity in the same fractions as those containing MIF, suggesting a molecular weight of 35,000 to 55,000.

Our finding has led to some interesting experiments. We have been able to use the same Sephadex fraction for comparisons of MIF activity, stickiness to glass, and cytotoxicity for mouse L cells and guinea pig fibroblasts. In work done with Rosenberg and Coyne, the cytotoxin destroys mouse L cells after 72 hours, just as the preparation described by Granger did. The decreased incorporation of amino acids is definite. But if one measures amino acid incorporation in macrophages, one finds a greatly increased incorporation with supernatants rich both in MIF and lymphotoxin. As for guinea pig fibroblasts, these cells are not at all affected by the guinea pig lymphotoxic factor.

These differences suggest two alternative possibilities. One is that we are dealing with another in vitro activity of MIF. Or, as is more likely, lymphotoxin may be a different substance but one that has differing effects because cell types vary in their susceptibility to it.

Another major question regarding lymphotoxic factor activity about which there is still a measure of disagreement can be traced back to the many investigations that seem to show that lymphocyte ability to kill a target cell depends on direct contact between the two. In this context, experiments performed by Brunner are particularly interesting.

In these experiments, lymphocytes were sensitized to a specific cell line, A cells; the lymphocytes were then incubated for 4 to 6 hours with mixtures of A cells, the target cells, and B cells, antigenically unrelated cells. In one mixture the A cells were labeled with chromium-51 and in another mixture the B cells were so labeled. Release of the Cr^{51} label, an indication of cell death, occurred only in the mixture in which the A cells were labeled. In experiments using lymphocytes sensitized to B cells the result was reversed, that is, only the B cells were killed and released the Cr^{51} label. These results indicate specificity of cell killing over a short period of time and cannot easily be explained by the production of a lymphotoxin; such a lymphotoxin, once produced, should kill both A and B cells in the mixtures as both cells were shown to be susceptible to killing.

However, this might be explained on the basis of temporal factors since the lysis of target cells by lymphocytes takes place in a few hours while the elaboration of a chemical factor requires 24 hours or more before the same cytotoxic effect can be expected. What remains uncertain is whether the so-called cell-cell effects are separable from the cytotoxic effects. It is possible that the early phase may be due to a cytotoxic factor that only works at close range and when the lymphocytes are present in high concentration relative to the target cells. Clearly, the fact that lymphocytes can directly kill target cells does not in itself explain how this is achieved, nor does it exclude a possible role for lymphotoxin in the process.

Growth Inhibitory Factors

Another group of lymphocytic mediators includes those that have been shown in vitro to inhibit the growth of target cells without necessarily killing them. A number of such factors have been described. There is the cloning inhibition factor produced by Lebowitz and Lawrence by incubating tuberculin-sensitive human lymphocytes with PPD as the antigen and HeLa cells as the target. This factor was reported to inhibit the cloning of

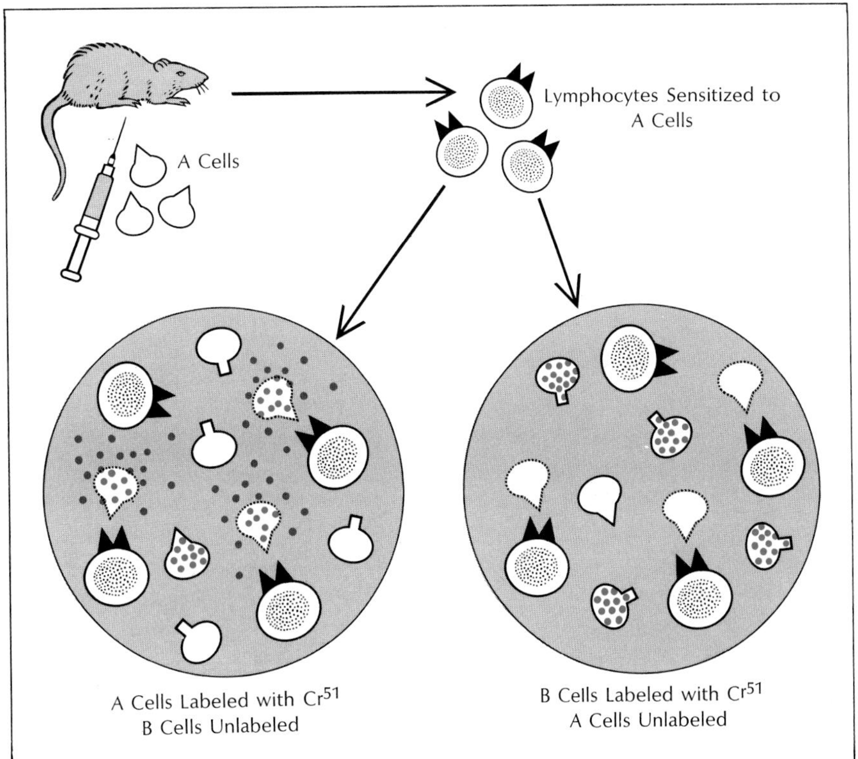

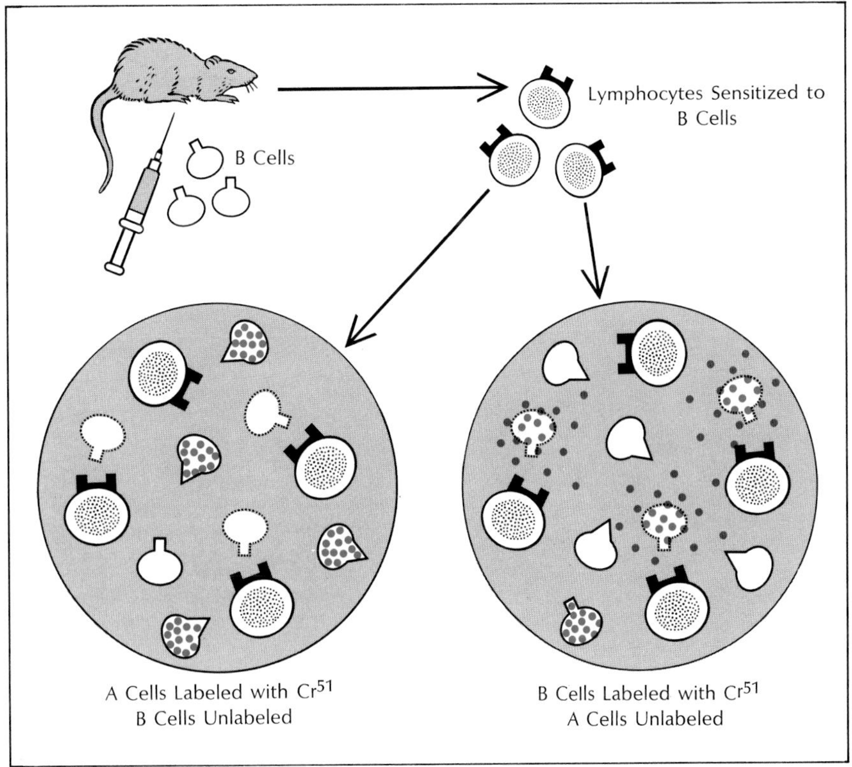

The possibility that lymphocyte killing of target cells depends on direct cell-cell interaction, rather than on mediator activity, cannot be dismissed. In these experiments by Brunner, in which cell lysis was shown by release of radioactive chromium (Cr^{51}), lymphocytes sensitized against one cell line (A) killed only cells of the same line, while those sensitized against B cells killed only B target cells. While this suggests direct cell-cell interaction since both lines were susceptible, time factors might be critical. The reactions schematized here take only a few hours, while elaboration of detectable chemical lymphotoxin requires a longer period of time.

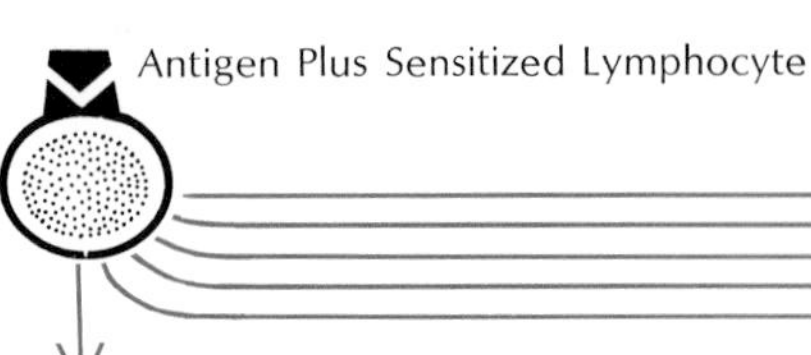

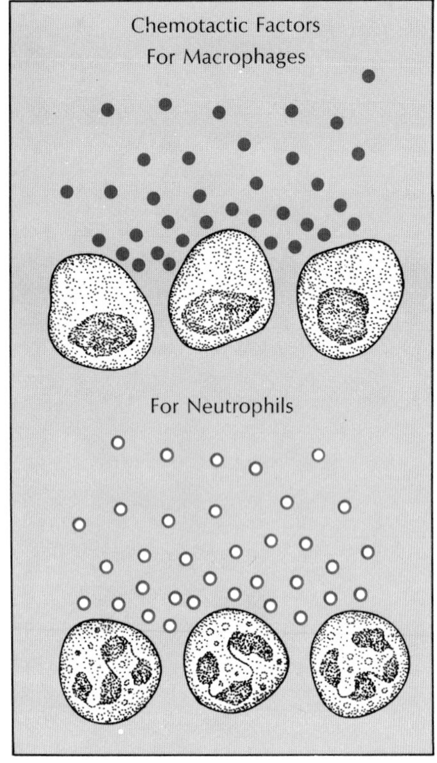

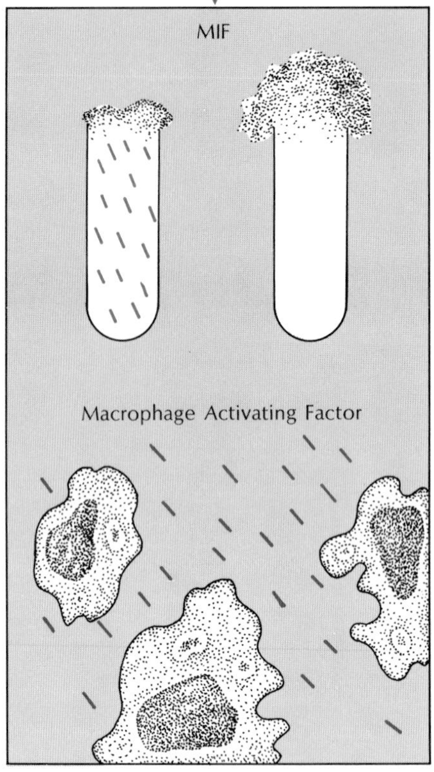

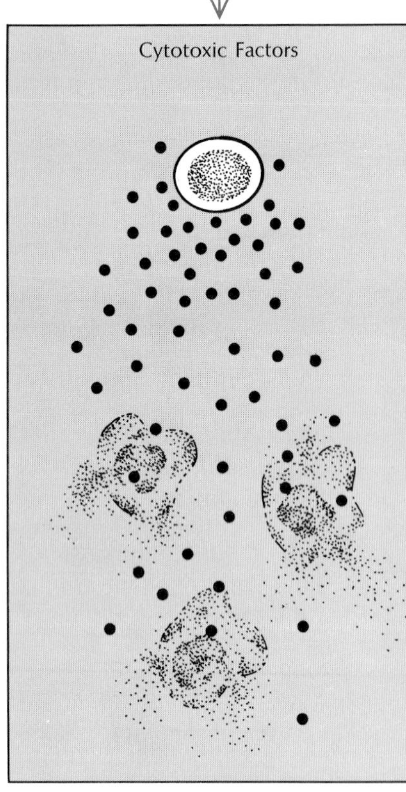

Some of the lymphocytic factors that have been studied and described are represented symbolically above. They include: chemotactic factors for both macrophages and neutrophils; migration inhibitory factor, which, when assayed for different parameters, may also be macrophage activating factor; a number of different cytotoxic factors; the growth inhibitors, cloning

the cells in a completely reversible manner. When the supernatant is removed, the cells again begin to proliferate. A second factor, described by Green and his colleagues, was derived from both PHA-stimulated and PPD-sensitized human lymphocytes. Upon sufficient dilution, this factor will prevent the growth of human cell lines (both HeLa and amnion). No effect is seen on such nonhuman cell lines as mouse L cells, the cells that, interestingly enough, are most susceptible to lymphotoxin. A significant observation concerning this factor is that it must be diluted before it inhibits growth; concentrated or neat, it will kill cells, suggesting, of course, a possible relationship with the cytotoxic factors.

Smith and his group in Florida have worked with another factor produced with PHA-stimulated lymphocytes and capable of preventing DNA synthesis in other lymphocytes used as target cells. With this material, the lymphocytes proceed as far as blast formation but then "abort" because of a failure of DNA synthesis. Again the effect is completely reversible.

Practically speaking, these growth inhibitory factors may have some significance. Certainly, the ability to inhibit DNA synthesis could be very useful in the in vitro study of lymphocyte behavior. And conversely, knowledge that one of the factors produced in the reaction between lymphocytes and antigen can inhibit DNA synthesis must be taken into account in any studies of lymphocyte kinetics in cellular immunity.

Mitogenic or Blastogenic Factors

Before concluding the description of the lymphocytic factors and turning in more detail to consideration of how they might function in delayed hypersensitivity, brief mention should be made of the several factors whose activity appears to be stimulation of normal lymphocyte division. These are the mitogenic or blastogenic factors that were described by Valentine and Lawrence and others. These factors are prepared by stimulating sensitized lymphocytes with specific antigen in culture. When the supernatant containing these factors is added to normal (nonsensitized) lymphocytes, it will cause these cells to transform into blast forms and take up increased amounts of H_3 thymidine. It is quite possible that these factors are important in vivo in recruiting nonsensitive lymphocytes and perhaps in stimulating the production of other mediators.

Having outlined some of the characteristics of the more important lymphocytic factors, it now becomes appropriate to attempt to relate these factors to their significant context, that is, the variety of events that constitute cellular hypersensitivity in vivo.

It is clear that one is dealing with a basically two-cell reaction involving

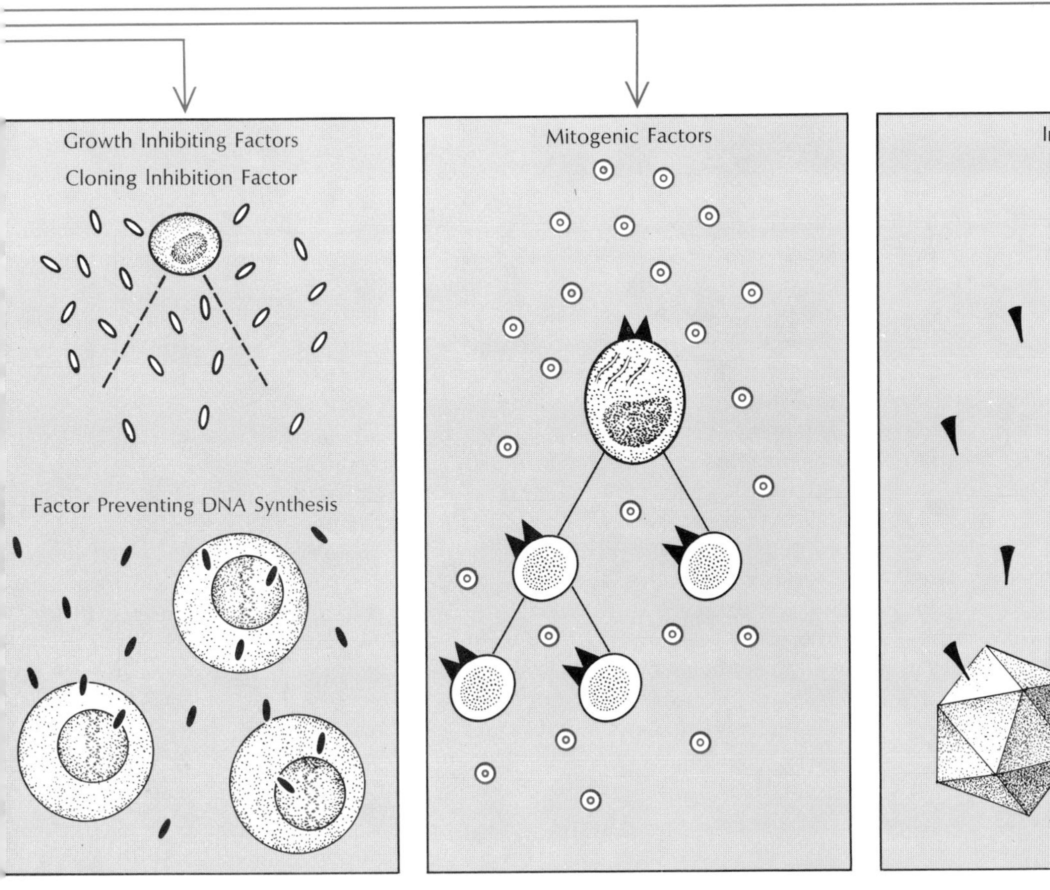

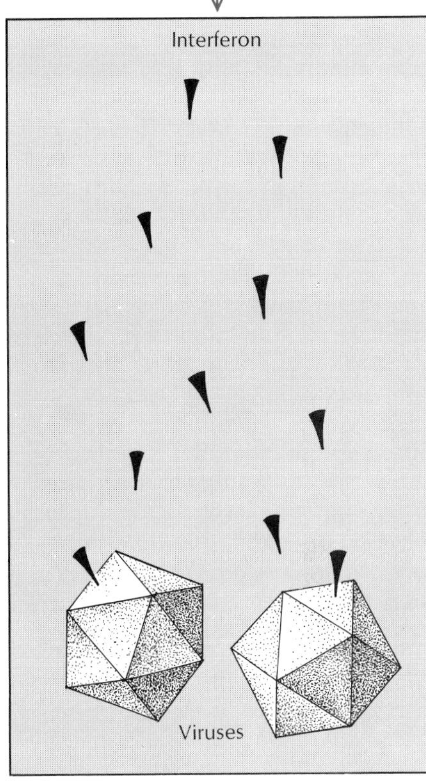

inhibiting factor, and the inhibitor of DNA synthesis; the mitogenic or blastogenic factors; and the antiviral substance, interferon. Not represented but also reported are transfer factor, skin reactive factor, macrophage aggregation factor. It remains to be learned how many of these are discrete factors, how many are different activities of similar substances under varied conditions.

sensitized lymphocytes and nonsensitized macrophages. How do these two types of cells interact with each other and what is the part played by chemical mediators in this interaction? A good starting point for the attempt to answer this question is studies performed by McCluskey and Benacerraf. In their experiments they administered tritiated thymidine to a normal guinea pig for several days so that the rapidly dividing cells of the animal would acquire the radioactive label. They then transferred sensitized lymphocytes from another animal into the test animal in order to create a delayed hypersensitivity skin reaction and took histologic sections from the reaction site. It was found that between 60% and 90% of the cells at this site were labeled, i.e., normal, nonsensitized cells, specifically macrophages derived from the rapidly dividing blood premonocytes within the bone marrow. Thus it was shown that in vivo as in vitro, cellular hypersensitivity is a two-cell reaction in which, quantitatively, the predominant cell type is the macrophage. Clearly the lymphocytes subserve an informational role in the interaction with antigen. Somehow – and the mechanism is still unknown – they get to the reaction site and there set off a chain of biochemical events that bring the reaction to maturity.

Hypothetically, one can assign roles to several of the previously described lymphocytic factors in this chain of events. Chemotactic factors, particularly the factor for macrophages but also that for neutrophils, mobilize the other cellular participants in the reaction. MIF not only keeps the macrophages in place but also serves as an activator to increase the metabolic activity of the cells and to increase their phagocytic capacity. The ingestion of bacteria early in the cellular hypersensitivity reaction has now been established as a major component in the host defenses against many infections, particularly against those caused by intracellular bacteria (as described by Mackaness). In this sense we have come a long way since the days when Arnold Rich and his followers felt that delayed hypersensitivity was essentially a destructive mechanism. We now know the importance of the mechanism against infections and strongly suspect an equally important role against tumors. Logically, then, any factor capable of increasing the phagocytic activity of macrophages, and perhaps the production of lysosomal enzymes, could be an important constituent of most defenses.

Cytotoxic Factors

To turn now to the cytotoxic factors, it may still be premature to pinpoint their role, largely because it has not yet been satisfactorily shown that their cellular targets are specific. If they were indiscriminate in their action, then their role might be anything but helpful. On the other hand, if, for example, lymphocytes sensitized by tumor antigens produced lymphotoxins that killed tumor cells more readily than other cells, this would have great importance. As has been pointed out, differential cellular susceptibility to lymphotoxins has been shown. One would also want to know the interrelationship between lymphotoxin and the other lymphocytic factors and the various other mechanisms that appear to function later on in the delayed or cellular hypersensitivity reaction, including those relating to the vasculature and to the blood coagulation systems. Are these fired off by lymphocytic factors?

Because we have not yet been able to show the in vivo functions of many of the lymphocytic factors, we pursue our efforts to purify and characterize them. When one is able to separate purified factors it should be possible to make antibodies to them (as they seem to be proteins) and use these antibodies to detect their presence in vivo and, perhaps, neutralize the effect of one or another. Obviously this would be a great help in defining their function as the functions of so many biologic substances have been defined by studying and clarifying the consequences of deletion.

Equally important, analysis of the roles of the different factors could provide an important means for "dissecting" the cellular hypersensitivity reaction in man rather than looking upon it as a single all-or-nothing phenomenon. An example of this approach can be seen in the experiments of Rocklin in our laboratory. He has been studying patients with diseases in which cellular hypersensitivity is suppressed – sarcoid, Hodgkin's disease, thymoma, etc. He has analyzed their cellular hypersensitivity using as parameters skin test reactions and, in vitro, MIF production and thymidine incorporation by lymphocytes. Some of the results reported from these experiments are interesting.

Rocklin divided his patients into three groups. The first comprised those who were positive with respect to all three of the parameters being studied – so that within the limits of these studies one can say they have normal cellular hypersensitivity mechanisms – and those who were negative or completely anergic to all three. The second group had negative skin tests and negative MIF assays but were positive for thymidine incorporation. Third, there were four patients who were negative on skin testing, so that by conventional criteria they were anergic, but had positive MIF assays and thymidine incorporation. Therefore, by in vitro criteria, they could be assumed to have sensitized lymphocytes. Perhaps they were not making the right mediator; perhaps they had a defect in their macrophages, or in the vasculature, or in their clotting mechanisms. The possibilities remain myriad, but it is significant that a beginning has been made in disassociating the various parts of the hypersensitivity reaction.

Another experimental approach in our laboratory that has interesting implications was taken by Rocklin and Lewis working with glomerulonephritis. The question asked was whether or not these patients made MIF. Using a glomerular basement membrane antigen derived from human cadaver kidneys, the investigators found that only 6 of the 14 glomerulonephritis patients produced MIF. By means of fluorescent microscopy, it was found that seven of the eight patients incapable of making MIF had either the "lumpy-bumpy" type of disease or no fluorescence [see Chapter 17, "Glomerulonephritis and Immunopathology," by Frank J. Dixon]. Those patients who produced MIF had linear deposits, i.e., they showed antibody to the glomerular basement membrane. We are now, of course, looking at the other side of the cellular hypersensitivity coin – the pathogenetic rather than the defensive side – and it seems likely that the lymphocytic factors are involved here too. These experiments also point to the utility of factor assays as a means of determining the presence or absence of sensitized lymphocytes and perhaps of differentiating between the roles of sensitive cells and humoral antibodies in these pathogenetic situations where both appear to be present.

It should be stressed that clinical applications of our knowledge of lymphocytic factors are still remote, but the possibilities are considerable. We are all interested in determining whether tumor antigens are capable of inciting cellular hypersensitivity, and our ability to detect or failure to detect MIF or chemotactic factors or cytotoxic factors could well provide information on this problem. Nor can the possibility be excluded that breakdown in host tumor defenses might involve a specific failure in the production of one or more of the lymphocytic mediators.

Similarly, the shortcomings of present means of immunosuppression are for the most part results of our inability to narrow the effects down to just the desired one. Here again, the dissection of the cellular defense mechanisms being sought through understanding of the lymphocytic factors might afford a solution. Just to mention another of the many possibilities, one could also speculate that in situations where cellular hypersensitivity is a pathologic mechanism, that mechanism could be thwarted by inhibiting the production of one of the factors while leaving all other aspects of host defense mechanisms intact. Most certainly the avenues open to students of the lymphocytic factors are multiple and many of them could lead to clinical destinations.

Section Four

Pathogenetic Mechanisms Involving Immunologic Factors

Chapter 16

Mechanisms of Immunologic Injury

FRANK J. DIXON
Scripps Clinic and Research Foundation

Antibody-induced injury is produced by circulating humoral antibody. Its character, localization, and severity are dependent upon the immunologic specificity of the antigen, the type of antibody involved, the mediators through which the immunologic reaction of the antibody is expressed, and the quantities of antibody and antigen reacting. Various cell types, most notably the polymorphonuclear leukocytes, may be called into the reaction subsequent to its immunologic initiation, but their role is a nonspecific inflammatory or phlogogenic one.

With the central role of the antibody in mind, it should not be surprising that the nature of injury has such wide variation. At one end of a spectrum is the damage resulting from antibodies of the IgE class, which are capable of producing largely reversible anaphylactic types of tissue changes. However, for purposes of this chapter, we are more concerned with those immunoglobulins that lead to destructive pathologic changes and more or less permanent alterations in physiologic function. Even within this stricture, the variation is broad. Thus, noncomplement-fixing antibodies, usually of the IgG class, will produce relatively mild tissue damage in which participation of the PMN leukocytes and other inflammatory cells is minimal, while complement-fixing antibodies, whether IgG, IgA, or IgM, are likely to produce severe, necrotizing injury.

The second parameter that has critical bearing on the severity of injury, and therefore on the course of ensuing disease, is the quantity of antibody. The greater the amount, the greater the reaction with antigen and the greater the pathogenic effect. If one has a large amount of complement-fixing antibody, the reaction can be explosive, with large amounts of tissue destroyed by an acute necrotizing response in which great numbers of inflammatory PMN leukocytes are mobilized. With very low levels of circulating antitissue antibody, the typical reaction would be a gradually developing, smoldering type of inflammatory response. In such instances it may take months or even years before the amount of tissue destroyed is sufficient to interfere with function and cause overt disease.

Whereas the type of injury and its severity are most influenced by such parameters as the quantity of antibody and its ability to activate mediators such as complement, the site of injury is largely determined by the immunologic specificity of the antibody, that is to say, by the antigen with which it reacts. If, for example, the antigen is a tissue-fixed component of lung, that is where the antigen-antibody interaction will eventuate and the affected tissue will be lung. If the antigen is one that circulates, then the antigen-antibody reaction will take place in the circulation and injury is likely to be at multiple sites. Such circulating complexes are likely to localize in and damage structures that function as physiologic filters, such as the glomerulus.

Antibody-induced injury may be either truly autoimmune or may represent an antibody response to exogenous agents that happen to be present in the host. True autoimmunity is involved if the antibody is reacting against tissue- or organ-specific antigens that are natural components of the body. As has just been noted, if the "self" antigen is an integral component of an organ, say basement membrane in the kidney or lung, or an endocrine product of a gland, such as thyroglobulin, the antibody-induced injury will result from an attack on the organ involved, as in kidney, lung, and thyroid in the examples given. The antigen may also be microbial, and evidence is accumulating that viruses may be the most likely agents to play this part. In such situations, the localization of the injury will depend on the tissue predilections of the virus or other agent. The microbes may be on the surface of the cells and present as a surface antigen, thereby inviting antibody and antibody-induced injury to its host cells. Alternatively, a viral genome may preempt the cells' synthetic machinery and actually direct the formation of abnormal cellular membrane antigens, with the same effect.

Up to now, we have been discussing for the most part injuries induced directly by the antibody that circulates until it reaches its antigen and in combining with that antigen initiates an attack on the tissue to which the antigen is fixed. The second major mechanism by which antibodies can produce injury is that of immune complex pathogenesis. This mechanism was alluded to in the situation of the circulating antigen that forms complexes with antibody in the bloodstream and then deposits within various organs and tissues, usually within filtering structures such as the glomerulus or other blood vessels. It is there that the injury is produced.

In this form of injury, the antigen must be in the circulation for a prolonged period, at least long enough to evoke an antibody response and be around when the antibodies are elaborated into the circulation. Such antigens may be self constituents like thyroglobulin or environmental antigens like foreign therapeutic serum or infecting viruses.

We can now exemplify the two basic forms of antibody-induced injury, those evolving from antibody directed against tissue-fixed antigens and those resulting from localization of circulating immune complexes. Parenthetically, it can be noted that both pathogenic mechanisms are involved in the clinical spectrum of glomerulonephritis; this will be more fully elaborated in the chapter following.

Much of our understanding of the ability of antibody to produce tissue or organ injury subsequent to interaction with fixed antigens comes from studies of an experimental disease, Masugi, or nephrotoxic, nephritis, produced by heterologous antibody. Typically, kidney from rat is injected into a rabbit, which makes antibody to it. This antibody is then harvested and injected back into a rat. Because the antibody is heterologous, it is relatively simple to observe and quantify its effect in vivo. In this system, the antibody made by the rabbit is directed against rat glomerular basement membrane (GBM). When this anti-GBM antibody is injected into the rat it circulates, comes into direct contact with the rat GBM, and fixes along the inner aspect of the membrane. It then activates complement, resulting in chemotactic attraction of PMN leukocytes [see Chapter 10, "The Immunologic Role of Complement," by Henry Gewurz]. The resulting inflammatory reaction produces injury to the GBM, which is expressed clinically by compromised renal function and proteinuria.

Another laboratory demonstration of this phenomenon is found in the work of W. O. Weigle and other investigators. They have produced necrotizing lesions of the thyroid by passively transferring antithyroglobulin antibodies to normal rabbits. In this system, the immunized donor rabbits have been previously thyroidectomized so that they lack target antigen to absorb circulating antithyroglobulin antibodies. If the antibodies are harvested and injected into a normal intact rabbit, the thyroid of the recipient animal will develop inflammatory lesions. The antibody is organ specific and capable of reacting phlogogenically with thyroid antigens. Similarly, antisperm antibodies can react with sperm in the excretory or conducting system of guinea pig testes to produce lesions.

It has also been clearly demonstrated that passively transferred antiviral antibodies can injure virus-infected cells in a number of animals. The situation here is somewhat different than in the prior examples, since the virus is, of course, not in itself native to the animal. However, virus apparently can dictate the formation of specific antigens on the surface of cells they infect.

Several mechanisms are involved. Some viruses leave cells by budding from the cell surface. During this process, the viruses actually become exposed so that the viral-envelope antigen is for a time on the surface of the cell. It is to this antigen that the viral antibodies direct themselves and, by complexing, initiate the events leading to cell injury. In other cases, the virus within the cell takes over its synthetic apparatus, which then forms antigenic proteins on the surface of the cell. These, apparently, are not native to the viral coat nor structurally related to the virus. They are, however, foreign to the host and capable of eliciting an antibody response. When the antibody called forth is complement fixing, as it often is, the resulting sequence in most mammalian cells eventuates in lysis and death and, of course, significant injury to the involved organ or tissue.

A large number of viruses have the ability to initiate these events. One that has been studied particularly intensively in the laboratory has been the lymphocytic choriomeningitis (LCM) virus, an agent found most often in mice but one that also can infect man. Immunologic damage invoked by LCM infection is most commonly found in liver cells, which are highly susceptible to infection. CNS cells are also involved frequently and are found to contain the virus or its antigens. In general, LCM's properties are closely akin to those of a number of chronic or slow viruses, including the chronic neurotropic viruses in man, such as kuru, the scrapie virus that affects sheep, and the Aleutian disease agent of mink.

The role of antibody in the pathogenic events seen with LCM virus has been clearly defined. If an infected mouse is immunosuppressed or made immunodeficient in some way, it will develop tremendously high titers of virus but no tissue injury. If one then passively transfers anti-LCM antibody, disease will occur. In both passive transfer experiments and active infection, the development of disease can be associated with circulating antibody.

The second major pathogenic mechanism through which antibodies produce injury can also be exemplified in a number of ways. While we have discussed virally evoked antibody injury in situations where the virus first invades cells and alters them antigenically to cause "tissue-fixed" injury, viral antigens can also encounter antibody in circulation and form complexes that, in turn, are the pathogenic agents. Certain iatrogenic agents – foreign serum and various drugs capable of combining with host protein – have also been implicated in complex-initiated injuries. Perhaps the best prototype of complexes involving purely self antigens is that formed in patients with systemic lupus erythematosus. In SLE, the patient has circulating nuclear antigens, the most pathogenic of which are DNA. The DNA antigens complex in the circulation with anti-DNA antibodies, which then lodge in various filtering structures, producing syndromes such as lupus nephritis. This, too, will be more fully discussed in the succeeding chapter.

The question of why immune complexes accumulate pathogenically in filtering structures has been investigated intensively in our laboratory. Normally, such complexes could be expected to be eliminated by phagocytic cells and other elements of the host defense mechanisms. We know that there is a relationship between the size of the macromolecular complexes and their susceptibility to phagocytosis, and that the very large complexes are more likely to be phagocytosed. We know, too, that the complexes that seem to be most frequently deposited in the glomerulus or in other filtering structures seem to be soluble and are larger than 19S and have a molecular weight of at least one million. In aggregate, however, they seem to be somewhat smaller than the complexes that will be phagocytosed most completely. Therefore, one of the possibilities we are now investigating is that the accumulation of pathogenic antigen-antibody complexes in vessels results from a relative failure of phagocytosis.

Whether this proves to be the case or not, the complex size appears to be critical. If the complex is small enough, it will be filtered through without hindrance and excreted. If it is large enough, it will be incapable of moving into interstitial fluids, will remain intravascular, and will be phagocytosed. Moreover, size is important, too, because very small complexes, such as those consisting of only one antibody molecule attached to two antigen molecules, do not have the ability to fix complement and to set in motion either humoral or cellular events eventuating in tissue injury.

In experimental models where quantitative studies may be undertaken, it has been found that the amount of complex localization in injured tissues is relatively small, that is to say, only

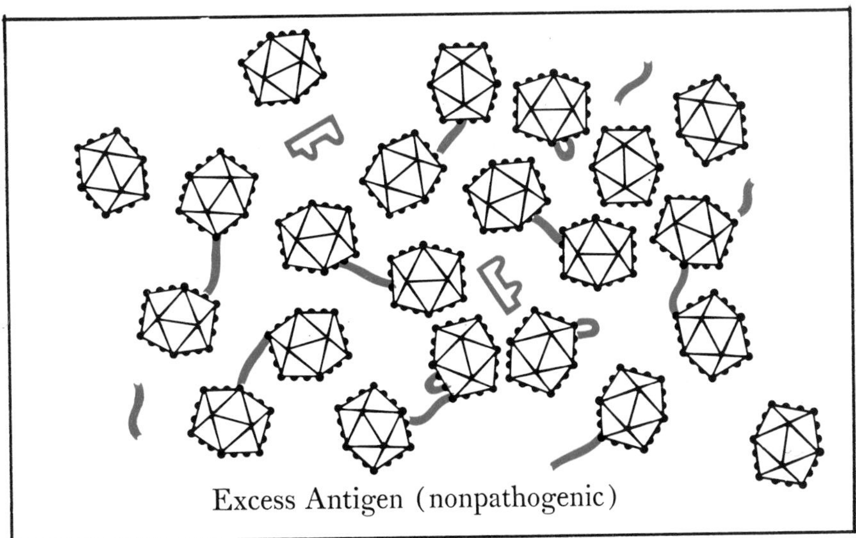

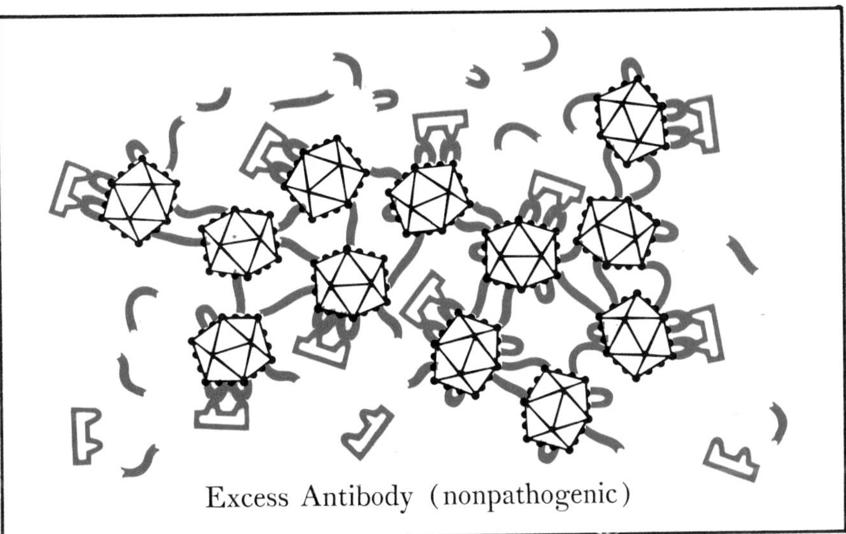

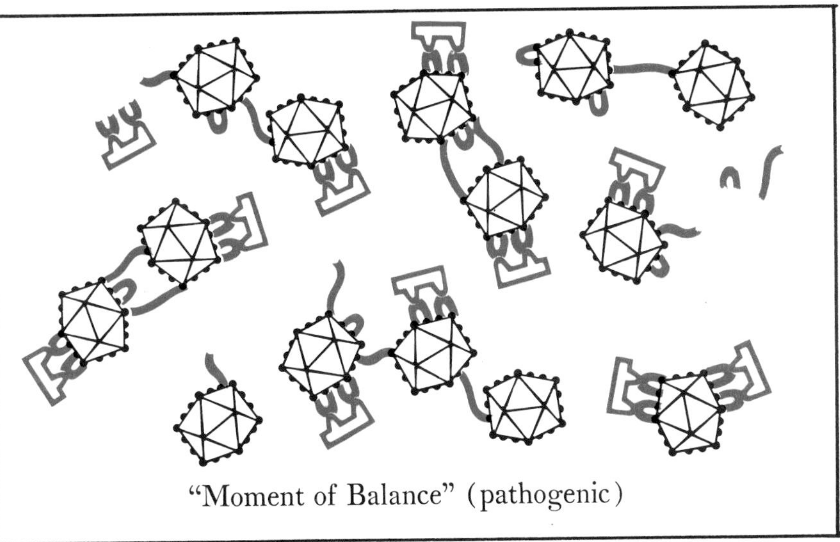

Hypothesis suggests antigen-antibody balance is needed for immunologic injury. With excess antigen, complex size is limited and complement is not activated; with excess antibody, very large complexes are formed and these do not circulate.

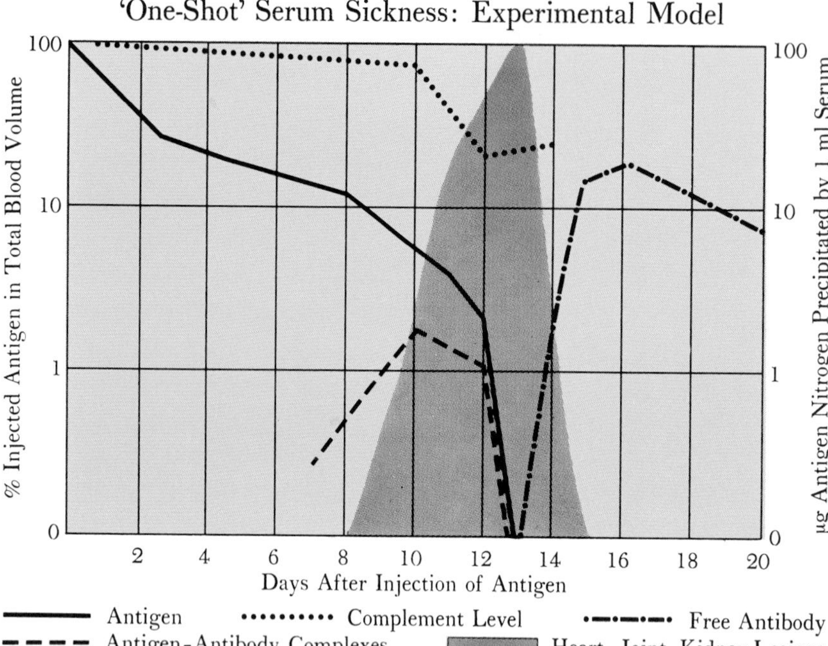

The sequence of events in classic "one-shot" serum sickness parallels the record of an experiment involving injection of I^{131}-labeled bovine serum albumin into a rabbit. As detectable antigen-antibody complexes appear in the circulation, complement drops to less than half normal values, morphologic lesions appear in heart, blood vessels, joints, kidneys. Shortly after all antigen-antibody complexes are eliminated, free antibody appears in circulation, and inflammatory lesions rapidly disappear.

a small percentage of the total antigen involved in complex formation is concentrated in the injured structures. The bulk of the material is actually picked up by phagocytic cells and degraded so that its phlogogenic potential is obviated.

The small quantities are, however, often quite sufficient to produce inflammatory or degenerative changes. With complement activation and the attraction of PMN leukocytes, the injury may be acute. But even when there is low, chronic deposition and little or no participation of PMN's or other cells characteristic of acute inflammatory reactions, one sees degenerative hyaline-type changes in vessel walls, with effects such as abnormal filtration by the kidney.

Much of our understanding of the immune complex pathogenesis of disease has been derived from the study of experimental (and clinical) serum sickness. This research had its origins in the prescient insights of C. F. von Pirquet, who at the beginning of the century undertook studies of the serum sickness that developed in patients receiving heterologous sera as part of the treatment of a variety of infectious diseases. He noted that after a latent period of a week or more the foreign serum disappeared rapidly from the recipient's circulation and was followed by the appearance of antibody to the heterologous material. He also observed the occurrence of a brief period during which serum and antibody seemed to coexist in the patient.

Von Pirquet perceived that, during this period of coexistence, a "toxic product" was being elaborated, and he attributed many of the symptoms that developed in the serum sickness syndrome to this "toxic product." Some of von Pirquet's assumptions were fallacious (e.g., he thought that the foreign serum contained a single antigen rather than the many antigens we now know to be present), but his conclusions were essentially correct and we now know that his "toxic product" is the antigen-antibody complex.

In studies of one-shot serum sickness we have been able to demonstrate that as an antibody response to the serum is evoked, complexing of the antibody with circulating foreign antigen begins. Then, over a period of several days, the amount of immune complex in the circulation rises. As the quantity of complex increases there is a corresponding diminution of circulating complement, reflective of the activation and fixation of the complement by the circulating complexes.

Once the complexes aggregate to the point where they are large enough to be removed from the circulation either by phagocytosis or localization in vessels, the antigen disappears from the circulation and free antibody reappears.

During the period when complexes are being formed and circulate, one sees allergic inflammation in the kidneys, heart, blood vessels, and joints. As the complexes disappear so do the lesions.

The one-shot serum sickness model has been extremely valuable in enabling investigators to prove conclusively that immune complexes are capable of lodging in certain tissues and causing injury. However, it did not provide us with a model analogous to most chronic clinical conditions involving antigen-antibody complexes in man. Its development was too rapid, its repair too prompt to permit such analogy. Therefore, the experimental design was altered so that foreign serum could be injected intravenously daily in smaller amounts over periods of many months. With this approach, the circulating complexes could be maintained in animals for prolonged periods at somewhat lower levels than those in the one-shot model. As a result, apparent disease developed only after a period of some weeks or even months. Complex accumulation, when it did occur, was largely in the glomeruli and was followed by the development of chronic glomerulonephritis.

In this model it was obvious that, in the early period of injections, the complexes that formed were being handled by host defenses. These defenses, other than the obvious participation of phagocytic cells, have yet to be fully defined. There is some evidence that the glomerular mesangia are able to eliminate small quantities of circulating complexes. However, that these defenses become insufficient is attested to by the fact that with a constant load of complexes over a period, the appearance of disease is rather sudden and does not seem related to any change in the quantitative aspect of the immunologic insult. Rather, one seems to find a breakdown in complex elimination.

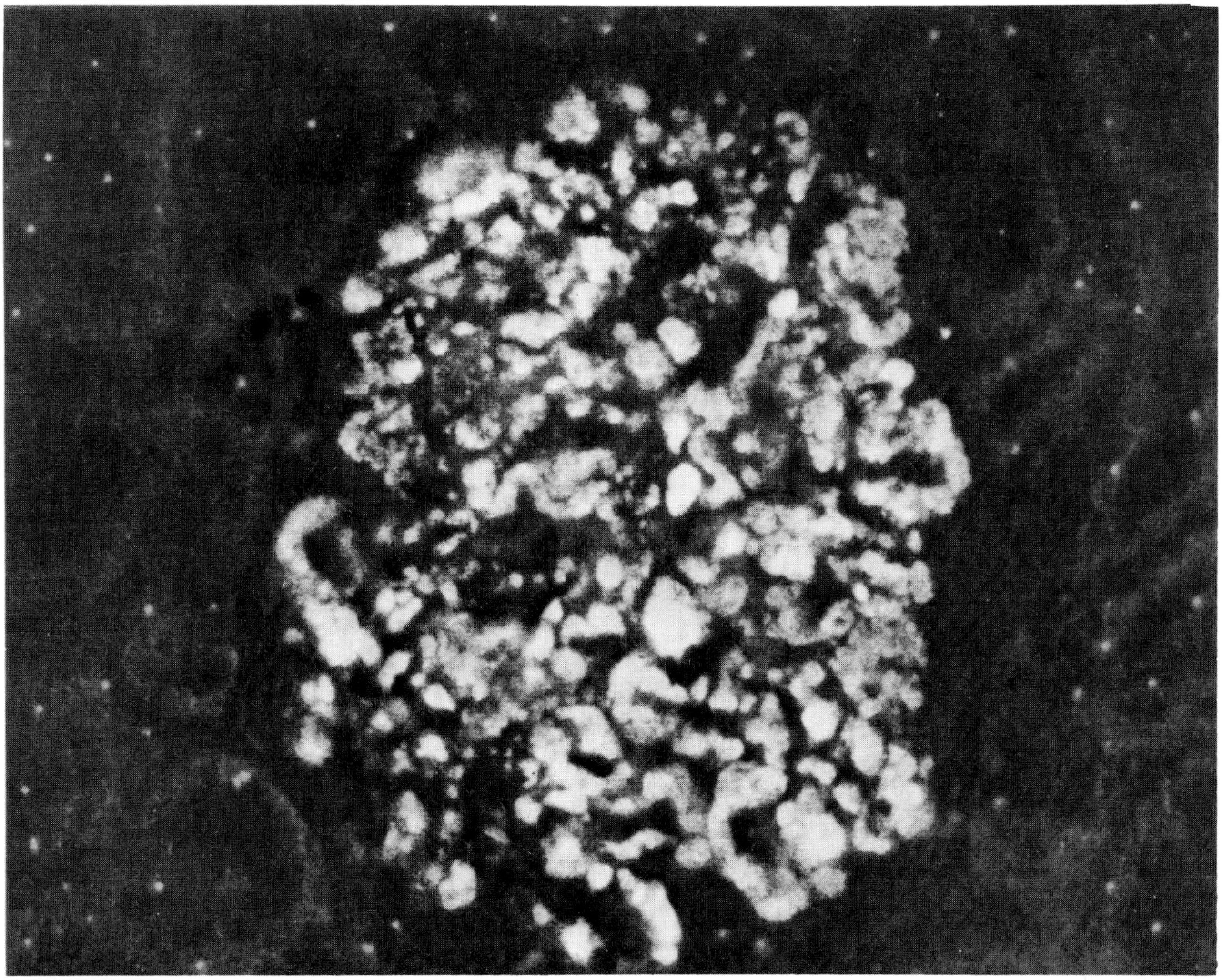

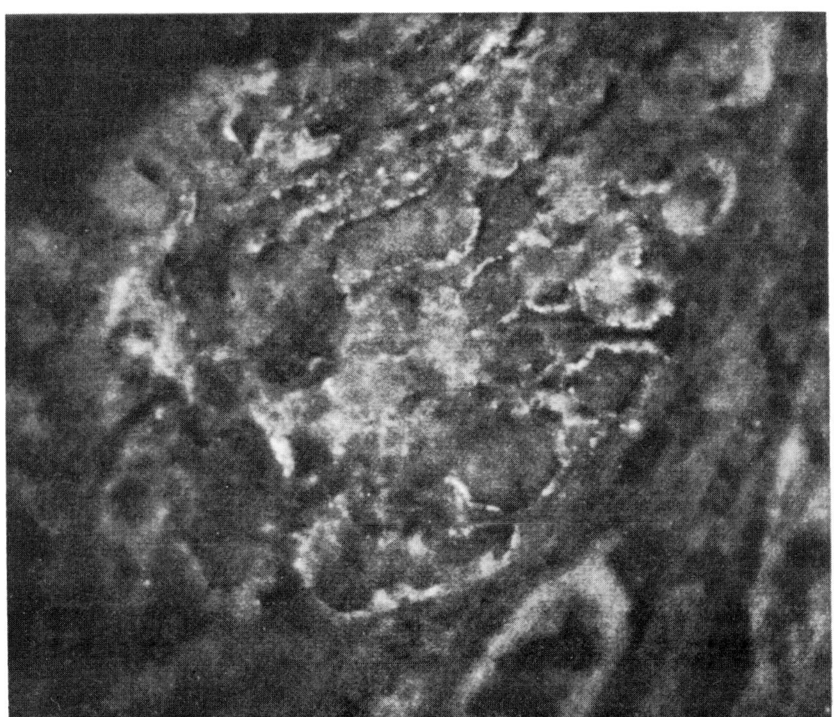

The immunofluorescent photomicrograph above depicts lesions similar to those of advanced chronic glomerulonephritis. It shows a rabbit glomerulus with chronic membranous glomerulonephritic lesions resulting from daily injections of small amounts of antigen. Lumpy fluorescent deposits are found on outer side of thickened basement membrane with scarring and endothelial proliferation. The deposits contain host gamma globulin, complement, and concentrated antigen. Deposits and renal malfunction may persist for a year after antigen injections are stopped.

The photomicrograph at the left shows a rabbit glomerulus in "one shot" serum sickness. In this case, deposits are present in a powdery form on glomerular capillary walls; there is no scarring. The disease is transitory and serves as a model for early stages of chronic progressive conditions like rheumatic fever or rheumatoid arthritis.

Early in the study of chronic serum sickness it became apparent that the quantitative relationship between the antigen and antibody was a significant parameter in the development of disease. One can postulate, with considerable experimental support, three basic situations of antigen-antibody quantitative relationship in the body.

First there is the situation in which antigen is plentiful but the amount of antibody is very small because of the incapacity of the host's immunoresponsive mechanisms. In such situations, there will be a great excess of antigen over antibody and the immune complexes formed are likely to be quite small, since the capacity of any one antibody molecule to interact with antigen is limited. Typically, a complex might contain two antigen molecules and one antibody molecule. These complexes would not be pathogenic because they are too small to be held back on filtering structures and also too small to fix complement.

At the other extreme, one has the situation in which there is a tremendous antibody response and a large excess of antibody over antigen. The complexes formed would be extremely large and also not pathogenic, since they would likely be phagocytosed from the circulation rapidly and not have the opportunity to lodge in the glomeruli or other filtering structures.

In between the two extremes, of course, would be the situation in which there is an approximate balance between antigen and antibody, usually in the region of slight-to-moderate antigen excess. It has been shown that when an animal has a slight antigen excess, sizable soluble complexes are formed – those with a molecular weight of over a million – that are capable of fixing complement, that are not completely phagocytosed, and that do lodge in filtering structures. These complexes that stay in the circulation for a few hours are the ones most often involved in vascular injury.

These kinetics tell us about the immunologic competence of those individuals most susceptible to complex injury. Such an individual would not be a particularly strong antibody-former, nor would he be unresponsive. It would be the individual who makes an antibody response *almost adequate* to neutralize all antigen, but not quite, who would be most likely to harbor the type of complexes most injurious to him.

Up to now, we have confined the discussion to conventional immune complexes – antigen and humoral antibody. There is, however, some evidence that other complexes might be equally phlogogenic, specifically, immunoglobulin aggregates without antigen. Ishizaka, who, with Germuth, had first shown that a state of slight antigen excess was the most likely situation for the formation of injurious immune complexes, also noted that whenever biologically active antigen-antibody complexes were formed, these complexes underwent a change in their optical rotation, suggesting an alteration in the tertiary configuration of the antibody molecules involved. He postulated that this change in configuration might, in fact, be responsible for the phlogogenic properties of the complexes. He therefore formed gamma globulin complexes without antigen, either by heat aggregation or by direct chemical bonding. And such aggregates did show a change in optical rotation similar to that seen with the Ag-Ab complexes, and they did have biologic activity. They were able to fix complement and to initiate inflammatory processes in animals.

These experiments, and others done subsequently that confirmed the results, have made necessary an expansion in our frame of reference with regard to immune complex pathogenesis. Certainly, the most important and common etiology in the type of disease we have been discussing is the complexing of antigen and antibody under the conditions we have defined. But we must also consider nonspecific aggregation of immunoglobulins. Such aggregation might occur in situations where circulating gamma globulin levels are extremely high, as in some forms of myeloma. Also, one would not want to exclude the possibility that drug reactions might ensue if the therapeutic agent involved had the ability to aggregate the gamma globulin molecules. Perhaps, most important, therapeutic gamma globulins as commercially prepared may contain large molecular aggregates, and these could account for the pain on injection and the other problems with which clinicians administering gamma globulin are all too familiar. Fortunately, the common route of administration, intramuscular, tends to localize the effects of aggregates in these preparations.

We have mentioned in passing some of the clinical situations in which immune complexes or antibodies induce tissue injury: those involving endogenous antigens, such as in SLE, immune thyroiditis, and glomerulonephritis; those involving exogenous iatrogenic antigens, such as in serum sickness and drug allergies; and those involving exogenous microbial antigens, such as chronic viruses. One that has not been previously discussed is that pertaining in rheumatoid arthritis. Here the pathogenic events are less clearly defined than in, say, SLE. It is known that immune complex formation occurs both in the circulation and locally in diseased joints. In at least some instances the complexes appear to consist of rheumatoid factor, usually 19S gamma globulin and 7S gamma globulin. In the joints these complexes appear to be involved in causing the acute inflammatory and necrotizing reaction characteristic of this disease. However, the pathogenicity of the complexes in the circulation is less well established. But it is known that rheumatoid arthritis patients with vascular complications do have immune complexes in their circulation.

Perhaps the best-documented clinical condition in which both immune complexes and tissue-fixed humoral antibody play decisive pathogenic roles is glomerulonephritis. Because of the importance of this disease clinically and because of the knowledge that has been gained from studying it, a separate chapter, immediately following, is devoted to the immunopathology of glomerulonephritis.

Chapter 17

Glomerulonephritis and Immunopathology

FRANK J. DIXON
Scripps Clinic and Research Foundation

Although only in the past decade has conclusive evidence for the immunologic etiology of most glomerulonephritis in man been established, suspicion that inappropriate host defense responses were involved dates back at least 60 years and probably longer.

The question of whether or not glomerulonephritis is an autoimmune disease is essentially one of semantics. Certainly it is autoimmune in the sense that the host is made sick by his own immunologic responses. But, as was discussed in the previous chapter, the stimulation for the aberrant response may be either endogenous or exogenous. In either case, the offending agent appears to be humoral antibody. There is little evidence for the participation of cellular or delayed hypersensitivity mechanisms.

The humoral antibody's role in the pathogenesis may subserve either of the two defined mechanisms for induction of tissue injury; that is, antibody may be directed at tissue-fixed antigens in the glomerular basement membrane (GBM), or it may combine intravascularly with circulating antigens to form complexes that reach and lodge in the glomeruli. A number of antigens have been implicated in human glomerulonephritis. The nuclear DNA antigens that circulate in SLE enter into complexes with antibody that lead to the classic lupus nephritis; thyroglobulin-antibody complexes have been identified in patients with the nephritis that occasionally accompanies autoimmune thyroiditis; streptococcal antigens are almost certainly involved in the formation of complexes that produce poststreptococcal nephritis; malarial antigens are probably involved in the formation of immune complexes that serve as the pathogenetic agents in the nephrosis commonly associated with quartan malaria, particularly in African children; iatrogenic agents such as foreign serum or hapten conjugates formed between certain drugs and endogenous proteins may similarly be responsible for initiating the sequence leading to glomerular nephritis; and, of course, the GBM itself may be the target of a host immune response and the focus of glomerular injury.

Clinically it is extremely difficult to differentiate between glomerular disease resulting from antibody reacting with fixed antigen and from circulating antigen-antibody complexes. Both mechanisms eventuate in disease with a similar range of clinical expression. Either may produce an acute, rapidly progressive glomerulonephritis at one extreme, a chronic, indolent disease with an obscure onset, at the other. The rate-determining factor is probably the amplitude of the antibody response, which, in turn, determines the number of phlogogenic complexes causing tissue injury.

One major reason for the clinical parallelism between the two types of immunologic injury to the glomerulus is that the results are the same: altered filtration and urine formation accompanied by degenerative alterations in the glomerulus. Later, scarring develops and, as the process continues, there is functional loss of kidney tissue, with consequent oliguria and rise in BUN. Differential diagnosis between the two mechanisms is dependent almost exclusively upon immunologic procedures, the most readily performed being fluorescent antibody study of tissue obtained by renal biopsy. The fluorescent antibodies usually are used to determine the presence of host gamma globulin or complement in the glomeruli. Distribution of these immune reactants in the glomeruli vary characteristically with the mechanism involved. If the gamma globulin is anti-GBM antibody, it will be found in a smooth linear distribution along the GBM, much as one would find a specific basement membrane stain. Complement, if present, will be distributed roughly in the same way. As might be expected, if the disease is caused by the trapping of circulating complexes, then both antibody and complement will be located in irregular concentrations at sites where they would accumulate from the circulation. These deposits, granular and lumpy in appearance, are concentrated along the wall of the glomerular capillaries.

Mechanism of Injury by Specific Antib

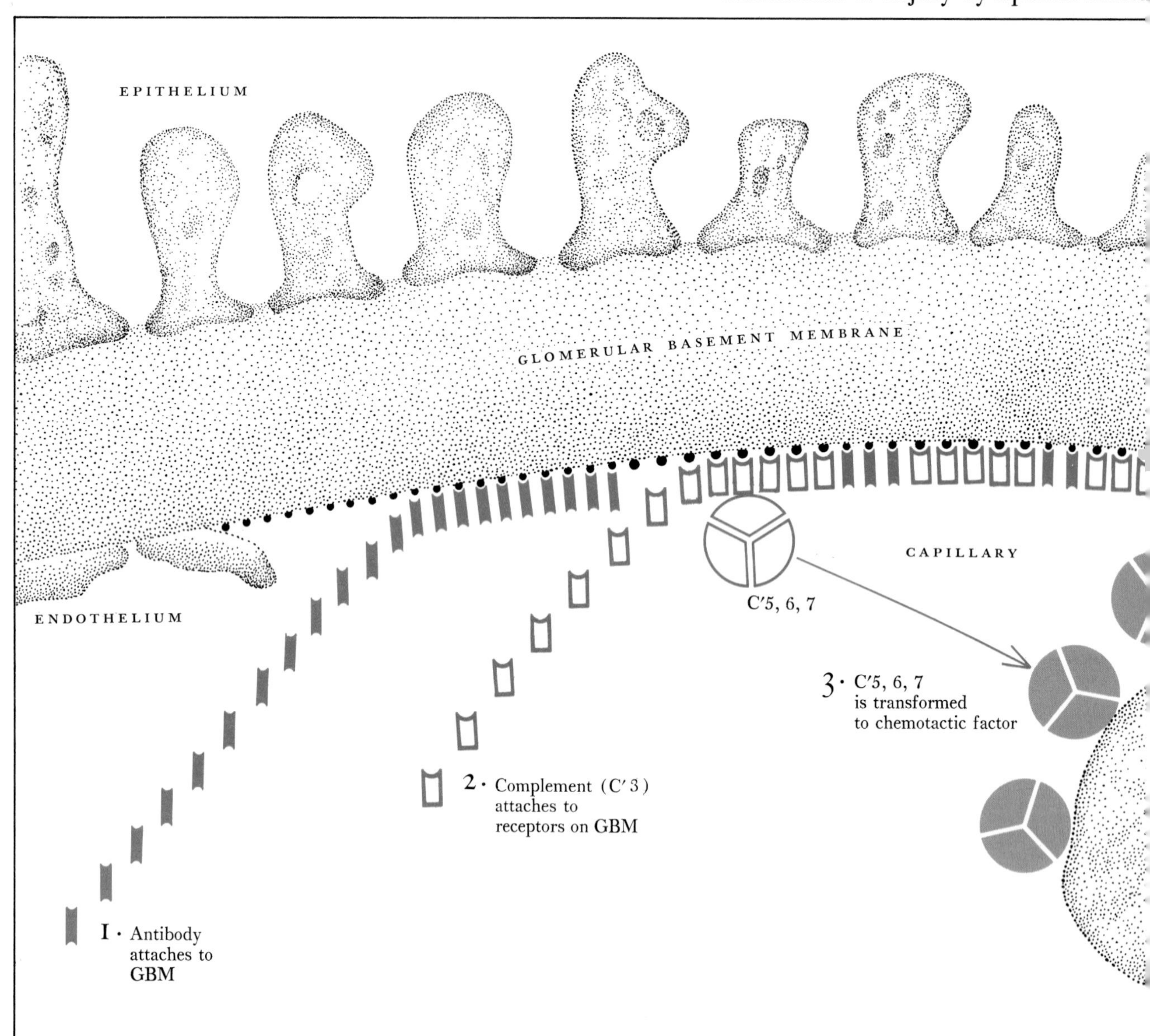

In the postulated mechanism of glomerular injury illustrated above (see also pages 170-171) the initiating factor is antibody specifically directed against glomerular basement membrane. Antibody attaches to inside of capillary along GBM. Then complement component three (at end of sequence C'1,4,2,3) attaches to receptor sites on basement membrane. C'3 activates next three complement components, which are transformed to chemotactic factor; this, in turn, attracts polymorphonuclear

Experimental studies have provided us with reasonably precise models of the events that occur clinically. In disease mediated by anti-GBM antibody, the first such model was provided by Masugi nephritis [see preceding chapter]. In this model, heterologous serum, usually an anti-rat kidney serum produced in the rabbit, is injected into the rat intravenously. The antibody fixes along the rat GBM and initiates a sequence of pathologic events, which can readily be observed since the heterologous antibody can be labeled and followed quantitatively and the precise amount of antibody involved in the reactions can be determined. With the aid of an electron microscope, similar precision can be attained with respect to the antibody's distribution. With these techniques, one can see that shortly after the injection of the anti-GBM antibody it localizes along the inner aspect of the basement membrane. At the same time, an abnormal separation between the epithelium and the GBM develops and the space thus created becomes infiltrated with light, wispy deposits.

The interaction between antibody and GBM is not in itself injurious to the membrane. However, the fixation of the antibody along the GBM is followed by activation and fixation of complement. This in turn is followed by the chemotactic attraction of polymorphonuclear leukocytes. The PMN leukocytes elaborate catheptic enzymes and basic proteins to induce actual destruction of basement membrane. The roles of both complement and the PMN leukocytes can be af-

Glomerular Basement Membrane

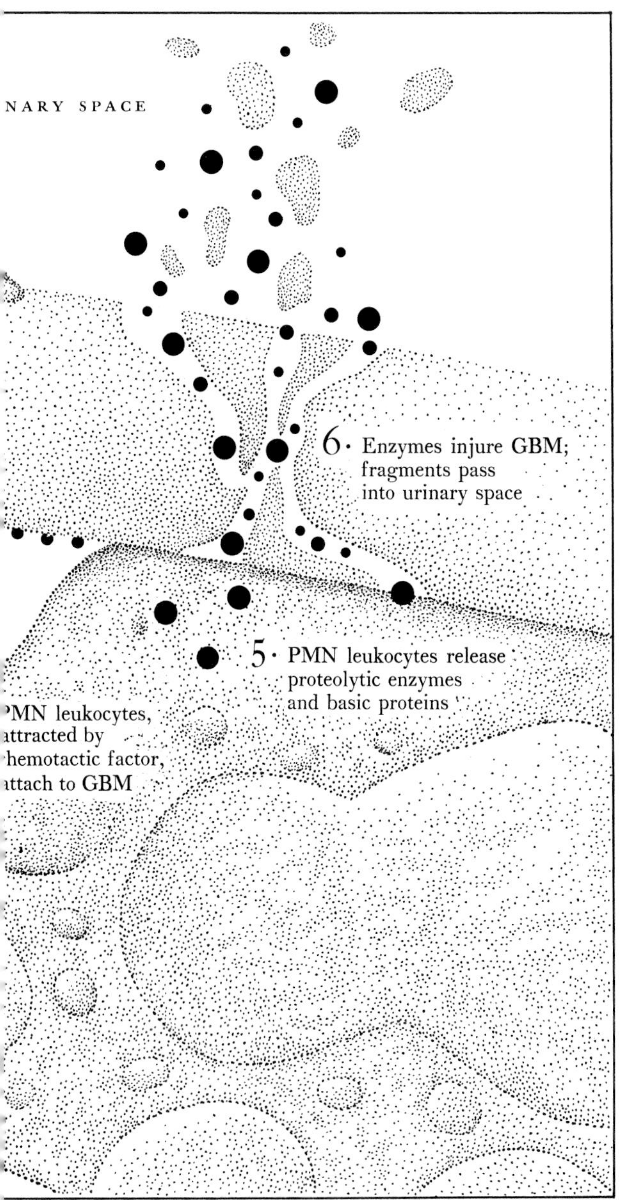

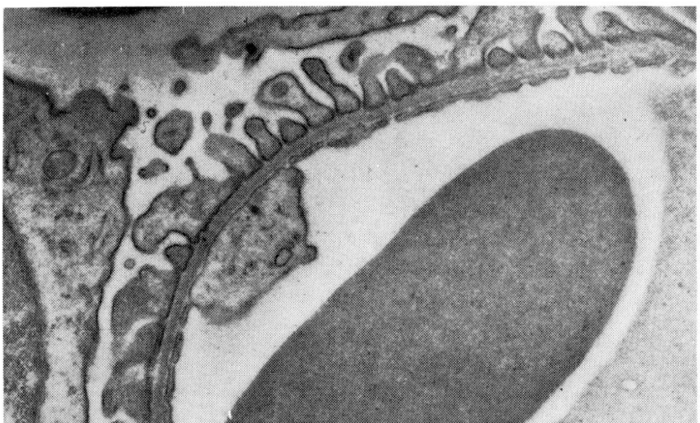

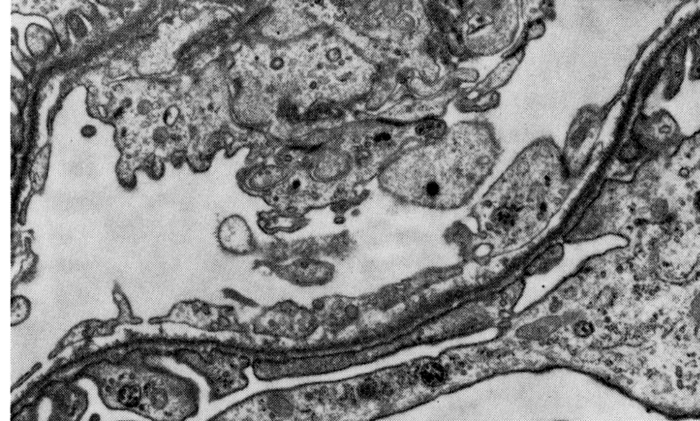

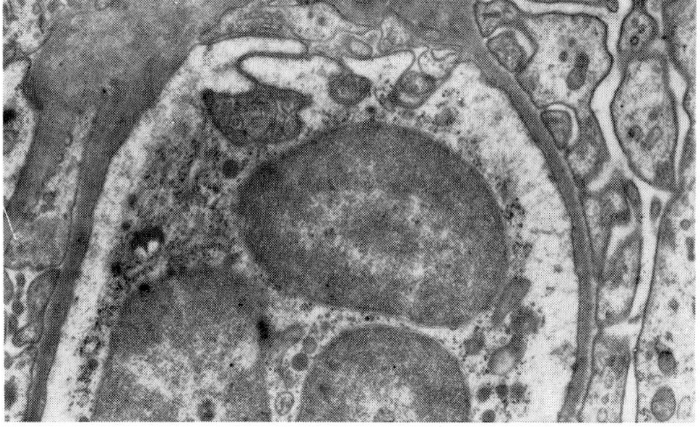

leukocytes, which attach to GBM and displace endothelium. PMN leukocytes liberate proteolytic enzymes and basic proteins, source of actual injury to GBM; fragments of GBM are released into urinary space. Right, top EM shows part of wall of normal glomerular capillary; center, glomerular capillary soon after fixation of antibody to GBM. Antibody has separated endothelium from GBM. Two hours later (bottom) capillary is filled with PMN leukocyte that has stripped off endothelium.

firmed by using animals depleted either of complement or of PMN's prior to administration of the antiserum. When these maneuvers are carried out, there is relatively little injury to the GBM and no subsequent dysfunction of the kidneys.

Although all of these events have been documented in the Masugi nephritis model, it was felt that the artificiality of this model made it precarious to extrapolate findings derived from it to human disease. However, a second experimental design for the induction of anti-GBM antibody nephritis was developed first in sheep, by Stebley, and then in rabbits and other "more convenient" laboratory animals. In this model, the glomerulonephritis is induced by the direct immunization of the animal with either homologous or heterologous GBM. The events observed are almost exact parallels of those in Masugi nephritis, and they provide an excellent indicator for the pattern that has now been observed in clinical disease.

The clinical studies have been greatly facilitated by the opportunities afforded by renal homotransplantation. In the various transplant series followed in the U. S. and elsewhere, it has been calculated that anti-basement membrane nephritis accounts for about 5% to 15% of all adult glomerulonephritis cases seen. It occurs in two forms, either as an uncomplicated subacute or chronic glomerulonephritis, or as a component of Goodpasture's syndrome, in which antibodies are directed against both kidney and lung basement membranes, causing glomerulonephritis and hemorrhagic pulmonary disease.

We observed the first case of anti-basement membrane disease in a patient being prepared for transplantation who had developed a completely typical subacute glomerulonephritis. This man had no anti-GBM antibodies in his circulation prior to bilateral nephrectomy. Shortly after the removal of his kidneys, while he was being maintained on dialysis, anti-basement membrane antibodies could be readily detected in his circulation and these persisted during the several weeks until renal transplantation. Within 24 hours after transplantation of a kidney, the antibodies disappeared from the circulation and were found fixed to the GBM of the newly grafted kidney.

One of the important facts derived from this intriguing case was that the kidneys are extremely efficient in removing anti-GBM antibody from the circulation. This understanding is important not only in itself but because it provides an explanation of why it is difficult to detect circulating anti-GBM antibody in some patients who have anti-GBM immunopathology.

The transplant experience has also afforded us an opportunity to obtain the actual human antibodies from kidneys removed at the time of operation and, therefore, to investigate the behavior of these antibodies both in vivo and in vitro. If kidneys are removed from individuals with the anti-GBM type of nephritis, antibody can be eluted from the GBM. When the elutes are examined immunoelectrophoretically, it is found that the only serum protein present in detectable amounts is gamma globulin. Immuno-

Mechanism of Injury by Circulating Non-Glomerular Antigen-Antibody Complexes in Syste

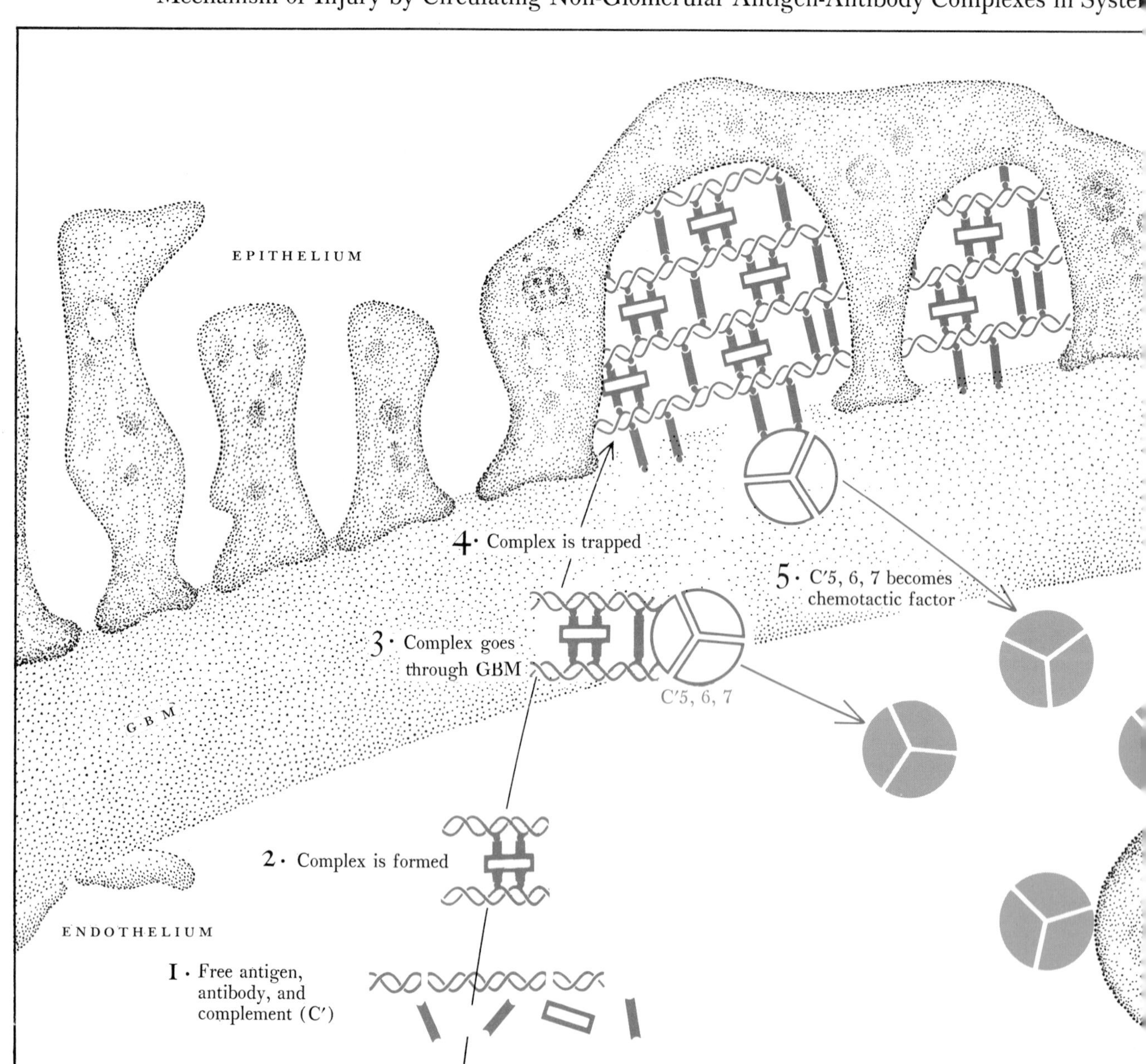

In the glomerular injury of systemic lupus erythematosus, the circulating antigen may be DNA, which complexes with circulating antibodies and complement. The complexes pass through the GBM and are trapped between the membrane and the epithelial cells; C′5-6-7 is transformed into chemotactic factor. This attracts PMN leukocytes, which become attached to GBM. Proteolytic

fluorescent studies with this gamma globulin shows that it will react specifically with GBM and to lesser extents with other basement membrane tissue, including nephron tubular BM, vascular BM, and the basement membranes from nonrenal organs. In our experience, anti-basement membrane antibodies from patients with Goodpasture's syndrome are more widely reactive with nonrenal basement membranes than those from patients with uncomplicated anti-GBM nephritis. The gamma globulin reacts in a much wider number of anatomic sites, perhaps accounting for the involvement of the lungs in this disease.

Finally, it should be noted that the antibody removed from patients with anti-GBM glomerulonephritis at transplantation has fulfilled one of Koch's major postulates. As little as 5 mg of gamma globulin removed from such patients will produce an acute proliferative glomerulonephritis in squirrel monkeys.

Clearly the ability of antibody to basement membrane to produce disease is well documented. But what about the nature of the etiologic agent or event that triggers formation of such antibody? The search for an environmental antigen that might conceivably cross-react with GBM and thereby serve as the necessary antigenic stimulus has been long and relatively unproductive. It has included studies of numerous microbial agents for such cross-reactivity. Some laboratories have reported cross-reactive antigens in certain streptococcal strains, but this observation has been far from universal. Moreover, even if such streptococcal cross-reactive antigens were to be identified definitely, this would in no way explain the pathogenesis of poststreptococcal glomerulonephritis as we know it. All evidence is that the poststreptococcal kidney disease results from the activity of immune complexes, rather than from antibodies to GBM.

In searching for an alternative to environmental or microbial antigens as the source of immunogenic stimulation, we have systematically investigated various endogenous materials that conceivably could provide or contribute to the initiation of an antibody response. Specifically, we looked for possible GBM-like antigens in the sera and urine of normal men and animals. Considerable such material was found in the urine and low levels were detected in sera. Since the amount of BM antigen in the serum increased after nephrectomy, it was suggested that it might originate in basement membranes throughout the body. Such "debris" might reach the urine because of normal excretion patterns.

After identifying these basement membrane antigens, we tested them for immunogenicity. Using normal rabbits, we made partially purified basement membrane antigen preparations and injected them back into the animals from which they had been collected. The animals responded with antibody formation and developed acute proliferative glomerulonephritis, which disappeared after a week or two but which could be revived by a second injection of a similar antigen. During the active stages of the disease, gamma globulin could be eluted from the rabbit kidneys. This antibody – again in quantities as small as 5 mg – was capable of transmitting an acute but nonlethal glomerulonephritis when injected into recipients of the same species. Further, we demonstrated that human urinary basement membrane antigens had a similar but not quite so potent nephritogenic effect when injected into rabbits. This clearly suggests that man has, in his serum and urine, basement membrane antigens that have the potential for initiating nephritogenic antibody response. However, it remains to be determined if endogenous antigens resulting from the catabolism of basement membranes are involved in the etiology of naturally occurring immunologic kidney disease. Even if they are, we would still have a considerable gap in our understanding of the etiology of anti-GBM antibody nephritis. The catabolic antigens seem to be universal in their occurrence; the disease certainly is not. One must postulate additional adjuvant events or substances – perhaps infections, perhaps other stimuli – that would make ordinarily tolerated antigens immunogenic. One possibility is genetic predisposition.

As was stated at the outset of this chapter, two pathogenic mechanisms are involved in immunologic injury to the glomerular basement membrane. The second mechanism involves the formation of circulating complexes in the vasculature and the migration of these complexes to the filtering structures of the kidney. Although these nephritides can be best classified according to the antigen involved, it must be quickly noted that in something like 70% or 75% of cases these antigens remain unidentified.

We have already mentioned several situations in which either an exogenous or endogenous antigen is clearly associated with nephritogenic immune complexes – poststreptococcal glomerulonephritis, in which the antigenic contributor to the immune complex is

...upus Erythematosus

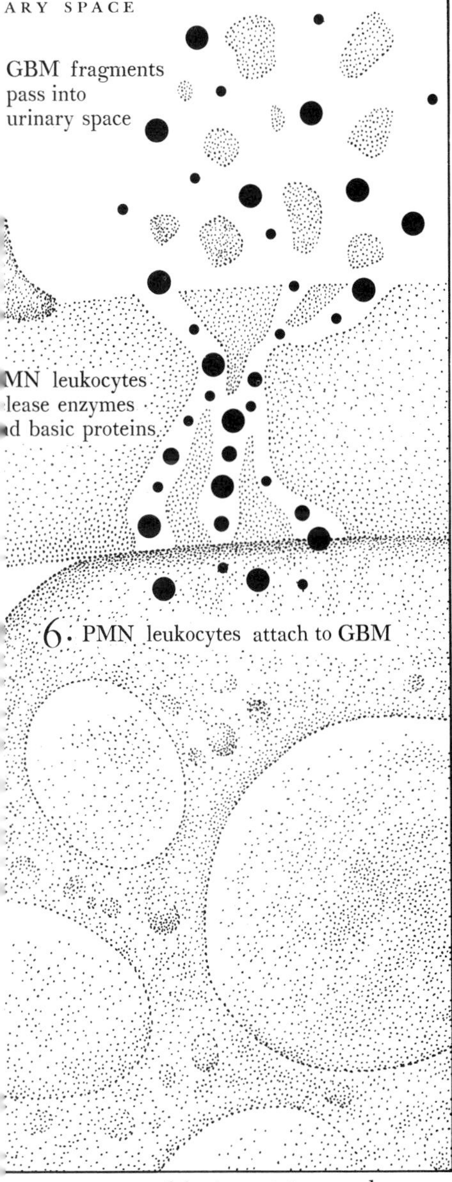

enzymes and basic protein complexes are then released. These "chew up" the basement membrane, releasing fragments.

streptococcal; nephrosis associated with quartan malaria and involving a malarial antigen; lupus nephritis triggered by nuclear DNA antigens in the circulation; thyroiditis-associated nephritis, in which circulating thyroglobulin-antithyroglobulin complexes are pathogenic.

Much attention in the effort to identify antigens for the remaining majority of cases of immune complex nephritis has focused on viruses. This concentration has largely been motivated by the fact that among nonhuman animal nephritides, virtually all appear to be immune complex diseases, many involving viral agents associated with chronic infections. However, to date, the definite establishment of any viral agent that serves in man as an antigenic stimulator of chronic immune complex disease remains to be achieved. There have been a few reports of finding immunoglobulin deposits in the glomeruli of patients with multiple myelomas, leukemias, and lymphomas. But this appears to be the exception rather than the rule. Nevertheless, even the exception is intriguing because in animals it is the rule, at least in the mice in which we have studied this phenomenon most intensively. Viral leukemias in these animals are quite uniformly accompanied by immune complex glomerulonephritis. Similarly, in Aleutian disease of mink, the symptom complex includes a lymphoma-like process and immune complex glomerulonephritis.

In the preceding chapter, the serum sickness models that have elucidated many of the characteristics of immune complex disease were described. It is appropriate now to review these models in relationship to what they suggest about clinical disease, specifically about immune complex glomerulonephritis in humans. With the one-shot serum sickness model, we have been able to trace quantitatively the fate of the injected foreign serum. In the rabbit, the heterologous serum injection leads to formation of circulating immune complexes in about a week. The complexes increase in size and there is depletion of serum complement. Once the complexes reach a sufficient size, they are rapidly eliminated from the circulation, and a few days to a week later the manifestations of disease in the cardiovascular system, joints, and kidneys, which had appeared when the complexes became detectable in the circulation, subside. We have been able to measure the antigen in the form of antigen-antibody complexes in the serum and in the glomeruli of the rabbits and have found that it takes 4 to 5 times 10^8 molecules of antigen per glomerulus to produce clinical disease.

While the clear picture of the immunologic events and their relationship to the clinical manifestations that we have for experimental serum sickness is not matched for any of the human immune complex nephritides, we do have considerable information with respect to several of the latter. In post-streptococcal glomerulonephritis, it has been shown quite definitely that the antigen is derived from the bacterial cell wall of the nephritogenic streptococci. This antigen can be detected in the irregular granular deposits along the glomerular capillary walls. The most definitive work in this area has been done by Lange and his associates, who have demonstrated that when the patient's own serum, containing antibodies to the inciting antigen, is employed in immunofluorescence studies, it is possible to detect the antigen in the glomeruli.

Parallel investigations have been carried out for lupus nephritis, in which the antigen is endogenous rather than exogenous. In patients who have been studied just prior to and during spontaneous exacerbations of renal disease, a sequence has been observed in which the presence of anti-DNA antibodies in the circulation is followed by the appearance of free DNA and then by the reappearance of anti-DNA globulins. From our experience with the serum sickness models, it seems obvious that DNA-antibody immune complexes would have to have formed simultaneously with the appearance and disappearance of free DNA and with the recrudescence of glomerular disease. Complement utilization is consistent with this.

In most clinical cases of presumptively diagnosed immune complex nephritis, we are ignorant of the nature of the antigen involved. We must rely primarily upon immunofluorescent delineation of the patterns of distribution of immunoglobulin and complement. However, we have taken one rather substantial step beyond this in demonstrating that antibodies eluted from affected kidneys have a strong affinity for that kidney or for a kidney from another individual with the same disease. This is strong evidence for immune complex pathogenesis, although it is noncontributory with respect to identifying the antigen.

Our very inability to identify antigen in the majority of immune complex nephritides in man has provided one of the most cogent teleologic arguments for suspecting a major role for viral antigens. Keep in mind that most cases appear to develop slowly, that they are often diagnosed quite incidentally subsequent to a physical examination unrelated to the nephritis, and that when they are picked up it is impossible to establish any definite relationship to an antecedent event. The etiologic agent would seem most likely one that acts slowly and inconspicuously over a prolonged period. Certainly we know no candidates that would better meet these criteria than chronic virus infectious agents, which may produce low-level infections over many months or years. Such a constant low-level antigenic exposure could lead to a parallel indolent pattern of complex formation, which, as in the case of the chronic form of serum sickness, would slowly induce a glomerulonephritis.

Having considered the mechanisms involved in both of the immunologic types of glomerulonephritis, we can now proceed to consider some of the therapeutic possibilities suggested by various aspects of these mechanisms. Certainly, the most obvious course is to proceed from the premise that if the disease is attributable to immunologic responses, then its cure might be achieved by immunosuppression, particularly the chemical immunosuppression that is immunologically nonspecific and would presumably interfere with the formation of any antibodies capable of causing nephritis. And some patients with nephritis have responded well to immunosuppression. However, this experience is still limited so that the argument for the value of immunosuppression needs to be bolstered by additional evidence. This is available from comparisons between the fate of identical-twin renal transplants and those done between allogeneic individuals.

In the identical-twin cases, the assumption was that no immunologic barriers to graft acceptance existed and therefore little or no immunosuppressive prophylaxis was used. In about 75% of these patients, who had had glomerulonephritis prior to nephrectomy and transplantation, glomerulonephritis recurred in their organ grafts within months after transplantation. Patients with similar pretransplant glomerulonephritis who received kidneys from nonidentical donors had a much lower rate of recurrence, and when glomerulonephritis did recur, it did so after a much longer time and at a much slower pace. These individuals, of course, were immunosuppressed after transplantation.

As an alternate to immunosuppression, one can consider not the inhibition of the antibody response per se but rather the inhibition of the various mediators of the immune injury: complement, the PMN leukocytes, histamine and serotonin, among others. Thus far, the evidence for the efficacy of this approach is almost entirely experimental. Complement inhibition, for example, can be achieved with a fraction of cobra venom, which exerts its effects through the inactivation of the third component of complement ($\dot{C}'3$). The cobra venom preparation has been successfully used in preventing the development of glomerulonephritis in animals treated with anti-GBM antibody. Unfortunately, cobra venom is not only currently in very short supply but is itself antigenic and unsuitable for clinical therapy.

The approach to limiting the participation of PMN leukocytes and their tissue-damaging enzymes in the immunologic reaction also rests primarily on techniques for inactivating complement, since the release of the chemotactic factor for PMN's is dependent on complement activity. With respect to vasoactive amines such as serotonin and histamine, the approach has been equally tentative. Animal experiments have shown that these amines are involved in localization of immune complexes, that they specifically increase vascular permeability to molecular aggregates of the size required for producing glomerular injury. In rabbits, antagonists in the amines were administered during procedures known to produce immune complex injuries. It was found that the antagonists prevented localization of complexes and largely inhibited the development of lesions. Depletion in rabbits of the major source of the vasoactive amines – platelets – had a similar effect.

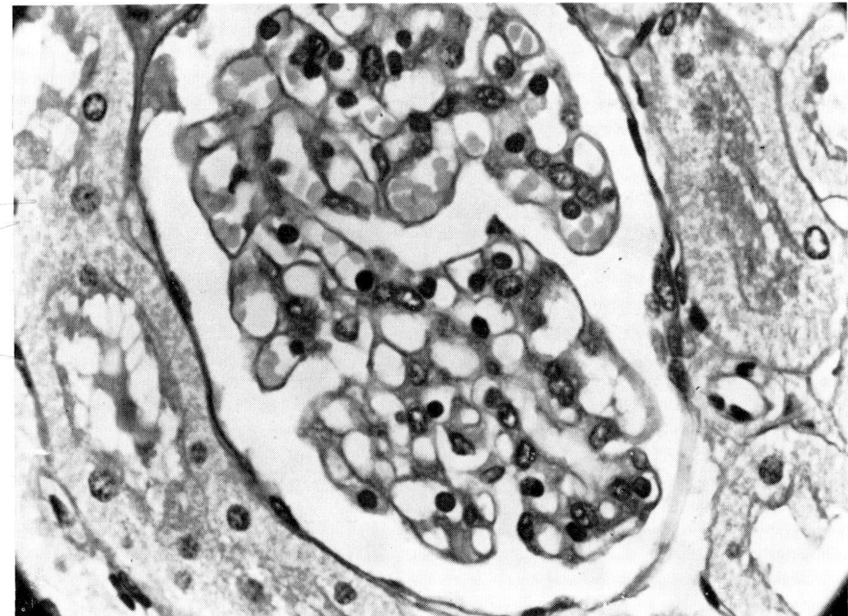

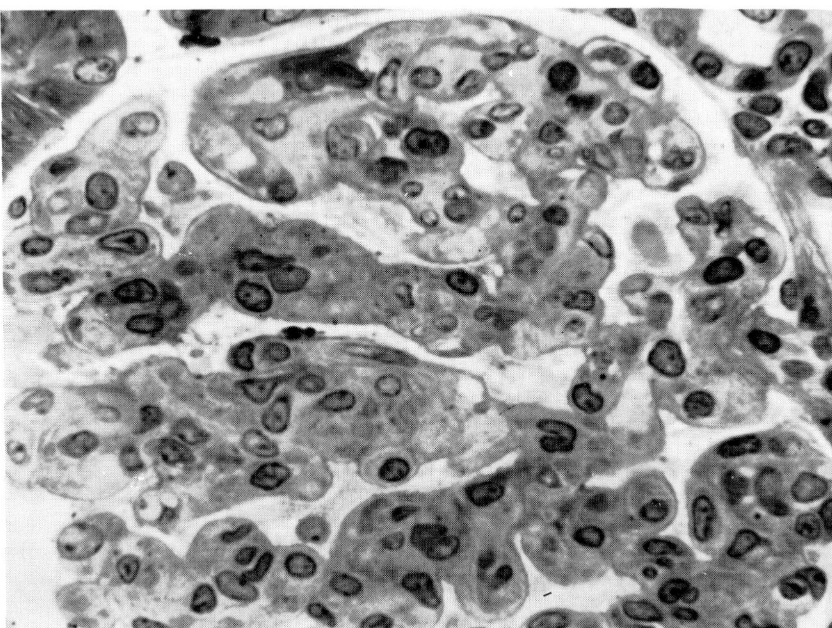

In contrast to normal rabbit glomerulus shown at top, lower photomicrograph reveals a proliferation of endothelial cells resulting from deposition of antigen-antibody complexes in the glomerulus. The structure's vascularity is greatly reduced, a pathologic change paralleling that of acute proliferative human glomerulonephritis.

Clearly our ability to treat immunologically mediated glomerulonephritis in humans is still very limited. Theoretically, however, there are a number of avenues that seem most worthy of exploration. For example, with respect to the disease resulting from antibody to specific GBM antigens, if we could identify the particular antigenic determinants involved in invoking the antibody response, we might use these determinants either to block the reaction with antibody or to induce specific tolerance. And in the realm of immune complex disease, a key development would be the clear-cut identification of one or more of the antigens, perhaps viral agents, commonly associated with such disease. Such identification could open the way to prophylactic immunization against the offending viruses.

Chapter 18

Are Autoimmune Diseases Immunologic Deficiency States?

H. HUGH FUDENBERG
University of California

As is abundantly shown by other authors in this text, the past decade has seen an unprecedented proliferation of discoveries in fundamental immunology. Important new data have been acquired about the morphology of immunoglobulin, the nature and size of antibody combining sites, and the sequence and heterogeneity of antibody responses to administered exogenous antigens.

During this time, however, our understanding of clinical diseases associated with immunologic aberration has not kept pace with the fundamental advances. This lag is due in part to the fact that the matrix in which clinical progress must be shaped is not yet complete. Perhaps, too, basic scientists have not devoted sufficient time and effort to human immunologic diseases.

One clinical area that seems to merit reexamination at this time is that of autoimmune disease (AID). An increasing number of diseases have been shown to fall into this category. These include warm- and cold-antibody acquired hemolytic anemia, lupus erythematosus, chronic membranous glomerulonephritis, Hashimoto's thyroiditis, rheumatoid arthritis, myasthenia gravis, and scleroderma.

An autoimmune disease can generally be defined as one in which an autoantibody or a sensitized lymphocyte reacts with host tissue. It must be stressed, however, that this definition does not mean the autoantibody or lymphocyte plays a causative role in the disease. Indeed, as will be pointed out later, in the current state of our knowledge it cannot be determined whether the autoantibody is causative, a consequence of human disease, or merely a concomitant; a causative role has been established in two experimental forms of renal disease, and the cytotoxic action of lymphocytes on host tissues has been demonstrated in vitro in other experimental forms of AID. But in the broader arena of clinical disease the classic concept that the autoantibody attacks tissue and causes disease remains to be proved. Equally unproved is the hypothesis that autoimmunity is a manifestation of immunologic hyperactivity.

Two concepts have dominated the thinking of investigators whose starting point is the belief that autoimmunity is a function of immunologic hyperactivity — the "sequestered antigen" and "forbidden clone" theories. Both these hypotheses owe their existence to the work of Sir Macfarlane Burnet. Considerably simplified, the sequestered antigen theory can be outlined as follows:

During embryonic life lymphocytes go through a stage in which they have not yet developed their ability to react immunologically to antigens but do have the capacity for future recognition of these antigens. Any antigens exposed to the circulation in the fetus will therefore "imprint" themselves on the lymphocytes' recognition system without eliciting an immunologic response, and the lymphocytes will ever after recognize these antigens as "self" and will not produce antibodies against them, i.e., they will "tolerate" the antigens. In contrast, antigens residing within the cells or in areas of the body which the blood supply does not reach (e.g., lens tissue, or thyroglobulin within the colloid of the thyroid gland) and not having contact with lymphocytes during embryonic life will not in the future be recognized as "self." If, in later life, infection or trauma disrupts the cells of, say, the thyroid and exposes these sequestered antigens (e.g. thyroglobulin) to the circulation, the lymphocytes will respond to them as they would to foreign proteins and produce an appropriate antibody—an antithyroid autoantibody.

Essential to understanding the alternative concept of the forbidden clone is the definition of the clone as a population of cells derived from a single parent. The theory starts from the premise that mutation is a constant phenomenon among lymphocytes and that most of the mutant lympho-

Forbidden Clone Theory

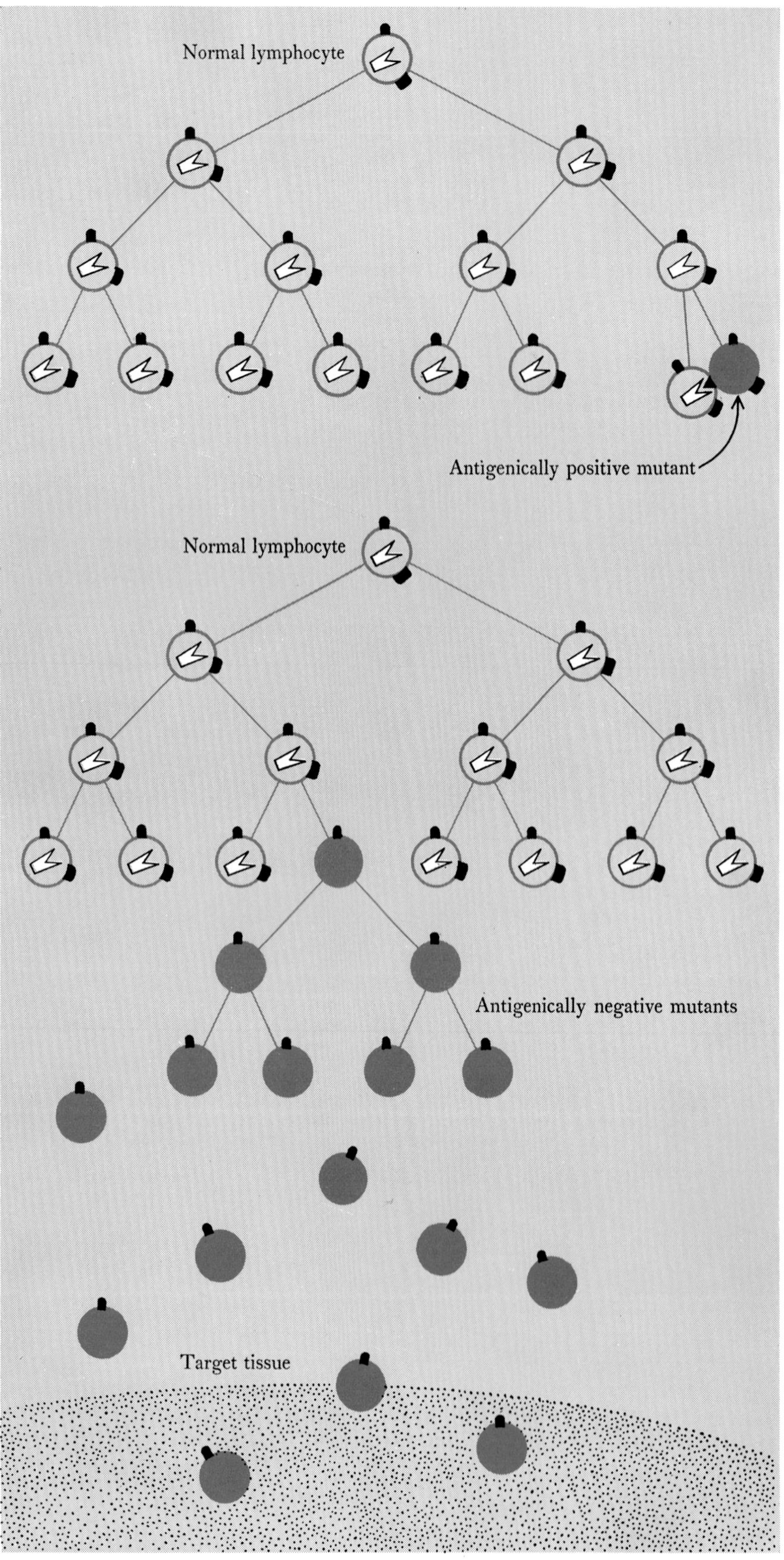

The forbidden clone theory presupposes lymphocytic mutations. When the mutant lymphocytes are antigenically positive in relationship to the normal population, the nonmutant lymphocytes eliminate the mutants immunologically. But if the mutant cells are antigenically negative, they proliferate and attack tissues.

cytes will carry "new" or "derepressed" antigens. The progeny of these lymphocytes will also carry the same antigens. Because these are "antigenically positive" in relation to the normal lymphocyte population, they will elicit an antibody response from the normal lymphocytes and be destroyed. Formation of mutant clones is therefore "forbidden" by normal immunologic processes involving cell-bound antibodies. But when a mutant is "antigenically negative" and does not call forth an antibody response from normal lymphocytes, such mutants proliferate and form clones capable of attacking normal tissue and of interacting with normal tissue antigens to produce pathogenic autoantibodies.

As noted previously, both of these hypotheses have as their critical premise the belief that autoimmunity stems from immunologic hyperactivity, leading to the production of autoantibodies capable of attacking tissue and causing disease. How can these concepts then be reconciled with a most significant clinical observation — that the prevalence of autoimmune disease is highest by far among persons with generalized immunologic deficiencies? Indeed, the person with agammaglobulinemia and an inability to form detectable antibody of any type, including autoantibody, has a far greater risk of developing an autoimmune disease than does one who appears to possess a normal gamma globulin profile. This and other observations have led us to hypothesize that autoimmune diseases are in fact manifestations of either generalized or selective immunologic deficiencies, and we can postulate pathogenetic mechanisms for this theory.

The first, applying to the person with a generalized immunologic deficiency such as agammaglobulinemia, presupposes, like the forbidden clone theory, the mutation of lymphocytes. But in this case, since mutation takes place in the absence of immunologic competence, the mutants *all* survive and reproduce, thereby creating a large population of lymphocytes capable of attack on normal tissue. The major appeal of this thesis is that it readily explains the prevalence of autoimmune disease in the agammaglobulinemic. For, if the thesis is valid, not only do all mutants survive but, equally significant, the established inability of the agammaglobulinemic individual to immunologically destroy many microorganisms in the circulation creates a vast source of agents having the capacity to induce lymphocytic mutation.

Before this hypothesis is accepted, however, there is some need for caution. For one thing, it makes only an assumption — logical, but thus far unproved — that the agammaglobulinemic person who by definition lacks circulating immunoglobulins is similarly deficient in intralymphocytic gamma globulins. Second, it fails to explain why, in any given patient, particular tissues are attacked by abnormal lymphocytes while others are spared. This is a defect it shares, of course, with the forbidden clone theory.

A second pathogenic mechanism underlying the thesis that autoimmune disease is secondary to immunologic hypoactivity is necessary to explain the occurrence of such disease in the person who appears to have normal titers of circulating gamma globulins. This concept of selective deficiency in its broad outlines suggests that an individual may have a genetically determined inability to respond immunologically to a particular antigen. Thus, in the genetically predisposed, a bacterium, virus, mycoplasma, or other microorganism that normally is handled readily by the immune system will be allowed to circulate freely and to attack tissues for which it has a tropism (even as certain adenoviruses, for example, selectively attack the mucous lining of the upper respiratory tract). As the microorganism damages the tissue, it may expose a new antigenic site previously protected from the circulation. As a result, the lymphocytes will interact with the new site and autoantibody will be produced. Alternatively, the microorganism may adhere to the surface of the tissue and combine with a previously existing antigenic site, forming a new haptenic antigen that, in turn, elicits the autoantibody response.

It should be noted that neither of these hypotheses, based on immunologic deficiency, requires assigning a pathogenic role to the autoantibody. One can, in fact, suggest that the more classic mechanism of pathogenesis — disease caused by an exogenous infective agent — is operative. One can also incorporate into this system the concept of transient immunologic deficiency, which would permit a previously latent virus or mycoplasma, or perhaps even a pleomorphic form of a bacterium, to become pathogenic. At any rate, it is important to note here that the autoantibody need not be the pathogen and indeed may even represent an inadequate effort by the host to counter the true pathogenic agent.

The clinical relevance of basing autoimmune disease on immunologic deficiency rather than immunologic hyperactivity should be readily apparent. Such an alteration in our thinking would suggest an entirely new look at the therapeutic approaches pursued to date without consistent success. In general, such approaches as adminis-

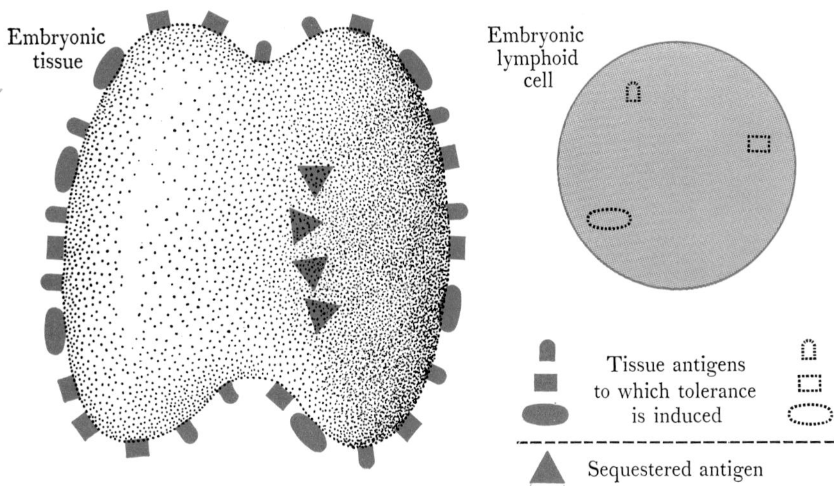

This autoimmunity hypothesis postulates that all antigens on cell surfaces during embryonic life come into contact with circulating lymphocytes and are ever after recognized as "self." But antigens below the surface, or to which lymphocytes are not accessible because of the nature of the vascular supply of a given organ, are not encountered in embryo and recognition is therefore not imprinted on the lymphocytes.

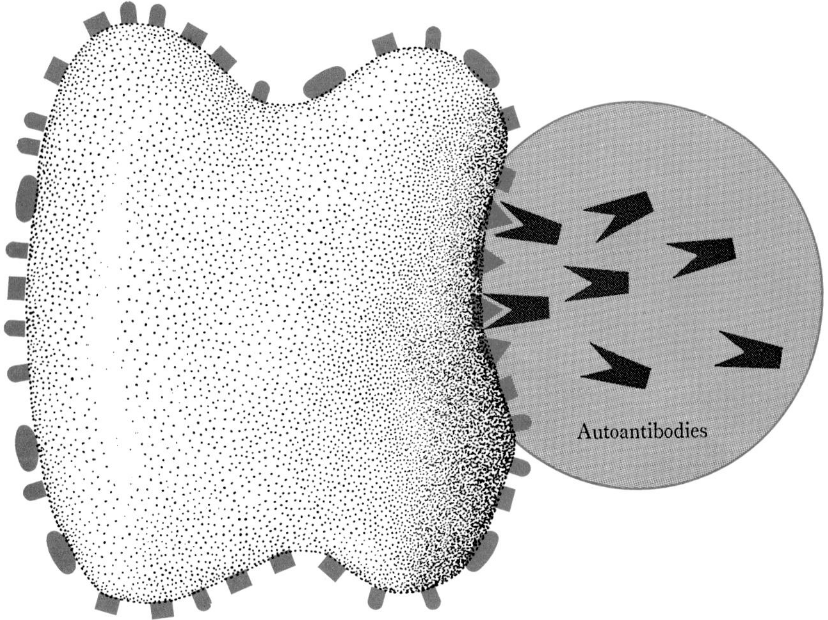

If such a previously sequestered antigen is later exposed by infection or trauma, lymphocytes react as to a foreign protein and autoimmune antibodies are produced. The recent finding of thyroglobulin in sera of all tested normal individuals has raised serious doubt of the theory's validity in regard to Hashimoto's disease.

General Immunologic Deficiency (Agammaglobulinemia)

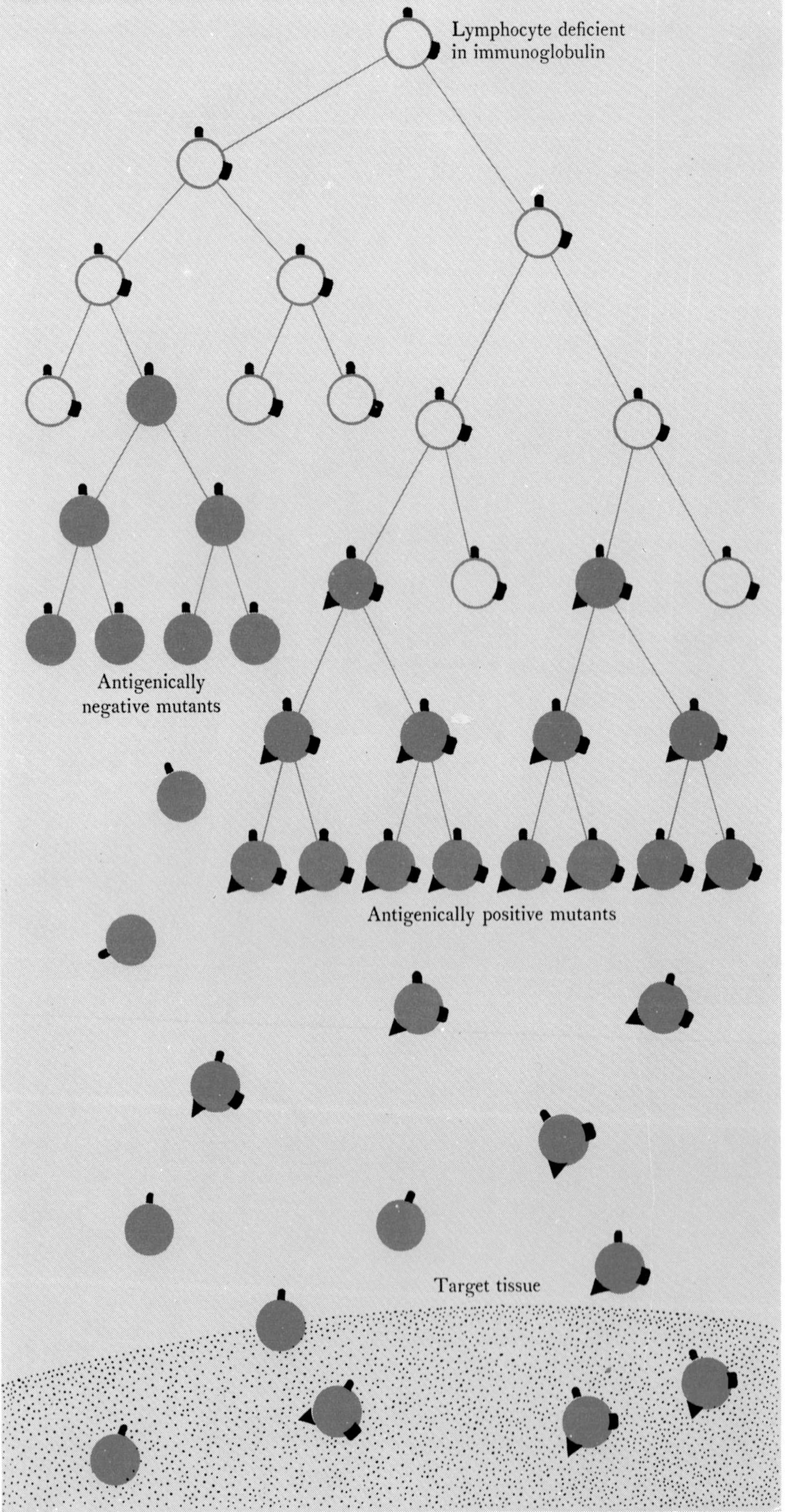

The high incidence of autoimmune diseases in individuals with agammaglobulinemia could be accounted for on the basis of the concept schematized above. If one assumes that the lack of circulating immunoglobulins is paralleled by lack of cell-bound globulins, then all mutant lymphocytes (antigenically positive and negative) can be expected to survive, proliferate, and become pathogenic.

tration of immunosuppressants like the corticosteroids might yield to modalities designed to bolster an individual's immunologic competence. Even more significant, perhaps, is the enhanced role proposed for the microorganisms. The therapeutic opportunities this suggests are obvious. Before therapeutic possibilities are discussed, however, it is necessary to take a closer look at another aspect of AID pathogenesis — the genetic factor.

Genetic predisposition to AID is now well documented in experimental animals. Although human data are more difficult to obtain and to evaluate, there are certain pedigrees in which a clustering of autoimmune serologic abnormalities is so marked that the phenomenon cannot be attributed to mere chance or to unidentifiable environmental factors.

The genetic mechanisms that affect autoimmune reactions are not known, but several possibilities exist. As previously suggested, there may be an inherited susceptibility to an infectious agent capable of attacking host tissues and causing an altered array of antigenic sites. Genetic factors may also allow alteration of host antigens in other ways – as in the degradation of normal tissue components. Further, genetic mechanisms may determine the presence or absence of tissue antigens cross-reactive with various bacterial antigens and thus permit or prevent formation of antibodies cross-reacting with host tissues. It might be noted that the proposal of antigenic alteration in autoimmune disease due to a purely somatic cause — i.e., by the liberation of previously sequestered antigen — now seems unlikely. There is recent evidence, for example, that the antigen thyroglobulin, to which the autoantibodies of patients with thyroiditis are primarily directed, is normally present in immunologically detectable amounts in the circulation. In other words, this so-called sequestered antigen is not sequestered after all.

As an alternative to genetic alteration of antigenic components, one may hypothesize genetic factors that affect immune responses. Such effects could underlie the immunologic hyperactivity implicit in the forbidden clone hypothesis. They could equally well explain the mechanisms proposed by the concepts of generalized and selective

Autoimmunity and Selective Immunologic Deficiency

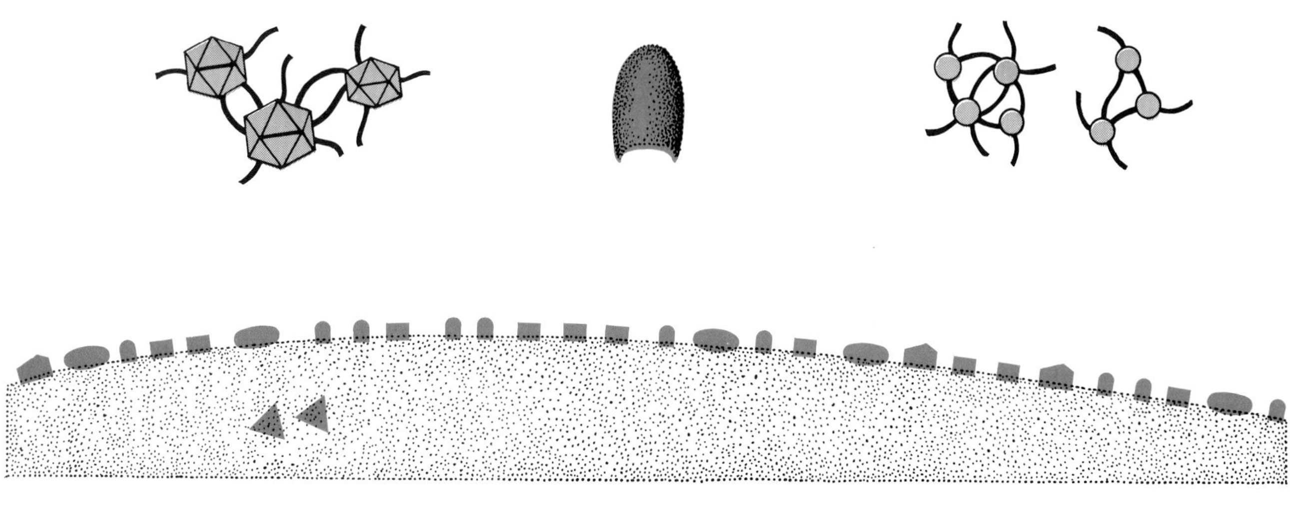

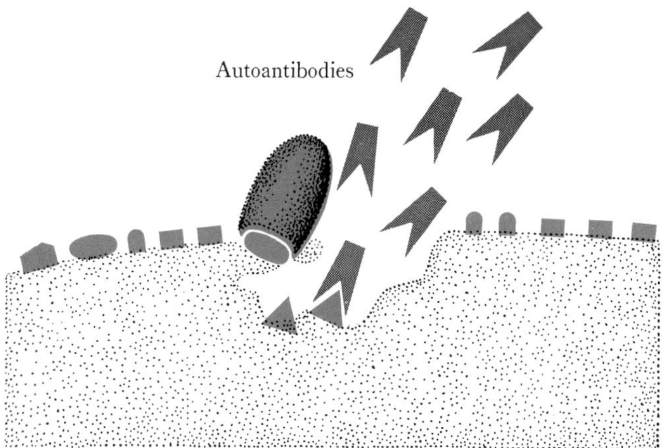

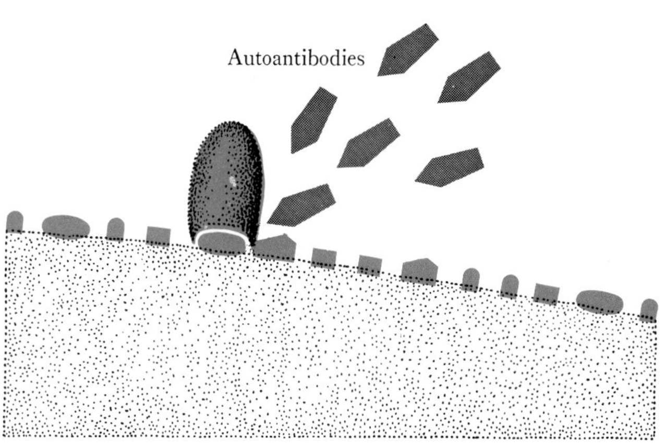

In individuals with a genetically determined inability to react to a specific antigen, a normally nonpathogenic microbe may escape binding by circulating antibodies (top drawing) and attack target tissue. In doing so, it may expose a previously covered antigenic site (left) and produce a circulating antibody response, or modify antigenic sites in tissue to produce new antigens. Or the new antigenic site could be a haptenic combination of the exogenous antigen and one previously existing on cell surface.

immunologic deficiency, which seem to us more likely mediators of autoimmunity. What are the specific data derived from both animal experimentation and clinical observation that tend to support this view?

The documentation of genetic susceptibility to AID has come from studies with several species. For instance, while mice of the New Zealand Black strain (NZB) invariably develop antibodies characteristic of hemolytic anemia, those of the New Zealand White strain (NZW) do not. Hybrid F_1 offspring of NZB/NZW matings, but not those of NZB with other strains, have a high incidence of severe renal disease analogous to that seen in human systemic lupus erythematosus (SLE), and 100% of NZB/NZW offspring eventually show positive tests for lupus cells or antinuclear antibodies.

Immunization of Hartley strain guinea pigs with low doses of guinea pig thyroid extract results in a high incidence of thyroiditis, whereas similar doses produce thyroiditis in only a small percentage of strain 13 guinea pigs; the frequency of this experimentally induced AID also varies in different strains of inbred mice. All of these findings point toward genetic control of autoimmune phenomena, at least in these two animals. Genetically determined "autoimmune" thyroid disease in chickens has also been recently documented in certain strains of obese chickens with thyroid autoantibodies.

It is characteristic of AID that several different types of autoantibodies and/or disease states occur in the offspring of those affected. This holds true not only for inbred experimental animals but for the human families we and others have investigated. To cite one example, we have studied the relatives of several patients with acquired hemolytic anemia and found a large number of autoantibodies of types other than those associated with this disease. Such discoveries suggest that if genetic mechanisms are operating, perhaps they predispose families to immunologic diseases in general rather than to just one particular condition.

It is important to point out that in both animals and man hereditary factors may be a necessary but insufficient cause of autoimmune disease. There is abundant evidence to support the belief that environmental precipitating factors such as infectious microorganisms may be required. For example, laboratory animals rendered immunologically deficient by neonatal thymectomy, appendectomy, or cortisol administration plus irradiation reveal some features that are indistinguishable from human autoimmune conditions — Coombs'-positive hemolytic anemia, rheumatoid-like arthritis, and renal disease closely similar if not identical to that seen in SLE and in the NZB/NZW hybrid mice. On the other hand, animals treated the same way neonatally but raised in a germfree environment either fail to develop autoimmune symptoms or do so at a much later stage in life.

Animals that harbor a virus in a chronic carrier state are also susceptible to AID. For example, those made tolerant to the virus of lymphocytic choriomeningitis (LCM) at birth subsequently have asymptomatic viremia and a high incidence of AID, and the association between specific viral infection and chronic hemolytic anemia has been documented in horses ("equine infectious anemia"). In human beings a close association has been found between Coombs'-positive hemolytic anemia in children and cytomegalovirus.

We attempted to provide evidence that immunologic deficiency, induced experimentally, can cause lesions identical to those of autoimmune disease. For that purpose, P.H. Guttman, K.D. Wuepper, and I studied mice rendered doubly deficient immunologically by neonatal thymectomy plus irradiation. These mice, by 60 days of age, developed renal lesions indistinguishable from those seen in the F_1 NZB/NZW hybrids and from those seen in lupus nephritis. Both gamma globulin and complement were bound to the glomerular tissue of these animals, as shown by immunofluorescence and also by electron microscopy with ferritin-conjugated antibody. We assumed that the disease was caused by a viral agent that could not be eliminated in these immunologically deficient animals. Daily injection of the antiviral agent interferon appeared to retard the occurrence of the renal lesions.

Indeed, Frederick D. Baker and J. E. Hotchin of the New York State health department have recently shown that the long-continued presence of LCM in mice who were made tolerant to the virus at birth causes deterioration of renal function and renal glomerular lesions similar to those seen in the NZB/NZW mice, thus proving that "slow" viruses can produce renal lesions of an autoimmune nature in animals immunologically capable of response to this viral agent. This is perhaps due to virus-antivirus antigen-antibody complexes similar to the DNA-anti-DNA antigen-antibody complexes responsible for the renal lesions in lupus nephritis. (Incidentally, M. Oldstone and F. Dixon have shown that the neurologic lesions in lymphocytic choriomeningitis are probably also due to antigen-antibody interaction.)

Robert C. Mellors and his associates at Cornell Medical College have demonstrated with the electron microscope that lymphoid tissue of NZB mice contains virus-like particles. Viruses have also been suggestively implicated in an autoimmune-like disease associated with renal lesions in the Aleutian strain of mink. Further, several lines of recent evidence indicate that rheumatoid arthritis is probably a slow virus disease, as are certain human neurologic diseases of obscure etiology.

The clinical evidence for the infectious basis of autoimmune conditions comes from several sources. Already noted is the extremely high incidence of autoimmune phenomena in patients with generalized immunologic deficiency. Approximately 20% to 30% of these agammaglobulinemic individuals, if they survive long enough, show clinical signs of AID. These patients are particularly prone to rheumatoid arthritis, dermatomyositis, or lupus-like syndromes, and in our experience they show an unusually high frequency of ophthalmologic findings that are immunologic in nature. We have also seen two agammaglobulinemic patients who developed classical ulcerative colitis.

Since they cannot make detectable amounts of serum antibodies to any antigen, patients who have both agammaglobulinemia and an autoimmune condition lack the appropriate autoantibody, i.e., rheumatoid factor, lupus factor, antibodies to colon tissue, and so on. This is very significant, for it suggests, as stated before, that antibodies themselves are probably not the cause of autoimmune disease. In fact, they may be part of a normal protective mechanism designed to help the body eliminate dead or damaged tissue. If this is so, a clinically normal individual whose serum contains an autoantibody may have such minor tissue damage that he does not have overt symptoms. Indeed, many of the parents, siblings, and children of these agammaglobulinemic patients have autoantibodies in their sera but show no signs of clinical disease.

A pattern of hereditary susceptibility has been found in a group of patients with rheumatic heart disease — an ailment that many investigators would add to the list of autoimmune diseases — with the precipitating agent presumed to be beta-hemolytic streptococci. A. Michael Davies and Eliahu Lazarov of the Hadassah Medical School in Jerusalem were able to study the disease in a controlled environment provided by a communal farm settlement in Israel in which children lived apart from their parents and were raised in buildings where they were housed according to age.

There were many asymptomatic streptococcal carriers in the community, but the carrier rate was the same among children with and without rheumatic heart disease. And yet the incidence of heart disease was 2½ times greater in children whose parents had the same illness! Upper respiratory infections of a streptococcal nature were also much more common among affected children than those free of rheumatic disease.

Here is an indication that genetic factors can predispose a population to a disease clearly not genetic in immediate etiology. While hereditary factors probably do not act directly to induce rheumatic fever, clinical disease seems to result from genetic susceptibility to the agent that causes streptococcal infection. We can only conjecture at this point whether the susceptibility reflects a selective immunologic deficiency for streptococcal antigens.

In addition to infectious agents, certain drugs have been implicated as precipitating autoimmune ailments. These include antihypertensive and anticonvulsant compounds, penicillin, isoniazid, L-dopa, and other drugs. It is conceivable that such medications, as well as agents like sunlight and other radiation, activate latent viruses in individuals with the appropriate genetic makeup. A possible example of this situation has been observed in the asymptomatic relatives of patients who develop drug-precipitated SLE. These relatives frequently reveal the stigmata of autoimmune conditions — autoantibodies in their sera, blood protein deficiencies, and the like.

Thus far, we have shown that there is a distinct possibility that autoimmune diseases have a hereditary foundation and that overt disease may result from the combination of genetic predisposition and exposure to the proper etiologic agent. But what is the evidence for the rest of the hypothesis — that these diseases result from a deficiency in the body's immune mechanism, allowing a causative agent to attack without the normal counterattack? And is there any immunologic evidence that genetic mechanisms control *individual* antibody response?

Evidence of such control, necessary

Genetically Determined Variation in Response to Antigen

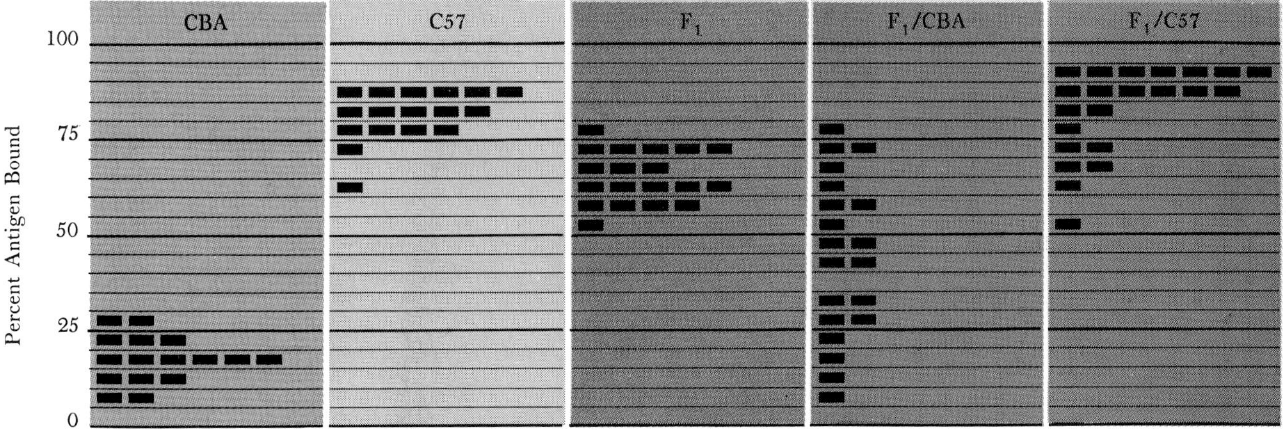

Experiments of McDevitt and Sela have clearly delineated a genetic basis for response to antigens. Using a branched synthetic polypeptide antigen, they tested responses of two inbred strains. They found CBA mice bound the antigen very poorly (each rectangle in drawings above represents one animal). C57 mice, on the other hand, bound from 65% to 90%. When the strains were crossed, their progeny (the F_1 generation) showed an intermediate binding capacity. Backcrossing F_1 animals with the low-responder strain produced a wide range of response, while backcrossing the F_1 with the high-responder strain produced mice with a range of response similar to that of the C57. Next the investigators changed just one residue at the tip of the polypeptide side chain, i.e., substituted histidine for tyrosine. This single change reversed the response pattern. The CBA mice were good responders, the C57's poor ones to the histidine-containing copolymer. Genetic study indicates that ability to respond to both antigens is a dominant trait.

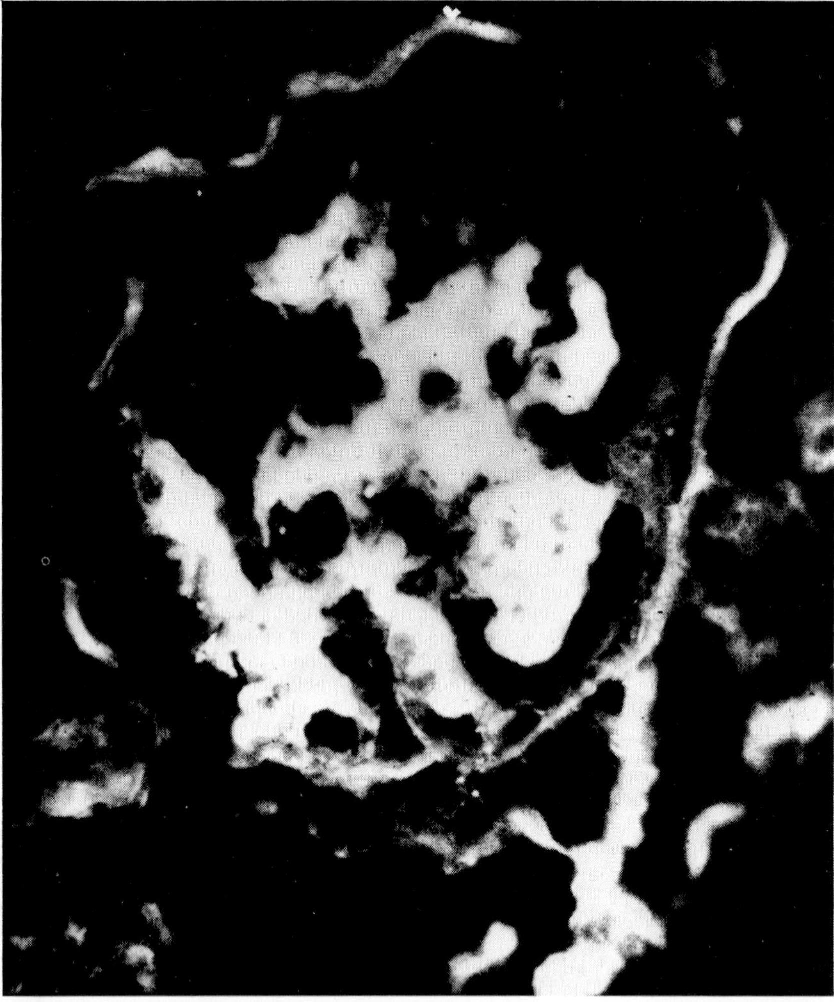

Binding of gamma globulin and complement to altered glomerular tissue can be seen in immunofluorescent photomicrograph above, made in mouse thymectomized and irradiated soon after birth. Similarity of lesions to those seen in human lupus nephritis provides evidence that experimentally induced immunologic deficiency can cause lesions identical to those of autoimmune disorders. Disease may have been caused by a viral agent the immunologically crippled animal could not eliminate.

if selective deficiency is involved in these diseases, has not been obtained in man, but there is convincing documentation from animal experiments with inbred strains. We can at least say that in such animals hereditary factors regulate the response of separate antibodies.

Bernard B. Levine, Baruj Benacerraf, and their associates at New York University showed that strain 13 guinea pigs were unable to respond immunologically to any of four different haptens conjugated with poly-L-lysine (PLL), whereas 100% of strain 2 animals responded to the same antigenic conjugates. All the offspring of breeding pairs composed of nonresponders failed to react to the hapten-PLL conjugates; in contrast, the vast majority of the offspring of responding animals also responded.

F_1 animals produced by mating responders to nonresponders reacted positively, suggesting the F_1 guinea pigs were heterozygous for a dominant gene; these, when mated with nonresponders presumed to be heterozygous recessives, produced offspring of which 50% were responders. Such experiments are consistent with the belief that response to hapten-PLL antigen is dependent upon a single, dominant Mendelian gene.

Studies by other workers have shown that inbred strain 2 guinea pigs produce antibodies against both PLL azobenzene-arsonate and portions of the insulin molecule but that strain 13 does not react to either. Further investigation of the F_1 hybrids of the two strains and their F_2 offspring provided data strongly indicating that genetic factors regulate antibody production against these specific antigens.

Hugh O. McDevitt, now of Stanford University, and Michael Sela of the Weizmann Institute of Science in Rehovot, Israel, carried out elegant collaborative studies of the effect of simple synthetic polypeptide antigens on two inbred strains of mice. C57 mice, for instance, responded very well to one branched, multichained compound (from 70% to 100% of the antigen bound), but CBA mice produced only about 10% as much antibody; CBA/C57 hybrids gave intermediate responses. When the F_1 hybrids were crossed back to the parental animals, a wide variety of response was found. These data can be interpreted to mean that a single, dominant gene is responsible for the different reactions to the same polymer in the two strains.

Even more interesting were the results of changing one residue that made up part of the side chain of the polypeptide. The original compound used contained a polylysine backbone and poly-D, L-alanine side chains tipped with two glutamic acid residues and one tyrosine residue. When the investigators substituted a histidine residue for the tyrosine on the copolymer, the antigenic effect of the polymer was reversed in the two strains of mice. These results indicate that the genetic control of the immunoresponse in these animals is specific for a given simple antigenic determinant, since changing just a single amino acid at the antigenic site of two simple molecules, constructed almost identically, alters a genetically determined immune response. Especially fascinating is the recent observation by McDevitt that at least one gene controlling response or nonresponse is genetically linked to the histocompatibility (H^2) locus.

All these investigations provide strong indications that genetic mechanisms at least control antibody production qualitatively. But do hereditary factors also regulate the amount of antibody in man? Experiments conducted by R. Kamin in our laboratories to demonstrate the genetic foundation of so-called acquired agammaglobulinemia seem to suggest an answer to this question. Our studies involved measuring the incorporation of labeled precursor into the DNA and RNA of peripheral lymphocytes growing in synchronous cell culture. Lymphocytes from patients who have adult-onset (so-called acquired) agammaglobulinemia synthesized only 3% to 30% of the DNA and RNA manufactured under the same circumstances by cells of normal individuals. Even more significant to us was the finding that seven parents of the six patients studied so far also had reduced lymphocyte DNA and RNA synthesis. Their cells produced from 20% to 35% of the normal amounts of nucleic acid.

These experiments with the patients and their parents provided for the first time direct evidence that acquired agammaglobulinemia is genetically determined. And since other immediate relatives of such patients show many of the serologic signs of AID, even though they have no clinical symptoms, our new findings lend weight to the suspicion that these autoimmune manifestations may also be due to genetically determined immunologic deficiencies. We may then perhaps hypothesize that parents, siblings, and children of agammaglobulinemic patients have a more selective immunologic deficiency than do the patients.

All of this is compatible with our picture of a genetic predisposition and an activating environmental agent. The increase in incidence of most autoimmune conditions with age is also in keeping with the deficiency hypothesis. We know that in mice, at least, the number and activity of immunologically competent cells decline as the animals grow older. William H. Hildemann and Roy L. Walford Jr. of the University of California at Los Angeles demonstrated in addition that the number of lymphoid cells producing autoantibodies increases with age. If the same is true in man, we would expect the body to lose its ability to reject mutant lymphoid cells that have antigenic features which are absent in normal cells. This would lead to an increase in lymphocytic malignancies in old age, a phenomenon observed in mice and men, and to autoantibody production by mutant lymphocytes.

The same mechanism could also explain the inordinately high incidence of lymphoreticular malignancies and other generalized immunologic deficiency states in patients with agammaglobulinemia and in diseases associated with defects in cellular immunity. Without an immune system capable of recognizing mutant lymphoid cells, the body permits these mutants to survive and proliferate.

But if autoimmune conditions result from selective defects in the immunologic machinery of the body and not from immunologic hyperactivity, how do we explain the role of the autoantibodies? As suggested earlier, the old view — that autoantibodies attack normal body cells — is probably naive, particularly in light of the fact that many normal individuals have autoantibodies in their sera but show no signs of clinical disease.

Investigation of the rheumatoid factor in our laboratory and elsewhere, and of acquired resistance to allergic encephalomyelitis by Philip Y. Paterson and his associates at Northwestern University, offers a possible answer. Perhaps circulating antibodies are signs of a special type of tissue damage. They may, in fact, help protect an organ from increased damage. This would explain in a somewhat paradoxical way why patients with AID occasionally benefit from treatment with immunosuppressive agents.

Robert S. Schwartz and his colleagues at Tufts University showed that 6-mercaptopurine enhanced instead of decreased formation of antibody during the secondary response. If autoantibodies help to prevent rather than cause tissue damage, we can expect the immunosuppressive drugs to improve the patient's condition because of an increase rather than a decrease in autoantibody production.

Should the hypothesis be proved that autoimmune disease results from immunologic deficiency instead of hyperactivity in the immune system, this could offer us as clinicians new avenues of attack on these puzzling and devastating conditions. Until now we have been grasping at straws for most of our therapeutic approaches. Hopefully, further information may soon lead us to solid therapeutic weapons.

Chapter 19

Organ Transplants and Immunity

DAVID M. HUME
Virginia Commonwealth University

If its major purpose were to provide the immunologist with a laboratory for the study of various phenomena related to his discipline, then organ transplantation could already be rated an unqualified success. As we probe the mechanisms of graft acceptance and rejection we become intimately concerned with the genetics of histocompatibility; primary and secondary immune responses; the relative roles of serum and cell-bound antibodies; the functions of complement, the thymus, lymphocytes, and immunosuppression; and the relationships between autoimmunity and the conditions that complicate management of the patient.

But of course the actual goal of clinical organ transplantation is to prolong and improve the quality of life. We do not perform human organ transplants simply to increase our knowledge of immunology; rather, we investigate the immunologic consequence of homotransplantation to improve our ability to provide patients, who otherwise would die, with durable and adequately functioning grafts. And although we must still regard transplantation as an experimental procedure, a considerable degree of success has already been achieved in its most extensive clinical application – kidney transplantation. At this time, it can be conservatively stated that an individual receiving a related donor renal transplant has an 85%, or better, chance of living with that graft indefinitely. And the possibility of his receiving a second transplant, should the first one fail, further enhances his outlook for survival.

Survival obviously depends on the patient's ability to pass through whatever rejection crises may occur. A substantial majority of all transplant patients undergo such rejection episodes at one time or another. Our own experience is that 75% of patients receiving kidneys from related donors have one or more crises, while 95% of those receiving cadaver kidneys undergo at least one rejection. Three different chronologies of rejection have been delineated; these episodes differ not only in time of occurrence but also in mechanisms that appear to be involved.

Hyperacute (acute humoral) rejection: This may occur within hours or even minutes of the transplant and can be quite startling. After the donor kidney is in place in the recipient and the clamps are taken off the vessels, the kidney fills with blood and becomes pink. It looks normal and blood flow is good. But in a very short time it becomes soft, blue, and mottled. The blood flow drops from 300 cc or 400 cc a minute down to as low as 30 cc a minute. If the kidney is left in place for several weeks it will undergo cortical necrosis, followed by progressive vascular changes leading ultimately to ischemic destruction of the entire transplant. Kissmeyer-Nielsen and colleagues were the first to demonstrate in man the presence of humoral antibodies to donor antigens in cases of hyperacute rejection.

This phenomenon has been investigated by sequential biopsies and selective arteriography. The biopsy specimens have been examined by light and electron microscopy, grown in tissue culture, and submitted to various immunologic tests. On the basis of studies by my colleagues, G. M. Williams, P. Morris, R. P. Hudson, R. Weymouth, J. C. Pierce, myself, and collaborators F. Milgram and K. Kano a hypothesis was formulated to explain the events.

As a consequence of preexisting antigenic exposure – through a previous transplant, blood transfusion, pregnancy, or perhaps certain bacterial antigens – antibodies have been formed. If a subsequent transplant is carried out from a donor whose antigens are similar to those producing the immunization, the transplant may be damaged by the antibody. The antibody becomes attached to the endothelium of the small blood vessels of the cortex within seconds after circulation to the transplant is restored. Complement is fixed and polymorphonuclear leukocytes adhere to the sticky antibody-complement layer on the endothelium. It is important to note that these are polymorphonuclear leukocytes, not the lymphocytes that would

The Mechanism of Hyperacute Rejection

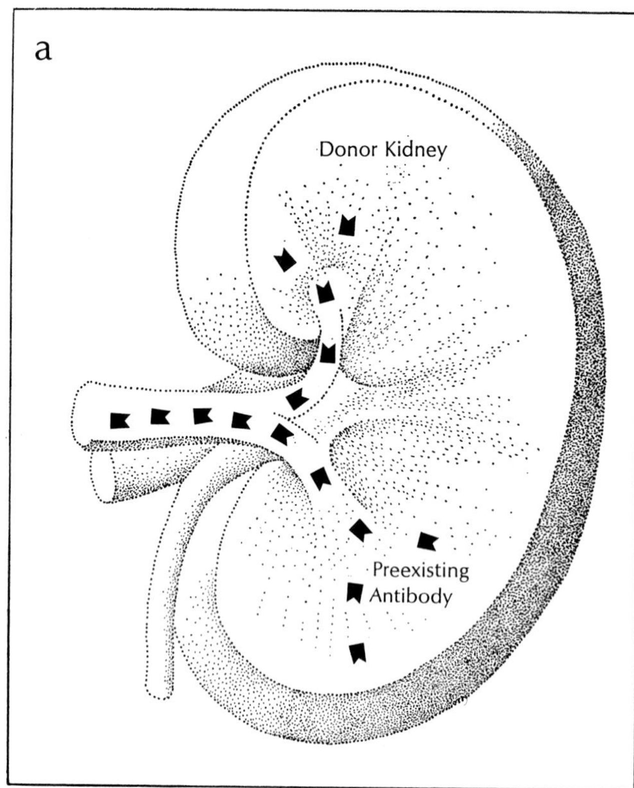

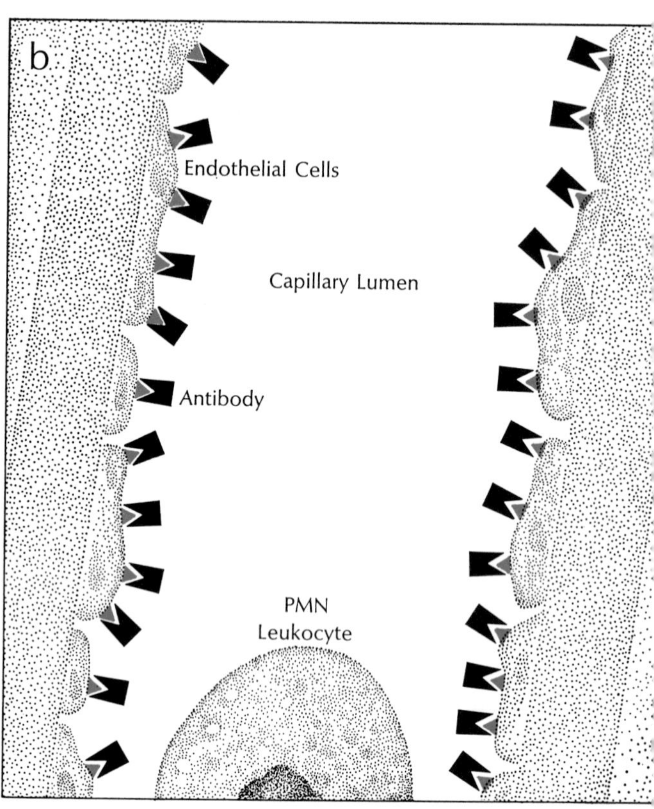

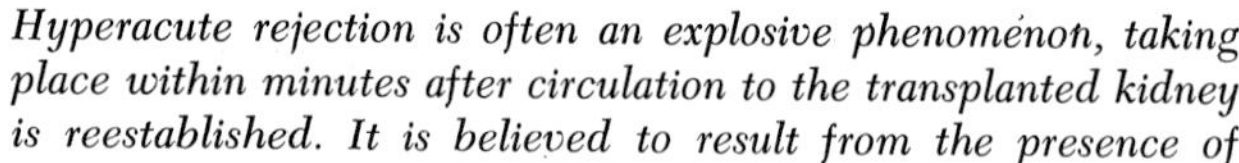

Hyperacute rejection is often an explosive phenomenon, taking place within minutes after circulation to the transplanted kidney is reestablished. It is believed to result from the presence of preformed antibodies to the donor kidney (a) Such antibodies, a result of bacterial infections, blood transfusions, or previous transplants, attack the graft by attachment to the endothelium

be expected to participate in primary immunologic reaction. Under the electron microscope one can see bridges formed between the polymorphonuclear leukocytes and the endothelial cells. The endothelial cells are destroyed. A raw surface is thereby created to which platelets adhere, producing a thrombus that occludes the vessels and leads to cortical necrosis.

It has been demonstrated that antibodies are present in the serum of the recipient prior to transplantation and that these antibodies react against lymphocytes of the donor and/or cells of the kidney transplant. Furthermore, it has been possible to elute the antibody from the rejected transplant.

Three steps are taken to avoid acute humoral rejection. First, the prospective recipient's serum is reacted against the lymphocytes of a panel of 40 to 50 donors to see if it contains preformed antibodies against a significant proportion of the population. Second, the serum is reacted against the proposed donor's lymphocytes (histocompatibility cross match), and third, the serum is reacted against kidney cells of the proposed transplant. The kidney cell cross match is sometimes positive when the lymphocyte cross match is negative, and we have several times seen hyperacute rejection under these circumstances. Although the donor lymphocytes and kidney cells presumably contain the same HL-A antigens, the concentrations of certain antigenic specificities may be greater on the kidney cells, thus leading to a positive test.

Acute and intermediate rejection: In related donor kidney transplants, the great majority of rejection episodes occur after the first week and within four months of grafting. In cadaver transplants, the danger period extends up to two years. The immunologic mechanism here appears to be cellular. This concept is strongly supported by our experience with local irradiation of the kidney, which has no systemic effect yet can be extremely effective in reducing or abolishing the rejection. Presumably, the radiation works through its ability to destroy lymphocytes, which are extremely radiosensitive. A dose of 150 rads is enough to damage lymphocytes but not enough to affect other cells. At least experimentally, and apparently also clinically, four 150-rad doses of radiation given to the transplant on the first, third, fifth, and seventh days after transplantation are sufficient to improve the survival of renal homotransplants. Apparently the events that must be interrupted to end an acute rejection crisis occur locally and relate to a cell moving into the kidney. Presumably this is the small lymphocyte.

The acute (cellular) rejection pattern is mediated by the small thymus-derived lymphocyte, which recognizes the foreign nature of the transplant antigens as it passes through the graft. The antigen is picked up by the lymphocyte, which becomes sensitized by it. The sensitized cell ("killer" cell) is then capable of destroying graft cells on contact without the need for complement or other serum factors. The ability of the sensitized cell

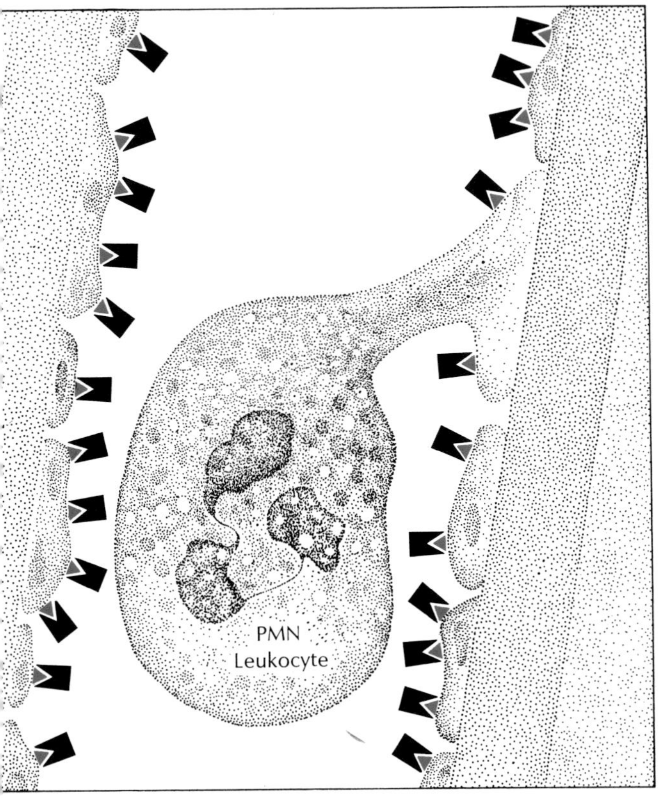

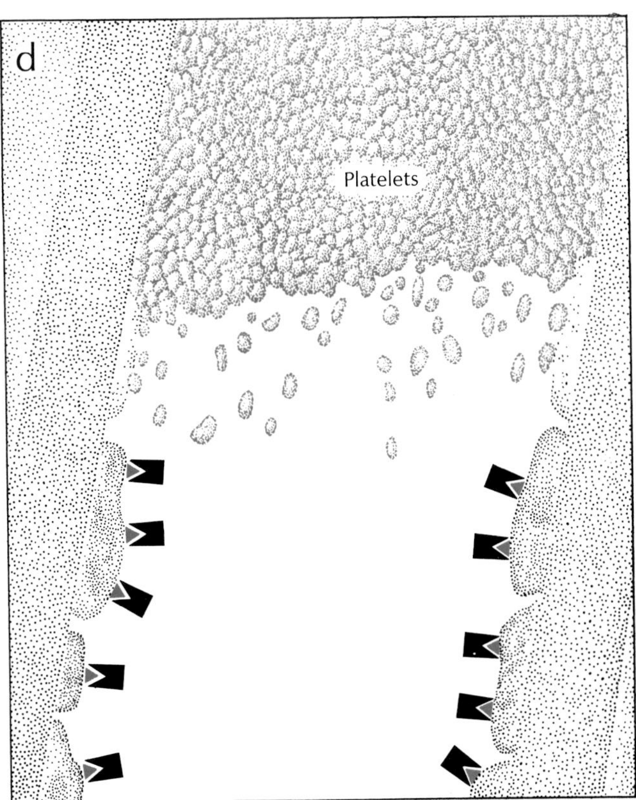

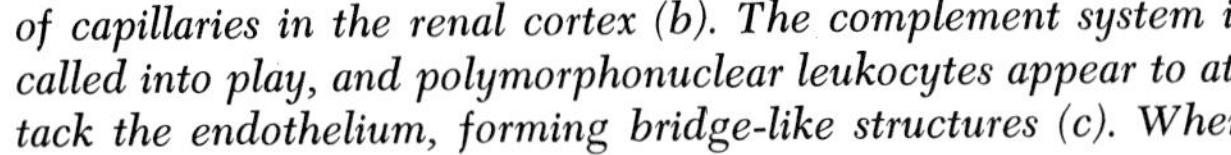

of capillaries in the renal cortex (b). The complement system is called into play, and polymorphonuclear leukocytes appear to attack the endothelium, forming bridge-like structures (c). When the endothelium is denuded a rough surface is exposed. Platelets are mobilized and a thrombus is formed, closing vessels and causing widespread cortical necrosis (d).

to destroy the donor cells has been demonstrated by J. S. Wolf in our laboratory by utilization of monolayer cultures of human donor kidney cells. While nonsensitized lymphocytes have no effect on the tissue cultures, sensitized lymphocytes are capable of destroying the donor cells in four hours.

Late, or chronic, rejection: The third major pattern of rejection generally is seen in patients who have been undergoing immunosuppressive therapy for prolonged periods. It seems to be an expression of an almost successful regimen of immunosuppression, and its histologic development is somewhat different from the earlier types of rejection. This pathway appears to involve primarily the glomerular basement membrane (GBM) and the endothelium of the blood vessels but not as destructively as in the early hyperacute rejection. Rather, extensive and progressive endothelial proliferation is produced, with progressive narrowing and ultimate occlusion of the lumen. This process appears to involve serum antibody. As vascular stenosis proceeds, the patient often develops the nephrotic syndrome, irrespective of whether he originally had glomerulonephritis or not. The hallmark of this is loss of protein in the urine. Once protein is being spilled in large quantities, one can be sure that the patient is either experiencing chronic rejection or has recurrent glomerulonephritis. The rejection will usually progress slowly and insidiously, sometimes over a period of years, until the kidney is finally destroyed. If late rejection is going to develop, its early stigmata will make their appearance within two years of transplantation and will be recognized on biopsies by proteinuria, by hypertension, and by some degree of depressed renal function. Final failure of the transplant may take as long as five years. Late rejection, once fully developed, can almost never be reversed. Thus, acute rejection is potentially reversible, while hyperacute and chronic rejection are not. Hyperacute rejection is explosive and complement dependent, while chronic rejection produces irreversible ischemic changes and permanent damage to the vascular system.

Glomerulonephritis

Although the development of glomerulonephritis [see Chapter 17, "Glomerulonephritis and Immunopathology," by Frank Dixon] has been a major cause of failure of identical-twin transplants, recurrent glomerulonephritis is seldom seen in non-twin transplants. The GBM antigen is not primarily a histocompatibility antigen but is similar in different individuals. Thus, if a patient develops glomerulonephritis as the result of autoantibodies (or antigen-antibody complexes) against the glomerular basement membranes of his own kidneys, these antibodies may persist after transplantation and attack the GBM of the transplanted kidney. Since identical twins with renal transplants receive no immunosuppression, the formation of GBM antibodies is un-

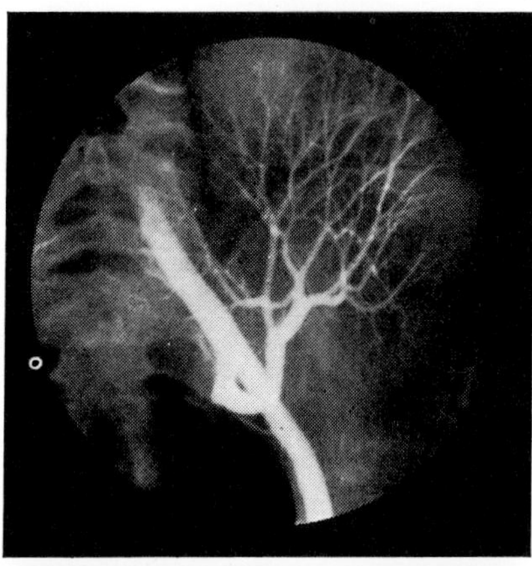

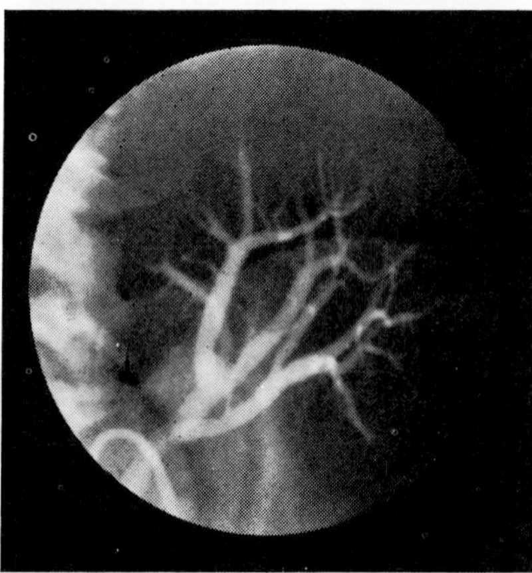

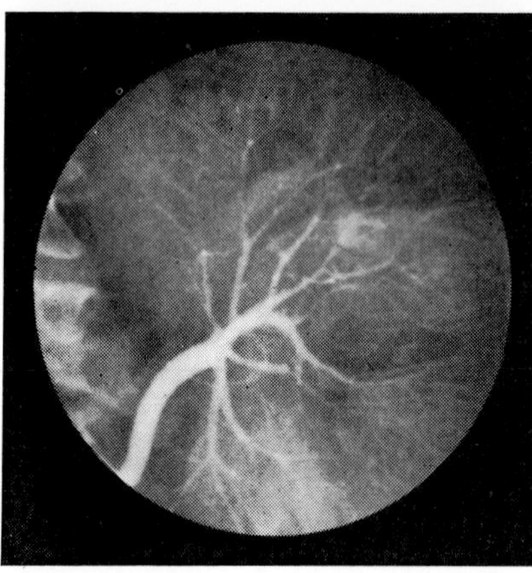

Normal renal artery graft arteriogram (top) shows fine vessels reaching all the way into cortex. In hyperacute rejection (center), the cortical vessels are completely obliterated. In chronic rejection (bottom), vascular narrowing is diffuse, but many of the smaller vessels remain patent.

opposed. It is presumed that the immunosuppression given to the non-twin renal transplant recipient to avoid rejection also protects, to some extent, against the development of glomerulonephritis by suppressing the formation of GBM antibodies.

Nevertheless, recurrent glomerulonephritis (as distinguished from the membranous glomerulonephritis of chronic rejection) does sometimes occur in the non-twin donor transplanted kidney even in the face of immunosuppressive treatment. In our own experience, this development is most likely to be seen in children with the nephrotic syndrome.

Prognosis and Clinical Course

While the kidney transplant that never experiences a threatened rejection is obviously better tolerated than the one that undergoes numerous episodes of rejection, the latter occurrence early in the course of the transplant is not incompatible with long-term survival and excellent renal function. If the excellence of histocompatibility matching of donor and recipient is to find an expression in the clinical course of the transplant, then the clinical events must be predictive of the ultimate outcome. In analyzing the transplants done in our series over the past nine years, it was found difficult to predict the ultimate outcome of cadaver donor (CD) transplants until the two-year mark was reached. At this time interval, however, the functional excellence of the transplant bore a very close relationship to its continued survival. There was a difference in the course of related living donor transplants (RLD) and CD. The RLD transplants showed a fall in the percentages of transplants with functional survival throughout the first year after transplantation but with very little loss after that time. The CD transplants, by contrast, continued to show a fall in the percentage of surviving transplants for the first two years after transplantation, followed by a leveling off with very little further loss. It does prove to be impossible to assess the likelihood of continued functional survival of the CD transplant until the two-year mark is examined.

The function of the kidney transplant at two years was used to divide the patients into two groups, those with excellent function (BUN less than 22 mg%, creatinine 1.5 mg% or less, and creatinine clearance 70 cc/min or more) and those whose function was less good. There were 61 patients whose transplants were functioning at two years and for whom follow-up was available 3½ to 8 years after transplantation. Of those patients showing excellent function at two years, 94% of the RLD transplants continued to function throughout the period of long-term observation, 3% subsequently died, and 3% (one patient) later rejected the transplant. In this instance, the transplant functioned for 4½ years, and there was evidence by biopsy at 17 months that the transplant was undergoing severe chronic rejection. Nevertheless, the kidneys still showed excellent function at two years. Of the CD transplants with excellent function at two years, 78% continued to demonstrate functional survival throughout the period of long-term observation. There were no rejections at all in this group, but 22% of the patients ultimately lost the transplant or died of some cause unrelated to rejection, such as recurrent glomerulonephritis, hepatitis, etc. Of those patients showing reduced function at two years, none ever achieved the degree of excellence seen in the first group. Nevertheless, 69% of the RLD transplants continued to function throughout the long-term observation period, 23% were ultimately rejected, and 8% of the patients lost the transplant or died from some cause unrelated to rejection. Of the CD transplants, 50% continued to show functional survival, 33% were rejected, and 17% ultimately failed or the patients died of causes unrelated to rejection.

It became apparent, therefore, that at least four degrees of histocompatibility could be established from the clinical course and that three of these could be identified at the two-year mark. The least compatible transplants were rejected prior to two years, while the next most incompatible group showed reduced function at two years and were subsequently rejected. The third most incompatible group showed reduced function at two years but continued to function at pretty much the same level throughout the subsequent 3½ to 8 years. The most compatible group showed excellent function at two years, with only one transplant subsequently rejected.

It is obvious that to relate the clinical course to histocompatibility, one must eliminate those transplants that are hyperacutely rejected and those patients whose transplants were lost through recurrent glomerulonephritis, as distinguished from the type of glomerulonephritis seen with chronic rejection. More will be said later on about the difficulties of making this distinction. The transplants undergoing hyperacute rejection may actually be quite well matched to the recipient but are destroyed on the spot by preformed antibodies and complement. It is, of course, impossible to analyze those transplants whose recipients die before two years of some event unrelated to rejection at a time when the transplant still shows excellent function. It is possible, however, to retain those patients for analysis whose transplants continue to show excellent function but who die after four or five years of an event unrelated to rejection, such as reticulum cell sarcoma.

We have lost only eight transplants after two years. Six of them were rejected and two were lost through recurrent glomerulonephritis. All eight patients are currently surviving on a retransplanted kidney. Only seven patients in our series have died after two years, from 31 to 76 months after transplantation. Three of them died of lymphoma, two of hepatic failure, and two of CVA's.

Selection of Donors

It is axiomatic that the successful outcome of a renal homotransplant is closely related to the degree of antigenic similarity that exists between donor and recipient. Since the antigenic make-up is determined genetically, similarity is more likely in a related living donor than in a genetically disparate cadaver.

While the most critical factor in the immunologic acceptance of a renal transplant is that of matching donor and recipient histocompatibility antigens, at least three other considerations are of major importance. One is the immunologic competence of the recipient. If a patient is immunologically crippled by his disease or by the immunosuppressive agents, he may accept a graft even from a donor not particularly well matched to him antigenically. Secondly, the question of preformed antibodies must be considered. While histocompatibility matching procedures may measure strong antigenic determinants on the leukocyte, they may not necessarily identify all the antigens of the kidney. Preformed antibodies, resulting from previous blood transfusions, prior transplants, or exposure to bacteria that share antigens with body tissues, may react against the grafted kidney and destroy it, even when donor and recipient matching is quite good. Thirdly, anti-GBM antibody may be present in the recipient and may react with the GBM of the transplanted kidney. The GBM antigen is not a histocompatibility antigen and would not be recognized by tissue typing.

The histocompatibility antigens can be determined by leukocyte typing with test sera that have a known antibody composition. The sera may contain either agglutinating or cytotoxic antibodies. Blood leukocytes from the prospective donor or recipient are added to the test sera. Then if the

The Mechanism of Primary Acute Rejection

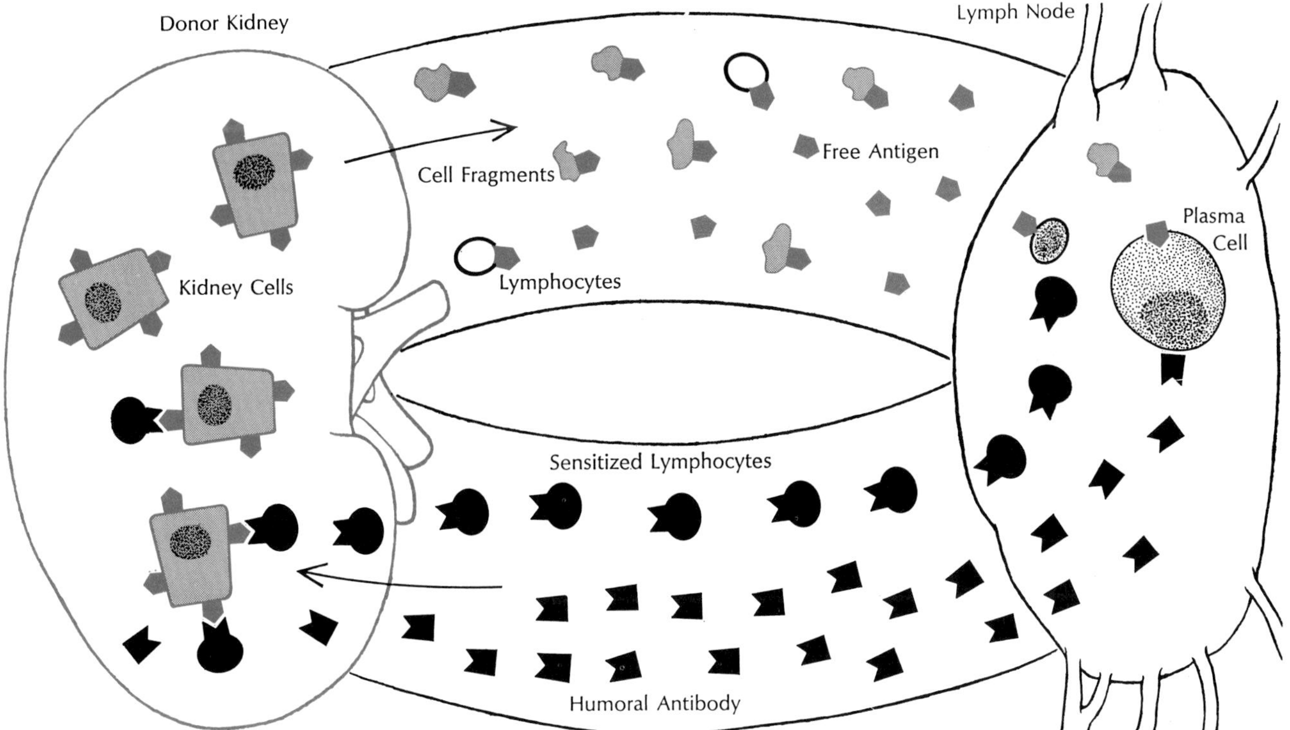

This mechanism usually accounts for rejection episodes in the first four months after transplantation. Antigens may escape from the donor kidney in soluble form, on cellular fragments, or attached to lymphocytes. The antigen migrates to the lymph node. There it encounters immunocompetent plasma cells, triggering production of humoral antibody and small lymphocytes, which become sensitized. Thus two forms of antibody may leave the lymph node and migrate back to the donor kidney. The initial immunologic attack on the kidney cells is believed to be a function of the sensitized lymphocytes.

cells are killed or agglutinated, the presence of the antigen recognized by that antibody is demonstrated. The cells of the donor and host are not reacted with each other. The donor and recipient are typed separately and the results then compared with respect to known antigenic groups. It is particularly important that the donor should not have antigens absent in the recipient, since these would tend to incite an immune response. It is also important to attempt to determine if the recipient possesses antibodies capable of reacting against the donor kidney. Such antibodies can be present even though the donor and recipient appear well matched with regard to antigens on their leukocytes. For this reason, we routinely test for recipient antibodies against both donor lymphocytes and kidney cells. We also test for the presence of anti-GBM antibody, which, though not related to rejection, could produce glomerulonephritis.

In the presence of preformed antibody that reacts against cells of the prospective donor, hyperacute rejection of the transplant is very apt to occur if that donor's kidney is used. The presence of gross antigenic incompatibility between donor and recipient is apt to lead to early or late rejection. But it is sometimes possible to have significant degrees of donor-host incompatibility and still have a successful outcome of the transplant in the immunosuppressed patient.

It should be emphasized that even "perfect" matches between, let's say, sibling donor-recipient pairs would not permit kidney transplant success in the absence of immunosuppression. This is presumably because histocompatibility testing by leukocyte typing recognizes only a few of the many antigens possessed by each individual, and some antigenic differences exist between any two individuals who are not identical twins. Weak antigenic differences can usually be overcome by immunosuppression, however, so that perfect matching of the strong antigens will almost always lead to a successful outcome of the transplant unless preformed anti-GBM antibody is present.

Immunosuppression

To some extent our shortcomings in determining the most appropriate donor for a kidney transplant – including the extreme narrowness of available choices – are compensated for by the great advances in suppressing the immune response. Since another article in this series deals entirely with immunosuppression [Chapter 24, "Immunosuppression: The Challenge of Selectivity," by Robert S. Schwartz] the discussion here will be limited.

It is worth while to point out that only three agents have been shown, at least experimentally, to prolong renal homograft survival indefinitely when used alone – azathioprine, prednisone, and antilymphocyte serum (ALS). Actually, it is very hard to achieve

The Mechanism of Primary Chronic Rejection

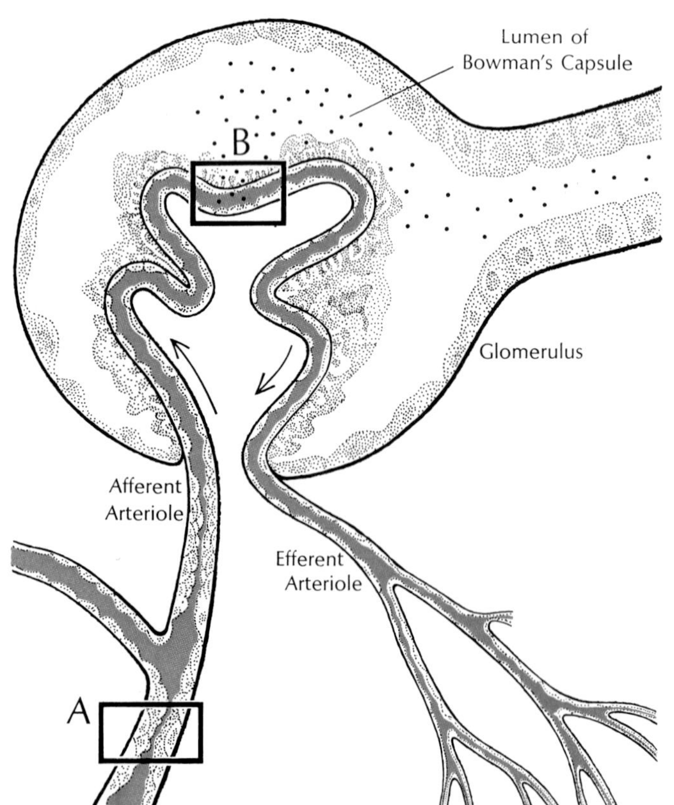

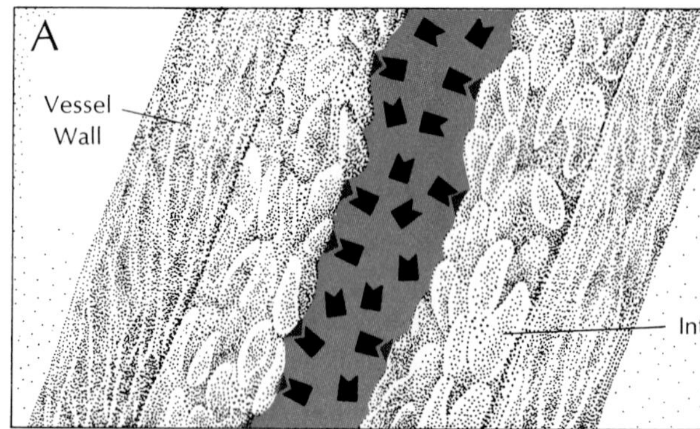

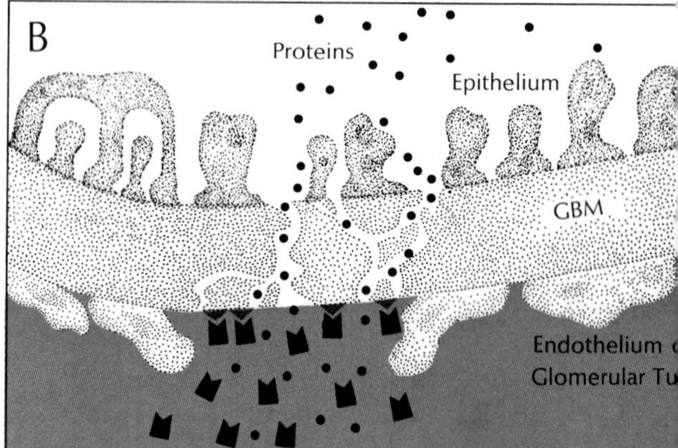

There are two foci of immunologic damage in chronic rejection. First, humoral antibody irritates the intima of the arterial tree (A and detail A) and produces endothelial proliferation, reducing distal blood flow. Second, in the glomerular tuft (B and detail B), antibody causes damage to the glomerular basement membrane It attaches to GBM where antigen-antibody complexes activate complement. The GBM becomes permeable to proteins, which leak into the urinary space. These characteristic changes of

such survival with prednisone alone, but this agent is the most valuable of all for the reversal of acute rejection episodes. Both prednisone and local irradiation of the kidney are of great value in coping with the mechanisms of rejection at the level of the kidney itself. Azathioprine is the primary immunosuppressant, and the introduction of its clinical usage coincided with the beginning of consistent long-term renal transplant survival in man. Lymphocyte depletion by thoracic duct drainage or blood irradiation has also been used.

Probably the most intriguing agent used for immunosuppression is antilymphocyte serum or antilymphocyte globulin (ALG). Interest in ALS for various immunologic studies has been considerable for a number of years.

For all its promise, work with ALS or ALG can be most perplexing. Among many variables are the kind of lymphocytes used to make the antiserum, the animal used to make the antiserum, the route of injection into the animal in which the antiserum is made, the dose of cells used, and the schedule of injections. All these are extremely important. For example, injecting small doses at long intervals may produce no immunization at all. On the other hand, injecting large doses at short intervals may produce tremendously high antibody titers, but then an additional booster shot may quite quixotically shut off antibody production entirely. Moreover, while the initial goal of ALS was to produce lymphopenia, it has been found that the degree of lymphopenia produced may not correlate with transplant survival.

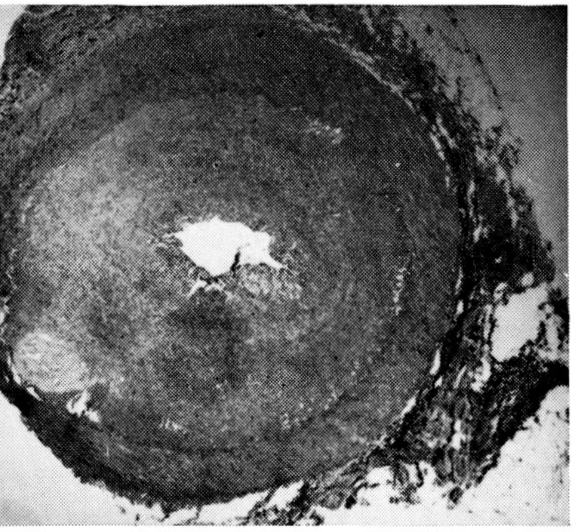

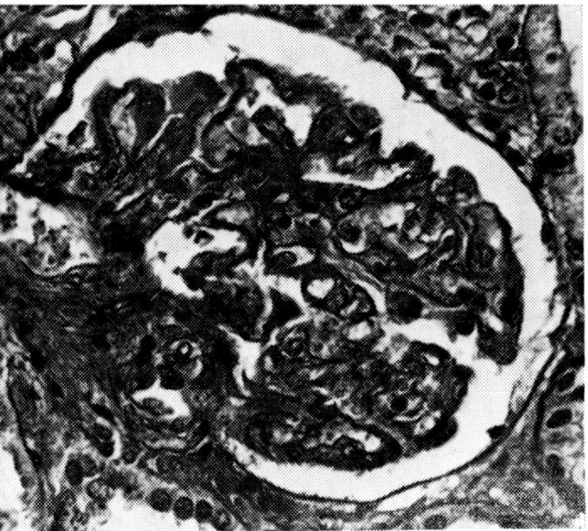

chronic rejection are apparent in the photomicrographs above, which show narrowing of the arterial lumen (A) and membranous glomerulonephritis (B).

Clinically of great importance would be the ability to make an ALS directed specifically against lymphocytes concerned with primary rejection but sparing cells needed to combat infection. Some types of ALS seem to be more selective in this respect than others. We are hoping that perhaps the answer to selectivity lies in a variant of ALS – antithymocyte serum (ATS). The rationale underlying this hope is the likelihood that the lymphocyte primarily concerned with transplant rejection originated in or under the control of the thymus. There may be a large clone, or population of lymphocytes, directed against bacterial and viral antigens and having its embryonic origin in structures analogous to the avian bursa of Fabricius [see Chapter 1, "Disorders of the Immune System," by Robert A. Good]. An antithymocyte preparation might spare these cells and "home in" instead on those lymphoid cells that at some time or another were related to the thymus, no matter where they now may be in the body. Experimentally, we have been able to make an antithymocyte serum that is much less toxic than ALS and very effective in prolonging transplant survival. Human antithymocyte globulin (ATG) has been prepared using thymocytes removed from young children undergoing open heart surgery. Its critical clinical evaluation is not yet complete.

All ALG contains antibodies, not only against specific lymphocyte antigens but also against the HL-A histocompatibility antigens on the lymphocytes. Since these latter antigens are present on all body cells, the effectiveness of ALG is thus decreased by its attachment to nonlymphoid cells. Attempts are being made to produce an ALG that has antibodies only against specific lymphocyte antigens and that should, therefore, be far more potent.

While ALS appears to add to the suppression of early primary (cellular) rejection, it has no effect on the cell already producing serum antibodies. It is thus ineffective in altering 1) hyperacute rejection, 2) chronic rejection, or 3) the development of glomerulonephritis.

Three other possible methods to attenuate homograft rejection deserve mention. The first is antigen pretreatment to "desensitize" the host or to provide antigen overloading or antigen competition. The second is to "enhance" the survival of the graft with enhancing antibody treatment, which may inhibit the production of host antibody. The third is to interfere with the actual destructive mechanisms by means of anticomplement agents or agents that destroy intracellular histamine.

Second Transplants

On a theoretical basis, a second transplant might well seem a futile maneuver. It will be recalled that Medawar's first contribution to the field of transplant immunology was his demonstration that when a skin graft from animal A was rejected by animal B, a second A-to-B graft would encounter the antibodies previously made and experience a markedly accelerated rejection. If the second graft was from animal C, however, graft survival was not greatly compromised.

It was largely against this experimental background that we undertook second transplants in man. We felt that if an initial transplant failed we should try a second transplant, and we were pleasantly surprised to find that in general the second transplant worked better than the first. Struck by this phenomenon in our own investigations, we studied all the second transplants that had been done elsewhere as well. By and large, we found that the impression of the efficacy of second transplants could be confirmed.

In our own experience, the difference in responses was often most striking. For example, one patient who rejected his first transplant very violently only four days after surgery had a second graft done. At the present

Why Second Kidney Grafts May Be Accepted

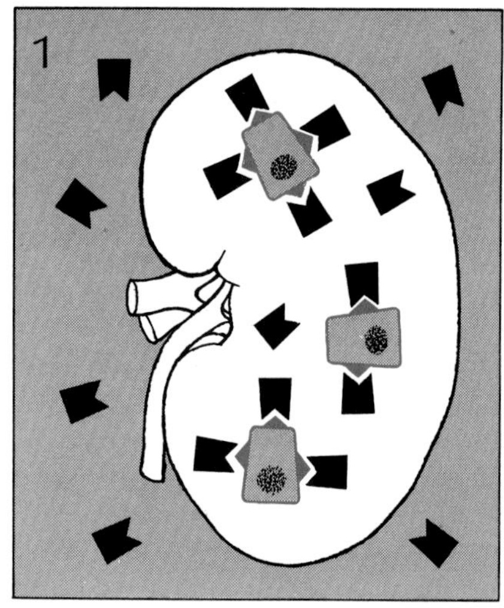

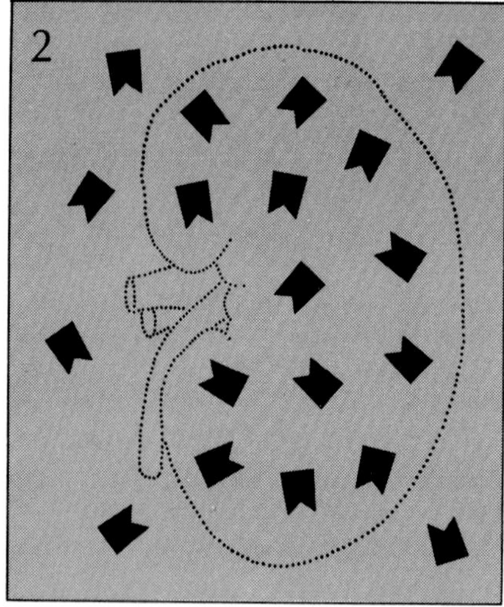

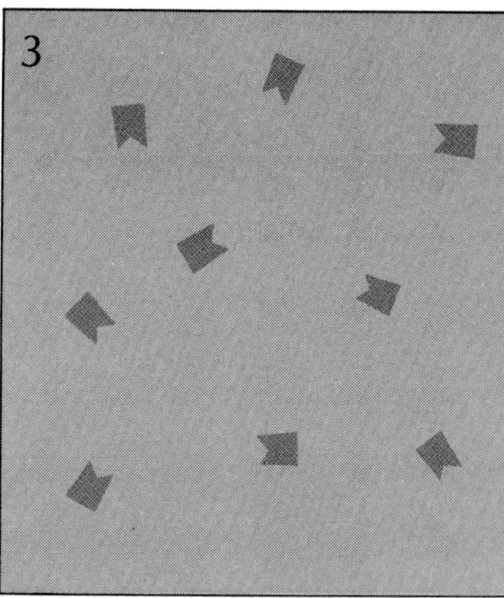

A hypothesis that may explain acceptance of second kidney transplants after rejection of first grafts is illustrated. When the rejected graft (1) is removed, circulating antibody is left behind (2). After a wait of at least 40 days, antibody titers fall; antibody may have become attenuated (3). An antigenically dissimilar kidney is transplanted from second donor (4). New cell-bound anti-

time, six years later, this cadaver kidney is providing completely normal kidney function. In fact, quite a long time elapsed before we encountered our first failure with a second graft. This occurred in a little girl who had received her initial transplant from her father. After 15 months, this kidney failed and had to be removed. The second graft was a cadaver kidney that lasted only three months. A third transplant was then carried out, and this is still functioning well, more than five years later.

Our first report of favorable experiences with second grafts was followed by reports from other investigators with contrary results. It was suggested that a favorable outcome was encountered when the first graft had failed for technical reasons but not when the first graft had been rejected. The argument was advanced that a second transplant should not be attempted if the first graft had been rejected. This challenge led us to a detailed analysis of second transplants. Our own results show that of 25 patients receiving second, third, or fourth transplants, 13 survived with functioning grafts. Most of the 12 failures had hyperacute rejection due to prior immunization of the recipient with a transplant that shared antigens with the second transplant. In our laboratories Pierce has shown that the incidence of hyperacute rejection of second, third, or fourth grafts taken from random donors can be accurately predicted mathematically from calculations based on the distribution of the various HL-A antigens. The success rate of retransplantation can be vastly increased, of course, by testing the recipient's serum for antibodies against the donor's cells and avoiding those transplants in which hyperacute rejection is inevitable. Thus, although we originally thought that the success of retransplantation might be due to "enhancing" antibodies as shown in the illustration (above and next page), it seems more likely now that it is due to what started as a fortuitous and has now become a planned avoidance of transplantation when there are host antibodies present that are capable of reacting against donor antigens.

Early in our series, we were fortunate in not encountering any patients with cytotoxic antibodies against the donors of their second transplants. However, several patients who received transplants later in the series did have such antibodies, and the result of one of these cases is extremely interesting:

The girl's first transplant was from her sister. It underwent chronic rejection and finally had to be removed after 4½ years. A second kidney, taken from a cadaver, was hyperacutely rejected in about two minutes, but we left it in place for three hours in the hope that it might extract the cytotoxic antibodies that we suspected were present. We then removed it and put in the second kidney from the same cadaver. Rejection again took only minutes. We left the kidney in place for about seven weeks. After removal of the transplant, the patient had very high titers of cytotoxic antibody; injections of as little as 6 cc of her serum produced fatal nephritis in squirrel monkeys. She had cytotoxic antibodies against many members of the lymphocyte donor panel.

The patient was given a two-month course of ALS, which did not reduce her antibody titers at all. About five weeks later, we happened to get another cadaver donor. The donor's lymphocytes were tested against the patient's serum, which did not show any cytotoxic antibody against the donor. We therefore carried out a fourth transplant, using the kidney from this donor. This transplant worked immediately and at three years continues to work well.

Recurrent Glomerulonephritis

When renal transplants are carried out between identical twins in circumstances where the disease of the host kidney has been glomerulonephritis, the incidence of recurrent glomerulonephritis is 67%. This finding raises a specter that recurrent glomerulonephritis may be a major deterrent to renal homotransplantation in patients with this disease. However, the inci-

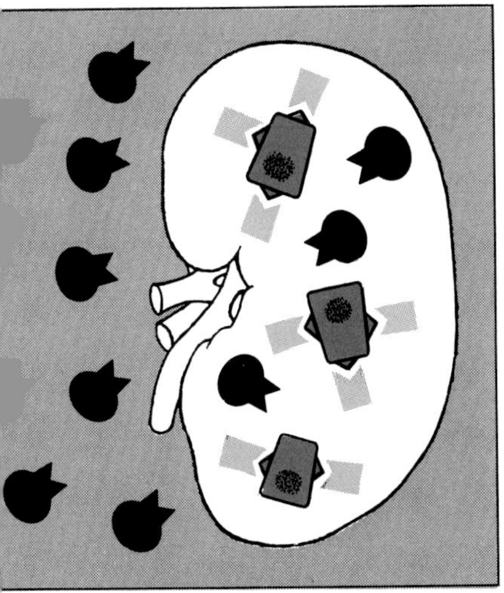

body cannot effectively attach to graft because "old" antibody has protectively covered combining sites.

dence of recurrent glomerulonephritis in non-twin transplants whose recipients are receiving the immunosuppressive drugs appears to be far less. The actual incidence is difficult to determine because chronic rejection produces a type of glomerulonephritis that is sometimes almost impossible to differentiate from recurrent glomerulonephritis. In our series, the incidence of recurrent glomerulonephritis appears to be 18%.

In a few cases where the recipient had high titers of anti-GBM antibody, recurrent glomerulonephritis was seen in a matter of days after transplantation, and all subsequent transplants to the same patient suffered the same fate.

In a study of the glomerular changes of the transplants in our series, it appeared that recurrent glomerulonephritis could usually be differentiated from chronic rejection nephritis on the basis of the following findings:

- The type of glomerular lesion in the transplant was generally similar to that in the host's own kidneys when the disease process was recurrent glomerulonephritis.
- There was more apt to be a relationship between the degree of protein loss and the function of the kidney early in the course of the transplant when chronic rejection nephritis was the etiology, whereas quite often there was a heavy protein loss from kidneys with recurrent glomerulonephritis while the renal function was still quite good.
- Deposits of IgG were characteristically seen on the GBM in recurrent nephritis, and these were in linear fashion in anti-GBM nephritis and in a coarse granular pattern in complex nephritis. In chronic rejection nephritis, one frequently saw deposits of IgM that tended to be finely granular. IgM was much more uncommon in recurrent nephritis.
- The thickening of the endothelial cells of the glomerular capillaries was more pronounced in chronic rejection nephritis than in recurrent glomerulonephritis. Furthermore, the electron-dense deposits in the basement membrane were more irregular with rejection nephritis, and although they tended to be positioned subendothelially they were often scattered throughout the markedly thickened basement membrane as well.

While none of these criteria proved to be absolute in distinguishing between the two types of nephritis, when taken in their entirety along with the clinical course and with knowledge of the original disease, a differentiation could usually be made.

Transplants and Cancer

As more and more transplants were done and more and more patients survived for longer periods of time, sporadic reports began to appear showing the development of spontaneous cancer in some of the patients. There have now been many cases reported, and it appears that the incidence of the development of cancer in transplant patients may be as high as 6% to 8%.

Many of the patients developed lymphoid cancer, often reticulum cell sarcoma, while others showed a wide variety of other types of spontaneous cancer. In our series of cases, four patients have developed cancer. One of these was cervical and three were reticulum cell sarcomas, two of which made their appearance more than six years after transplantation.

The mechanism for the development of reticulum cell sarcoma appears to be related both to the immunosuppressive agents and to the transplant itself – patients receiving such agents without transplants almost never develop lymphatic cancer. The continued presence of the transplant provides an antigenic stimulus to the lymphocyte that increases the likelihood it will undergo malignant degeneration, and the effect of the immunosuppressive agents on the lymphocyte probably increases this likelihood. The nonlymphatic types of cancer seen in transplant patients probably result from the decreased cancer surveillance brought about by the immunosuppressive agents and the decreased resistance to oncogenic viruses seen in such patients.

While the incidence of cancer in patients with transplants is not high enough to contraindicate the procedure, it is a factor to be reckoned with and will become more important as transplant patients live longer.

Although it is true that most of the clinical data accumulated on the immunobiology of transplantation is referable to experience with kidney transplants, no current article on any aspect of homotransplantation could fail to mention the results of transplantation of other organs.

As of the present date, 170 heart transplants have been carried out in man and 24 patients continue to survive, two more than a year, six more than 18 months, and 11 over two years. The longest surviving heart transplant is in a patient who was operated on at our hospital by Richard Lower; at this writing it is of 30 months duration. The function of the heart is excellent, and the patient lives a normal life.

There have been 102 orthotopic liver transplants and of this group 12 survive, three of them over a year, one over 18 months, and two over two years. The longest survival at this writing is 31 months and is in a patient operated on by Thomas Starzl in Denver. No heterotopic liver transplants survived.

Of 25 lung transplants and 23 pancreas transplants, none survive at this writing.

Although transplants of hearts and livers are more difficult technically than kidney transplants, there is no real barrier to their success other than the immunologic resentment of the recipient common to all transplant situations, particularly those in which cadaver donor organs are used. As the mechanisms for dealing with the immunologic barriers become more refined and develop in the direction of avoidance of rejection rather than suppression of it, heart and liver transplants, and probably those of many other organs as well, will become standard clinical procedures.

Clearly, the field of organ transplantation is one in which, despite great progress, many problems are still to be solved. But probably the most exciting aspect of transplantation today is that never before in history have there been so many tools to work with, so many opportunities to find the keys to the remaining problems. While ALS is useful clinically, its greatest potential may be in delineation of the specific cellular mechanism involved in graft rejection. Fruitful approaches may be developed toward modifying the graft's antigenicity as well as the host's ability to respond to the graft. Histocompatibility typing will be further refined. Progress has been made toward preconditioning the host so that he will be less likely to react against the graft. All these approaches remain for the future, but the future does not seem to lie too far ahead.

Chapter 20

The Current Status of Liver Transplantation

THOMAS E. STARZL
University of Colorado

Treatment of terminal liver disease by transplantation was founded on the encouragement and knowledge provided by the steadily improving experience in renal transplantation. The liver, however, is a far more complicated organ, and its derangement leads to vastly more complex physiologic impairments. Liver patients are further handicapped, as are heart patients, by the lack so far of a satisfactory means of artificial support comparable to renal dialysis that could take over the organ's compromised functions during the wait for a suitable donor, or during the critical immediate postoperative period. Live donors, of course, are not feasible, timing is of the essence, and the circumstances for obtaining an optimal homograft are rarely if ever ideal. The transplanted liver must function efficiently practically from the moment of anastomosis or the patient is lost.

Despite these and other formidable difficulties, the past 10 years have furnished enough progress in the laboratory and clinic to let us state that liver transplantation is now a feasible and legitimate, albeit imperfect, form of treatment, one that may in certain cases be considered as a last best hope. Human survivals for up to two and one half years have been achieved. A great deal has been and is being learned – at a pace suggesting that the next phase, when liver transplants will have at least as much a chance as kidney grafts now have, is not far off. Eventually much more than that will need to be accomplished, of course, but rather than engage in speculation it would appear more useful here to record how far we have come and to identify the major hurdles immediately ahead.

When research in liver transplantation was in its early stages, it was hoped that as the liver played a significant role in graft rejections, hepatic homografts might enjoy a better fate than other transplants because presumably the grafted liver would not participate in rejecting itself. The case for this rather mystical view seemed even strengthened by certain experiences with laboratory animals. When immunosuppression in canine recipients was stopped after four months a surprising number of animals continued to thrive, with no signs of rejection or with rejection episodes that waxed or waned remittently. One such dog is still alive, with stable liver function seven years after the transplant. This phenomenon of "graft acceptance" had been noted in dogs with renal transplants, but less frequently.

If the liver thus seemed to be an immunologically more favored organ in dogs, its status in pigs – as observed by Garnier in Paris, Terblanche in Bristol, Calne in Cambridge, and in our own laboratory – was even more noteworthy. In some experiments with pigs not treated with immunosuppressive agents, identifiable homograft rejection did not occur. In other experiments, rejection was indolent and spontaneously reversed. This state of affairs applied only to a minority of animals. Nevertheless, these results had to be attributed to some special privilege of the liver, since porcine skin and kidney grafts were regularly rejected in the usual way.

These observations in both dogs and pigs (and now in other animals) invited certain hypotheses in addition to the one stated above that the new liver helped create an internal milieu favorable to itself. There were the possibilities that the liver was inherently less antigenic than other organs, that its relatively great antigenic mass was a beneficial factor, that its enormous regenerative capacity made it less susceptible than other tissues to the effects of chronic rejection, or (Calne) that it possessed or released some special factor promoting the induction of specific immunologic tolerance.

Whatever the explanation, overstatement of the case

for the liver's privileged status could lead to erroneous conclusions about the practical requirements for immunosuppressive therapy following hepatic transplantation in man. At a research level, another danger could stem from the notion that hepatic transplantation, especially in the pig, is somehow qualitatively unique. The fallacy of such a contention is obvious from the fact that even in the "easy" pig model the majority of untreated liver recipients die from acute rejection. In dogs and humans, control of hepatic rejection may be difficult or impossible in spite of very heavy immunosuppressive therapy.

It is my opinion that liver homografts differ from other organs only in the degree of host immunologic response they evoke in all species, including the pig. In this context, two key observations first made with kidneys have been extended to the liver, and there is little doubt that they apply to other tissues as well. The first is the reversibility of rejection, which has been well documented in canine, porcine, and human recipients of hepatic homografts. In patients, reversal usually requires intensification of treatment, but it has sometimes been noted without any change in the preexisting therapy, suggesting that such recoveries had an element of spontaneity. As mentioned earlier, "spontaneous remission" of rejection in the absence of all therapy has occurred both in dogs and pigs, particularly the latter. The reactions of the liver in all three species are undoubtedly expressions of the same phenomenon, differing only quantitatively.

The second observation of overriding practical and theoretical interest concerns what has already been referred to as "graft acceptance." In many of the human kidney recipients treated almost a decade ago, it was shown that a melting away of host resistance to the homograft occurred surprisingly early after transplantation, often following an acute rejection crisis. This was manifested by eventual declines in the doses of immunosuppressive agents necessary to retain stable graft function. In many patients, the level of chronic immunosuppression has proved to be less than that which at the outset failed to prevent the onset of a severe rejection.

It is probable that all treatment could be stopped in some of these human renal recipients whom we have now followed for seven or eight years, but we have not dared to take such a drastic step. However, as described earlier, therapy has been successfully discontinued in dogs after kidney transplantation and even more consistently after liver replacement, indicating that graft acceptance may become complete. In pigs, the barrier of natural host resistance is apparently low enough so that the cycle of hepatic graft acceptance can be completed without any immunosuppression at all. Viewed in this way, the curious pig liver experiments become only a special example of, rather than an exception to, a general principle of transplantation. Recently, Perper has provided evidence to support both this concept and the original idea that there is a slight but limited biologic advantage in transplanting the liver rather than the kidney. Perper showed that a three-day course of heterologous antilymphocyte globulin (ALG) treatment (or other short-term therapeutic maneuvers) in pigs permitted long-term acceptance of kidneys in precisely the same way as it does with the liver in the absence of all iatrogenic intervention.

It is indisputable that some element of acceptance of various kinds of grafts occurs often in humans under the appropriate conditions of immunosuppression and that the degree to which this develops is a prime determinant of the long-term prognosis. Unfortunately, the reason for the change in the host-graft relationship is not known. More than one immunologic pathway may be involved. Schwartz and Talmage first called attention to the possibility that the continuous presence of a transplanted organ in a host being treated with immunosuppressive therapy could lead to a selective loss of responsiveness to antigens. The suggestion here is that specific lymphocyte clones, induced to replicate by the graft antigens, are thereby rendered more vulnerable to the killing effect of immunosuppres-

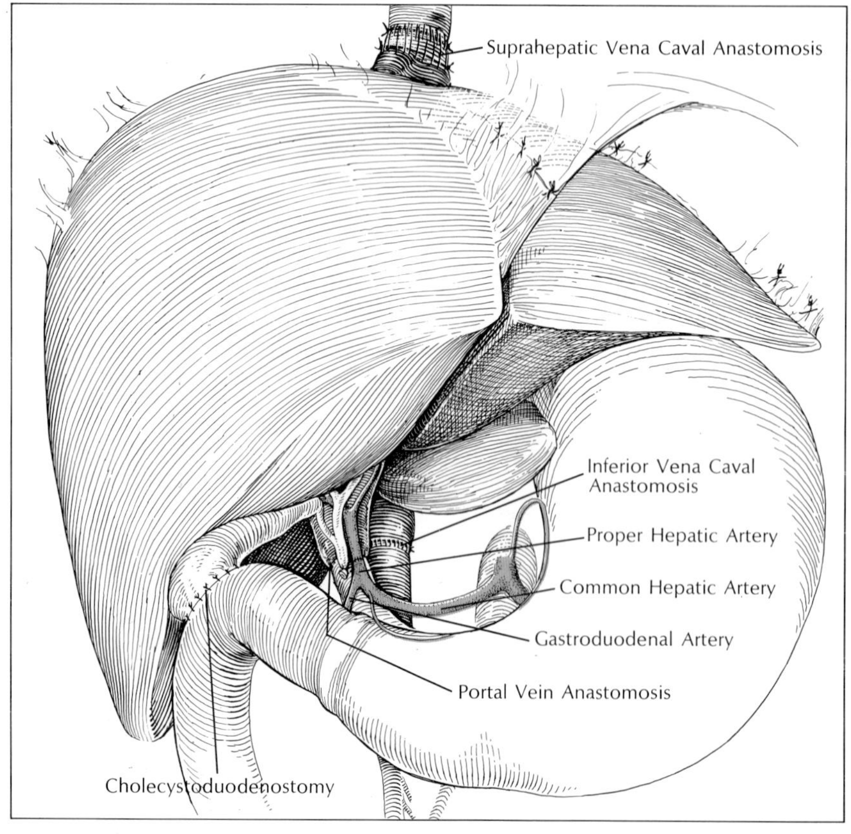

Insertion of second homograft in child pictured opposite proceeded as shown above, with cholecystoduodenostomy performed for biliary drainage and the donor celiac axis attached to the recipient proper hepatic artery. Note that a cuff of the first homograft's inferior vena cava was left to lengthen the suprahepatic connection.

sive agents than is the rest of the lymphocyte population. Inasmuch as the maintenance of such activated cell lines appears to be thymus-dependent even in adult life, at least in some experimental animals, it is reasonable to be curious about the effect of thymectomy as an adjuvant immunosuppressive measure. The results of thymectomy in a series of our human renal transplants were inconclusive; though those with thymic excision did not have better survival or superior renal function, there were fewer and less severe histopathologic abnormalities when the grafts were examined long after transplantation.

At any rate, the concept of specific, differential tolerance through "clone stripping" can partly explain the characteristic cycle of rejection and reversal that occurs after whole organ transplantation both in treated animals and man and in the weak, self-resolving crises in the untreated pig. Moreover, this concept is consistent with the fact that a wide variety of agents that are capable of general immunologic crippling can also provide specificity of action under the stipulated conditions of immunosuppressive treatment during presence of the antigen.

To date, few investigations to establish the presence or absence of classic immunologic tolerance to donor tissue have been carried out in human recipients of chronically functioning renal homografts. It would be interesting to know if skin from these donors would be accepted. One of the reasons why such a test has not been carried out in patients is the potential

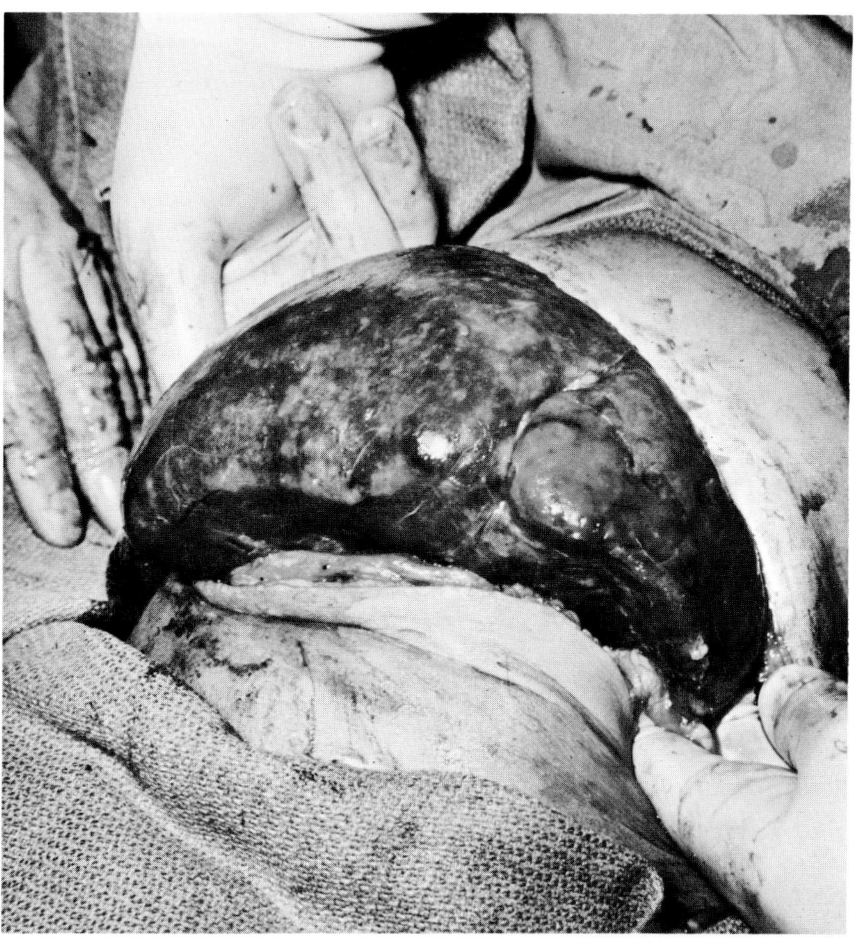

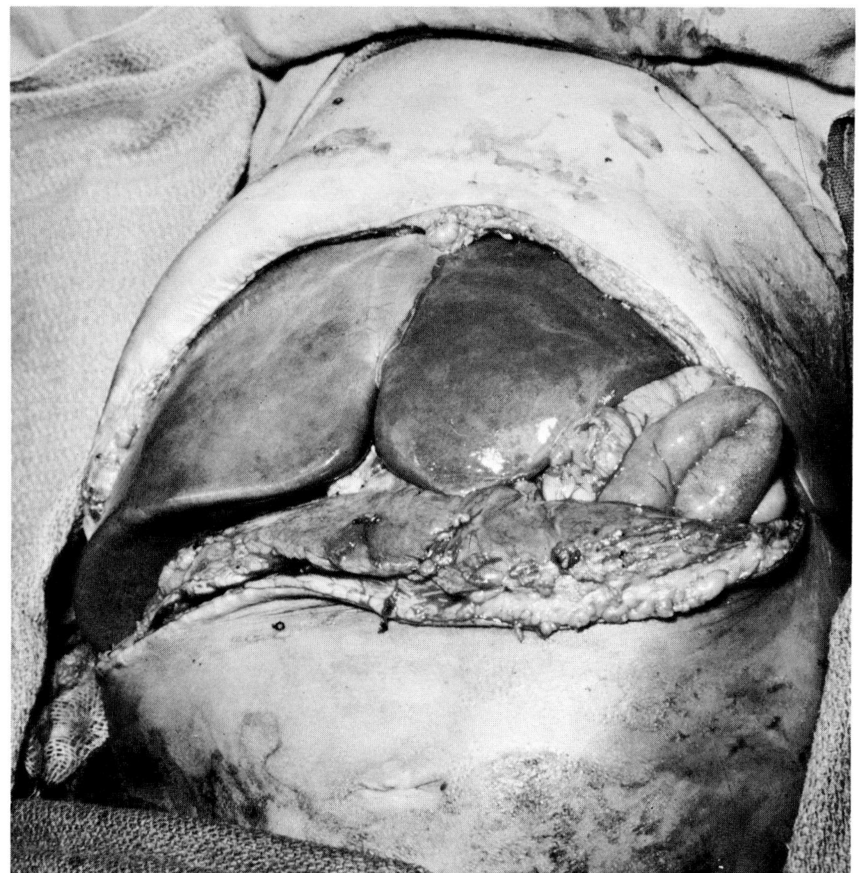

A rejecting homograft in a two-year-old child treated by transplantation for extrahepatic biliary atresia is shown at top at the time of its removal, 68 days following insertion. (The liver weighed 250 gm at insertion, 880 at removal.) The child received a second homograft (lower photo); his subsequent course was extremely complicated, in part because of the large size of the second liver (which came from a seven-year-old donor), which severely crowded the abdominal cavity. Fortunately, swelling due to rejection was delayed for a month and eventually the child was able to eat a full diet. Although jaundiced, the child lived for one year after the second transplant and died of hepatic failure. (For gross appearance of first graft on pathologic examination see next page.)

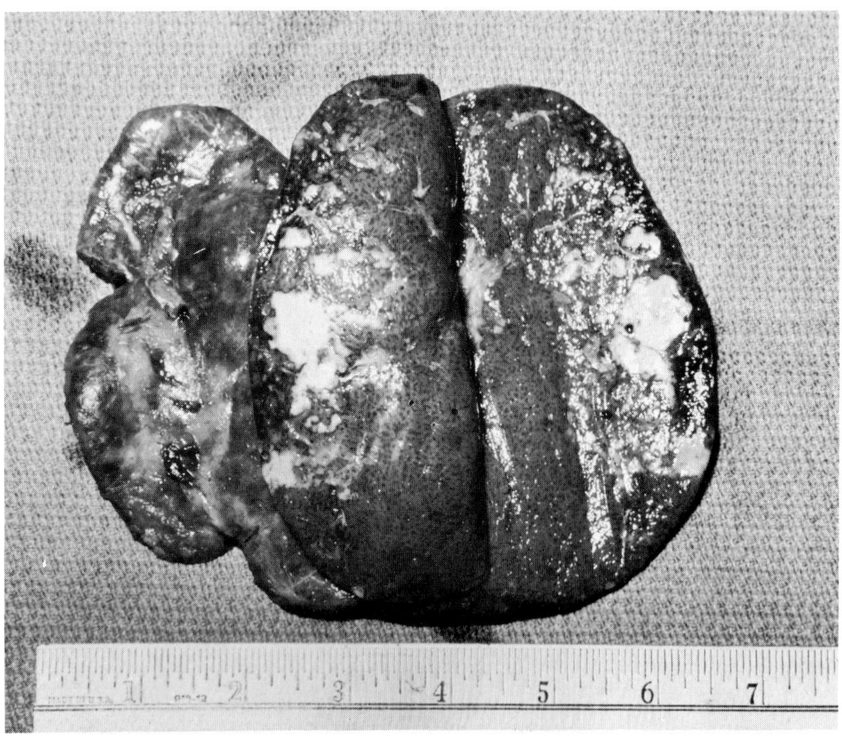

Gross subcortical infarcts were easily seen in the rejected homograft removed from the patient described on pages 196-197. Some necrotic areas revealed by slicing seemed to have been devitalized very recently, others seemed to be older, and both types tended to be near the surface. The major blood vessels were found free of clots.

risk of precipitating an immune reaction that could damage the kidney. Of course, the liver recipient's viable donor tissue is not available for such an experiment even if this were a desirable undertaking.

Fritz Bach has provided evidence that at least some kidney recipients develop true tolerance to their donors. Dr. Bach performed mixed lymphocyte cultures with peripheral blood from a number of our renal recipients and their donors two to four years after transplantation. He was able to demonstrate in some cases that recipient lymphocytes no longer developed blast transformation when exposed to killed donor white cells, although they reacted vigorously to third-party cells. It is important to note that this was not always the case and that animal experiments with skin transplants similarly showed mixed results.

These ambivalent findings do not disprove tolerance through clone stripping so much as they suggest that at least another mechanism of graft acceptance is involved. One such mechanism, termed enhancement, has been envisioned as a process in which immunoglobulins synthesized by the activated lymphoid tissues return to the target tissue and coat it or protect it in some way that is not yet understood. Antigraft antibodies, selectively capable of being absorbed by the nucleated cells of the original donor, have been detected in patients carrying well-tolerated renal transplants. Extensive immunoglobulin deposition has been demonstrated by immunofluorescence techniques in long-functioning kidney homografts, but this finding usually has an adverse connotation rather than a favorable one.

An understanding of the means by which grafts are accepted may hold the key to improvements in therapy. When we come to know more about these mechanisms it may prove possible to arrange the conditions required for graft acceptance in advance of the arrival of the homograft rather than to rely on their development while fighting the battle of rejection. The result might well be the prevention of rejection with far less immunosuppressive crippling of the immune apparatus in the critical postoperative period. In this connection it is heartening to refer to the experiments of Stuart and his colleagues at the University of Chicago. When enhancing antibodies were combined with tolerance induction by donor-specific antigen pretreatment, rat renal transplants functioned 18 months and longer, even in the presence of strong histocompatibility barriers, the absence of immunosuppression, and the retention of immunologic reactivity to most antigens.

Another way to improve clinical results might be by effective donor-recipient matching of histocompatibility (HL-A) antigens. Unfortunately, the state of our knowledge about human histocompatibility systems is still primitive. While a good match between siblings appears to provide a more favorable prognosis after renal transplantation than a poor match, our experience with unrelated subjects provides no such correlation and has led us for the moment to the possibly heretical practice of ignoring the question of HL-A matching altogether in cadaveric cases. In liver transplantation, in which nonrelated cadaveric sources must be utilized exclusively, we have had some excellent results with poor histocompatibility matches and some discouraging results despite close matches. Not only has a correlation with tissue typing been absent with regard to clinical outcome but K. A. Porter of London has found no connection between the quality of the match and the appearance of the hepatic homograft at subsequent histologic examination. Until the discrimination of the matching methods is improved in nonrelated cases, we see no justification for denying a patient an available organ solely on the basis of poor serologic histocompatibility. Nor do we even use most favorable matching as an instrument of selection among candidates for transplantation. At the present time, a more valid criterion may be: Who has the most pressing need?

None of this should be construed as denigrating the ultimate value of histocompatibility determination in the transplantation of the future. What is at issue today is acceptance of the fact that typing between nonrelated individuals with serologic methods is imprecise, incomplete, and incapable of consistently predicting the extent of the antigenic confrontation in individual cases or the effectiveness with which immunosuppression may be used. The mixed lymphocyte culture method of Hirschhorn and Bach may be more discriminating and its findings more relevant for the selection of recipients. However, the procedure takes the better part of a week to perform, much too long for practical application in most cadaveric cases at the present time.

Here we turn to the question of logistics, for the problem of obtaining a fresh, functioning, nonischemic liver is paramount and provides the strongest correlation with success or failure. A major advance in one technical aspect of logistics, that of organ preservation and banking, would not only reduce the present inevitable waste of cadaveric organs but would also make more feasible the use of tissue typing when these techniques become more predictive. Selection on the basis of favorable histocompatibility would then become far more realistic and meaningful.

In the meanwhile, the most favorable prognostic thing that can be done for the hepatic transplantation candidate is to assure him an undamaged liver.

In discussing homograft quality, the technical details of organ preservation become interwoven with, or even distinctly secondary to, ethical considerations about the conditions for the pronouncement of donor death and problems of cooperation by the medical and lay community. Unquestionably, one of the most important advances in transplantation has been social in nature – acceptance by the public of the concept of cadaveric organ removal. In turn, this was made possible by a willingness of many in the medical profession to identify potential donors, approach family members at the time of their bereavement, or indicate in other ways their belief in the propriety of these efforts. The consequence has been a major contribution to our transplantation program by a well-informed community.

I believe that the transplantation team's style of community relations is a vital factor in determining the success of a cadaveric program. The difficult decisions required by the several parties to organ replacement cannot be made objectively in the atmosphere of a fishbowl. I have the impression that securing donors is less of a problem where transplant teams deliberately keep the matter in its proper perspective as a private concern between doctor and patient. The general public, quite naturally, is keenly interested in the drama and medical achievement represented by transplantation, and it is likewise important to transplantation that the public be informed of legitimate progress. This can and has been done in many areas impersonally, with restraint, without exaggeration, and without infringing on the personal right to privacy of the individuals involved.

After the donor has been identified and made available, an effort is made to maintain good liver perfusion up to the last possible moment in order to minimize the ischemic damage that even a short unperfused period may wreak under normothermic conditions. The extraordinary efforts required to prevent circulatory depression in the donor in the face of a hopeless prognosis usually require explanation to relatives and represent a problem of emotional substance to all parties.

Ultimately, a final decision to discontinue supportive measures must be made after all is in readiness to proceed with the recipient. During the first years of liver transplantation at the University of Colorado a considerable physiologic penalty was accepted because of criteria that insisted on both brain death and cessation of heartbeat before organ removal. The price of this insistence was the loss of critical time and the occurrence of

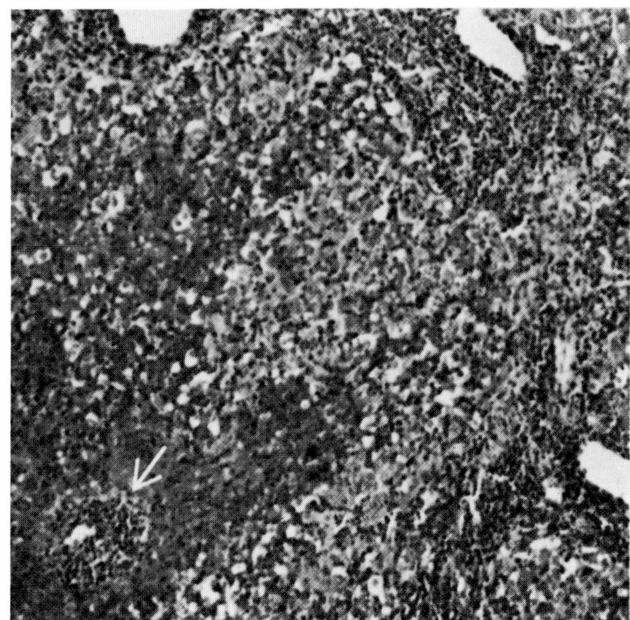

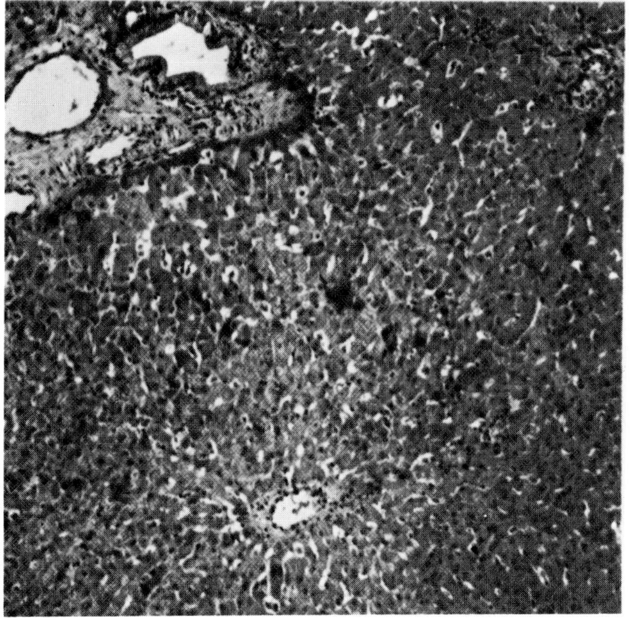

An untreated canine hepatic homograft is shown six days after transplantation (left). Portal veins (clear spaces) and central vein (arrow) are surrounded by dense cellular infiltration and there is centrilobular necrosis with hemorrhage (hematoxylin and eosin stain, x30). Photo at right shows normal liver architecture in another canine homograft one year after transplantation. This dog received azathioprine for four months, no additional therapy. It is still alive after some seven years.

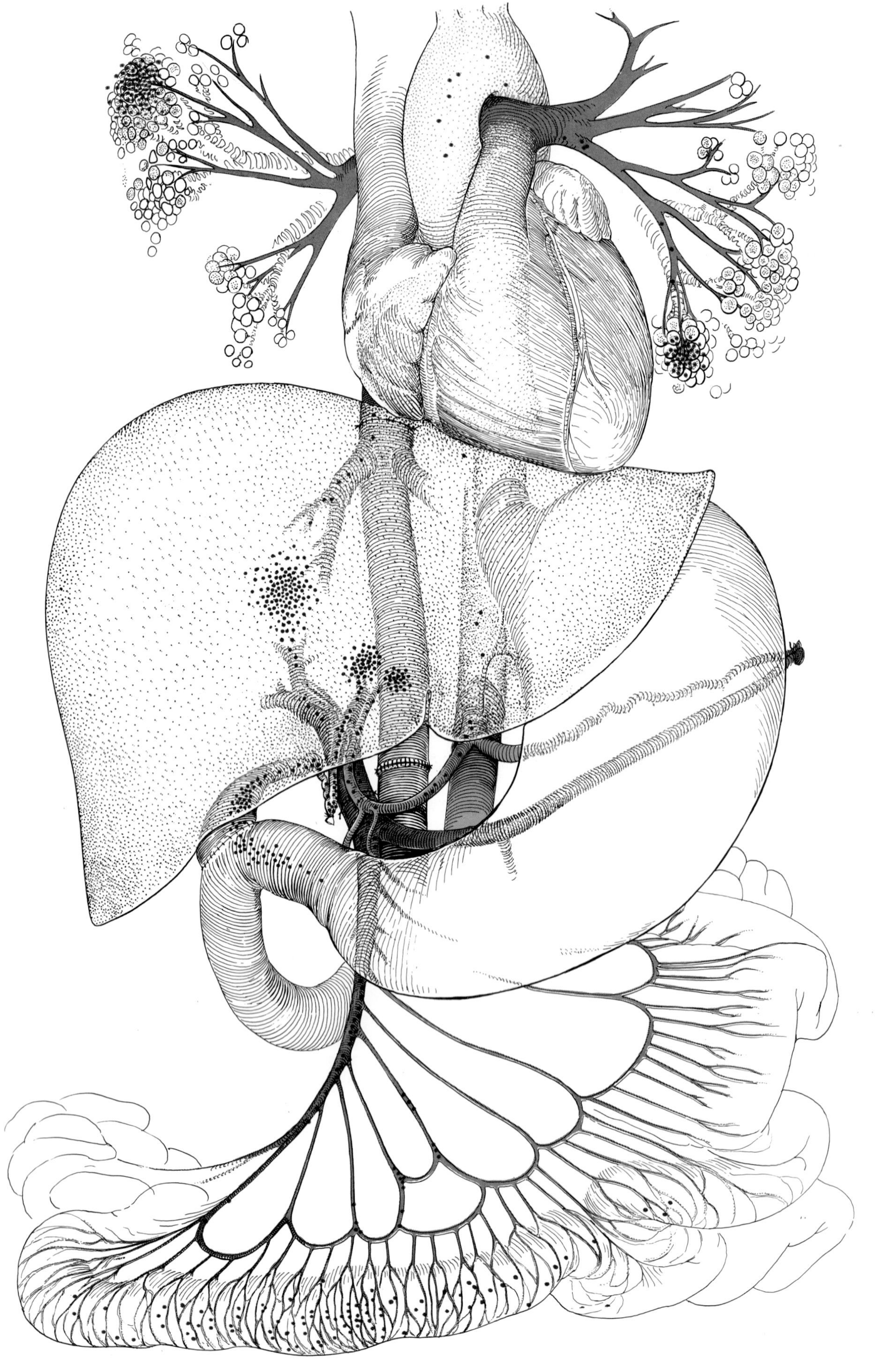

ischemic damage during both the agonal stages of circulatory failure and in the minutes after cardiac arrest. The reason for accepting these conditions was the fear that the quality of terminal care for the donor might be compromised by the pronouncement of death while there was still a heartbeat.

In 1968 we liberalized our criteria in accordance with the concept of irreversible brain injury as it was first outlined and applied at the University of Louvain, Belgium, by Alexandre and later defended by the Harvard ad hoc committee. Our experience since then has convinced us that anxieties about terminal care were unfounded. Acceptance of the brain death concept alleviated one of the most serious problems in liver transplantation, for it virtually eliminated the interval of normothermic ischemic injury and permitted the organ to be taken in the presence of an intact and effective circulation.

The subsequent preservation of the liver is also of vital importance and at our center we use one or more preservation modalities, depending on circumstances and always including organ hypothermia. With the acceptance of brain death as a criterion, it is often possible to maintain a naturally perfused liver in situ practically up to the moment of its excision. After removal, the liver may be quick-cooled by running a chilled electrolyte solution through the portal vein, thus lowering its temperature to about 10° or 15° C, which is sufficient for adequate preservation during the hour or so required for the vascular anastomoses in the recipient. Should the donor's heart stop before the recipient is ready, it is possible to employ the procedure used before 1968 (when cardiac arrest was required); by means of a heart-lung machine, circulation in the cadaver is reinstituted in combination with cooling. When longer periods of preservation and storage are needed (which has not been the case at this center since 1968) the liver may be removed and placed in a chamber such as that devised by Brettschneider, which combines perfusion, refrigeration, and hyperbaric oxygenation – this last process having an empiric favorable effect for reasons not clear. Conceivably, one could add to the perfusate a variety of metabolic inhibitors such as those reported by Webb, Fonkelsrud, and others. In one of our cases, the perfusion chamber permitted preservation of a liver without undue damage for nine hours, long enough for the recipient to make a transcontinental flight to Denver and to be prepared for surgery.

The above methods are still a far cry from the objectives of organ banking, and it must be conceded that there has been less progress in this than in any other aspect of transplantation. The importance of effective organ storage over the long term is obvious not only for reasons already noted but also to make it possible by portable devices to bring suitable and available organs to patients on a national exchange basis. Fresh ideas about organ preservation, either with solid state or perfusion techniques, are badly needed, for existing protocols seem to have reached the limit of their effectiveness. The importance of this problem has been acknowledged by a one-day "think tank" recently sponsored in Bethesda by the NIH, the Veterans Administration, and the National Research Council to smoke out some innovative ideas as well as to promote the funding with which to test these ideas.

Now, let us consider a few interesting aspects of the liver replacement operation. This procedure was first attempted in dogs by Francis Moore of Boston, and independently in our laboratories a short time later. As might be expected, the transition from animal experimentation to clinical application required some major technical adjustments and at least in one important and unexpected way demonstrated the need to be alert to the special requirements of human physiology. With removal of the host liver it is necessary to cross-clamp temporarily the great veins draining the intestines and the lower half of the body. In dogs, if provision is not made for decompression of the distal venous pools during the anhepatic phase, the animals either die of shock on the operating table or expire at a later time because of irreparable damage to the mesenteric vessels. It was assumed that the same precaution would be necessary in humans and this was accomplished in the first five human recipients by plastic tube bypasses from splenic and/or femoral veins to the external jugulars. There was a dismaying incidence of pulmonary emboli that caused or contributed to the death of at least two of the recipients. It was suspected that the clots either originated within the bypasses and were actually carried to the lungs during the operation or were formed a short time later at or near the site where the femoral catheter had been inserted. To our relief, the omission of the venous decompression procedure in later patients did not produce any serious or long-lasting circulatory effects, including hypotension. Although a slight duskiness of the intestine developed in some recipients, it immediately disappeared when blood flow was restored through the reconstructed venous channels. One can explain the ease with which portal and vena caval cross-clamping was tolerated by man's inherently richer network of potential collateral channels for return of blood to the right heart. Presumably, also, the size and ramifications of these vessels are further increased as a result of the disease in the liver. Venous decompression with bypasses has not been used in any recent case. The ability to omit this step has been a major technical advantage.

In planning a liver transplantation, the surgeon must be prepared for a high incidence of anatomic variations of either the graft or host structures. These have been noted in almost 40% of our cases. Multiple arteries have been the most frequent anomalies. When the recipient has had these, we have usually connected the graft celiac axis to the host aorta. When the multiplicity has been of the transplant vessels, multiple arterial anastomoses or other variant procedures have been used. There is no question that the need to improvise in these situations imposes an extra risk, particularly in very young recipients whose arteries are quite small and thin-walled. In pa-

The location of the orthotopic liver homograft, between the bowel and the heart, helps explain the predisposition of these patients to graft sepsis and eventual gangrene. As the drawing opposite suggests, invading microorganisms (brown dots) may enter via portal vein or through the reconstructed biliary tract; the lungs also are at high risk.

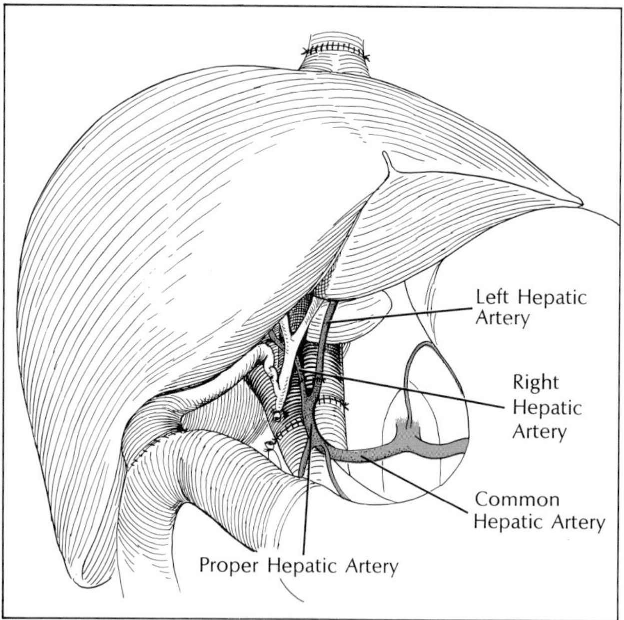

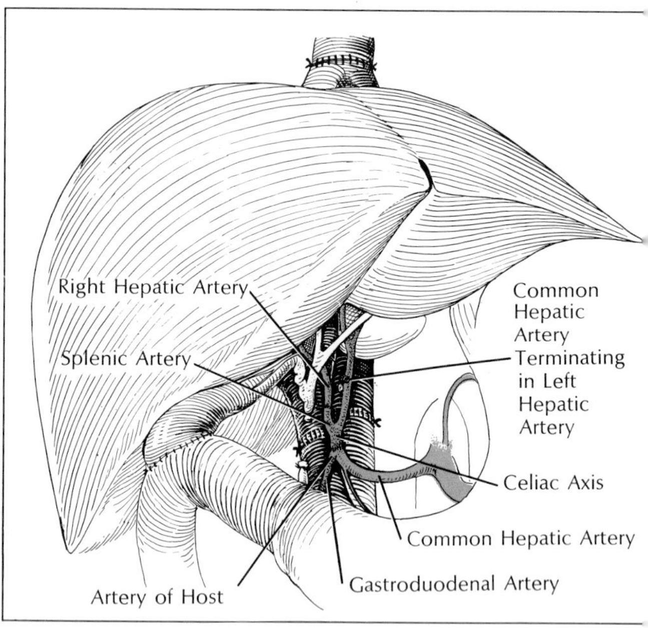

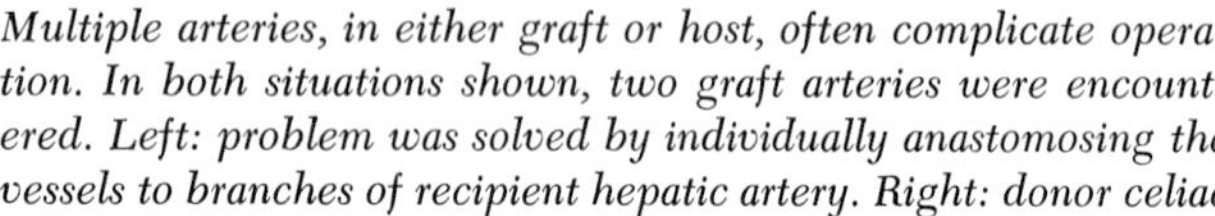

Multiple arteries, in either graft or host, often complicate operation. In both situations shown, two graft arteries were encountered. Left: problem was solved by individually anastomosing the vessels to branches of recipient hepatic artery. Right: donor celiac axis was first joined to recipient common hepatic artery. After blood flow was restored through larger left branch, other (right) donor artery, which had originated from superior mesenteric artery, was revascularized by being attached to donor splenic artery.

tients with biliary atresia, anomalies may be so complex as to make it virtually impossible to succeed. Two of our infants with biliary atresia had a curious type of malrotation in which the portal vein passed in front of the pancreas and duodenum, the arterial blood supply issuing from the superior mesenteric artery rather than from the celiac axis, which was absent as was the retrohepatic inferior vena cava. In both cases corrective maneuvers to overcome the structural deficits were unsuccessful and the patients died within a few days.

The critical problem of obtaining adequate bile drainage and avoiding technical errors that may lead to leakage or obstruction may also be complicated by biliary tract anomalies, and the surgeon must be prepared to tailor his procedures to the individual case. An end-to-end anastomosis of the common duct, if it were normal, would have the advantage of preserving the sphincter of Oddi, thus providing drainage through a normal distal channel and reducing the chances of reflux of food or bacteria. This method, which of course is not available in the case of biliary atresia, is considered the procedure of choice by some surgeons. However, from our experience this anastomosis involves too high a risk of leakage and infection. We consider it undesirable to leave a T-tube prosthesis and a drain in an immunosuppressed patient when the duct reconstruction is in close proximity to the portal venous and hepatic arterial anastomoses. Further, there may not always be an adequate blood supply to the distal portion of the homograft common duct, which normally receives its principal arterialization from retroduodenal sources but now must depend on retrograde flow from arteries in the central hepatic hilum. Therefore, when feasible, we use the safer if somewhat less elegant technique of anastomosing the gallbladder directly to the duodenum and ligating the common duct.

Some dangers attend ligation of the transplant common duct if certain anomalies go unrecognized. Communication between the cystic and common ducts may not always be at the point of their apparent juncture. In one patient the ducts were externally fused but separated by an internal septum; in another, the homograft cystic duct passed behind the common duct and descended for almost two inches as one compartment of a double-barreled lumen. In both cases biliary drainage was inadvertently obstructed when the common duct ligature closed both parallel passages, a technical error subsequent surgery failed to correct and that proved fatal.

Some of the vascular and ductal anomalies could have been predicted, resulting either in better planning for surgery or in a decision not to operate at all. These earlier cases did not, however, have the benefit of the extensive arteriography and cholangiography that we now use routinely in the donor and sometimes in the recipient as well.

Other problems during and after operation may be caused by derangements in the coagulation mechanism that may result either in hemorrhage or thrombosis. As one would expect, acute bleeding can be particularly troublesome during the actual liver transplantation. To begin with, the very nature of the underlying hepatic pathology produces a portal hypertension in nearly every patient and the mechanics of the operation tend to exaggerate it. The usual consequence is mechanical bleeding that can rapidly assume nightmare proportions during the procedure. Many normal coagulation factors that might help control this unpleasant situation are dependent on the liver and are therefore defective in the diseased recipient. These coagulation factors may be even more deficient during the anhepatic phase, or they may subsequently

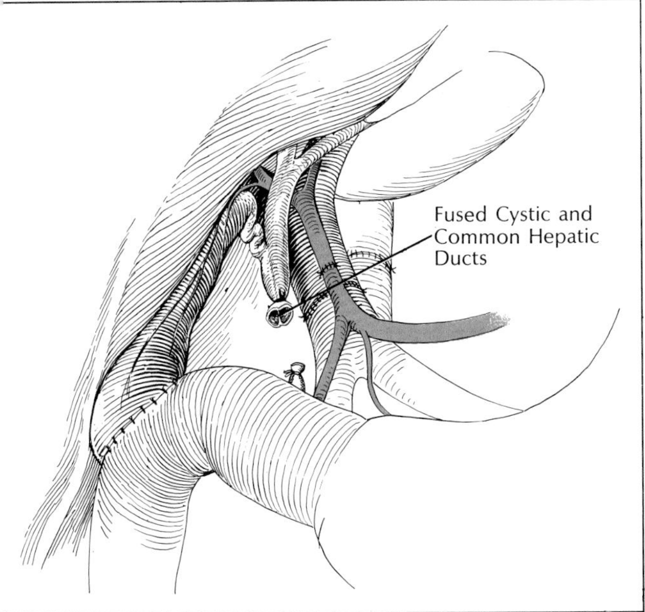

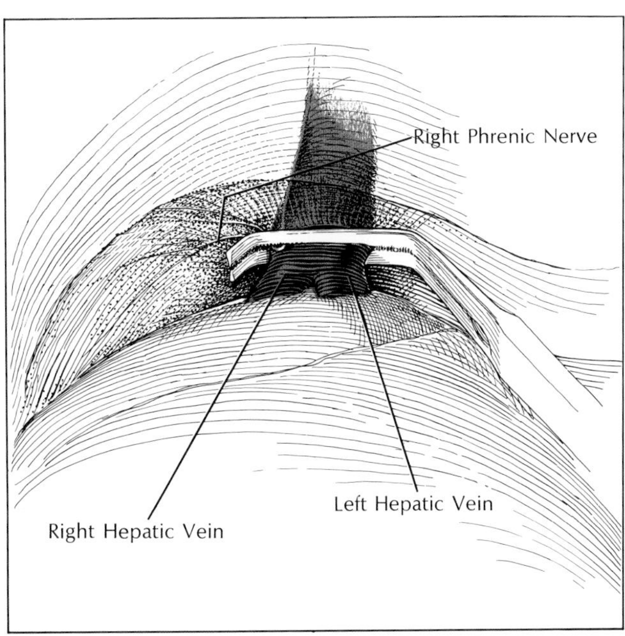

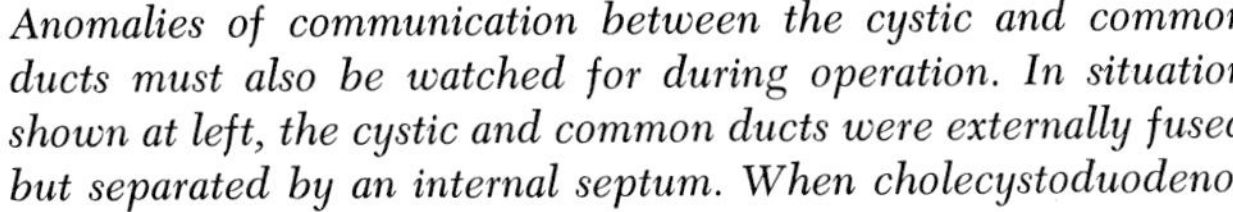

Anomalies of communication between the cystic and common ducts must also be watched for during operation. In situation shown at left, the cystic and common ducts were externally fused but separated by an internal septum. When cholecystoduodenostomy and common duct ligation were carried out, the result was total biliary obstruction. At right, right phrenic nerve is inadvertently included in clamp occluding suprahepatic vena cava, as is a piece of the diaphragm. Temporary phrenic paralysis resulted.

be of dubious quality, depending on the state of preservation of the homograft – how much ischemia it has suffered and how much immediate functional capability it has retained.

When hemorrhage occurs, the surgeon must use any and all available hemostatic tactics – ligating, suturing, cauterizing – until the revascularized homograft can participate in what is hoped will be appropriate coagulation function. With our earlier patients, whose homografts were generally of less than optimal quality for the reasons previously stated, we attempted to meet bleeding problems by administering thrombogenic agents. However, hypercoagulability was caused in some instances. The unacceptable incidence of pulmonary embolism in these patients led us to abandon this approach.

In retrospect, it is possible that the coagulability induced by exogenous thrombogenic agents might be prohibitively additive to the clotting brought by the homograft, which, when it begins to function, conceivably overreacts. Indeed, the better the condition of the transplant, the greater the risk of unwanted coagulation. Almost every series of liver transplants, including our own, has at least one example of thrombosis of the hepatic arterial circulation to which the rebound phenomenon may have contributed. The use of anticoagulants to forestall this emergency is dangerous. Proved intravascular clotting during the operation would be an indication for heparin, but such proof is hard to come by. Moreover, heparinization is a double-edged maneuver: depressed clotting can have devastating effects on patients submitted to such major trauma and with so many potential bleeding sites.

In general, we now believe that it is advisable to avoid the manipulation of the clotting process either with thrombogenic or anticoagulant agents. Instead, our current approach is to leave correction of coagulation abnormalities to natural processes, intervening only under special circumstances and for very specific indications.

During operation, there are other metabolic abnormalities than those concerned with coagulation. Perhaps anesthesia deserves a comment here; it, too, is a complex problem in liver transplantation. Not only is the procedure long and difficult but, even more important, it is an operation on the very organ involved most in the metabolism and detoxification of most common anesthetics. At any point during the operation the liver is either inherently impaired, absent, or untried in its new setting. Hence the task in anesthesia is to administer correctly drugs that, first, are not hepatotoxic and, second, do not depend primarily on the liver for their degradation. The anesthesia in most of our early cases was administered by J. Antonio Aldrete. He has tended to rely mainly on such volatile agents as fluroxene added to a nitrous oxide–oxygen mixture in nonexplosive concentrations below 4.4%. This combination permits use of electrocautery, gives flexibility in lightening or deepening anesthesia, and allows anesthesia to be abruptly stopped if the changing physiologic circumstances require it.

So much for some of the more important technical difficulties associated with liver transplantation. There is, of course, a long list of other technical pitfalls: adrenal venous infarction, air embolism, crushing of the right phrenic nerve by too high a clamp on the upper vena caval cuff, to mention but a few. The reader interested in a more detailed discussion of these and other surgical problems is referred to in the book *Experience in Hepatic Transplantation* [see Selected Readings]. These technical matters have played a major role in the mortality encountered in our first cases. However, as deaths from such causes are highly avoidable, surgical technique is of less critical signifi-

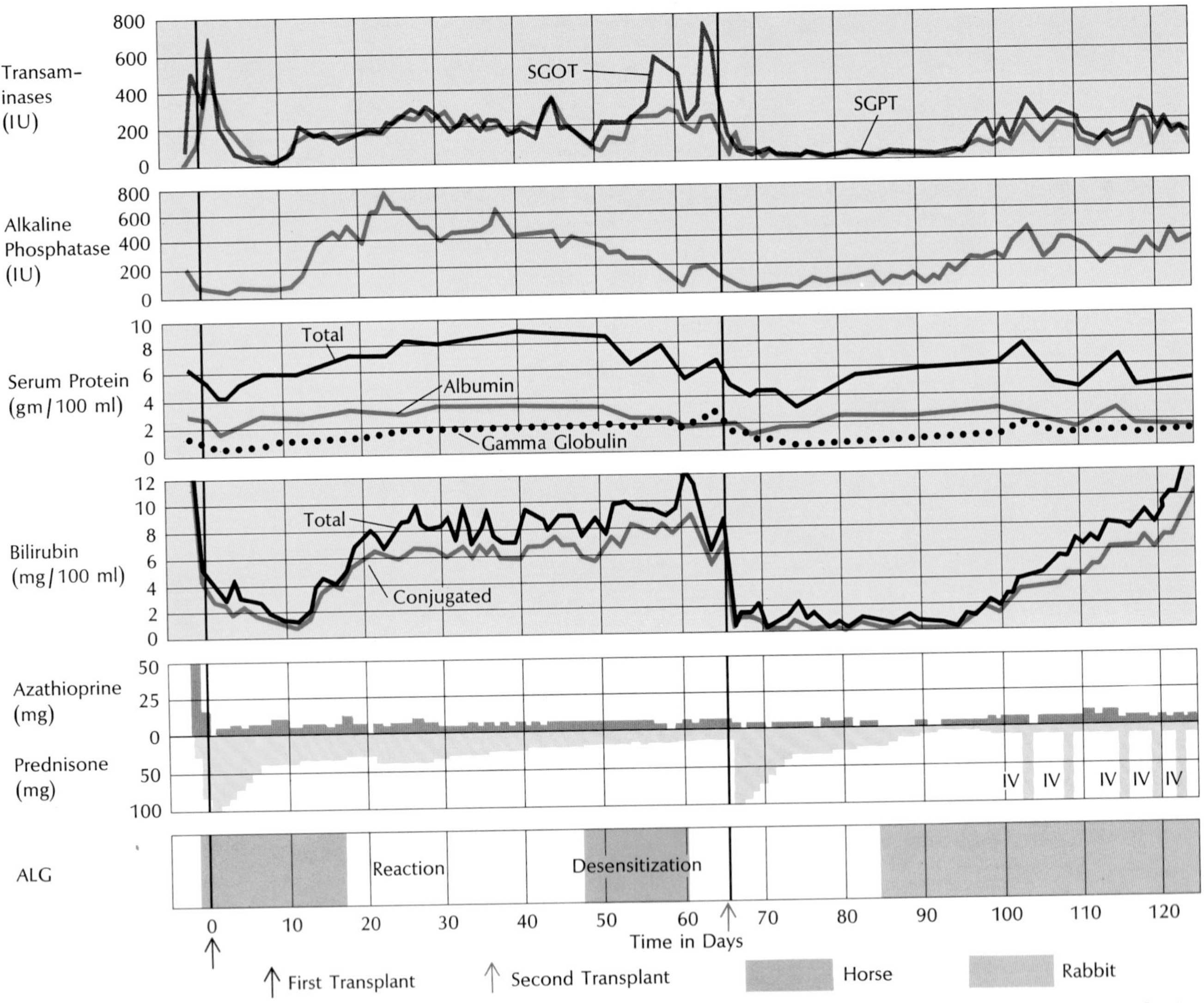

An "indolent" type of rejection characterized the clinical course of the child who received two homografts (see page 197); this proved to be the type most difficult to treat. Rejection of the first transplant began on the 13th postoperative day and progressed slowly; horse ALG had to be stopped after 18 days because of severe local reaction. Jaundice then developed; other measures of liver function were maintained for many weeks despite the fact that the child was extremely ill. Desensitization was attempted in the hope of resuming horse ALG treatment but was eventually abandoned. Note hypergammaglobulinemia toward end of second month. Onset of rejection after second transplant was delayed about a month; by this time rabbit ALG was available for treatment

cance to the future of transplantation than are the immunologic problems. The most important factor in successful transplantation remains the prevention of graft rejection by the host.

Immunosuppressive therapy in liver transplantation has borrowed heavily from the experience gained with human renal transplants. Two general treatment programs were evolved with the simpler kidney model and then applied to the liver recipients. The first protocol that was used from 1962 to 1966 for all organ recipients at the University of Colorado consisted of double-drug treatment with azathioprine and the synthetic adrenal cortical steroid, prednisone. Evolution of the use of these two agents together, appreciation of their marked synergism, and demonstration that rejection could be readily reversed by increasing the steroid doses were among the advances that made clinical transplantation practical and introduced what is known as the modern era of this field. But in spite of moderately satisfactory results with renal transplantation, the double-drug therapy either did not prevent rejection of hepatic homografts or else proved too toxic to permit host survival. Six patients so treated in liver transplantation from 1963 to 1965 died in a month or less.

In 1966, heterologous antilymphocyte globulin (ALG) was introduced clinically at our center as a third immunosuppressive agent, added to the drugs mentioned above. Since then, this triple-drug therapy has been given to all our renal, hepatic, and cardiac recipients. In our experience, rejection has been more easily and regularly controlled, and the risks and morbidity imposed by the necessity for high-dose steroid therapy have been reduced. It must be admitted that not all transplant surgeons concede the need for ALG. However, those most familiar with its use have enthusiastically confirmed the value of the triple-drug regimen, beginning with Traejer of Lyon, France, and including most recently Simmons and Najarian of Minneapolis. The latter authorities advocate raising the heterologous serum with cultured lymphoblasts as the antigen rather than mature lymphoid tissue and recommend administering the subsequently refined ALG by the intravenous rather than the originally employed intramuscular route. All of our human liver recipients who achieved chronic survival were treated with the combination of azathioprine, prednisone, and intramuscular ALG. In the event of a rejection episode, it is the steroid component that has proved most amenable to quick adjustment of dosage.

We will not review here the various hypotheses explaining the actions of these immunosuppressive drugs (see "Antilymphocytic Serum: Its Properties and Potential," HOSPITAL PRACTICE, May 1969). But, as was stated earlier, the method by which these agents are used in conjunction with the actual transplantation may permit selective abrogation of the host rejection response. Were this not true, there would be little hope of returning patients to life in an unrestricted environment since each of the individual agents can cause general immunologic crippling more or less in proportion to the dose used. The most obvious penalty of a depressed immune system is heightened susceptibility to infection. However, it has also become obvious that chronically immunosuppressed patients have an increased vulnerability to de novo malignancies. In our own series of chronic survivors after renal transplantation, more than 5% have developed either mesenchymal or epithelial malignant tumors. Almost all other major transplantation centers have recorded this complication, which is presumably due to failure of the depressed immunologic surveillance mechanism to identify the tumor tissues as alien.

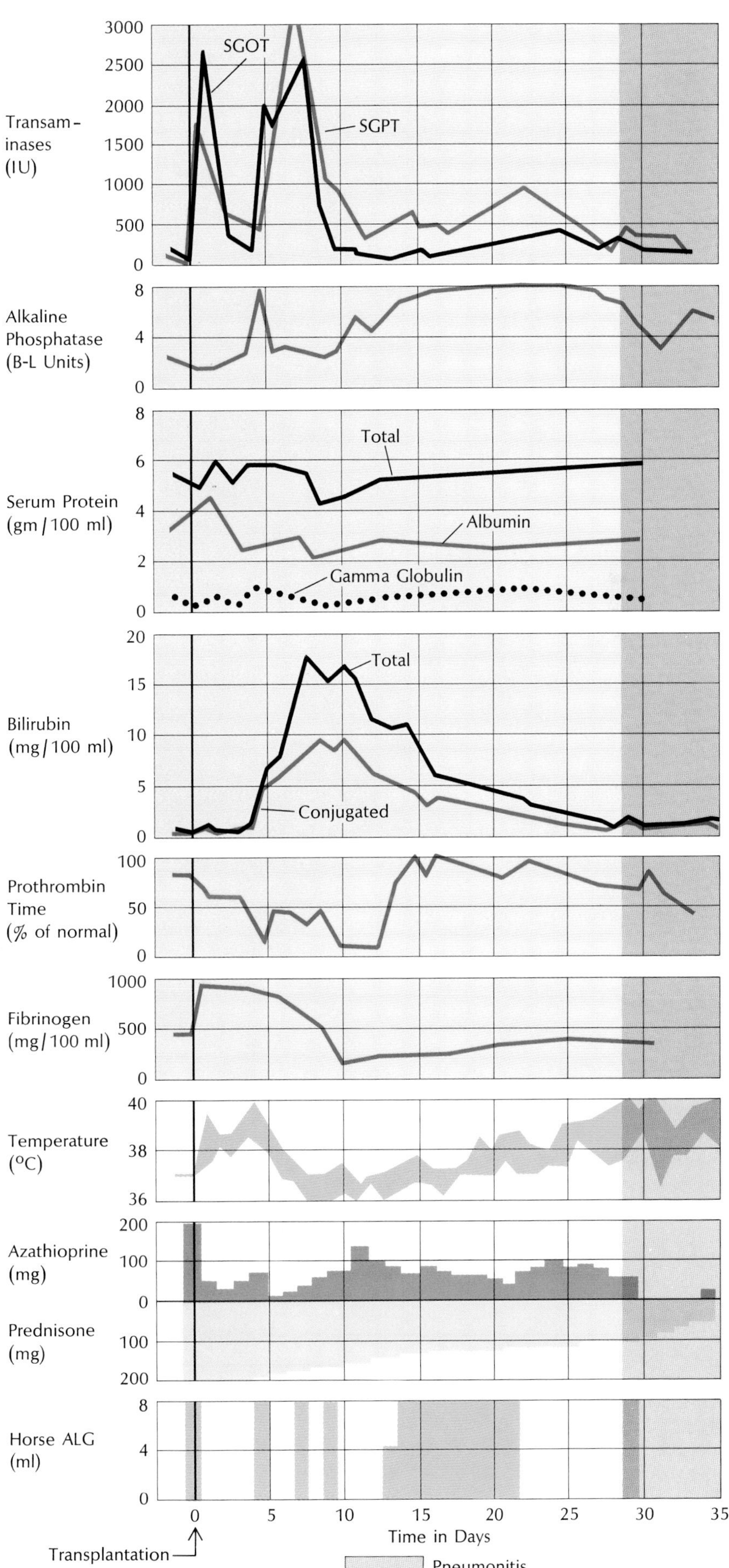

The course of an acute rejection is shown at right in record of a 23-year-old woman who underwent transplantation for hepatoma. Although the rejection crisis was overcome promptly, she died of pseudomonas pneumonia after 35 days. Even before the onset of jaundice her course was markedly febrile and she had severe bleeding problems: note marked depression of prothrombin time and fibrinogen concentration on days 10 through 13.

Orthotopic Liver Homotransplantations in Denver

Patient Number	*Disease*	*Date of Operation*	*Survival (days)*	*Age (years)*	*Donor Age (years)*	*Cause of Death*[°]
1	Extrahepatic biliary atresia	3-1-63	0	3	3	Hemorrhage
2	Hepatoma, cirrhosis	5-5-63	22	48	55	Pulmonary emboli, sepsis
3	Cholangiocarcinoma	6-24-63	7-1/2	68	69	Sepsis, pulmonary emboli, GI bleeding
4	Hepatoma, cirrhosis	7-16-63	6-1/2	52	73	Pulmonary emboli, ? hepatic failure, pulmonary edema
5	Hepatoma, cirrhosis	10-4-63	23	29	64	Sepsis, bile peritonitis, hepatic failure
6	Hepatoma	11-9-66	7	29	73	Hepatic failure, sepsis
7	Extrahepatic biliary atresia	5-21-67	10	11/12	1	Hepatic failure, sepsis
8	Hepatoma	7-23-67	400	1-7/12	1-6/12	Carcinomatosis
9	Extrahepatic biliary atresia	7-31-67	133	1-9/12	4	Septic hepatic infarction, hepatic failure
10	Extrahepatic biliary atresia	9-5-67	186	1-1/12	1-6/12	Septic hepatic infarction, hepatic failure
11	Extrahepatic biliary atresia	10-8-67	61	1-2/12	1-8/12	Septic hepatic infarction
12	Extrahepatic biliary atresia	11-24-67	105	1-4/12	1-2/12	Septic hepatic infarction
13	Extrahepatic biliary atresia	2-9-68	901†	2	3 10	Peritonitis
14	Hepatoma	3-17-68	432‡	16	27 17	Carcinomatosis, peritonitis
15	Hepatoma, cirrhosis	4-14-68	339	44	20	Carcinomatosis
16	Extrahepatic biliary atresia	5-26-68	407§	1-11/12	3 7	Hepatic insufficiency
17	Hepatoma	6-18-68	35	24	22	Pneumonitis
18	Extrahepatic biliary atresia	6-29-68	4	1	1-9/12	Hepatic artery thrombosis
19	Extrahepatic biliary atresia	7-20-68	915‖	4	10	(Alive)
20	Posthepatitic cirrhosis and cholangiectasis	8-13-68	1/2	8	10	Nonthrombotic occlusion of hepatic artery
21	Extrahepatic biliary atresia	8-20-68	1/2	2	5	Portal vein thrombosis
22	Laennec's cirrhosis	10-24-68	10	33	25	Biliary duct obstruction, hepatic and renal failure
23	Hepatoma	10-26-68	143	15	6	Carcinomatosis
24	Extrahepatic biliary atresia	11-10-68	11	3	2	? Hepatic arterial insufficiency, hepatic failure
25	Hepatoma	2-11-69	39	45	20	Bile peritonitis, sepsis, hepatic failure
26	Intrahepatic biliary atresia, hepatoma	5-11-69	76	11	17	GI hemorrhage, intraabdominal sepsis, metastases left lung
27	Wilson's disease	7-15-69	560‖	11	11	(Alive)
28	Laennec's cirrhosis	7-26-69	13	39	22	Bile peritonitis, disrupted choledochocholedochostomy
29	Intrahepatic biliary atresia	9-20-69	378	5-1/2	10	Hepatic insufficiency, chronic aggressive hepatitis
30	Extrahepatic biliary atresia	9-24-69	37	11/12	2	Partial biliary obstruction, cholangitis, pneumonitis
31	Juvenile cirrhosis	1-8-70	9	15	19	Massive homograft necrosis
32	Laennec's cirrhosis	1-16-70	3	46	17	Unexplained coma
33	Extrahepatic biliary atresia, hepatoma	1-22-70	370‖	3-10/12	7-11/12	(Alive)

° *In actuality, most of these patients had other potentially lethal complications besides those listed. The term "sepsis" is used loosely*

† *Died 901 days after first transplantation, 19 days after retransplantation*

‡ *Died 432 days after first transplantation, 52 days after retransplantation*

§ *Died 407 days after first transplantation, 340 days after retransplantation*

‖ *Alive as of Jan. 26, 1971*

In addition to the foregoing general liabilities of immunosuppression, there are some special risks for the liver candidate. One is the fact that hepatic injury in all kinds of organ recipients has commonly been produced by the agents, individually or in combination, of the therapeutic regimen. In some instances, viral hepatitis, apparently made chronic by the partial immunologic invalidism of the host, has been a plausible explanation; but in others, hepatotoxicity of the drugs was probably responsible. With liver malfunction, dose control of some of the agents may become difficult since the liver participates in their pathways of action. These hepatic factors are obviously important in any situation requiring immunosuppression, but plainly they have heightened significance for a traumatized, transplanted liver fighting for survival in a new and hostile environment.

Though infection is a major risk to any immunosuppressed patient, for the liver recipient postoperative sepsis of the graft itself has proved to be a special problem – partly because of the anatomic location of the orthotopically placed organ, interposed so to speak between the intestinal tract and the heart. Bacteria from the bowel, particularly of the gram-negative variety, can be brought into contact with the transplanted liver via intestinal veins draining into the portal vein, or, alternatively, by retrograde spread up the duct system after passage through the biliary anastomosis. In either event, the presence of nonviable hepatic tissue provides a perfect medium for bacterial growth. Eventually, piecemeal gangrene of the transplant can result, with characteristic nonvisualizing areas on the liver scans, gram-negative bacteremia, and all the findings of generalized sepsis.

Early in our clinical series, the above findings of graft and systemic infection led us to consider the essential problem to be that of bacterial invasion and prompted us to reduce the immunosuppression. This decision was tragically incorrect and was followed by necrosis and infection of large parenchymal areas. Experience soon taught us that ischemia of portions of the liver was the initiating event, and that the basis for the ischemia was rejection. Consequently, immunosuppression should ordinarily be increased rather than reduced if this complication is thought to be impending. When this was done by giving substantially higher doses of prednisone (as noted, the only highly dose-maneuverable component of the immunosuppressive triad), the incidence of regional hepatic gangrene fell to zero. It should be added that our prophylactic treatment protocol includes heavy antibiotic treatment for the first postoperative week, including agents effective against gram-negative bacteria, after which this therapy is stopped.

With the acquisition of experience, other important issues have also been clarified, including that of the indications for liver replacement. A brief summary of our first 33 consecutive recipients, treated from March 1963 to 12 months ago, can be used to illustrate these indications.

The 33 patients were aged 11 months to 68 years. The indication for 12 of these transplants was hepatoma, and an additional unsuspected hepatoma was found in a four-year-old child treated for intrahepatic biliary atresia. The latter is the only one of this group still alive; now 12 months after the operation she shows no evidence of recurrence of neoplasia. As for the other hepatoma patients, seven died within 39 days. Badly damaged homografts were a major cause of failure in five who were among our early patients in the period before the criterion of brain death was applied, while technical accidents, with subphrenic abscesses and bile peritonitis, were the major causes of death in the other two. Of the five hepatoma patients who had more prolonged survival – 76, 143, 339, 400, and 432 days – metastases developed in all, and in four instances the recurrences were directly responsible for death. Because of this high rate of recurrent carcinoma, it has become our policy to consider liver replacement for hepatoma only under the most exceptional circumstances, even though our experience and that of Calne have demonstrated the possibility of an occasional tumor cure.

Far more desirable candidates are those without neoplasms, even though the technical difficulties in benign hepatic disease are more severe because the patients tend to be sicker

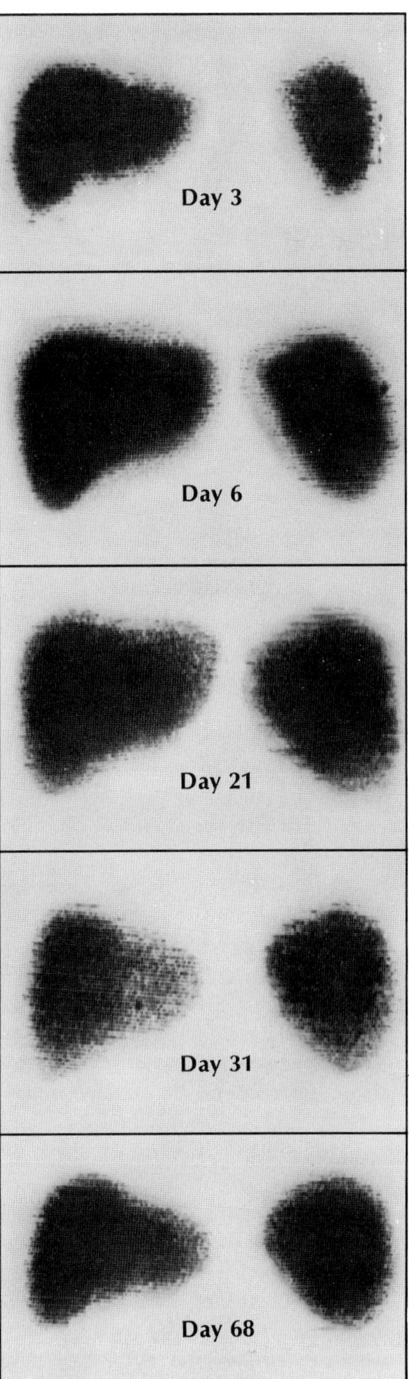

Scans using TC^{99M} were made in 15-year-old boy treated for hepatoma. Rejection began about a week after operation, as swelling on day 6 indicates, and lasted about two weeks. By day 68 anteroposterior scan returned to about the same dimensions as had been present shortly after the transplantation, but the lateral view showed that the liver mass was increased. Liver function at this time was completely normal. The pickup of the isotope remained homogeneous through the period of observation, except possibly at 31 days. The homograft was eventually destroyed by tumor recurrence and the boy died 143 days after the transplant operation.

and to have more advanced portal hypertension. Moreover, if the diagnosis is biliary atresia, an increased incidence of vascular anomalies can be expected to compound the difficulties together with the small size of the structures to be anastomosed in these young patients. Nevertheless, the longest survivors of liver transplantation in the world are those who had this disorder. Of our own series of 15 patients with biliary atresia, treated a year or longer ago, including the child with the incidental hepatoma mentioned above, five lived longer than one year and two are still surviving with completely normal liver function, one year and two and a half years, respectively, after operation. The three late deaths after 13, 13½, and 30 months were from recurrent hepatic insufficiency caused in two instances by chronic rejection and in the third probably by indolent viral hepatitis. Another four children survived 61 to 186 days, all expiring from regional hepatic gangrene for which the apparent cause was too little immunosuppression in the early posttransplantation period. The six other recipients with biliary atresia died within the first 40 days, two from hepatic necrosis probably attributable to ischemia of the donor organ, two from thrombosis of the hepatic artery or portal vein, one from a nonthrombotic occlusion of the hepatic artery, and the remaining one from generalized infection and pneumonia.

Six patients were treated for cirrhosis a year or longer ago, with the disappointing record of five early deaths. Reasons for the heavy acute mortality included the wretched physical condition of the recipients, major hemorrhage due to portal hypertension and depressed coagulation, and technical or metabolic mishaps. The survivor is an 11-year-old child whose cirrhosis was secondary to Wilson's disease. After liver replacement the child suffered an extremely severe rejection crisis, but the process was eventually reversed, with normal liver function now continuing 18 months after the operation. Moreover, the new liver, which was biopsied at 6 and 17 months, has not reaccumulated copper and it appears to have corrected the genetic error in copper metabolism – a finding that may be important in the search for the etiology of this disease.

Undoubtedly, one reason for the bad experience with cirrhotic patients has been a reluctance to recommend such therapy except in the agonal stages of the disease. But now that the feasibility of long-term survival and rehabilitation has been demonstrated, transplantation at an earlier time probably should be considered, particularly in postnecrotic cirrhosis in which the maximum value of medical management and of abstinence from alcohol has already been realized.

With another of our patients – one not in the series described above – there have been exceptionally interesting circumstances of transplantation. A 28-year-old woman with chronic active hepatitis, she was operated on August 9, 1970. For at least two years before the operation, as well as on the day of the transplantation, immunodiffusion tests for the Australia antigen were positive. This gave us an opportunity to examine the thesis that this antigen has an essentially hepatic source. The argument for this proposition was supported by the immediate disappearance of the antigen from the bloodstream after the operation. Almost two months later it reappeared, and within a few days there followed an attack of acute serum hepatitis with joint pain, anorexia, jaundice, and evidence of hepatic necrosis by transaminase determinations. Fortunately, her liver function abnormalities have regressed nearly completely, but she is still Australia antigen-positive, now five months posttransplantation. It remains to be seen whether the virus will doom the new liver to the same fate as the old one, whether the long-term pace of the infection will be affected by the chronic immunosuppression, and whether the patient will continue to be a virus carrier. The case has other interesting implications. It is customary to think of the incubation period of infectious diseases in terms of the host immune defenses. In this patient, the immune apparatus was retained but systematically weakened. Yet, the latent period of the disease was about that to be expected with a fresh infection, indicating that the incubation period in this patient was primarily concerned with the target organ.

Thus far, I have confined discussion strictly to the kind of operation (termed orthotopic transplantation) in which the diseased host liver is removed and replaced. The alternative to this procedure in patients with benign disease is auxiliary hepatic transplantation, in which the native liver is not disturbed and the hepatic homograft is placed in some abnormal location such as the paravertebral gutter, splenic fossa, or pelvis. Special technical and metabolic problems that have been encountered with auxiliary transplantation cannot be reviewed here but they have been detailed in *Experience in Hepatic Transplantation.* The results with the auxiliary procedure in animals and in limited clinical trials have not been particularly encouraging.

In summary, orthotopic liver transplantation has led to the prolongation of useful life. Among our first 33 recipients, 9 lived a year or longer, and their chances for survival rose with the increase in our experience. The longest survival to date exceeds 2½ years. With more experience, with successful efforts to reduce the toxicity of immunosuppressive agents, with improvements in histocompatibility typing, and with advances in preservation and storage techniques, the record can be expected to improve. Even now, patients with nonmalignant terminal liver disease and with no other hope for recovery can be candidates for liver transplantation.

Chapter 21

Immunologic Defenses Against Cancer

KARL ERIK HELLSTRÖM *and* INGEGERD HELLSTRÖM
University of Washington

The concept that cancer is a disease sequential to immunologic derangement has intrigued investigators for more than 50 years. Animating this work has always been the possibility that once the immunologic responses to tumor growth and invasion were identified and understood, means could be devised for altering the balance against the tumor in favor of the host, thereby preventing cancer or curing it. In recent years, a new dimension has been added to the problem. As techniques for suppressing immunity have been developed – for the most part in aid of organ transplantation – a fear has arisen that the utilization of the immunosuppressive techniques may facilitate neoplasia. Indeed, there have been reports that transplant patients maintained on immunosuppressive drugs show a marked rise in the incidence of tumors. Among the most fascinating of these reports have been those suggesting that cancers that develop and spread under cover of immunosuppression can rapidly regress and be eliminated when immunosuppressive regimens are suspended.

For the most part, however, these reports have been equivocal. The question of whether the observed malignancies arose spontaneously in the graft recipient or whether they were transplanted with the donor organ has often been unanswered. This ambiguity represents an important historical extension of a problem that has confronted the tumor immunologist since the beginning of the century: to differentiate between normal transplantation or histocompatibility antigens, present in both neoplastic and normal tissues, and transplantation antigens, unique to the tumor and therefore the logical targets for immunotherapeutic attack.

The claim that there are tumor-specific antigens dates back at least to the first years of the century. By the late 1920's a review of the subject was able to cite over a hundred published papers containing this claim, including reports of immunoprophylactic successes against tumors. Retrospectively one can, however, recognize the confusion in these papers between tumor-specific antigens and the still-to-be elucidated histocompatibility antigens. It wasn't until the 1940's that work by Little, Snell, Gorer, and others firmly established the tissue transplantation antigens and set out the immunologic "rules of transplantation." Even today a possible confusion between normal transplantation antigens and tumor-specific transplantation antigens (TSTA) must be considered in evaluating experimental findings. This problem is greatly eased, however, by our present ability to work with inbred lines of mice and rats in which histocompatibility differences are almost totally eliminated.

Possibly the first milestone in the identification of tumor-specific antigens was the report by Ludwik Gross in 1943 that mice immunized against tumors from syngeneic animals would not accept tumor transplants from these animals. Because the amount of material studied by Gross was limited and there was a scarcity of controls in his experiments, his findings were largely ignored at the time of their publication. Subsequently, however, Gross's work was confirmed and extended by others, most notably by E. J. Foley. Skepticism, however, was still prevalent in 1957 when R. T. Prehn and J. M. Main showed that not only could one immunize a mouse against a chemically induced tumor but that the mouse which rejected a tumor graft would accept a skin graft from the same animal in which the tumor had originated. This was the first well-controlled demonstration that the antigens involved in immunization were tumor specific. An important finding was that different methylcholanthrene-induced sarcomas had individually distinct tumor antigens that did not cross-react according to transplantation tests.

Even this clear-cut demonstration was not universally accepted. The possibility of heterozygosity in the inbred strain was raised by some critics. For that reason, George Klein's group in Stockholm performed experiments aimed at identifying immunologic reactions against an animal's autochthonous tumor. The possibility of genetic variability was thereby eliminated. What Klein did was to induce a sarcoma in the leg of a mouse, amputate the leg, and transplant the sarcoma to another mouse of the same strain. He then took cells from this tumor and irradiated them, gave the original animal in which the sarcoma had been induced multiple injections of the irradiated tumor cells, and attempted to reimplant the tumor in the "immunized" mouse. In fact, a very substantial immunity was demonstrated.

Up to this point the bulk of the work had been done with chemically induced tumors, using carcinogenic agents such as methylcholanthrene. A major advance came with the experiments reported by H. O. Sjögren et al. in which the antigenic behavior of polyoma virus–induced tumors was studied. Working with inbred mice, Sjögren showed that mice could be immunized either with the virus or with tumor cells so that under proper conditions a good resistance to transplanted polyoma tumor cells could be established. Moreover, not only could this be done with a single tumor but one could immunize mice with cells from tumor A and have resistance to tumor B. In contrast with the chemically induced tumor, these viral tumors have cross-reacting antigens.

Subsequent work confirmed the findings from these early experiments by Sjögren's group and from parallel studies by Karl Habel of the National Institutes of Health. It showed that all virus tumors studied possess antigens common for tumors induced by the same virus and different for tumors induced by different viruses. The common antigenicity appears to be determined by the virus; it crosses host species lines so that, for example, tumors induced by the polyoma virus in mice, rats, and hamsters have a common antigen. Tumors induced by related viruses sometimes cross-react. For example, tumors induced with adenoviruses 3, 7, 12, 14, and 18 show antigenic cross-reactivity.

Quite obviously, the cross-reactivity of virus-induced tumors in animals has an important bearing on efforts to establish the viral etiology of certain cancers in man. It is tempting to assume that if one finds a common antigenicity between tumors in humans, as has been shown for Burkitt lymphomas by Klein and for malignant melanomas and osteogenic sarcomas by D. L. Morton and R. A. Malmgren at the National Cancer Institute, one has evidence of a viral etiology. Such an assumption may prove valid, but it is important to sound a note of caution. First, tumor cells (as well as normal cells) can develop new antigens following superinfection with a virus, without the implication that the virus induced the neoplastic transformation. For example, Moloney virus–induced mouse leukemias can develop the polyoma tumor antigen following infection with the polyoma virus. Furthermore, studies by P. Gold and S. O. Freedman of Montreal have shown a common antigen in human colonic carcinomas that is absent from normal human colon but present in fetal gut epithelium. The presence of such a carcino-embryonic antigen may be interpreted as a sign of genetic derepression and does not necessarily imply that a virus is involved.

The demonstration that chemically induced tumors have individually distinct tumor antigens while those of a known virus origin have common antigens at first suggested a difference in etiology between the two groups. But this difference may be less striking than it appears to be. If one assumes a tumor virus widely distributed in a mouse population, one would also assume that this virus will have infected many animals by the time of their birth. The mouse population could then be expected to develop a high degree of immunologic nonresponsiveness to the virus and the antigens induced by it. Thus, if the action of a chemical carcinogen is, as has been suggested, to activate latent virus, it would be expected that the chemically induced tumors would have, in addition to the unique antigens, common antigens that might be hard to detect.

Studies performed by Morton, Weiss, Vaage, Heppner, and others have shown that mice which carry the mammary tumor virus from birth are immunologically nonresponsive to antigens of their spontaneous mammary carcinomas. However, the mammary tumors have individually distinct antigens in addition to common ones. If

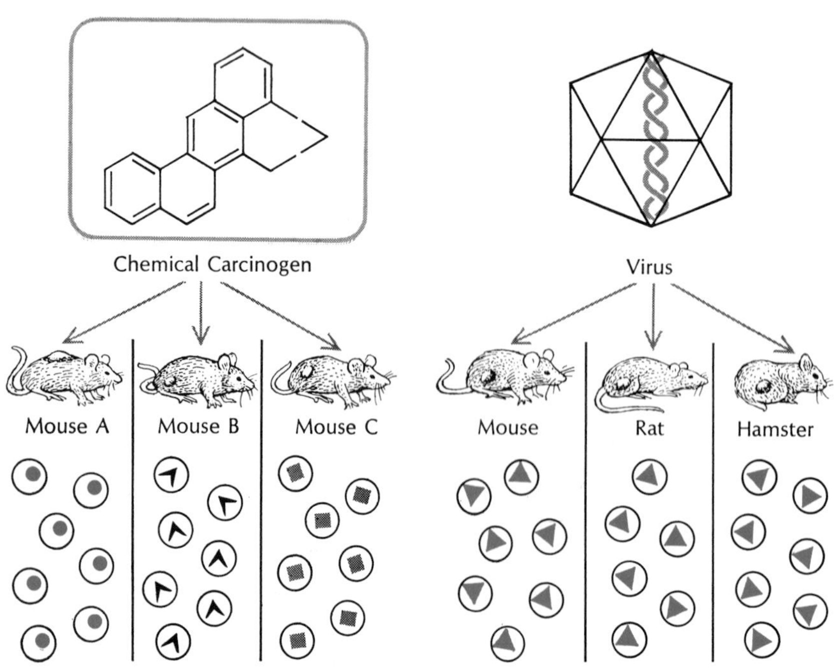

Animal tumors induced by chemical carcinogens have individual antigenic specificity, as symbolized above. In contrast, virally induced tumors appear to carry antigens common to all tumors induced by the virus even in animals of different species. However, recent studies indicate some virus tumors have unique antigens as well as common ones, some chemically induced tumors common antigens.

an investigator were to come to conclusions concerning the etiology of these tumors on the basis of having detected the unique antigens only, he might conclude that they were chemically induced. On the other hand, if he had studied mice of the same strain taken by cesarean section before they had developed "tolerance" to the virus, he would have detected their ability to become immunized against the common antigenic determinant of the tumors. The tumors would then behave like the virally induced neoplasms they are. Most likely, the unique antigens represent genetic differences between different mammary tumor lines.

Some evidence supporting the concept that chemically induced tumors may have a viral etiology with antigenic cross-reactivity has emerged from the work of Old, who found Gross virus–determined antigens in a number of chemically induced tumors. Studies by McKhann and Harder and by our group have similarly found cross-reactions among certain methylcholanthrene-induced sarcomas detectable by in vitro assays. The Gross virus is a C-particle RNA virus. Such viruses have recently been suggested by Huebner as a possible causative agent of many spontaneous tumors.

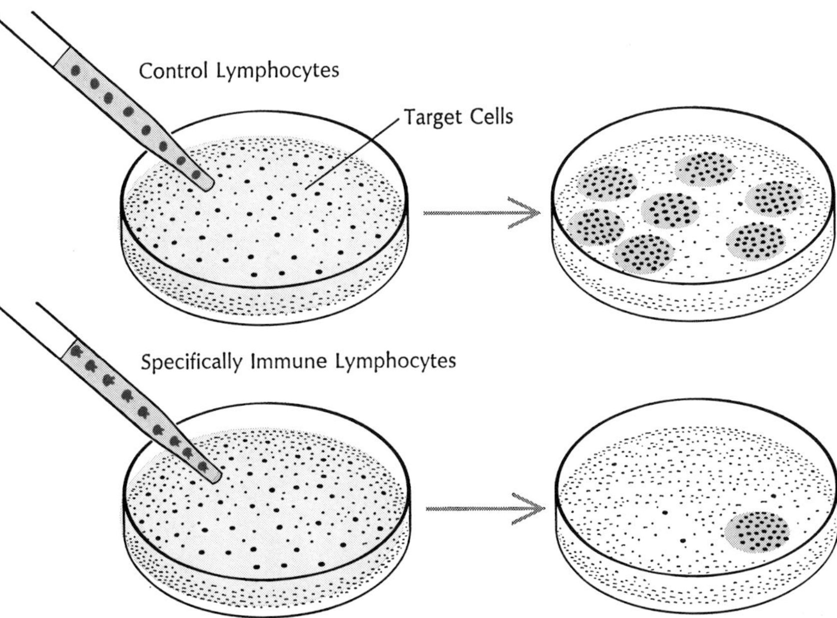

The colony inhibition test is predicated upon killing or growth inhibition of tumor cells by specifically immune lymphocytes. By comparing the number of colonies formed when immune lymphocytes are used with the number when control lymphocytes are used, the percentage of tumor cells killed or inhibited by the immune lymphocytes can be derived.

Immunologic Responses to Tumor Antigens

Up to now, this article has focused on the evidence for the existence of tumor-specific antigens. Nothing has been said about the host immunologic responses to these antigens. Obviously, to the clinician it is these response mechanisms and their possible manipulation that are of prime concern. For background we must once again go back to work done with normal tissue transplantation antigens. In the mid-50's, N. A. Mitchison in Great Britain showed that the immunologic response to normal transplantation antigens is primarily mediated by lymphocytes, and that one can adoptively transfer lymphocytes from an immune animal to a nonimmune animal and make the latter immune. Shortly afterwards, H. J. Winn developed a neutralization procedure in which he mixed tumor cells in vitro with lymphocytes that were immune to their normal H-2 histocompatibility antigens and showed that the lymphocytes could kill the tumor cells. Then, in 1960, Klein and colleagues showed that in the Winn neutralization system, lymphocyte-mediated immunity to tumor-specific antigens occurs in a manner similar to that against normal tissue transplantation antigens.

A number of other experimenters subsequently established the primary role of cellular immunity in response to tumor-specific antigens. It is interesting that their studies provided an experimental structure to support the insights of a number of scientists, among them Sir Macfarlane Burnet, who had postulated that the "physiologic" raison d'être of cellular immunity was as a surveillance system against neoplastic mutations continually occurring in the body and continually suppressed by lymphocytic action. It should be stressed, however, that while most evidence to date establishes the immune lymphocyte as the major responder to tumor antigens (as it is to homograft antigens), an important role for circulating humoral antibodies cannot be excluded. In fact, as we shall see later in this article, there is excellent reason to believe that humoral antibodies do participate, albeit in a rather disconcerting manner.

In the early work designed to define the immunoresponsive mechanisms to tumor antigens, investigators were somewhat handicapped by a lack of techniques sufficiently sensitive and definitive for the complexity of the knowledge needed. We believe that this need has been met by the colony inhibition test largely developed by one of the authors [I. H.].

The colony inhibition (CI) technique is shown schematically above. In principle it is based on plating a dilute suspension of tumor (or normal) cells in an appropriate culture medium onto Petri dishes and measuring the effect of humoral antibodies or lymphocytes on the ability of the target cells to form colonies, which are stained and counted (under coded designations). Colony counts are compared in experimental groups, receiving specifically immune serum or lymphocytes, and in controls, receiving the same dilution of serum or the same dose of lymphocytes, nonimmune to antigens present in the target cells. The colony inhibition test can also be used to study the combined action of lymphocytes and serum from the same (or different) donors.

Among our first applications of the colony inhibition system was an effort to demonstrate cellular immunity to primary (autochthonous) methylcholanthrene-induced sarcomas in highly inbred mice. We found that pooled lymph node cells from a mouse whose

Experiments are summarized in which the colony inhibition assay was used to demonstrate that a serum factor, or factors, was decisive in determining whether a Shope papilloma would persist or regress spontaneously. In this scheme, tumor cells are obtained from a rabbit with a persistent papilloma. To the cell culture, various combinations of immune lymphocytes and serum from normal, persistor, and regressor animals are added. It can be seen that only when persistor serum is used (1 and 2) are the tumor cells protected against killing by the immune lymphocytes. If either normal serum or regressor serum is used, the immune lymphocytes, derived from persistor or regressor animals, are able to kill tumor cells and inhibit colony formation (3-6).

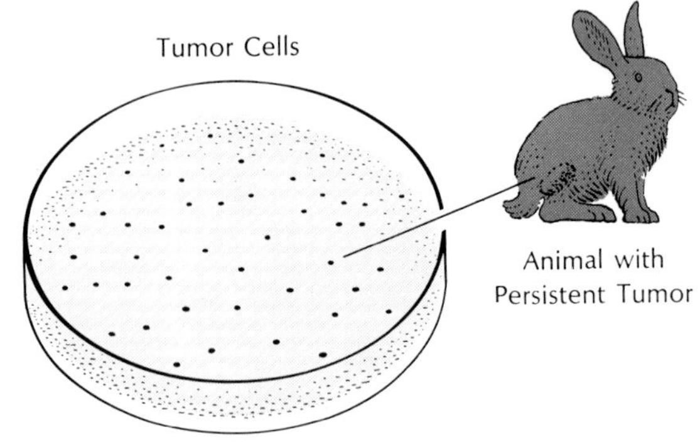

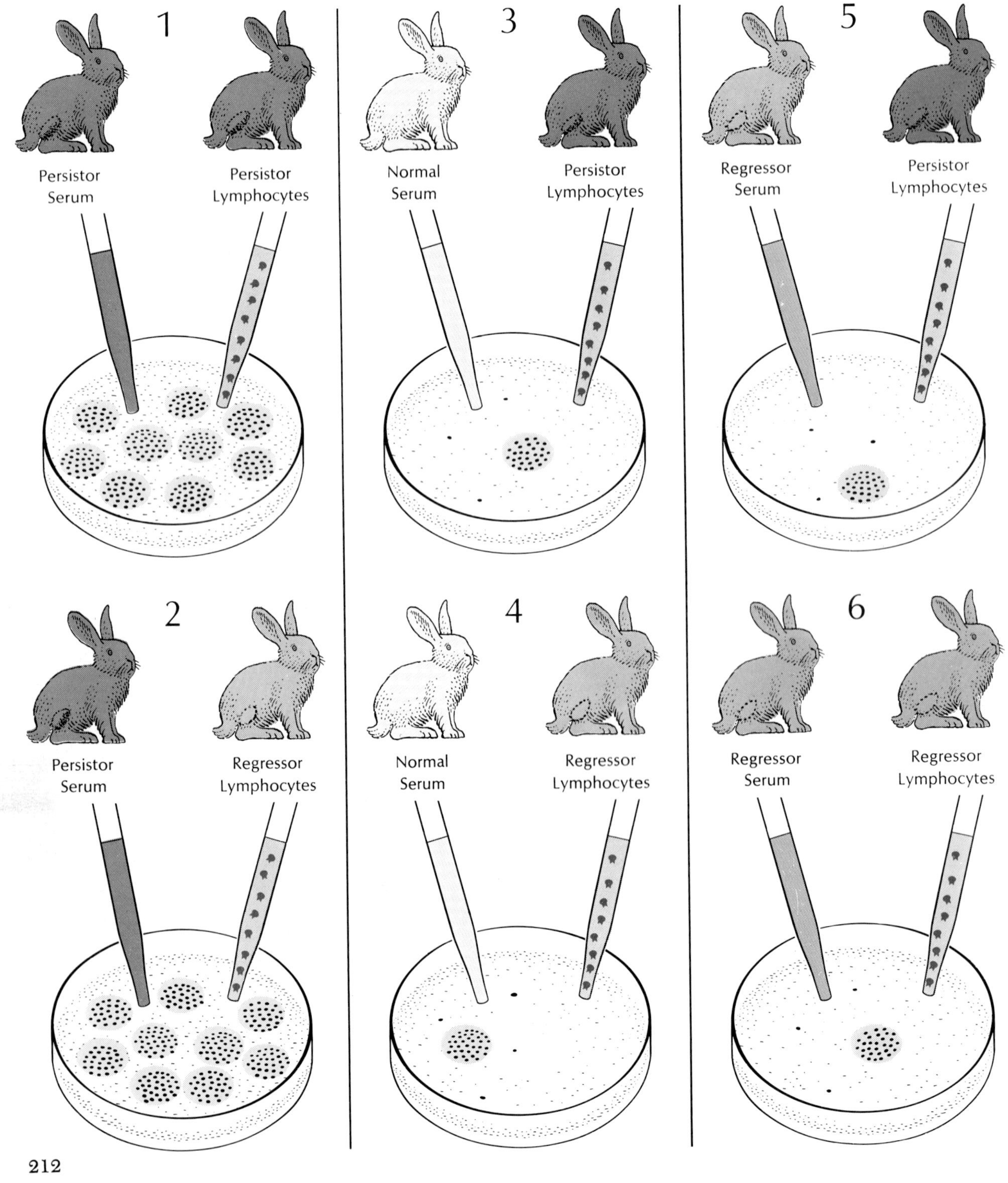

tumor had been removed and explanted could inhibit by approximately 60% the colony formation of tumor cells from the same mouse. Lymph node cells from a mouse from which another methylcholanthrene-induced tumor had been removed were used in the controls because of the fact that different methylcholanthrene-induced sarcomas have individually distinct tumor antigens.

The first experiments had been performed after amputation of the mouse leg bearing a tumor. We were then faced with the question whether cellular immunity against a tumor was operative in an animal in which the tumor was still growing. This question was answered by the demonstration that lymphocytes from tumor-bearing animals were able to kill tumor cells in our system without any significant decrease in efficiency. This was something of a surprise, since one of the premises of the lymphocyte surveillance theory is that tumor growth is permitted because of immunologic deficiency.

At the same time we were also working with Shope papillomas. Here the situation was somewhat closer to what confronts one in dealing with human neoplasia, since the animals (rabbits) represent an outbred population. Moreover, while Shope papillomas will generally progress to carcinomas and kill the animals, they will sometimes regress spontaneously. So far as ability of lymphocytes to kill tumor cells in vitro was concerned, we could not find any difference between animals with growing tumors and animals in which tumors had been present but had regressed. This was very disappointing in the light of work done in the early 1960's.

Evans and Ito had documented a clear-cut immunologic difference in vivo between rabbits whose Shope papillomas had regressed and those in which the tumors had persisted and developed into carcinomas. In one set of experiments, they injected the DNA from the Shope virus into each of the two types of animals – the regressors and the persistors. The DNA induced new tumors in the persistors but did not do so in the regressors. The latter appeared immune. We therefore expected to find an equally distinct difference between the lymphocytes of the two types of animals.

What kept us from writing off these experiments was the interest that had developed in immunologic enhancement and our feeling that perhaps our findings in the Shope papilloma experiments might relate to this phenomenon.

The concept of immunologic enhancement goes back some 30 years to the work of Casey with what he termed the XYZ effect – the ability of humoral antibodies to protect transplanted (mostly neoplastic) cells and permit them to grow without rejection in antigenically foreign hosts. This idea was more fully developed by N. Kaliss at Bar Harbor, who introduced the term "immunologic enhancement." He found that by transferring humoral antibodies to allogeneic animals, acceptance of a homograft could be achieved under circumstances that would otherwise mandate immunologic rejection. Kaliss also found that mixing of humoral antibodies with tumor cells in vitro made possible their development into tumors under conditions that otherwise preclude such events.

In what circumstances does a humoral antibody perform in the rather paradoxical manner required for immunologic enhancement? Many investigators have sought to define the enhancement phenomenon. An essential component is that such protective action of humoral antibodies is likely to take place in situations where host defense is primarily mediated by immune lymphocytes. Beyond that, the requirements for enhancement, as outlined by Möller in particular, for H-2 histocompatibility systems are that all foreign antigens be covered by humoral antibody either in vitro before transplantation or in vivo when humoral antibodies encounter transplanted cells. This scheme would account for one of the two types of enhancement proposed by Gorer, Kaliss, Snell, and others. This is the efferent form, in which the antigenic receptors of the graft are blocked so that immunized lymphocytes do not recognize the antigens of the putative target cells and therefore do not attack them. It has also been demonstrated that enhancement may take place on the afferent limb of the cellular immunity system. That is, the humoral antibodies may encounter the foreign antigens from tumor tissue transplants before these antigens reach lymph nodes or other immunologic centers where they would normally induce sensitization. Specifically, by preempting the antigenic combining sites, humoral antibodies prevent the antigens from sensitizing lymphocytes.

It should be emphasized that almost all of the early work on enhancement – and such work had evolved in many laboratories over more than a decade – involved normal histocompatibility rather than tumor antigens. However, a few reports by Möller, Bubenik, Weiss, and others indicated that certain hyperimmune sera to tumor-specific antigens could enhance the growth of transplanted tumor cells. This was one reason that motivated us to see whether immunologic enhancement might not play some part in the anomalous results we had noted with the lymphocytes of persistors and regressors in the Shope papilloma experiments. If our observations were correct and there were no discernible differences in the behavior of the lymphocytes derived from animals differing in immunologic reactivity in vivo, was it not possible that the factor or factors that led one tumor to regress while another progressed could be found in the sera of the rabbits?

To test this possibility we took tumor cells from the persistent papillomas and seeded them in tissue culture. With serum from the persistor animals present, no colony inhibition, i.e., no killing of tumor cells, was observed with persistor lymphocytes, and neither was there any inhibition when the lymphocytes were derived from regressors. Then normal serum was substituted for persistor serum. Normal (nonimmune) lymphocytes were, as seen before, incapable of killing tumor cells, but with both types of immune lymphocytes – regressor and persistor – colony inhibition was manifest. Finally, regressor serum was used, and the results were essentially the same as with the normal serum: no killing with nonimmune lymphocytes but killing with both regressor and persistor lymphocytes.

In short, immune lymphocytes in our system were capable of attacking and destroying papilloma cells without regard for the in vivo behavior of the tumor source (i.e., whether the animal was a regressor or a persistor) except in the presence of serum from persistor animals. Obviously, some factor resident in persistor serum afforded protection to the tumor cells.

Was the factor humoral antibody?

For our next experiments we decided to employ BALB/c mice and Moloney virus–induced sarcomas. The choice of the mouse was dictated by the experimental advantage of using inbred animals, that of the Moloney sarcoma by the knowledge, particularly from the work of Dr. A. Fefer, that here, too, was a neoplasm that in some instances progressed, in others regressed spontaneously. With the BALB/c mice, it has been shown that tumor regression is usual if a standardized Moloney sarcoma virus is administered to animals more than one month old, while if the animals are younger the tumors will not regress even though cellular immune mechanisms are intact. The system thus permitted us to know in advance whether each subject was to be a persistor or a regressor. Our goal was to determine whether the persistor animals had blocking factors in their serum. Our experiments showed not only that they had but that the blocking factors exerted their protective effect by coating the target cells.

While this evidence indicated the presence of an antibody, it did not prove such presence. Some previous reports had suggested that tumor-bearing animals may have in their sera nonspecific factors that diminish cellular response. This possibility had to be excluded in our systems before any conclusions about the presence of blocking antibodies could be supported. We therefore took sera from animals of the same strain with primary methylcholanthrene-induced tumors and primary mammary carcinomas. These sera did not afford any protection to Moloney sarcoma cells in the colony inhibition system, evidence militating against the concept of a nonspecific antilymphocytic factor in the sera of tumor-bearing animals.

Next we did absorption experiments in which we found that the protective factor in progressor serum could be specifically removed with Moloney sarcoma cells but not with the same dose of mammary carcinoma or methylcholanthrene-induced tumor cells. Such specific absorption with the target cells certainly supported the antibody hypothesis. Even more definitive was our experience when we mixed our persistor serum with a goat anti-mouse immunoglobulin preparation and found this would specifically remove the protective effect of the serum. Furthermore, fractionations of the persistor sera have shown that the protective effect is in the 7S fraction, additional evidence that it may be inherent in serum antibody.

Not only has the same type of antibody-protective phenomenon been identified in Shope papilloma and Moloney sarcoma systems but Gloria Heppner, working in our laboratory, got similar results with spontaneous mouse mammary carcinomas. She observed that mice with such tumors were immunologically nonreactive against the common viral antigens of the mammary tumors but maintained their ability to react against the antigens unique to each tumor mentioned earlier in this article. Lymphocytes from mice carrying primary mammary tumors could kill tumor cells from those tumors in tissue culture but did not act against tumor cells taken from other animals. They thus appeared to be tolerant to the common antigens but not to the unique ones. Sera of primary tumor–bearing animals had blocking antibodies against the unique antigens.

We have recently confirmed the presence of a parallel constellation of similar immunologic phenomena in another system, primary methylcholanthrene-induced tumors, and Sjögren has similar data for primary polyoma and Rous virus–induced tumors in rats and adenovirus-induced tumors in mice. A possibly analogous finding is that of Isaac Witz from Israel who could elute from tumors in vivo IgG antibodies which electrophoretically migrated with the IgG gamma 2 fraction. This is of great interest because in the H-2 histocompatibility system, enhancing antibodies very often belong to that fraction.

In our view, the similarity of these findings in different systems can hardly be coincidental and indicates that certain humoral antibodies may play a major role in counteracting the defenses put up by immune lymphocytes against oncogenesis. There are also indications that this occurs in human cancer situations, but before we get to this it is necessary to refer briefly to some of the evidence that human neoplasms possess tumor-specific antigens.

Human Tumor Immunity

In 1965, Gold and Freedman published the first clear-cut demonstration that carcinomas of the colon in man had antigens capable of eliciting immunologic response. This work was followed by several studies utilizing the fluorescent antibody technique to demonstrate humoral immunity to other human tumors, a technique previously used by Klein, Rapp, Tevethja, Malmgren, and others with good success in the demonstration of tumor-specific surface antigens in animal tumors. The first of these studies was performed by Klein's group with Burkitt lymphomas. The fluorescent antibody technique has also been used by Morton and Malmgren and their colleagues to show that malignant melanomas elicit a humoral antibody response in patients and also to identify cross-reactions between different melanomas. Cross-reactions were also demonstrated among osteogenic sarcomas, while no such reactions were detected between different groups of human cancers.

For our own work with human tumor material we have extended the colony inhibition system and used it to study a variety of cancers, including neuroblastomas, lung, colon, and breast carcinomas, malignant melanomas, fibrosarcomas, and osteogenic sarcomas. We have focussed our attention on cellular immune reactions, largely because of findings in animal experiments that the host defense against tumors is primarily mediated by immune cells.

It was possible for us to show that almost every patient tested had a strong cellular immunity to antigens present in his own neoplastic cells and absent in detectable amounts from his normal cells. Our most extensive efforts have involved neuroblastomas in children. We chose this tumor for a number of reasons. Prominent among them was that in some cases this tumor (which can appear very early in childhood or even before birth) regresses spontaneously, while in others it progresses rapidly and lethally. Thus, we saw an analogy with the

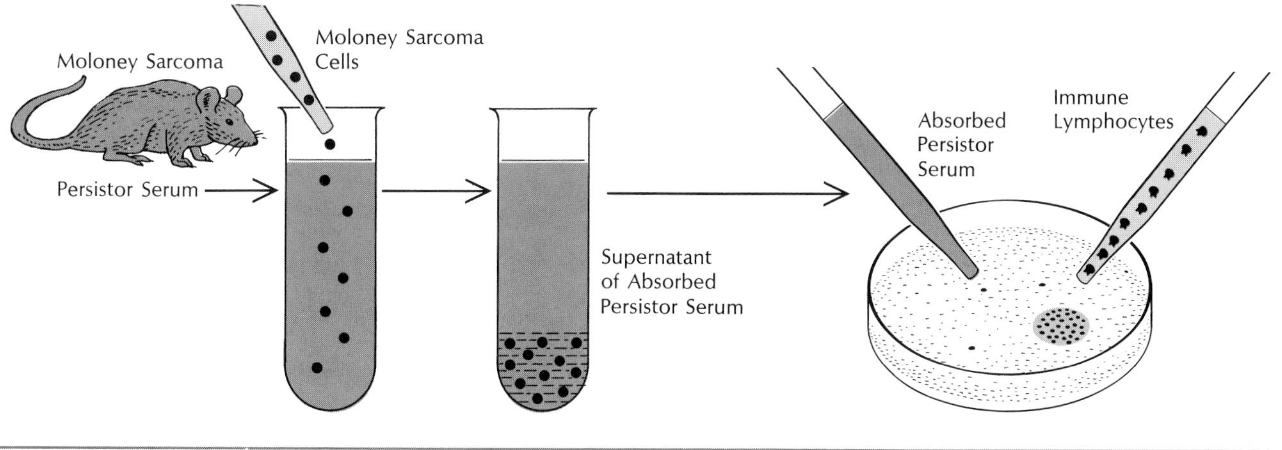

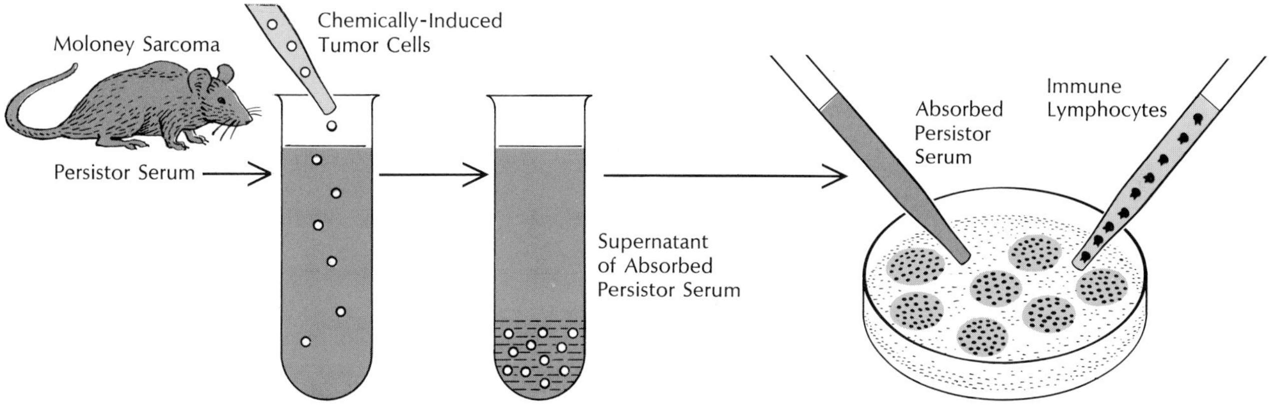

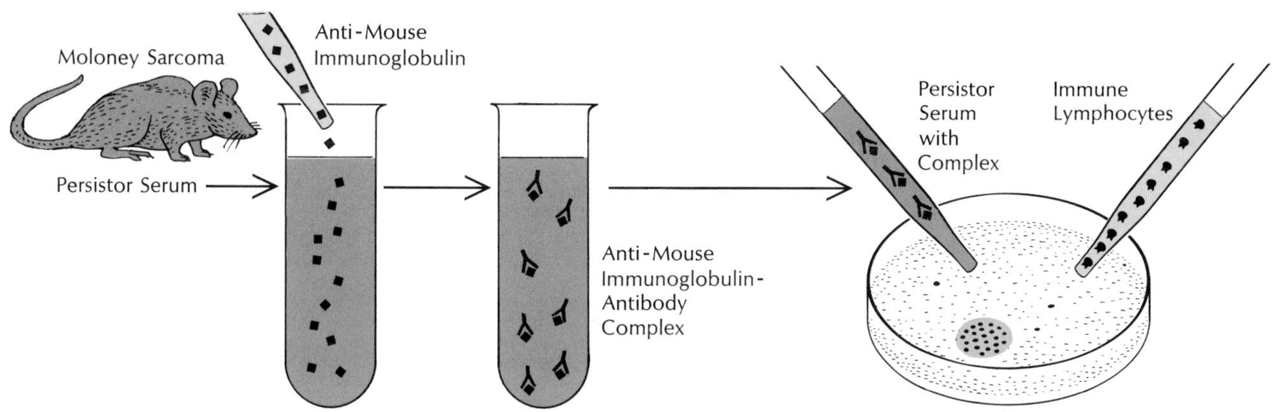

Two types of experiment provide evidence that the serum factors protecting persistent tumors are specific antibodies. When persistor serum from an animal with a Moloney sarcoma is absorbed with Moloney sarcoma cells, the serum loses its ability to protect tumor cells (top). When cells from a different type of tumor (chemically induced) are used, protective effect of the serum is unchanged (middle). Protective effect is also lost when goat anti-mouse Ig is added and complexes with serum antibody.

regressor-persistor situation studied experimentally with the Shope papillomas and the Moloney sarcomas. Also, the Children's Hospital here in Seattle is a center for the management of neuroblastoma cases on the West Coast. We were thus able to establish a rewarding collaboration with Dr. Alexander Bill, chief of surgery at the hospital, as well as with Drs. George E. Pierce and James P. S. Yang at the University of Washington.

In all studies of human cancers, we endeavor to obtain both a sample of tumor and one of normal tissue from the same patient – lung for lung carcinoma, colon for colon carcinoma, skin fibroblasts for fibrosarcoma. For the neuroblastomas, we use skin fibroblasts, since neural tissue cannot be regularly obtained and grown. We then cultivate both the tumor and the normal tissue so that the colony inhibition method can be used. Circulating lymphocytes rather than lymph node preparations are employed.

Our findings have been that lymphocytes from children with neuroblastomas not only can kill autochthonous tumor cells but also can cross-

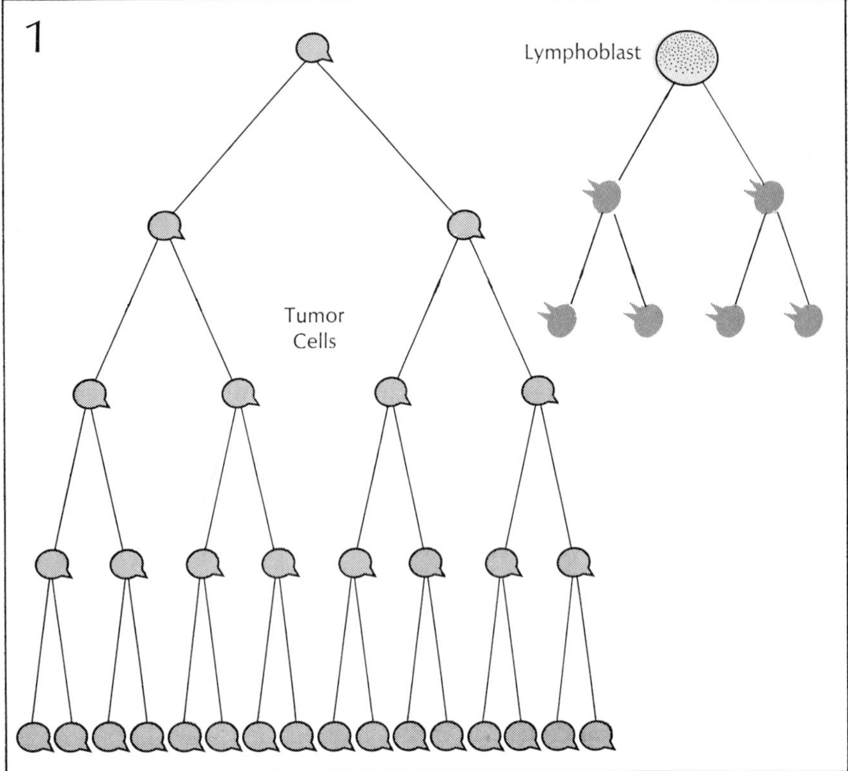

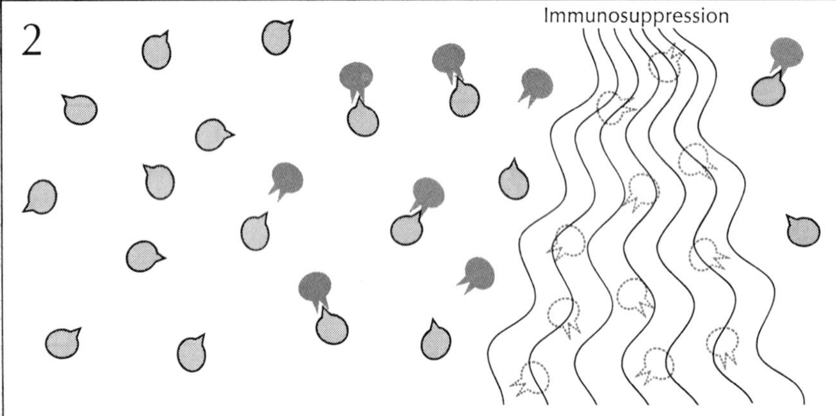

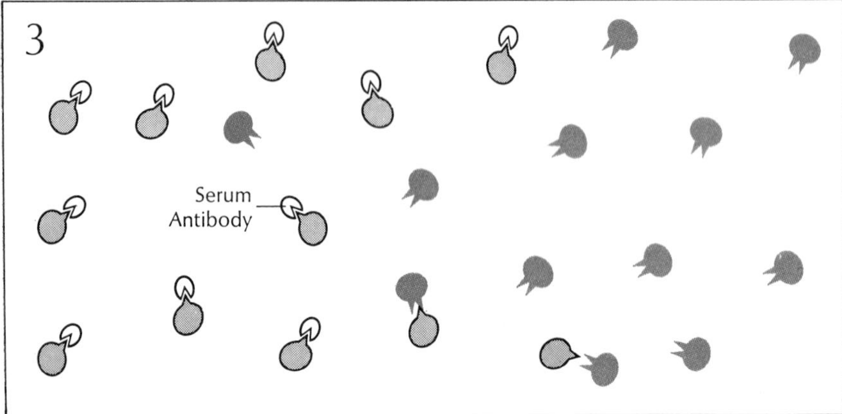

Three ways in which cellular immunity against cancers might be rendered ineffective are depicted. It could be a matter of simple cellular kinetics; the tumor cells might proliferate more rapidly than the lymphocytes (1). Or immunosuppression might reduce the number of sensitized lymphocytes to the point where they are too few to destroy the tumor cells (2). Or protective humoral antibodies might prevent an originally adequate number of lymphocytes from attaching to and destroying the tumor cells (3).

react and kill tumor cells from other children with neuroblastomas. On the other hand, these lymphocytes do not inhibit colony growth of normal cells.

In work further paralleling that done earlier in animal systems, we also sought to compare the effects of lymphocytes from children apparently cured of their neuroblastomas with those of lymphocytes from children with growing tumors, even with tumors that had already metastasized to the bone marrow. No major difference could be detected in the ability of the lymphocytes from these two groups of patients to kill tumor cells. In fact, we have also shown that the ability to kill neuroblastoma cells also applies to the lymphocytes of their mothers.

This last finding was all the more surprising because the mothers' lymphocytes behaved very much like those of their children, being able to kill not only the tumor cells taken from their children but also neuroblastoma cells from other children. Furthermore, the maternal lymphocytes showed no inhibitory effect on either normal tissue cells or cells from tumors other than neuroblastomas. More recently, we have found that lymphocytes from some other relatives – notably brothers and sisters – also have the capacity to kill neuroblastoma cells. These data suggest that a virus may be associated (not necessarily causatively) with human neuroblastomas.

Most pertinent to the main line of our research have been the investigations of enhancing or blocking antibodies in certain human tumors. These studies have been carried out in patients with carcinomas of the colon, malignant melanomas, carcinomas of the lung, retinoblastoma, and neuroblastoma. We were stimulated by the findings that lymphocytes from patients with progressive neoplastic disease gave approximately as much colony inhibition as did lymphocytes from patients whose tumors had been removed and who were considered to be clinically symptom-free. Serum from patients with a progressively growing tumor almost invariably was shown to contain blocking antibodies able to abrogate the inhibitory effect of the same patients' immune lymphocytes on their tumor cells. No such effect was seen with serum from patients apparently cured of their disease (whose lymphocytes were still reactive). These data tend to suggest, therefore, that prophylactic as well as therapeutic effects can be achieved by nonspecific bolstering of cellular immune reactions to tumor antigens. Studies by Eddy, Deichman, Girardi, Hilleman, and others indicate that specific stimulation of the immune response also may be of value in preventing development of certain viral neoplasms in animals.

Even on the basis of this brief and certainly far from inclusive summary of studies on the roles of cellular immunity and blocking antibodies, it is clear that a beginning has been made in the dissection of the relationships between cancer and the immunologic mechanisms. At this time, it is safe to state only that the interactions are highly complex. The evidence for the existence of tumor-specific antigens in animal systems and at least in some human cancers is strong. One can construct a number of hypothetical models for the responses to these antigens.

By way of example, one might cite the "sneaking-through" hypothesis advanced several years ago by Old and Boyse, which postulates that at any given time the immune response of the host may be inadequate to keep pace with a developing tumor. If it is assumed, on the basis of considerable evidence, that the killing of a single tumor cell requires a one-to-one confrontation with an immune lymphocyte, then this inadequacy could eventuate in a number of ways. It could be a matter of simple cellular kinetics – the tumor cells dividing more rapidly than lymphocytes can be recruited by immunization and division. Thus if a subject's thymus is removed, or if antilymphocytic serum or radiation or drugs are administered, the depletion in the lymphocyte population may leave the balance in favor of the tumor. Or if the number of immune lymphocytes is adequate, the role of the blocking serum antibodies may become paramount – there are enough lymphocytes but they cannot do their job because their ability either to recognize antigen or to engage it has been compromised. Obviously, these possibilities aren't mutually exclusive.

Almost without exception our investigations have involved manipulation of various elements in vitro. This

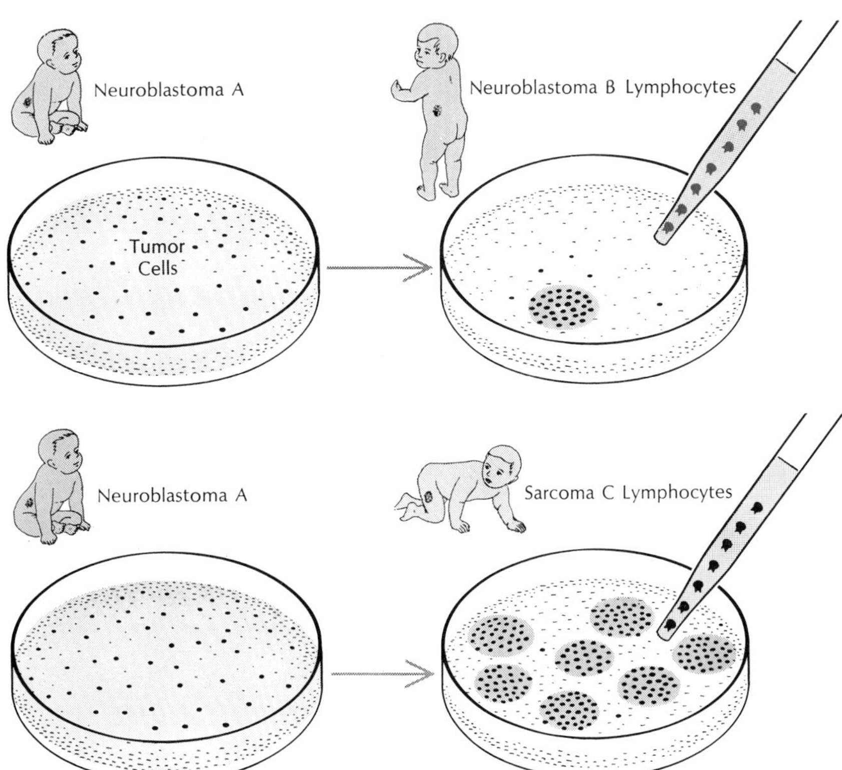

Specific antigenic cross-reactivity has been demonstrated between patients with neuroblastomas. In colony inhibition assay, neuroblastoma cells from child A are killed by lymphocytes from child B, who also has a neuroblastoma (or by his own lymphocytes), but not by lymphocytes from child C, who has an unrelated type of tumor.

is one reason why some workers question their applicability to the major problem confronted clinically – that of spontaneous oncogenesis in man – and feel that there is either a complete immunologic tolerance in human patients to their tumor antigens or that the antigens are masked in vivo and only show up after manipulation during the procedure of cell cultivation. Hence the observations by Starzl in Colorado, by Good in Minnesota, by a group in Texas, and others involved in organ transplantation are of particular significance, showing that patients submitted to immunosuppression have an increased risk of getting cancer. Similar findings, obtained in animal studies by Law, Allison, Vandeputte, and others, show that immunodepressed mice and rats are at increased risk from oncogenic viruses.

There is also a growing body of evidence that increasing the immunologic response serves to impede the emergence of primary tumors. Almost 10 years ago Old et al. and Weiss showed that nonspecific immunologic stimulation by BCG administration increased immunologic reactivity of mice to weak histocompatibility antigens and extended somewhat the latency period for chemically induced tumors. In the past year G. Mathé in Paris has reported exciting clinical trials indicative of some immunotherapeutic success with BCG treatment of certain leukemia patients. Furthermore, Sjögren and J. Ankerst have published results of experiments in which adenovirus induction of tumors could be impeded by inoculation of BCG.

Since the blocking antibodies are able to protect against the inhibitory effect of specifically immune lymphocytes in vitro it appears likely that these antibodies play an important role in vivo. Some recently obtained findings may be worth mentioning to support this view. We have found that mice injected with the Moloney sarcoma virus when more than 30 days old contain blocking antibodies as long as their tumors are still growing actively, but this is no longer so when the tumors start regressing. The regressors contain cytotoxic, nonblocking antibodies. Admixture of regressor serum with serum from mice with progressively growing Moloney sarcomas decreases the blocking effect of the latter, probably because both types of antibodies have affinity for the same target cell antigens.

These data suggest, therefore, that administration of nonblocking antibodies in vivo might be of therapeutic value. Mice transplanted with syngeneic methylcholanthrene-induced sarcomas develop both a cellular immunity and blocking antibodies within approximately a week following transplantation. Appearance of blocking antibodies precedes the development of palpable tumors. In some animals in which transplanted small doses of syngeneic methylcholanthrene-induced tumors were rejected, cellular immunity but no blocking antibodies was detected. This suggests that interference with the formation and action of blocking antibodies in vivo may be therapeutically beneficial.

Experiments done with Drs. Pierce and Fefer about a year ago may throw some further light upon this problem. We attempted to treat animals that had progressively growing Moloney sarcomas by giving them immune lymphocytes or serum from syngeneic animals in which Moloney sarcomas had regressed spontaneously. It was possible to cure approximately 30% of mice that way. The data were originally interpreted as suggesting that the regressor lymphocytes had improved the cellular immunity of tumor-bearing hosts by adding to the number of immune cells. However, some regressions were induced with as few as five million regressor lymphocytes, too small a number to be likely to play a role by just increasing the amount of cytotoxic lymphocytes present in the animals. (Lymphocytes from the persistor mice are inhibitory themselves in CI tests, as already discussed.) It would be easier to understand these findings by postulating that the injected immune lymphocytes (and cytotoxic antibodies) from the regressors acted by interfering with the blocking antibodies present in the mice, allowing the immune lymphocytes already there to go to work.

How close are we to exploring whether nonspecific immunotherapy and specific replacement immunotherapy have any potential against human tumors? Realistically, it seems likely that in vitro methodology is now adequate enough to allow investigators to trace the immunologic events sequential to the development of cancer and to our efforts to treat the disease. We should be able to learn whether surgery, irradiation, and chemotherapy influence immunologic response, whether they decrease it by disabling the lymphocytic system, or increase it by removing blocking antibodies, etc.

Animal experiments have shown that by bolstering immunologic responses we can cope with small foci of neoplastic cells. This indeed may be the eventual role of immunotherapy in cancer therapy. Once having gotten rid of the primary mass by conventional means, we may be able to call upon immunotherapeutic techniques to rid the body of the few remaining malignant cells that give rise to late metastases. Clearly, if we could bolster the cellular hypersensitivity system sufficiently to eliminate the "last" tumor cell, or if we could remove blocking antibodies, we might be in a better position to change the prognosis in certain types of cancer.

On the other hand, it does not seem realistic to hope that patients who arrive at a terminal stage of disease, with tumor masses widely disseminated, will be curable through immunotherapy. We know of no case in the literature of animal experimentation where this has been achieved. For a clinician the problem is a delicate one. If immunotherapy is attempted in patients whose prognosis with conventional therapy is reasonably good, the danger that enhancement rather than inhibition will occur looms large. If immunotherapy is reserved for the patient near death, failure is inevitable and could easily lead to unwarranted skepticism about such therapy.

For these reasons we believe that the definition of the situations in which immunotherapy is appropriate and the task of designing such therapy to ensure that it is beneficial and not harmful are for the time being still within the province of the laboratory worker using animal systems. Obviously, there must be a day when clinical trials should start. It may not be too far off. Even now, there are occasional situations in which some clinicians with a highly critical approach and with appropriate laboratory background could justifiably undertake immunotherapy. Probably the most suitable cases would be patients whose prognosis is extremely poor but in whom the tumor mass is still small. Then it might be worthwhile to attempt therapeutic techniques such as administration of BCG or of immune lymphocytes, if these were available, or cytotoxic, nonblocking antibodies, or perhaps to test specific absorption procedures if it could be determined that blocking serum antibodies had been elaborated.

From such small beginnings and from continuing collaboration between clinic and laboratory we will reach the point when immunologic manipulation can take its place in preventing and treating cancers in man.

Infective DNA and Immunity

The chapter by Dr. Kornberg, which follows, does not, strictly speaking, deal with studies in immunobiology. However, a number of factors have militated in favor of its inclusion here. All current theories concerning the elusive mechanism that underlies antibody synthesis and immunity require understanding of the intimate relationships of DNA replication, RNA production, and protein synthesis. Both instructional and selective theories of antibody production now view this process in terms of the conventional avenues of protein synthesis and secretion. Obviously, central to these processes are the DNA molecule and its replication.

Many of the profound abnormalities and perturbations of the bodily defenses are genetically determined. The need to correct such abnormalities in protein synthesis requires increased understanding of and enhanced ability to manipulate the DNA molecule. Indeed, basic to the entire concept of molecular engineering is the capacity to synthesize functional DNA. This capacity has already been attained in the synthesis of functional viral DNA, as reported by Dr. Kornberg. His fundamental achievement affords us major insights into the process of multiplication and into the function of DNA molecules. As such it represents a major step toward an ultimate goal of molecular engineering. It is not yet clear just how this advance can be used to manipulate immunologic and other human diseases, but the chapter includes some intriguing suggestions. It seems certain to us that this giant step in the basic science of the control of the first biologic language will ultimately have the greatest practical significance.

Out of growing knowledge of the specific details of DNA-RNA and protein synthesis and function, we can expect a most fundamental understanding of autoimmunity, specific and nonspecific defenses against microbial invasion, the nature of primary and secondary immunodeficiency diseases, the mechanisms of immunologic assault, and of allergy and cancer. Dr. Kornberg has brought into the realm of reality the hope that we will one day be able to prevent, treat, and manipulate disease by fashioning "desirable" DNA and introducing it at will and in functional form into mammalian cells. All of this, we believe, has special relevance to future progress in controlling infection and the immune response and its consequences.

R.A.G.

Chapter 22

The Synthesis of Infective DNA and Its Implications

ARTHUR KORNBERG
Stanford University

Ironically, the main danger in attempting to predict the future significance of a new scientific development is not that of being transported by enthusiasm to intemperance. Rather, the character of discovery is that we eventually derive so much more from it than we can anticipate. Thus it seems likely that real benefits to clinical medicine will eventually accrue from the synthesis of biologically active deoxyribonucleic acid reported by Mehran Goulian, Robert L. Sinsheimer, and me in the December 1967 *Proceedings of the National Academy of Sciences*.

But before these benefits can even be measured, much more biologic knowledge, particularly that relating to the chemistry of DNA, will have to be obtained. Perhaps the best way to look at the problems that lie ahead is to review those that have been encountered to date, that is to say, to review the investigative activity that has brought us to this point.

In searching for a start to the research line, one can go back to before the turn of the century when Eduard Buchner first showed that pressed-yeast juice could carry out alcoholic fermentation. This was revolutionary in terms of the thinking of Pasteur and the scientists of the time, who believed that live yeast cells were essential for fermentation. During the first half of the century, most biochemists focused on problems related to such energy-producing reactions as glycolysis, amino acid and fatty acid oxidation, and alcoholic fermentation. Since 1950 the emphasis has shifted to biosynthetic problems.

My initiation into biosynthetic studies came between 1948 and 1954 with efforts to determine how coenzymes, the simplest of the nucleotide condensation products, were assembled from glucose, ammonia, carbon dioxide, and amino acids. From this work we came to realize what form of nucleotide would be the most likely building block for assembly of nucleic acids. In the case of DNA these are the nucleotides containing adenine, thymine, guanine, and cytosine. We found that by incubating these building-block chemicals in certain cell "juices," we obtained some nucleic acid synthesis — very little, to be sure, but enough to encourage further work. We then set about purifying the enzyme or enzymes responsible for the conversion of these low molecular weight materials into an integral part of a big nucleic acid molecule.

The enzyme was purified and named DNA polymerase because its function was to polymerize monomeric material into something with the gross features of DNA. We also learned that the capacity of DNA polymerase to assemble the four building blocks into DNA absolutely required the presence of DNA to serve as a template. The product of the enzymatic assembly has the precise chemical composition dictated by the particular DNA put into the system. This precision appears to be very great. The polymerase follows instructions from the template without regard to the source of the DNA or to the relative concentrations of the nucleotides available to it in the synthetic mixture. Taken together, these attributes of DNA polymerase make it unique among enzymes.

We learned from these and subsequent experiments that the polymerase assembles the monomeric building blocks one at a time and that the resulting synthesized DNA has the familiar base-pairing architecture described by Watson and Crick, with adenine paired complementarily with thymine, guanine with cytosine. But there were three anomalous facts about the DNA synthesized in this system, three troublesome differences between it and native DNA:

- The synthetic DNA was branched.
- Unlike native DNA, which will denature (i.e., the two strands of the helix will come apart and remain apart)

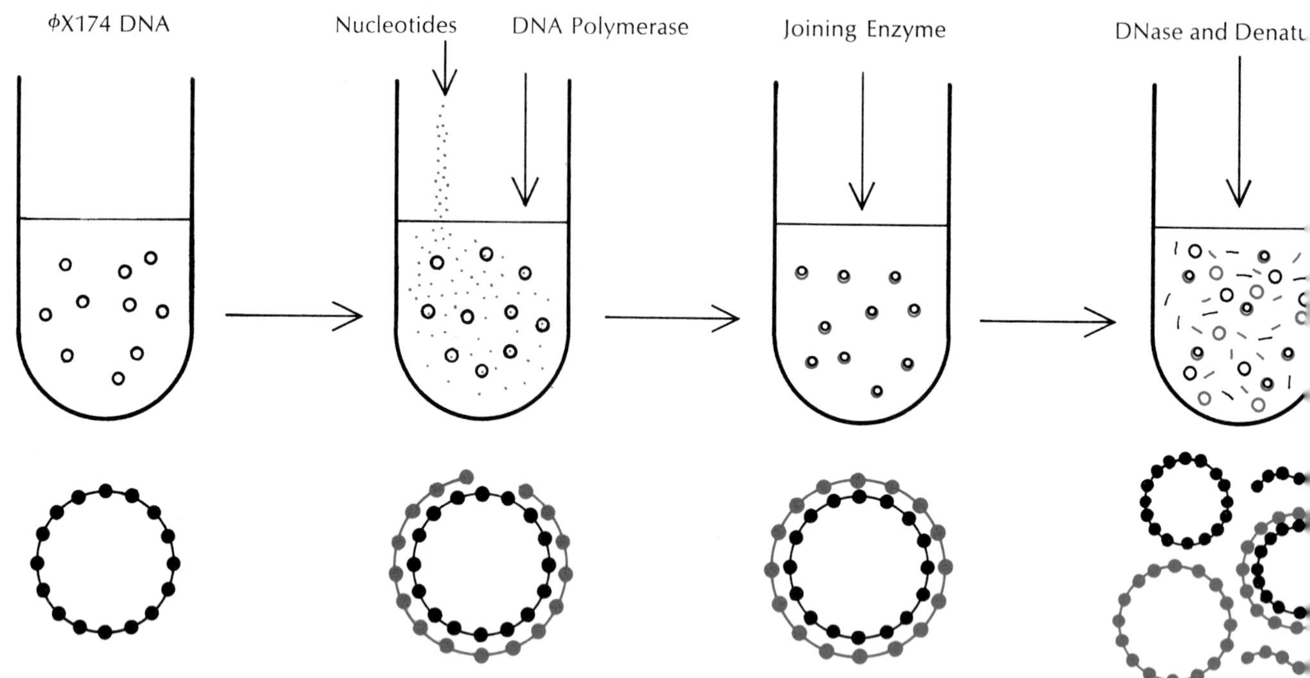

The various steps in the synthesis of complete, biologically active, viral DNA are schematically represented here. The circular DNA of ϕX174 virus is used as a template. Nucleotides containing adenine, thymine, guanine, and cytosine are then added, along with DNA polymerase. The enzyme causes formation of a synthetic polypeptide circle complementary to the template DNA. However, the synthetic circle is incomplete and therefore not biologically active. Completion of the complementary circle is accomplished by the polynucleotide joining enzyme, and a semisynthetic covalent duplex circle is formed. DNase treatment and denaturation permit separation of the two circles and of linear forms of both template and synthetic origin. Various techniques have been employed along the way to create density differences and exploit shape differences so that the template and synthetic linears, the template and synthetic circles, and the semisynthetic duplexes can be segregated as shown on facing page. The synthetic circles can then be employed as templates for the formation of a second complementary synthetic circle, using the same procedures as before. The result is a completely synthetic viral DNA in its biologically active replicating form.

under the influence of heat or extremes of pH, the synthetic DNA strands came apart but immediately snapped back together again.

• The synthetic DNA lacked biologic activity.

This last anomaly was in some ways the most troublesome. It can be demonstrated by using as a parameter for biologic activity the transforming activity of *Bacillus subtilis* DNA. The DNA from a strain of *B. subtilis* resistant to streptomycin, for example, can convey that trait to a strain of the organism previously susceptible to the antibiotic. However, synthetic DNA, made on a template of *B. subtilis* DNA from a resistant strain, did not increase the transformation to resistance. There was a chemically demonstrable increase of DNA, but the synthetic DNA appeared to lack the ability to transform bacteria, that is to say, biologic activity.

To better understand this biologic inactivity we sought explanations for the physical anomalies — the branching and the non-denaturability. These we were able to account for at least hypothetically. We knew that the two strands in a double helix have opposite polarity. At one end of a strand is a 3′ hydroxyl terminus, at the other 5′ phosphate. We theorized that the DNA polymerase could copy the DNA strand from the 3′ end but not from the 5′ end. Thus one strand at each end was left "unattended" by the polymerase. As synthesis proceeds up and down the strands from the 3′ ends, the unduplicated bases contiguous with the 5′ ends could "switch in" and themselves serve as new templates for synthesis. The result could be the branching observed under the electron microscope. As a secondary consequence, one would then have a synthetic DNA with a pleated structure which would be expected to re-form after denaturing. This hypothesis had limitations, to be sure, but it served to direct us toward the desirability of continuing our efforts to synthesize biologically active DNA on a template of a single-stranded DNA. Presumably a single-stranded DNA would not present the complication of the differential ability of the DNA polymerase to copy the 3′ and 5′ ended strands.

Another consideration motivated our interest in single-stranded DNA. Many infectious viral DNA's are single-stranded circular molecules which become duplex circles, "replicative forms," after they invade and infect cellular hosts. Therefore, work with such a viral DNA would offer insights into the process of multiplication of viral and other DNA molecules of circular structure.

We obtained circular single-stranded DNA from the bacterial viruses M13 and ϕX174. It should be noted that much of what we know about ϕX174 comes from the work of Sinsheimer at the California Institute of Technology. In undertaking an investigation of circular DNA we could foresee basic roadblocks. Perhaps DNA polymerase requires a 3′ hydroxyl ended strand to initiate synthesis; obviously, a circular DNA has no endings at all. We were pleasantly sur-

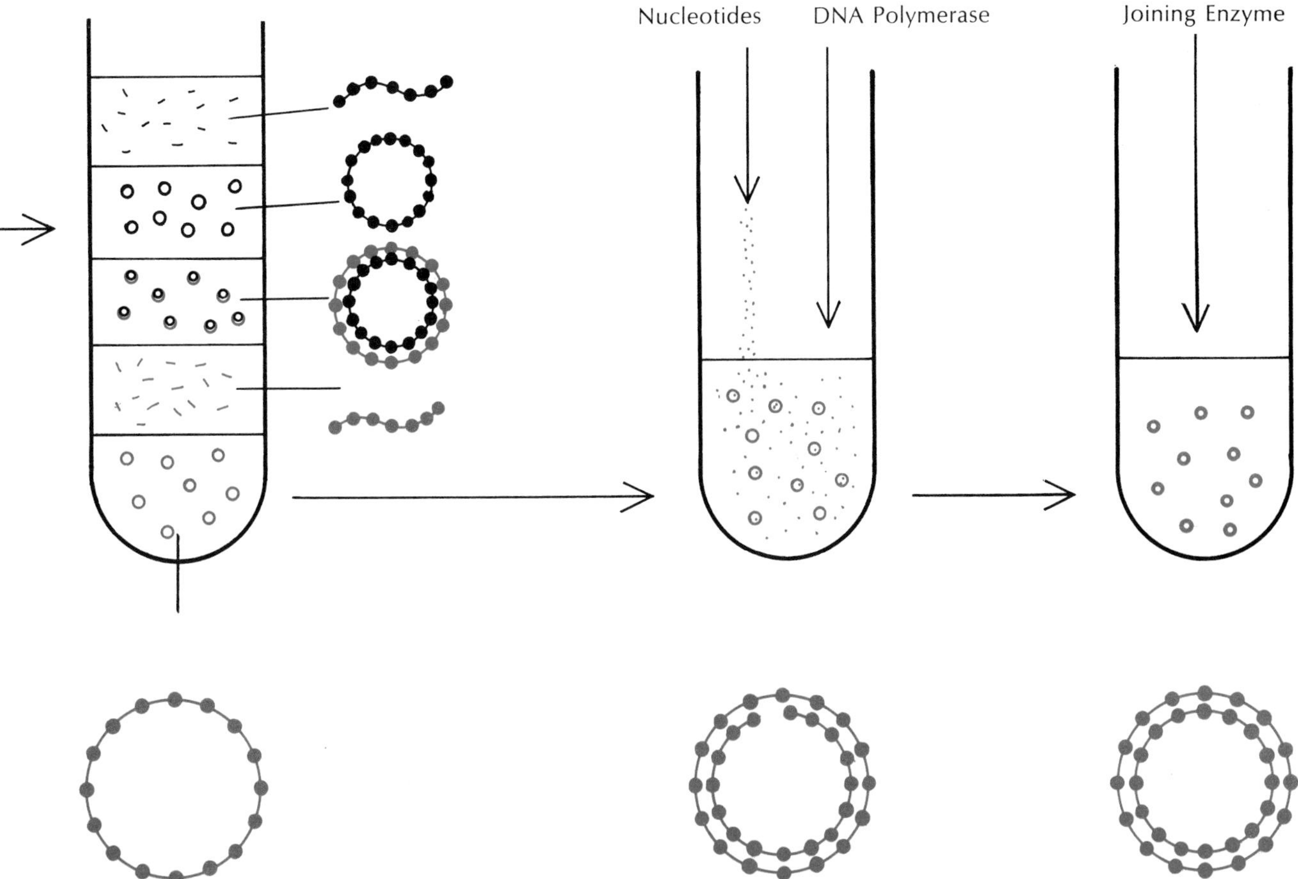

prised to find that the polymerase would work on the circular DNA. We then wondered if, despite electron microscopic appearances, the ϕX DNA was really just a simple circle. Perhaps, as had been suggested by other workers, it is really more like a necklace with a clasp, the clasp consisting of materials unrelated to the nucleotides we were supplying. Finally, we were aware from Sinsheimer's work with circular DNA that such DNA had to be a completely closed circle to be infectious. And polymerase could catalyze the synthesis of linear DNA molecules only.

At this stage we were able to show electron microscopically that starting with the ϕX DNA circle we could produce a complementary DNA strand to form a helical fiber without branches. Morphologically, the synthesized duplex gave the appearance of a full circle but, as expected, it was not a truly closed circle. When denatured (and it denatured in exactly the manner of native DNA) the newly synthesized DNA broke away as a linear coil with two ends. We were therefore still missing either the clasp-like component or an enzyme to close the circle (or both).

Fortunately, the missing factor was supplied to us by work carried on independently in five different laboratories. The discovery of a polynucleotide joining enzyme was made almost simultaneously by Martin Gellert and his coworkers at the National Institutes of Health, by Charles C. Richardson and Bernard Weiss at Harvard, by Jerard Hurwitz and colleagues at the Albert Einstein College of Medicine, by I. Robert Lehman and Baldomero M. Olivera at Stanford, and by Nicholas R. Cozzarelli in my research group. It was the Lehman-Olivera preparation that we employed in our further experiments.

The polynucleotide joining enzyme has the ability to repair "nicks" in the DNA strand. These nicks occur because of the cleavage of the diester bridge between the nucleotides of the nucleic acid strand. The enzyme can repair a break only if all the nucleotides are intact and if what is missing is the covalent bond in the backbone between a sugar and the neighboring phosphate. Given the joining enzyme, we were now in a position to find out whether it could work in conjunction with DNA polymerase to synthesize a completely circular and biologically active phage DNA. Incidentally, use of phage DNA offered us one other critical advantage. With a noninfective DNA as template we would have had to assay the activity of a product on the basis of transforming ability, along the lines suggested previously in the *B. subtilis* example. But even if we were to synthesize DNA with transforming activity, this would still be of relatively limited significance. For we could then say only that a restricted section of the nucleic acid – perhaps as few as 20 nucleotides – had been assimilated as the cell replaced a comparable section of its chromosome, substituting a proper sequence for a defective or incorrect one. However, Sinsheimer had demonstrated with ϕX phage DNA that a change in even one of 5,500 nucleotides is sufficient to eliminate phage activity or infectivity. Therefore demonstration of infectivity in completely synthetic phage would effectively prove that we had carried out virtually error-free synthesis of this large number of nucleotides, comprising five or six genes that do an integrated biologic job.

The steps in the synthesis can now be summarized. Template DNA was obtained from ϕX174 and labeled with tritium. This tritium would thereafter provide a continuing template tag. To the template were added DNA polymerase obtained from *Escherichia coli* and highly purified, joining enzyme and its cofactor (DPN), and the four nucleotides containing adenine, thymine, guanine, and cytosine. One of the latter was labeled with radioactive phosphorus. The P^{32} would, of course, provide a tag for synthetic material analogous to the tritium (H^3) tag for the template. The interaction of the reagents then proceeded until the number of nucleotide monomers polymerized was exactly equal to the number of nucleotides in the template DNA. This equality can, of course, be discerned by calculation and comparison of the radioactivity emanating from the tritium in the template and the radiophosphorus in the nucleotides provided for synthesis. Such calculation showed that the experiments had progressed to the formation of complementary circles of synthetic DNA, arbitrarily designated as (−) circles, on the (+) template circles; the result: partially synthetic forms of duplex covalent DNA with all the morphologic characteristics of the replicative forms of viral ϕX174 DNA.

Knowing that the ingredients we had used were capable of achieving this result was highly reassuring to us. We could now exclude the possibility that some "clasp" material different from the nucleotide-containing compounds we were using was involved in closing the viral DNA circle.

The critical questions remaining were whether the synthetic (−) circles possessed biologic activity, i.e., infectivity, and whether the synthetic circles could in turn act as a template for the formation of completely synthetic duplex covalent DNA analogous to the naturally occurring intracellular replicative forms.

To answer the first of these questions we had to isolate the synthetic DNA strands from the partially synthetic duplexes. For reasons which will be apparent shortly, we substituted bromouracil, an unnatural but biologically active thymine analogue, for thymine. We then introduced just enough pancreatic DNase to produce a single scission in one strand of about half the population of molecules, and we carried out the additional procedure of denaturing. We found we were left with a mixture that contained (+) template circles, (−) synthetic circles, (+) template linear forms, (−) synthetic linear forms (all in about equal quantities) and full duplex circles. The linear forms were those derived from the DNA circles that had been cut by the prior treatment with DNase.

It was at this point that bromouracil substitution for thymine became useful. Because bromouracil contains a bromine atom in place of the methyl group in thymine, it is heavier than thymine. Therefore, a bromouracil-containing molecule can be separated from a thymine-containing molecule by the density gradient techniques perfected by J. Vinograd at the California Institute of Technology.

After centrifugation, the material containing the various DNA forms was fractionated by equilibrium density gradient sedimentation in cesium chloride. In this system, the more dense a substance the lower down in the tube it will sediment. Thus, from top to bottom we obtained the fractions containing the light single strands of thymine-containing (+) template DNA, the duplex hybrids of intermediate weight, and finally the single-stranded synthetic (−) DNA "weighted down" with

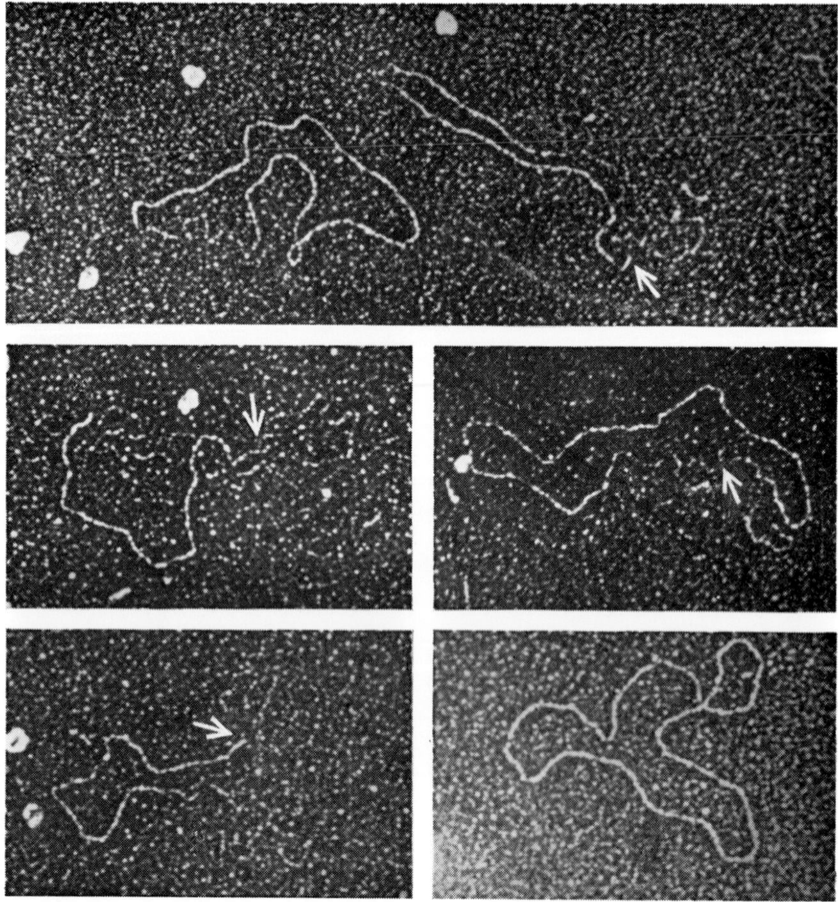

These electronmicrographs of M13 viral DNA replicated on a natural template show the degree of synthesis that could be achieved before the discovery and use of polynucleotide joining enzyme. The arrows note breaks in continuity in one strand of the duplex circle, specifically the synthetic strand. Only an occasional duplex circle appears complete (lower right). Elsewhere one sees stretches of material which are poorly resolved and probably consist of single-stranded template DNA.

bromouracil. The reliability of this fractionation was confirmed by three separate peaks of radioactivity corresponding to each of the fractions. Further reassurance was gained from observations that the mean density of each fraction corresponded almost exactly with the mean density of standard sample viral DNA containing bromouracil or thymine.

Still another physical technique involving density gradient sedimentation was used to separate the synthetic linear forms from the synthetic circular forms. The latter could then be used in tests of infectivity, employing methods previously developed by Sinsheimer to demonstrate the infectivity of circular ϕX174 DNA. We tested our (−) circles by incubating them with *E. coli* whose walls had been removed by lysozyme action. Infectivity is determined by the ability of the phage to lyse these bacteria in a plaque-assay system on agar plates. Our synthetic circles showed almost exactly the same infectivity patterns as had their natural counterparts. Their biologic activity had now been demonstrated.

One further set of experiments remained in which the (−) synthetic circles were employed as the template to determine whether we could produce completely synthetic duplex circular forms analogous to the replicative forms found in cells infected with natural ϕX174 virus. Since the synthetic (−) circles were labeled with P^{32}, we this time added a tritium tag to one of the nucleotide-containing building blocks (i.e., the cytosine). The remaining procedures were essentially the same as those described above, and we did indeed produce fully synthetic covalent duplex circles of ϕX174. The (+) circles were then separated and were found to be identical by all parameters to the (+) circles of natural ϕX virus. Their infectivity could also be demonstrated. Since, under the assay conditions employed, Sinsheimer had previously shown that a change in a single nucleotide of this virus produced a mutant markedly lacking in infectivity, this correspondence between the infectivity of our synthetic forms and their natural counterparts attested to the precision of the enzymatic operation.

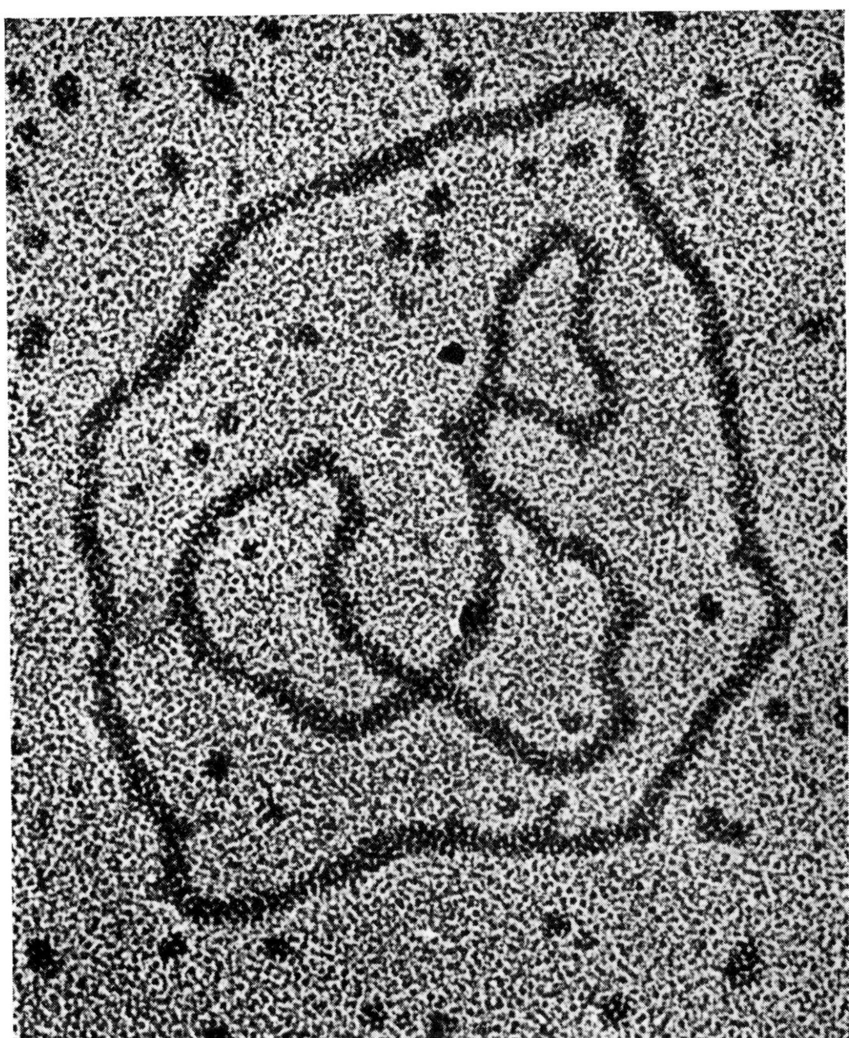

Two duplex circles of partially synthetic ϕX DNA are shown in electronmicrograph (310,000x); one duplex happens to lie inside the other. Each consists of a template of natural virus with a complete synthetic complementary circle.

In turning now to the possible applications of this research to clinical medicine it must be emphasized that we are entering a completely speculative realm. Perhaps the most obvious subject for investigation would be polyoma virus, which is known to induce a variety of malignant tumors in several different rodent species. Polyoma virus in its infective form is made up of duplex circular DNA, and it presumably replicates in this form upon entering the cell. On the basis of our experience it would seem quite feasible to synthesize the polyoma viral DNA. If accomplished, many opportunities would seem to exist for modifying the viral DNA and then determining where in the whole chromosome its oncogenicity resides. With this knowledge it might be equally practicable to begin modifying the virus to control its tumor producing potential.

But our speculations need not be limited to the viral DNA's. An active polynucleotide with some 5,500 bases and a contour length of about 2 μ having been synthesized, there seems to be no insurmountable obstacle to synthesis of larger DNA molecules. The DNA of mitochondria, also circular and with a contour length of 10 μ, might then be produced in a test tube. The major problems at the moment would seem to reside more in the ability to test for biologic activity than in the ability to achieve synthesis. However, let's carry our speculations to a somewhat more remote time when, for example, it might be established that a single mitochondrial gene is responsible for control of an enzyme necessary for normal cellular respira-

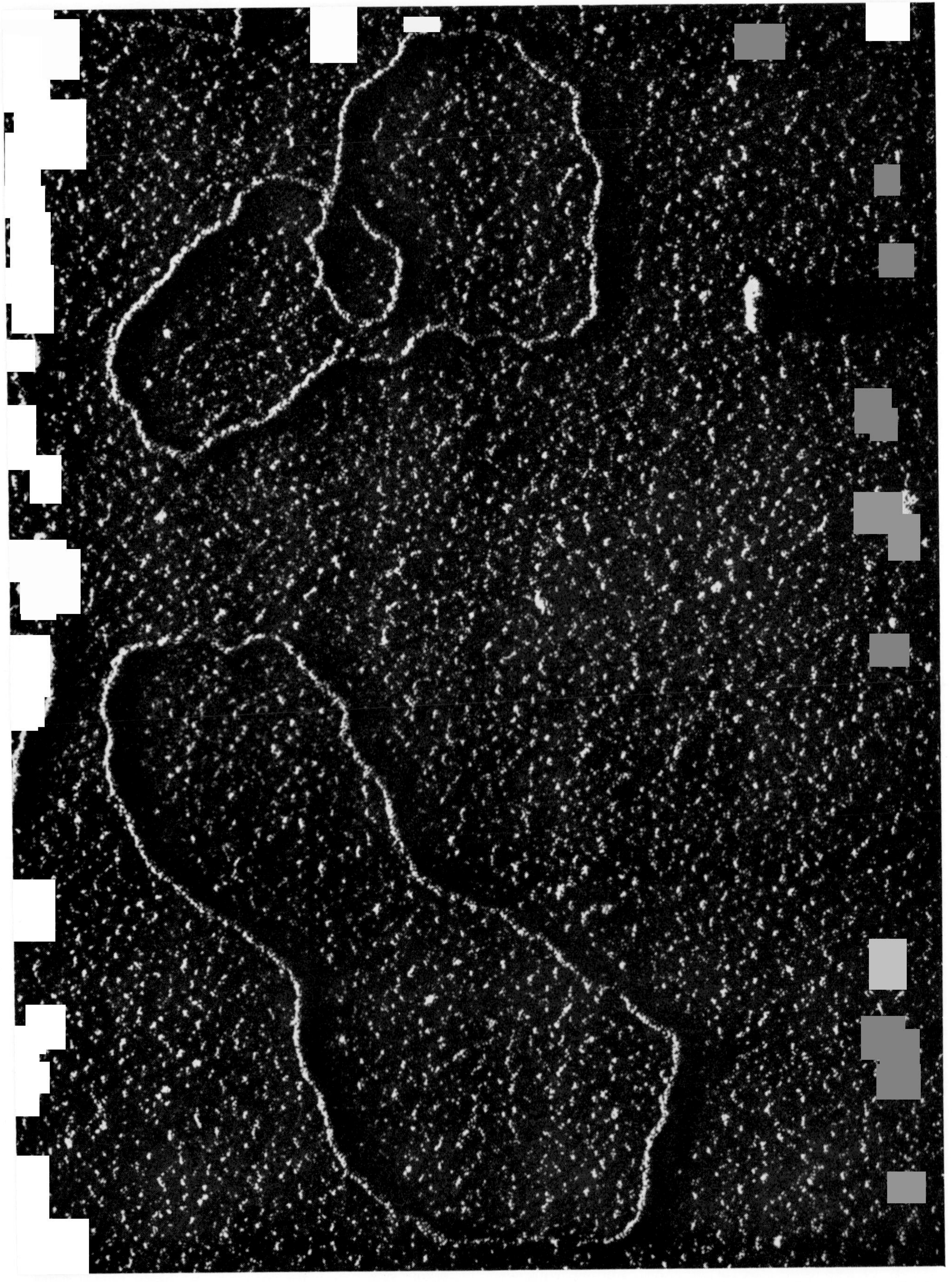

The synthesis of biologically active DNA was achieved with the φX174 bacteriophage virus. Here the phage virus is shown in its natural replicating form as duplex circles or loops. The electron-micrograph was made from a Kleinschmidt preparation by Dr. Humberto Fernandez-Moran, professor of biophysics, in his laboratories at the University of Chicago.

tion. In individuals lacking this enzyme, there would be a defect in cell metabolism. Knowing this and knowing which gene in the mitochondrial DNA is responsible could make it possible to normalize cell metabolism by replacement of the defective gene within the mitochondrial DNA. Or if failure in insulin production was an expression of another genetic deficit then administration of the appropriate unimpaired DNA might possibly afford a cure for diabetes.

Of course, a system for delivering corrective DNA to the patient's cells would also have to be available. But even this does not seem inconceivable. The extremely interesting work of Stanfield Rogers at Oak Ridge National Laboratory suggests a possibility. Rogers had shown that the Shope papilloma virus, nonpathogenic in man, is capable of inducing arginase production in rabbits at the same time as it induces tumor formation. Rogers found that among laboratory investigators working with the virus there is a significant reduction of blood arginine levels, apparently an expression of enhanced arginase activity. Might it not be possible then to use similar nonpathogenic viruses to carry into man pieces of DNA capable of replacing or repairing defective DNA genomes?

Obviously, all these speculations are well beyond our present investigative reach. Just how much beyond? A part of the answer to this question may depend on how soon we pass through what appears to be the greatest bottleneck in genetic research – the dearth of effective studies in nucleic acid chemistry. We have barely scratched the surface in seeking understanding of how DNA is organized into chromosomes. We use the term chromosomes for the DNA's of viruses and bacteria, but clearly these genomes are far smaller and less complicated than animal chromosomes. We are just beginning to fractionate chromosomes from one another. There is still no easy way to separate a given chromosome from the human karyotype. We do not know whether human DNA is circular or linear. Whereas great progress has been made in mapping the amino acid sequences in proteins such as myoglobin and gamma globulin, virtually nothing is known about the sequential arrangement of nucleotides in DNA. And we don't know where any particular gene sits on a chromosome, nor which genes are specifically related to a given disease state. Without knowing the parts, we can't hope to identify the flaws.

This is a contribution that must come from the chemist. The biologist has neither the tools nor the disposition to solve such problems. And regrettably our support for the chemist has lagged woefully behind our support for the disease-oriented biologist. We have done little or nothing to persuade chemists working in other areas of the great need and intellectual challenge that lies in nucleic acid chemistry. Obviously such persuasion must be backed by assurances of support.

To sum up, synthesis of biologically active viral DNA would appear to have significance for future medical progress provided it can be translated into basic understanding of the mechanisms subserved by DNA in the genetic control of both normal and aberrant physiologic functions. Such translation will depend on our ability to mobilize resources, particularly those encompassed in the discipline of nucleic acid chemistry, for the development of methods of analysis and modification of animal and human metabolic and biosynthetic processes.

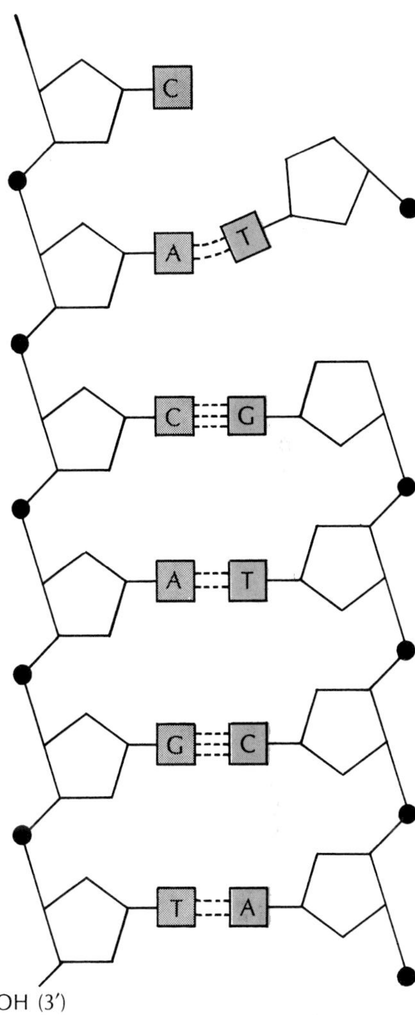

The above diagram indicates how synthesis of DNA proceeds on a single-stranded template, following the familiar base-pairing scheme of Watson and Crick – thymine with adenine, guanine with cytosine.

Section Five

Clinical Applications of Immunology in Prophylaxis and in Therapy

Chapter 23

Immunologic Reconstitution: The Achievement and Its Meaning

ROBERT A. GOOD
University of Minnesota

When Dr. Jerome A. L'Heureux telephoned from Meriden, Connecticut, we at the University of Minnesota were given an opportunity to test a concept of treatment which had evolved from basic experiments in our own and many other laboratories, as well as from our previous unsuccessful clinical efforts. As a result of this telephone call and the sequence of events it set in motion, we believe that a way may have been opened to treat a wide range of heretofore incurable and often fatal metabolic diseases. This belief is reinforced by a related and virtually simultaneous therapeutic experience reported by Dr. Fritz H. Bach and his colleagues at the University of Wisconsin.

Dr. L'Heureux's call was for the purpose of referring a four-month-old child with sex-linked lymphopenic immunologic deficiency. This rare condition, characterized by gross deficiency in both the cell-mediated and humoral antibody systems, had over three generations claimed the lives of 11 male children in the one family. All died in early infancy of infections with which they had been unable to cope because of their immunologic nullity. Dr. L'Heureux's young patient had already shown signs of following the same course, exhibiting a persistent pyoderma and low serum gamma globulin levels. On the basis of this, the history, and various other signs, a diagnosis of sex-linked immunologic deficiency had been made. In consultation with Drs. Gatti, Hong, Meuwissen, and Allen, a decision was made to bring the child and his parents and four sisters to Minneapolis. The reason for this "mass pilgrimage" will become apparent later on in this discussion. But before we reach that point, it is necessary to elaborate somewhat on the nature of the disease and on previous investigations that permitted both the characterization of the condition and the development of the therapeutic rationale we were prepared to test in this infant.

Sex-linked lymphopenic immunologic deficiency is one of about 20 separable and definable immunologic deficiency diseases. In this particular condition, the child is born lacking both of the major immunologic response systems: the thymus-dependent lymphocyte population upon which cell-mediated immune responses are based; and the thymus-independent lymphocyte population, the system analogous to the bursal-dependent system in birds, which accounts for the production of plasma cells, immunoglobulins, and the humoral antibodies required for defense against most bacterial, viral, and other infectious pathogens. In this specific disease, the deficiencies occur only in the male offspring, who, in a given family, have about a 50% chance of being born with the defect. The pattern obviously is one of an X-linked recessive genetic condition.

These children generally come to medical attention because they start very early in life to manifest susceptibility to infection. They develop persistent thrush. Similarly they do not get over virus infections in anything like the usual time. Measles infection is likely to lead to overwhelming and fatal pneumonia. Vaccination will lead to progressive vaccinia and vaccinia gangrenosa. And they are susceptible to clinical infection with a host of low-grade pathogens – fungi normally resident in the gastrointestinal and respiratory tracts (*Pneumocystis carinii*, etc.). It is interesting to note that in Sweden where BCG vaccination for tuberculosis is mandatory, these children will actually contract and succumb to BCGosis. Of the more than 10 million BCG vaccinations, there have been about a dozen deaths, all related to this immunologic deficiency.

If the physician alerted by the frequency and persistence of infection does a blood count on one of these patients, lymphopenia will be revealed. Further studies will reveal a lack of ABO group antibodies, a failure of response to antigenic stimulation, a failure to reject skin grafts, and the absence of the thymic shadow usually prominent on posterior-anterior chest x-rays in infants. In our experience, another very real problem with these children is that ordinary blood transfusion may be fatal. This was particularly well defined by Dr. Michael E. Miller, now at the University of Pennsylvania. Dr. Miller, formerly an associate at the University of Minnesota, clearly showed that transfusions in these infants produced fatal graft-vs-host (GVH) reactions. This is, of course, reasonable since the infants are unable to defend themselves against any foreign proteins and the transfused blood cells are able to mount an attack against the endogenous hematologic constituents.

Along the same lines, it is noteworthy that a number of investigators have considered the treatment of these children by replacement therapy with bone marrow transplants, thymus transplants, spleen cells, etc. These efforts to correct lymphopenia have in some instances had a measure of immunologic success, only to founder because of fatal, overwhelming GVH reactions. For example, Humphrey Kay of England supplied Dr. Hong and me with fetal liver as a stem cell source with which to treat one of these cases. We corrected the immunologic apparatus but the patient died of a GVH reaction. To date, it should be added, no treatment has been effective for severe GVH reactions either in experimental animals or in man.

The problem of GVH reactions might have proved insurmountable if it weren't for advances made in several of the laboratories dedicated to studies of transplantation biology. The first of these advances was the development of techniques for typing white blood cells, which can be credited to Dausset in France, Ceppellini in Italy, van Rood in Holland, Amos and Terasaki in the United States, among others. It was found that by matching leukocytes between donors and recipients, kidney transplantation was greatly abetted. Dr. Bach at Wisconsin then did a series of extremely meticulous family studies which confirmed earlier work by Ceppellini showing that multiple genes determining histocompatibility in humans operated at a single genetic locus.

Space does not permit detailed description of all of the relevant studies in this area. Suffice it to say that in our own studies we found that if mice were matched at this single locus – the H-2 locus in mice which corresponds to the HL-A in man – then one could achieve truly remarkable successes in homografting. But even more important for our purposes we confirmed the findings of a number of other scientists (Simonsen in England, Hasek and Ivanni in Czechoslovakia, Silvers and Billingham in Philadelphia) that when animals were matched at the major histocompatibility locus, the danger of fatal GVH reactions was obviated. Mild reactions did occur, but they were transient; the mice recovered and the homografts remained viable. The realization that this security stemmed from matching at the major histocompatibility locus was to prove vital to our subsequent clinical success.

With this knowledge, we now had all of the pieces required to solve the puzzle. Sorting them out in our own minds, we became convinced that, using Bach's technique for leukocyte matching, we should be able to match up siblings, and if the family were large enough, the chances would be good that the stem cells from one of the siblings could be used to cure the lymphopenic agammaglobulinemia syndrome without destroying the patient through a GVH reaction. The conviction was sufficiently deep so that with Hong and Gatti, I contributed an editorial to *The Lancet* which described the dangers of transfusion and

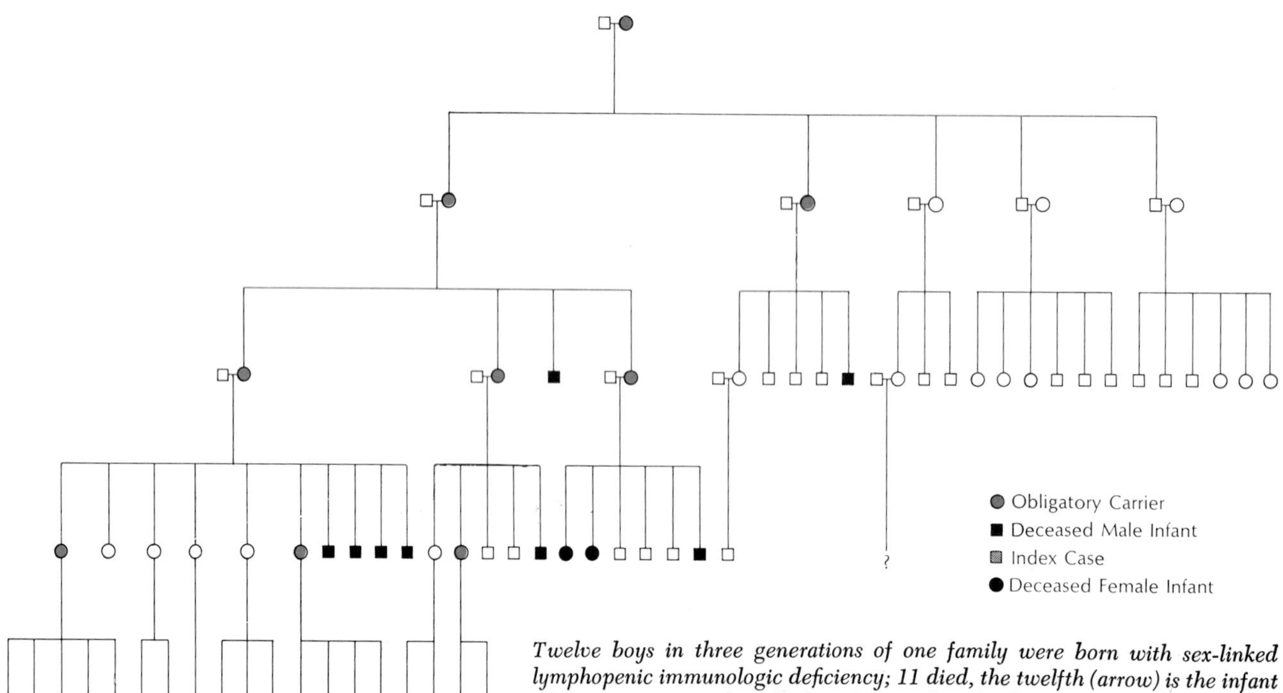

Twelve boys in three generations of one family were born with sex-linked lymphopenic immunologic deficiency; 11 died, the twelfth (arrow) is the infant whose treatment is described in this article. The deaths of two female infants indicated in this pedigree were unrelated to the disease.

went on to outline stem cell transfusion as a potential treatment for lymphopenic immunologic deficiency. I also suggested to a number of my colleagues that if they happened to get one of these patients, this approach should be considered. With this background in mind it should be easy to understand the excitement we felt when Dr. L'Heureux described his patient and told us that the little boy had four sisters. It seemed almost too good to be true since the genetically determined odds for siblings to match up at the HL-A locus are one in four.

When the child arrived in Minneapolis with his family, we immediately confirmed the diagnosis. The chest x-ray indicated absence of a thymic shadow. Hematologic study confirmed lymphopenia, immunochemical analyses the complete absence of IgM and IgA globulins and the presence of only a very small amount of IgG, probably largely attributable to the previous administration of exogenous gamma globulin. The child entirely lacked antibodies against the heterologous blood group, nor did he make antibodies against several antigens such as diphtheria toxoid and typhoid antigen. He also failed to develop any cellular immune responses. Finally, we were unable to find tonsils or adenoids or peripheral lymph nodes in this infant. As we have already mentioned, the child had begun to show the pattern of repeated infections that had always eventuated in death in patients with lymphopenic agammaglobulinemia. When he came to us, the baby was in the midst of a bout of pneumonia.

With the help of Dr. Paul Terasaki in Los Angeles, who carried out the leukocytotoxic typing of the blood cells, we checked the four sisters to see if any of them matched their little brother at the HL-A locus. And indeed, one of them proved to be a good but not perfect match, i.e., her blood was type O, her brother's type A. This mismatch worried us from the beginning, but because we were dealing with a progressive and fatal disease, we decided to attempt immunologic reconstitution.

We took 350 ml of peripheral blood from the matched sister, heparinized it and mixed it with 30 ml of 5% dextran. After sedimentation, the supernatant plasma was centrifuged and

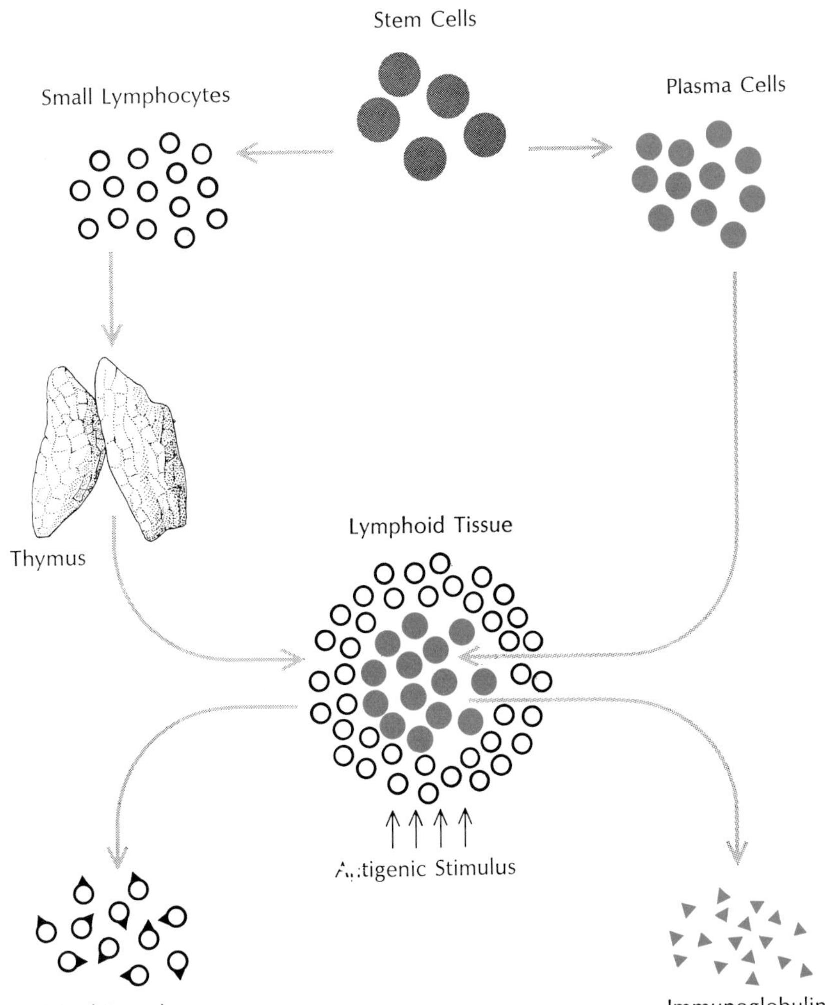

Normal differentiation of stem cells into thymus-dependent small lymphoctes, the mediators of cellular immunity, and into plasma cells capable of producing humoral antibodies is schematized above. In sex-linked lymphopenic immunologic deficiency, stem cells with the ability to differentiate in either way are apparently lacking.

leukocytes were resuspended in 70 ml of donor plasma at a final concentration of 5 x 10^6 lymphocytes/ml. From the same donor, 48 ml of bone marrow was aspirated from eight puncture sites around the iliac crest and the tibial bones. The total number of nucleated cells in the marrow aspirates was approximately 10^9. Both the leukocyte and bone marrow preparations were administered intraperitoneally.

Only a week after the bone marrow transplantation, we were confronted with what we could recognize as a "moment of truth." The baby began to vomit and became febrile. He developed a coarse, maculopapular erythematous rash over his back and face. We knew from our own experience and from previous reports that the rash was characteristic of a GVH reaction, the result of an attack by donor lymphocytes on the baby's skin – as if it were a whole-body skin graft. This was confirmed histologically. At the same time, the child developed hepatosplenomegaly and had some evidence of hemolytic anemia, which was apparently related to the ABO mismatch.

We now had to make a tough decision: whether to treat the GVH reaction or to gamble that in man, as in mouse, the reaction would be mild and transient so long as donor and recipient were matched at the major histocompatibility locus. Treating the reaction would have been tantamount to sacrificing the marrow transplant. The immunosuppressive measures required would destroy any donor stem cells that might be reconstituting the

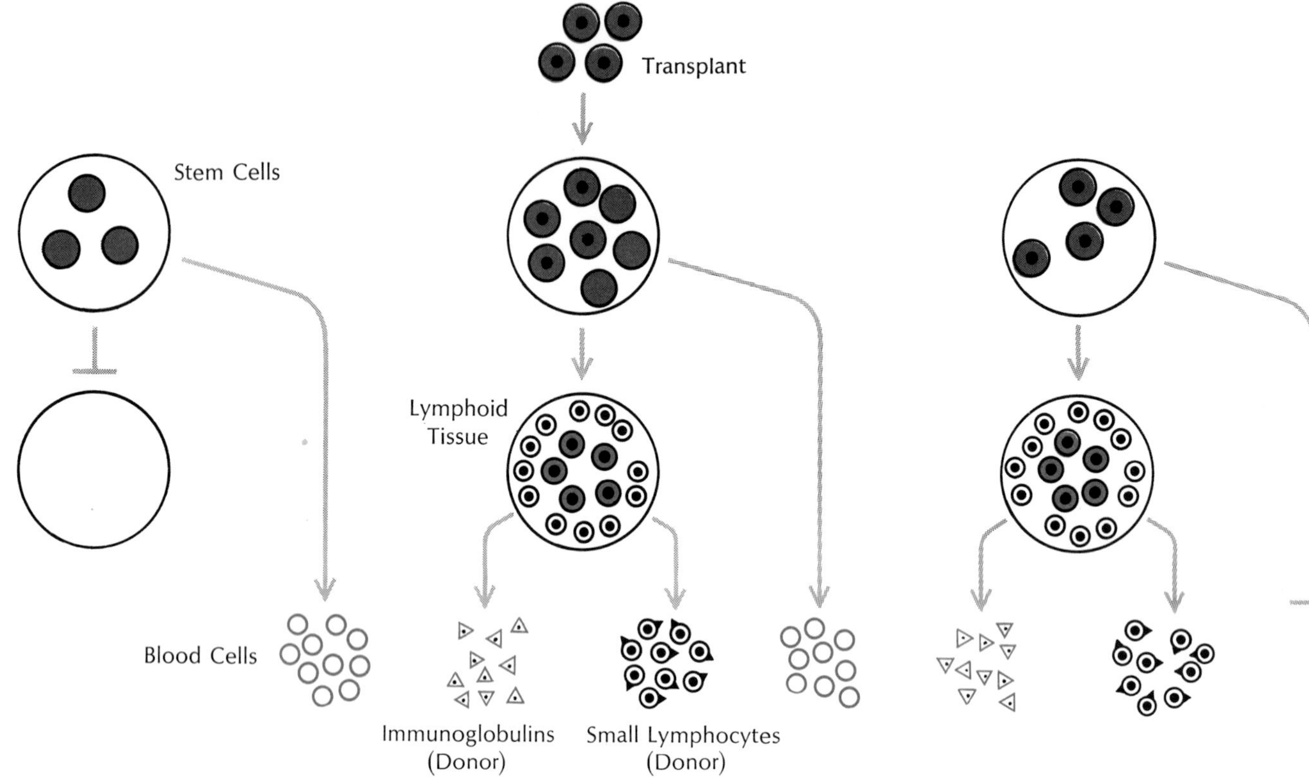

The treatment of the infant with lymphopenic immunologic deficiency is shown schematically. Before treatment, child's bone marrow contained stem cell precursors for all normal hematopoietic elements but completely lacked stem cells able to undergo lymphoid differentiation. A transplant of his sister's bone marrow provided a source for both immunoglobulins and small lymphocytes. However, the transplanted blood-forming stem cells attacked and destroyed the host's blood-forming stem cells (GVH

immunologic systems of the infant. We knew too that no methods of treating the GVH reaction had proved permanently effective to date. We chose to gamble. We restrained our impulse to intervene and waited for the reaction to subside. It did. In about a week, the fever and rash disappeared, as did the hepatosplenomegaly.

About the same time, evidence of immunologic reconstitution became manifest. By squash preparations and chromosomal analysis, we were able to determine that female cells were populating the little boy's marrow. Very rapidly, the child developed each of the classes of immunoglobulin. IgA appeared in secretions as well as blood; IgM appeared in the blood; IgG levels began to rise. In short, the child developed an ability to form circulating antibodies which was essentially like that of a normal infant. Moreover, a small lymphocyte population developed, and these cells showed a normal response to phytohemagglutinin (PHA) – a response which has been shown to reflect immunologic competence in the cell-mediated immune system. A thymic shadow was discernible on the chest x-ray. When we tested for immunity, the patient demonstrated that he could mount a delayed allergic response. Nor could the source of these new response capacities be doubted. We found that all of the responding peripheral lymphocytes and about 25% of the bone marrow cells could be identified as having a female karyotype.

The achievement was, of course, deeply gratifying. Not only had we accomplished a degree of immunologic reconstitution never previously observed in this type of disease but also we had learned something from the speed and extent of the response. It seemed to us that our findings bespoke a state of readiness in these patients. Although totally lacking in the effector mechanisms of immunity, the "factory sites" required for manufacture of immunologically competent cells and antibodies appeared to be completely adequate. All we had to do was to provide a line of stem cells capable of differentiation into lymphocytes and into antibody-producing plasma cells.

But neither our young patient nor we were out of the woods yet. Even as we were preparing an article describing our experience for *The Lancet*, the child's blood picture was becoming extremely disturbing. His white count started to fall and his platelet count to rise. As time went on, the platelet count turned down, the white count fell to very low levels, and he became severely anemic. When the marrow was closely studied, it was found that the pancytopenia could be traced to lack of cells forming erythrocytes, leukocytes, or platelets. In other words, he had an aplastic anemia which could be associated with the destruction of the recipient's A cells by the O-type donor cells. We look upon this as a GVH reaction, comprising a primary assault on blood-forming tissue and the peripheral blood. Experiments undertaken by Dr. Meuwissen in our laboratory showed that the reaction was related to the development of a specific cytotoxic antibody in the child's blood.

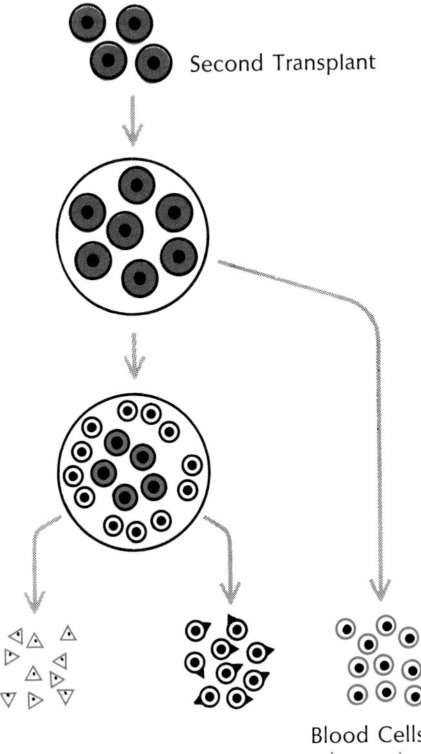

reaction) and the infant developed aplastic anemia. This was corrected by a second transplant of bone marrow, containing stem cells, from the same donor.

At this point, we were confronted with a situation in which we had taken a child who was immunologically virtually null but who had normal blood-forming capacities, and changed him into a child who was immunologically normal but had severe pancytopenia and aplastic anemia. It seemed to us, however, that while we had a new problem we already had a solution.

If an individual who was devoid of stem cells capable of differentiating into immunocompetent cells would so readily accept a transplant of such stem cells, we reasoned that an individual who had been made essentially devoid of blood-forming stem cells might be equally accepting of a transplant of those stem cells. This would hold, of course, only if there was no immunologic barrier to such a take. Acting on this rationale, we gave the child a second bone marrow transplant from his sister. This time there was no GVH reaction at all, indicating that a state of specific immunologic tolerance had already been induced. And very quickly, the child began to form red cells, white cells, and platelets, predominantly of O type and female karyotype; they had developed from the precursor cells of the sister.

Certainly, this experience afforded strong support for our theory that the defect in these patients is in their stem cells rather than in their ability to differentiate cells. In each of the two phases of our treatment, we placed normal stem cells into empty "factory sites," and each time the stem cells differentiated into the types of cells previously lacking. More important than the confirmation of our theory was that we had started with an infant whose prognosis for survival was nil, and ended with a child who, by many parameters, is now normal. All of his cell lines are normal; his immunologic capacity is normal; his lymphoid system is normal. All of the identifiable cells in his bone marrow are karyotypically female, and the predominant cell type in his peripheral blood is the O type of his sister rather than his own A type. That at least is the situation as this article is written four months after the second transplant.

Our satisfaction with the dramatic results of this treatment was compounded by Dr. Bach's simultaneous success in a patient with another immunologic deficiency disease, the Wiskott-Aldrich syndrome. This condition is characterized by thrombocytopenia and by a deficiency in the processing of antigen. As a result both cell-mediated and humoral-antibody responses are defective. As with lymphopenic agammaglobulinemia, the disease is sex-linked and confined to infant boys. The problem of Dr. Bach and his colleagues differed from ours in that the immunologic deficiency in Wiskott-Aldrich cases is not absolute and a bone marrow transplant could be expected to be rejected. He circumvented this problem by stimulating the patient to get both his cell-mediated and antibody-mediated immune responses going and synchronized. When this was done, he administered a massive dose of the cytotoxic drug cyclophosphamide. In this way, he succeeded in eliminating all host marrow function. Then he was able to undertake the bone marrow transplant. As in our case, the transplant of marrow from a female sibling, matching at the major histocompatibility locus, proved successful. The child is now thriving,

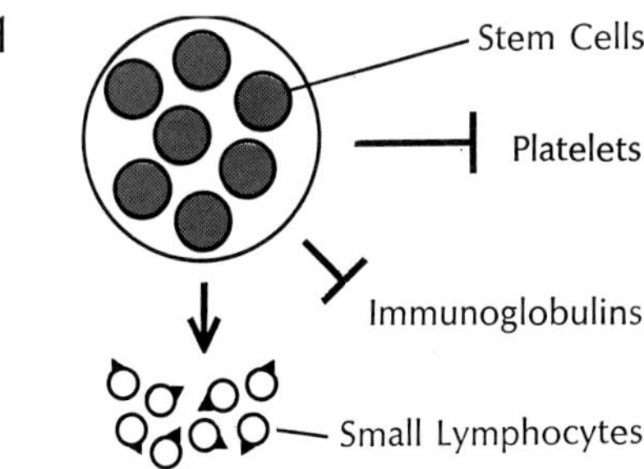

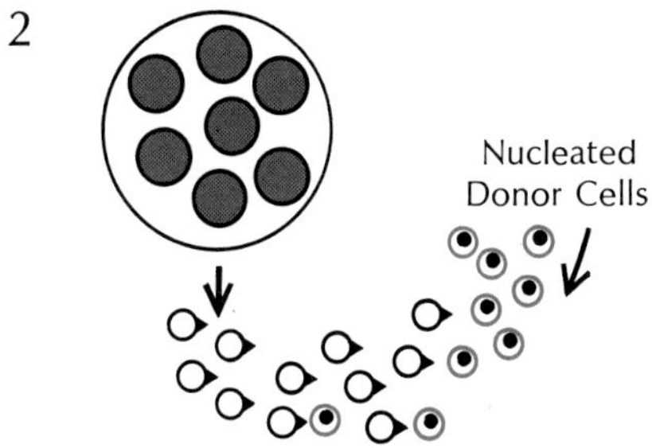

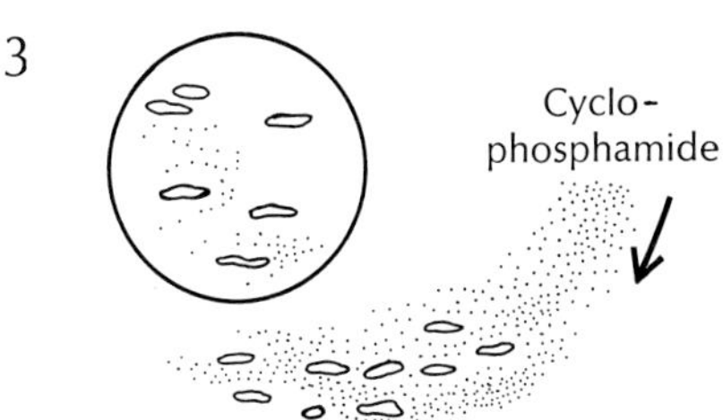

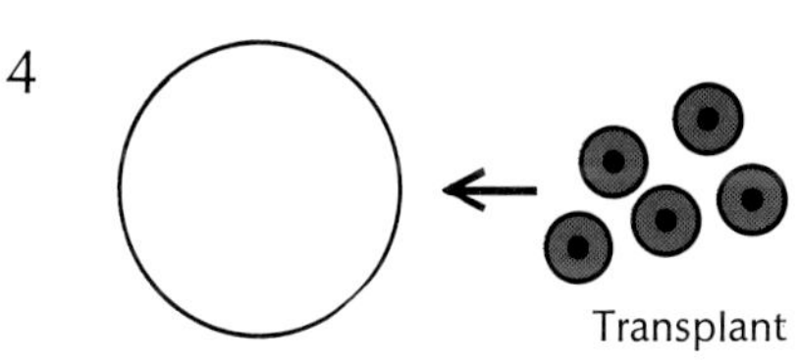

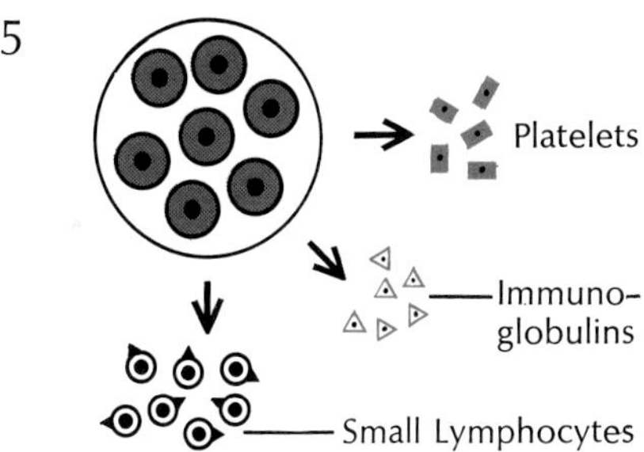

Prior to treatment by Bach et al at Wisconsin, child with Wiskott-Aldrich syndrome was deficient in platelets and in circulating immunoglobulins (1). Because his cell-mediated immune responses could cause rejection of a marrow transplant, donor cells were injected to elicit a lymphocyte response (2). Then cyclophosphamide was given to abolish cell-bound antibody response (3). A bone marrow transplant (4) then brought about normalization (5).

Summary of Minnesota Case: Specific Effects of Sequential Bone Marrow Transplants fo

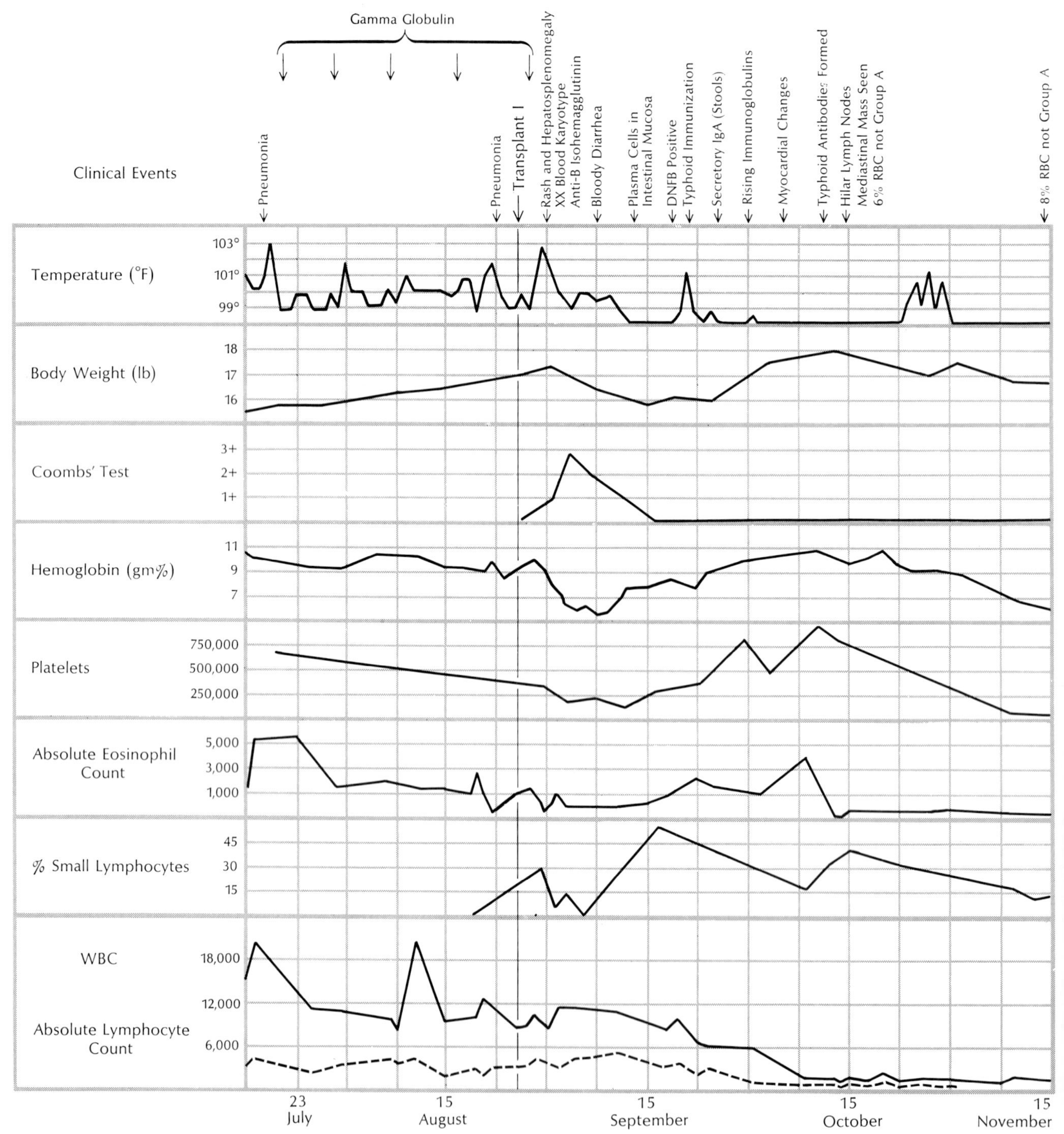

his platelet count is up and the bleeding problems consequent to thrombocytopenia have been eliminated.

In a very real sense, I believe that the Wisconsin case and ours provide complementary information. In that case, the problem was elimination of a defective system before "installation" of a normal one. This clearly raises the possibility of treating many inborn errors of metabolism – molecular diseases, if you will – on a cellular basis. In this sense, our problem was less difficult, since it should be easier to replace something that is lacking than it is to supplant something that is present but functionally deficient or aberrant. On the other hand, the fact that we were also confronted with ABO incompatibility gave us an opportunity to open a new avenue which may eventually lead to effective therapy for aplastic anemia – perhaps even for such genetically determined diseases as sickle cell anemia and thalassemia, for fatal granulomatous disease, and the leukemias and lymphomas. In other words, the sort of therapy that the molecular biologist would like to place on a molecular

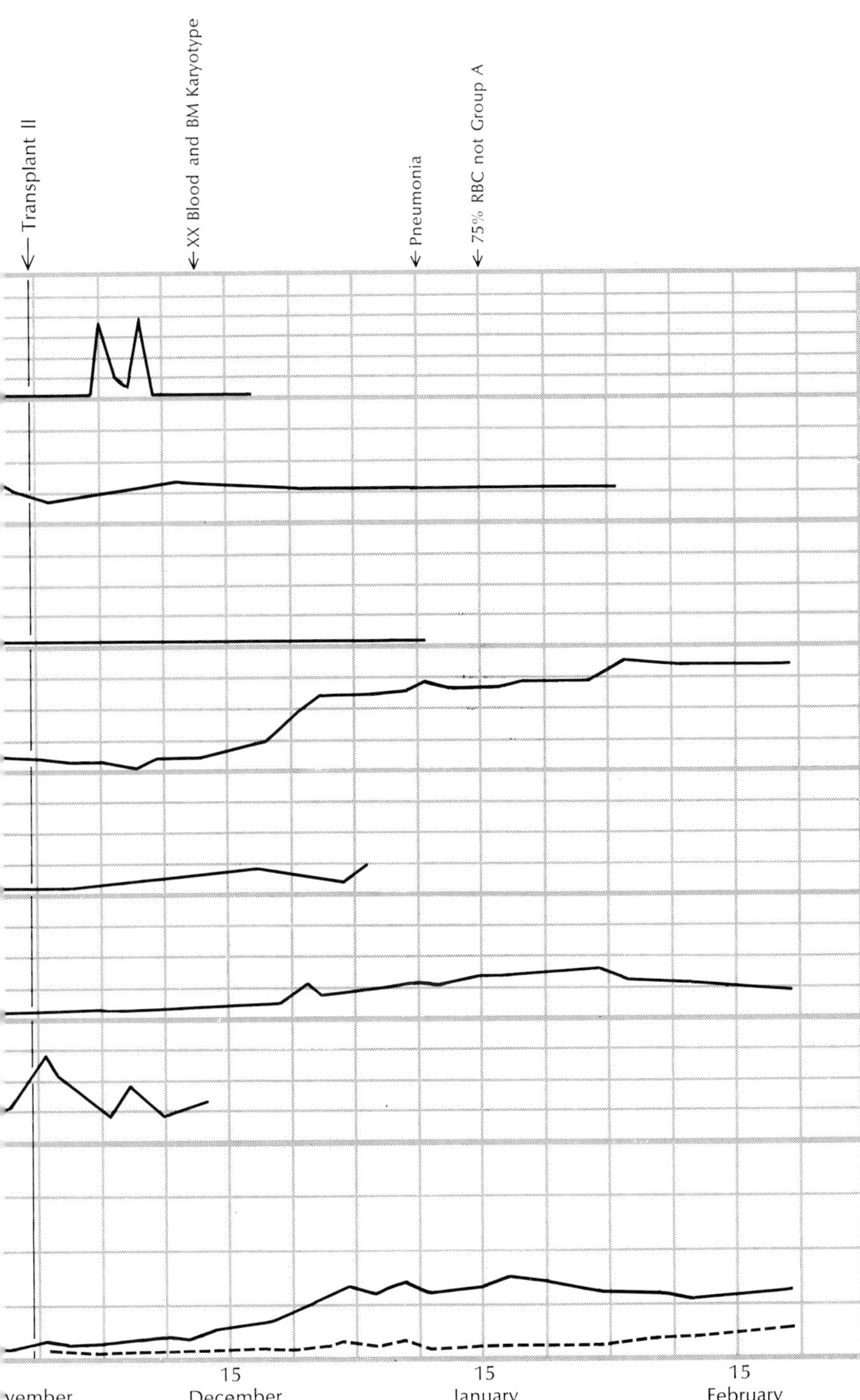

basis may actually be achievable through the manipulation of cells.

We have been able to follow our patient for nearly three years following the second successful marrow transplant. In this time, his immunologic systems have remained functionally normal. He has continued to produce in normal fashion both humoral-antibody and cellular responses to primary and booster antigenic stimulation. He was discharged from the hospital five months after his initial marrow transplant and has lived at home, reacting just as the other members of the family do to the usual environmental pathogens. His hematopoietic system and all of his peripheral blood cells have remained at normal levels. The youngster recently experienced an infection with EB virus, the agent associated with infectious mononucleosis. He developed the atypical transformed lymphocytes (Downey cells) that are characteristic of this infection. And, in a completely normal manner, he developed a vigorous antibody response to the virus, permitting control of the abnormal lymphoid cells. Four months after the onset of disease, his lymphocyte morphology was back to normal.

However, in one way this little boy remains different. All of his functioning lymphoid cells possess only female karyotype markers, clearly establishing their derivation from his sister's donated stem cells. All of his replicative bone marrow cells are also identifiable as derived from donor cells. By contrast, John Kersey in our laboratory has typed the child's fibroblasts and epithelial cells and these are entirely of male karyotype. Moreover, they have been shown to have the histocompatibility profile of the child with 1,7 HL-A markers. This is in distinction to the lymphocytes and hematopoietic cells, which are of the 1,3,7 HL-A type and identical to the histocompatibility pattern of the sister.

Since the boy was originally of blood group A and was converted to group O by his second marrow transplant from his sister, we have carefully studied the survival of group A cells in his circulation. It appears that the immunocompetent cells from his sister now tolerate the A cells as if there was no histocompatibility barrier between the two cell populations. When radioiodinated group A cells were injected, they survived as they would in a normal group A individual. A collaborative study with Yunis and Swanson in Minnesota and Cutbush-Crookston in Toronto showed that the child's group O erythrocytes have group A antigens on their surfaces. These appear to be products of his original A genes acting in concert with the Lewis genes of the donor cells and his original secretor genes to produce this antigenic anomaly. Thus, the surface of the patient's circulating red cells reflects two separate genetic origins.

By itself, this extraordinary case suggests many lessons. However, it does not stand alone as a harbinger of the future of cellular engineering.

With Hong and Amman, we in Minneapolis have already completely reconstituted a second child with a severe dual system immunodeficiency. And reports of successful immunologic reconstitution have also come from Leyden, Holland; Bern, Switzerland; Boston; and Los Angeles. The succésses to date have been limited to situations in which well-matched sibling donors were used. Mismatches across the strong histocompatibility locus have thus far failed in clinical practice because of the inability to overcome severe and fatal graft-vs-host reactions. But methods already have been developed to permit transplantation across the major HL-A barrier in mice, dogs, and even monkeys. If cellular engineering fulfills the promise of these initial experiments, many hematologic diseases in addition to the severe dual system immunodeficiencies and immunologically induced pancytopenias could be treated with hope for success.

Mention has been made of applying this approach to malignant diseases such as leukemia or Hodgkin's disease. In such situations, of course, one would have to cope with an additional problem – how to prevent the transplanted cells from themselves undergoing malignant change. One would have to be particularly cognizant of this danger if one accepts the postulated role for viruses and other infectious agents in oncogenesis.

There is some evidence that this is not an insoluble problem. Attempts have been made in the past to treat leukemia by knocking out the hematopoietic system with huge doses of radiation or cytotoxic drugs and then repopulating the marrow by transplantation. This was first done between identical twins, and in each case the procedure was temporarily successful. This success was limited, however, since eventually the newly transplanted synergeneic cells seemed to "catch" the leukemia. Barnes and Loutit demonstrated that in mice, while this would happen with synergeneic cells (such as these of identical twins) it did not always happen with allogeneic cells. In fact, Mathé has reported comparable clinical success in patients treated for leukemia by the transplantation of allogeneic stem cells, but his cases ultimately succumbed to GVH reactions.

It now becomes clear from the patients described in this article that it might be possible to utilize major histocompatibility-locus matching to reduce the risk of fatal GVH reactions. One would then employ allogeneic cells to take advantage of the genetic differences that appear to affect susceptibility to leukemia and then to utilize immunologic reconstitution to replace a "failed" anticancer surveillance system with one still competent against cancer. In this way, one might hope to attain immunologically what chemotherapists have sought unsuccessfully to do, getting rid of the "final" leukemic cell. This possibility must be seriously considered if one regards transplantation defenses as a system which has evolved over 300 million years as a means for the body's ridding itself of "foreigners."

All this is, obviously, highly speculative. But even without these speculations we regard our experience with this single case of lymphopenic immunologic deficiency as particularly satisfying. The agammaglobulinemias are relatively rare experiments of nature. In the past they have permitted us to dissect and understand how the normal body functions immunologically, simply because the understanding of any physiologic function is greatly aided by the opportunity to see what happens when it is deleted. Thus these patients have taught us a tremendous amount about how the body defends itself against infection, against neoplasia, against foreign tissue. For us who have used these patients in this way it is a very exciting event to be able to return something to them by way of treatment.

Chapter 24

Immunosuppression: The Challenge of Selectivity

ROBERT S. SCHWARTZ
Tufts University

Among the many recent advances in immunology must be counted those in the field of immunosuppressive therapy. The progress to date has brought us into lines of investigation that appear to converge on what must be regarded as the ultimate goal – the ability to suppress the response to a single antigen, or constellation of antigens, while leaving all other immune responses intact. And we have come far enough to be confident that this objective can be achieved – most probably by antigenic manipulation of the patient.

It is the purpose of this chapter to review the various modalities that have been employed to suppress immune responses, to describe briefly the several classes of immunosuppressive agents, and to place these agents into their clinical context, a context that includes organ transplantation, autoimmune disease, and malignant disease. The momentum of such a review can quite easily carry us into the future and into discussion of the induction of specific immunologic tolerance.

For purposes of systematic review, it is perhaps most convenient to divide immunosuppressive agents into four classes – radiation, the corticosteroids, cytotoxic chemicals, and antilymphocyte serum (ALS). While these are generally considered to be the four main groups of agents, there is a fifth, most fascinating class of immunosuppressants – antibodies themselves. Discussion of these along with discussion of the role of antigen in determining immunosuppressive specificity will lead naturally into what may well be the most intriguing and promising phenomena in the field, tolerance and enhancement.

Radiation: Radiation is the oldest known immunosuppressive agent, its properties in this regard having been

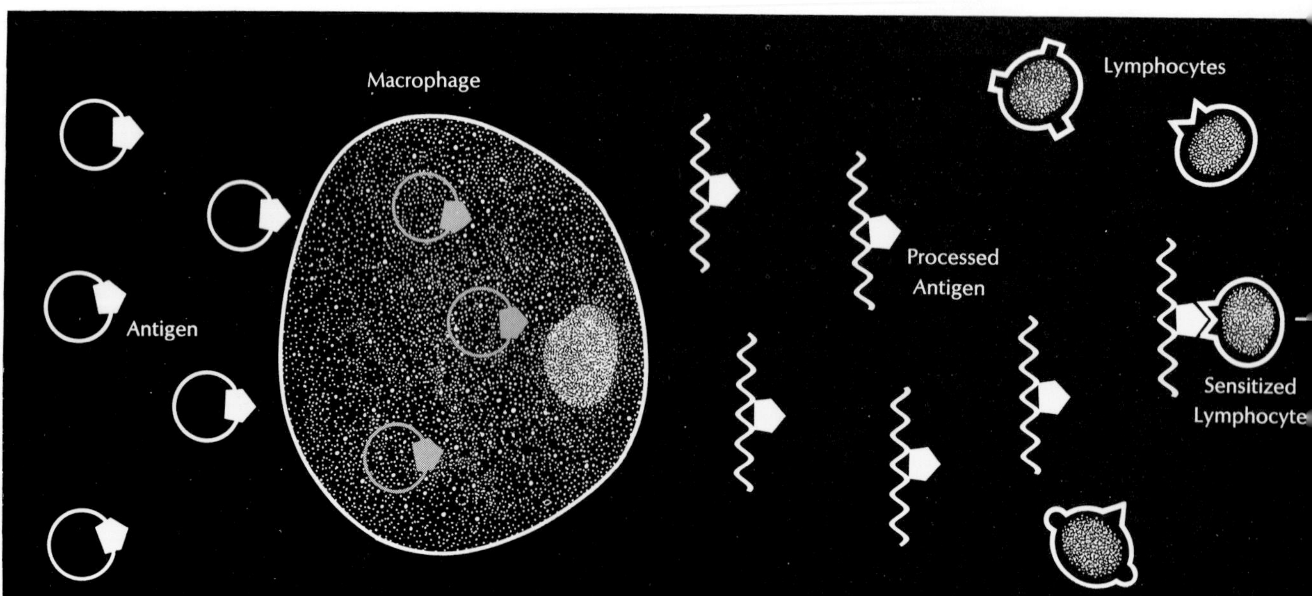

As a basis for understanding the sites of action of various immunosuppressive agents, the steps in immune response from antigenic stimulation to creation of the immunologic lesions are schematized above. The antigen is processed by the macrophage, then encounters and sensitizes the small lymphocytes. As a result, the lymphocytes differentiate into cells rich in polyribosomes. Eventu-

described in the last century. There can be no question about the ability of high doses of whole body irradiation to abolish all immunologic responsiveness in the animal. However, at this time, such irradiation has no role in clinical medicine. It will be recalled that in the early days of organ transplantation, whole body irradiation was used. But the dangers of the approach far outweighed any benefits and the method has now been abandoned. There is one possible exception to this statement: the work being done by some transplant groups with extracorporeal irradiation of the blood, which is of course tantamount to whole body irradiation but carries considerably reduced risks to the patient. By and large, though, extracorporeal irradiation has proved cumbersome and difficult to manage in human beings and is far from perfected. About all one can say at this point about the practical role of whole body irradiation in transplantation is that it may eventually prove to have some adjunctive value when employed in combination with other immunosuppressive modalities.

While radiation has not proved to be a clinically useful immunosuppressant, it has served to elucidate much about the mechanisms of action involved in the inhibition or abolition of immune responses, both its own mechanisms and those of other agents that, immunologically speaking, are radiomimetic. The corticosteroids fall into this category. Radiation inhibits antibody synthesis by destruction of small lymphocytes, and its mechanism is undoubtedly the depletion of these antigen-sensitive cells. This results in depriving the antigens of cellular components with which to interact. The problem with radiation is simply that it requires lethal or near-lethal doses to destroy all of the antigen-sensitive cells in the body.

Corticosteroids: With corticosteroids, the problem is different. In some species, depletion of small lymphocytes by adrenal corticosteroids is relatively simple. Rats, mice, and rabbits are extremely sensitive to the immunosuppressive activity of the corticosteroids. However, there are other species – among them man – that are resistant, or at least whose small lymphocytes are resistant, to corticosteroids. In point of fact, there is no really valid evidence that corticosteroids are immunosuppressive in man. Most relevant studies have failed to demonstrate that antibody synthesis is suppressed in human beings by steroid treatment. Here, it should be noted, is an area that requires a great deal of new investigation. Most of the studies on the relationships between immune competence and steroids were carried out years ago and the doses used were the "old-fashioned" amounts now generally recognized as homeopathic, e.g., 300 mg of cortisone a week. It is time that new investigations were undertaken employing newer steroids at clinically effective levels, e.g., 60 mg of prednisone a day in an adult patient.

Obviously one cannot ignore the fact that in clinical practice the corticosteroids have proved most important in the treatment of immunologic disorders and in facilitating homograft acceptance. If one discounts cortisone as an immunosuppressive agent, how can this experience be explained? One must appreciate the complex activities that adrenal corticosteroids produce in the body. Most notably, in relationship to transplants one must take into account the ability of these hormones to act as anti-inflammatory agents and to disrupt phagocytosis.

In graft rejection the central biologic event is of course the interaction between antibody and antigen, which in itself often evokes a strong inflammatory reaction. The possibility therefore exists that corticosteroids may en-

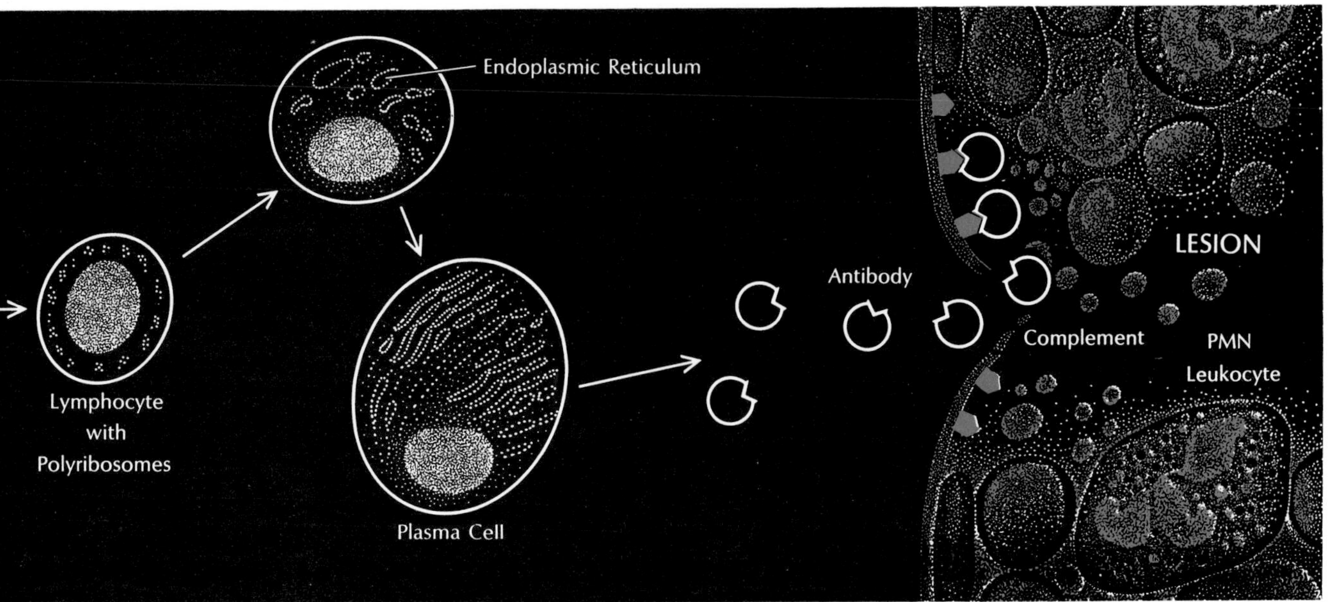

ally, the polyribosomes organize along the endoplasmic reticulum (ER). The ER-containing cells are the immediate precursors of the antibody-producing plasma cells. Antibodies, after complexing with their corresponding antigens, then activate complement and this attracts polymorphonuclear leukocytes, thus producing the inflammatory phase of the immunologic lesion.

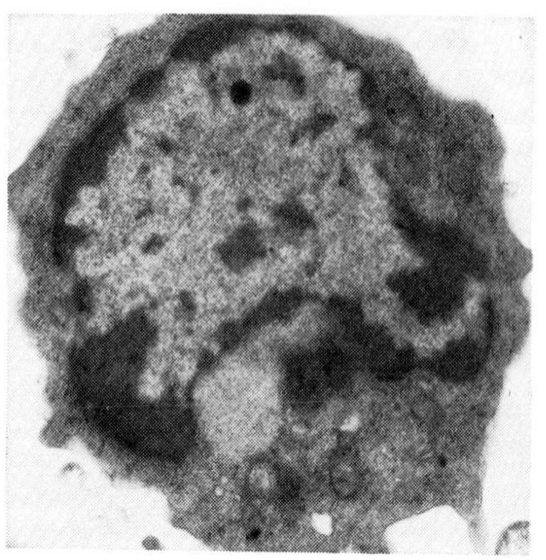

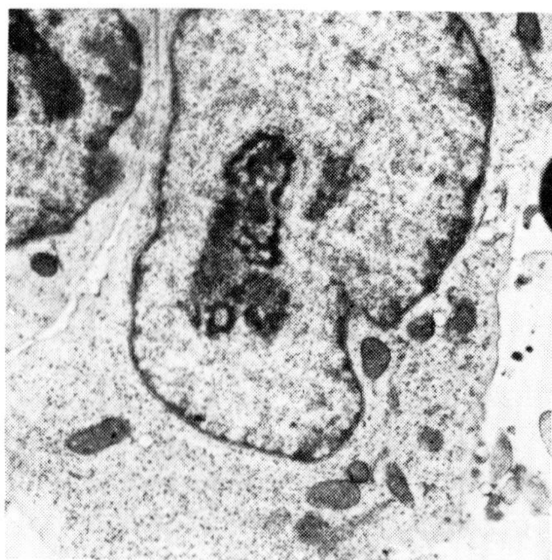

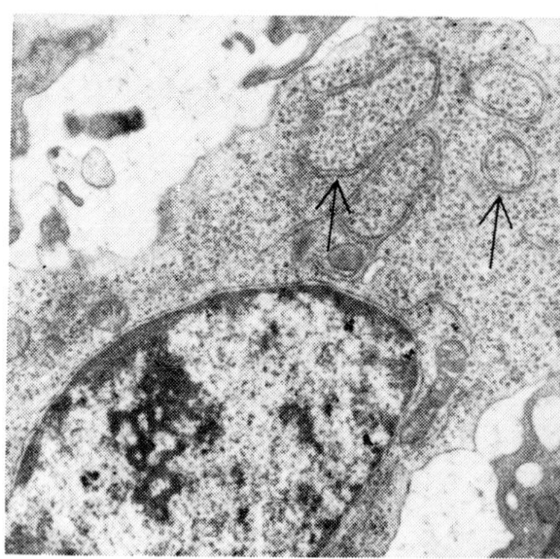

Four of the cell types involved in the immune response scheme that appears on the two preceding pages are illustrated in these electronmicrographs by Dr. Janine André-Schwartz. At the left is the resting lymphocyte, which becomes sensitized after encountering processed antigen. Next is the lymphocyte, which has begun its metamorphosis into an antibody-producing cell by ac-

hance the chances of graft acceptance by suppressing inflammation and thereby improving the host environment for the graft. Similarly, the known ability of corticosteroids to evoke or enhance infections by a number of bacteria is explicable on a nonimmunologic basis. For example, corticosteroids inhibit various aspects of the phagocytic process, including the release of lysozymes from granulocytes. In short, we must be on guard against falling into the simplistic assumption that all effects on processes in which immunologic responses participate are necessarily immunologically based, particularly when multifaceted substances such as the corticosteroids are involved.

Cytotoxic chemicals: As a general rule, almost all of the known antileukemia and anticancer agents have been shown to be immunosuppressive in one system or another. The following discussion is confined to those groups that either have been effective clinically or that hold some promise of such efficacy.

As a starting point we might consider the alkylating agents, whose prototype is nitrogen mustard. The most recently developed and clinically most useful alkylating agent is cyclophosphamide, which appears to be an extremely active and powerful immunosuppressant. Next come the classical antimetabolites, exemplified by such purine antagonists as 6-mercaptopurine (6-MP). In terms of current clinical practice the most significant of these agents is azathioprine (Imuran), which is 6-MP modified by the addition of an imidazole ring. The purpose of this chemical maneuver was to inhibit the biologic oxidation of 6-MP in the hope that this would smooth out its biologic processing. While there is evidence in mice that the therapeutic index of azathioprine is greater than that of 6-MP, there is not as yet any such evidence in man. Nevertheless, azathioprine appears to be enjoying great popularity as an immunosuppressive agent.

Next are the folic acid antagonists, typified by methotrexate. Extremely active both biochemically and immunologically, methotrexate may be a drug whose full potential has not yet been tapped. One possible reason is that the drug is excreted by the kidney so that its use in patients with any degree of renal impairment is contraindicated, and obviously this precludes its employment as an immunosuppressant in kidney transplant procedures. But methotrexate has been impressive when administered as treatment for dermatomyositis and systemic lupus erythematosus, and this drug might prove of major importance in transplanting organs other than the kidney.

Antilymphocyte serum: Certainly no other agent has caused as much excitement — some of it, to be sure, generated by nonconstructive press publicity, but some of it certainly justified — nor more intensive research than has ALS. The rationale of ALS is simple. By raising a specific antiserum against the human lymphocyte in an animal that is an effective antibody producer — the horse, for example — one should be able to direct an immunologic attack against those cells known to participate in delayed hypersensitivity reactions, including reactions against organ transplants. ALS undoubtedly has a vast potential. It is a powerful biologic agent that approaches the objective of immunosuppressive specificity defined in the first paragraph of this article. But, as will be seen, it falls far short of this goal and has inherent problems associated with its foreign-protein origin.

Taking these problems one by one, one must note that ALS shears off the entire delayed hypersensitivity response capacity, and not just the response to the particular delayed hypersensitivity reaction one wishes to combat (homograft rejection). Since cellular immunity is of particular importance in the defense against viruses, it comes as no surprise that ALS has a tremendous potency for inhibiting host responses to these infective agents. ALS will greatly enhance deliberate infection with viruses in experimental animals. This has been demonstrated not only with classic infectious viruses such as vaccinia but also, most importantly and most ominously, with oncogenic viruses.

When one gives mice leukemia viruses and at the same time injects ALS, the result is a marked acceleration in the appearance of malignancies associated with these viruses. Obviously, this phenomenon could be of major clinical importance and must greatly encourage conservatism in the use of ALS. Another warning sign with regard to ALS stems from the recent experience with cardiac trans-

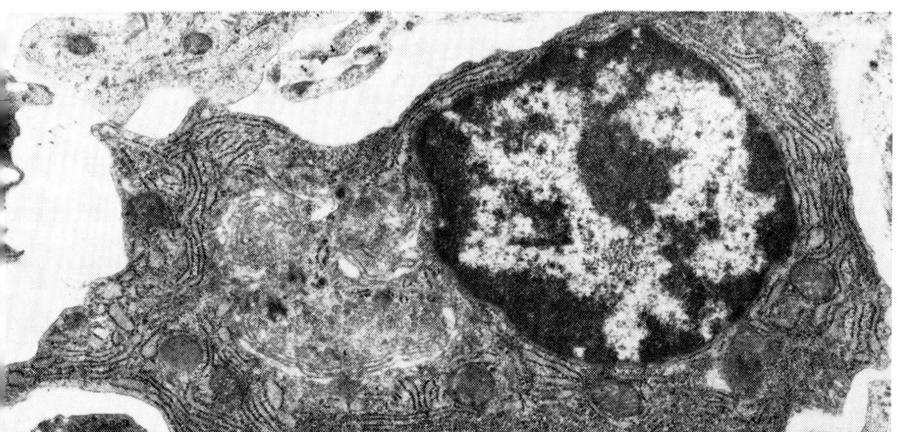

quisition of polyribosomes. The organization of these polyribosomes into rough endoplasmic reticulum (arrows) is visible in the third electronmicrograph. Finally one sees the fully developed plasma cell, which is capable of producing specific antibody.

plantation. There have been several cases of pneumonia caused by herpes simplex in transplant recipients, at least two of them fatal. Since these patients were treated with ALS and since herpes is an extremely rare cause of viral pneumonia under conventional conditions, the possibility of a causal relationship looms large.

The inherent toxicity of ALS as a foreign protein is an equally challenging and thorny problem. Ironically, the ALS-treated patient is likely to respond to the foreign protein just because his circulating antibody mechanisms are left intact while his delayed hypersensitivity responses are effectively suppressed. One therefore is confronted by risks such as serum sickness or anaphylaxis. Starzl, who is the transplant surgeon with the greatest experience with ALS, has reported that many of his transplant patients at the University of Colorado have had allergic reactions to ALS. Other investigators have reported situations in which ALS reactions have been lethal, and I believe that at least two heart transplant recipients have died of anaphylactic shock, probably in response to ALS.

One approach to the solution of this major problem has been to combine ALS administration with that of Imuran. According to recent reports, the combination works well in rats, but this does not necessarily mean that it will be useful in man. Among other objections, this double-agent regimen obviously constitutes the very pan-immunosuppression that should be avoided, with one agent attacking the circulating gamma globulins, the other directed against the delayed hypersensitivity mechanism.

The problem of specificity has recurred repeatedly in this article and, indeed, has been characterized as a keystone of all efforts to develop more effective immunosuppressive substances. The ability of ALS to inhibit delayed hypersensitivity while having relatively slight effect on humoral anti-

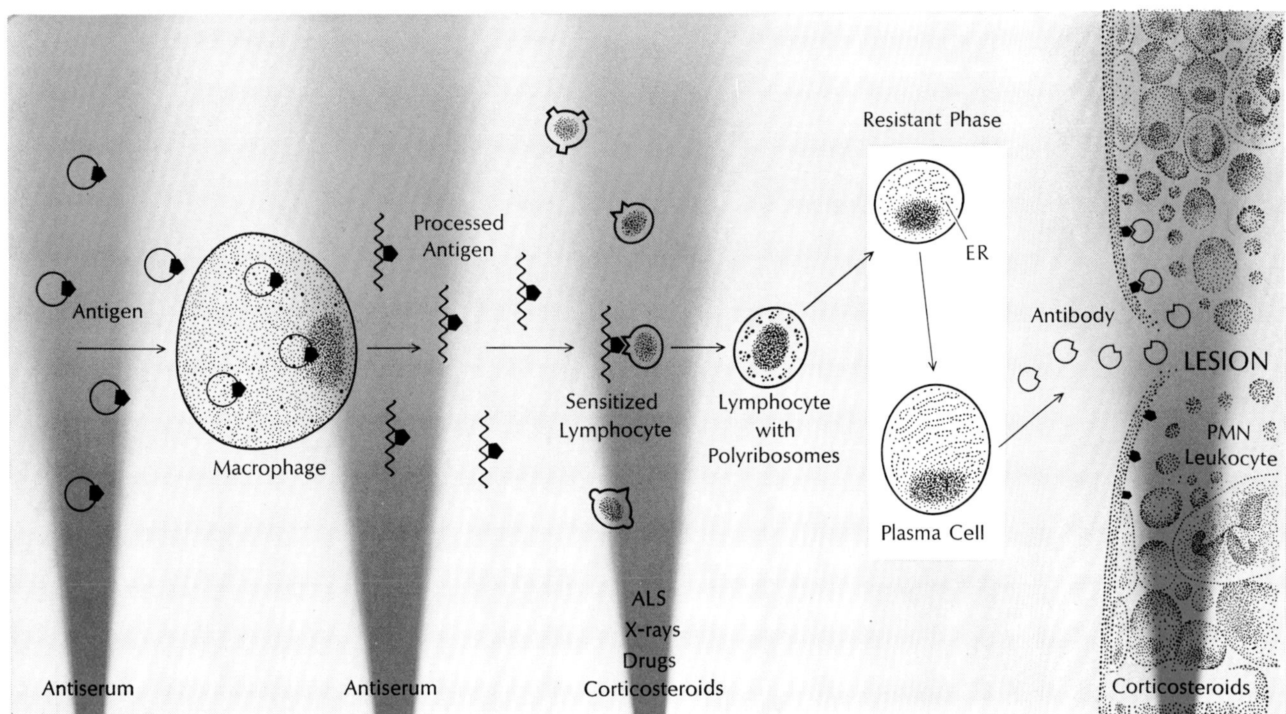

The "sites" of action of various immunosuppressive agents: Specific antiserum binds and nullifies the immunogenicity of antigen either before or after its processing by the macrophage. Cytotoxic drugs, x-rays, ALS, and (in some species) corticoids all act upon lymphocytes before the development of the endoplasmic reticulum. The corticoids may also exert their effects by inhibiting phagocytosis or by curbing inflammation. A phase of resistance to immunosuppression is also suggested.

bodies is a rough approximation of the type of selectivity being sought. It is also known that other agents – radiation, corticosteroids, and cytotoxic chemicals – block IgG synthesis much more successfully than they do IgM production. This is the probable explanation for the great resistance of cold agglutinin disease, which is mediated by IgM antibody, to immunosuppressive therapy. There may be some instances in which this immunosuppressive "gradient" among the classes of antibody will prove adequate to permit safe and effective therapy. We'd be very pleased, for example, to have an immunosuppressant that attacked only the IgE antibodies now known to be responsible for hay fever. The problem is that while the necessary specificity can be set up under precisely determined experimental conditions, in actual clinical situations the overlap is too great. Thus even ALS, with its predilection for cellular immunity, cannot select between the undesirable cell-bound antibodies, those responsible for homograft rejection, and the cell-bound antibodies necessary for immunity against viruses and possibly against oncogenesis.

Immunosuppressive antibody: Before we discuss more fully the laboratory manipulations involved in the effort to achieve real selectivity it is important to turn to a fifth class of immunosuppressive agents, one in which specificity is inherent – antibody. The most striking example of antibody itself being immunosuppressive is seen in the prevention of erythroblastosis fetalis by anti-Rh antiserum. Here one has the perfect immunosuppressive agent – a nontoxic, highly specific biologic substance that inhibits one and only one kind of immune response.

The exact mechanism by which antibody acts in this capacity is still somewhat in dispute. Originally, investigators termed antibody blockade of immunologic response the enhancement phenomenon. Most of the work in this area was done with tumors. Animals were immunized with lyophilized tumor extracts, provoking a circulating antibody response. A tumor graft was then placed on an animal immunized in this manner, and the animal did not reject the graft. It has now been shown that similar results can be obtained in systems other than the tumor graft situation and that there is a feedback type of mechanism applicable to immune responses in general. One can inhibit the response to a foreign protein by passively immunizing the animal with antiserum. In our own laboratory we employ sheep red cells and we can block the immune response to these erythrocytes by giving anti-sheep red cell serum to a recipient animal.

Two recent papers by Rowley and Fitch of the University of Chicago reported that a specific antiserum can inhibit delayed hypersensitivity in the rat and, perhaps more significantly, that antiserum against the donor kidney will markedly prolong the survival of kidney grafts in the rat.

It is thought by some that antibody acts as an immunosuppressant by preempting the immunogenic sites on the antigen. This bars recognition of the antigen and therefore nullifies the immune response it would provoke ordinarily. However, our own experimental data in the system that we have studied favor an interference at the level of the macrophage. This presupposes a scheme, not yet entirely proved, by which antigen is picked up by the macrophage and processed there into an immunogenic unit. This then comes in contact with the lymphocyte and provokes antibody formation. Our concept is that "enhancing" antibody binds to the macrophage-processed antigen and blocks its interaction with the next cell in the series, the lymphocyte. A third possibility, involving transplants, is that antibody coats the graft and prevents access of lymphocytes to its antigens.

Having touched on the role of antibody in immunosuppression, it is appropriate to turn now to the role of antigen. Perhaps we could introduce this discussion with a question: How can we engineer immunochemical specificity into a cytotoxic compound?

The day may well come when a compound with the ability to confer such specific tolerance can be found or synthesized. At this time, however, the only substance known to have this capacity is antigen. We know that to some extent immunosuppression can be achieved by desensitization with antigen. What we are now trying to do is to combine cytotoxic compounds – which are highly specific at the molecular level but anything other than specific at the cellular or immunologic levels – with antigens, in an effort to steer the cytotoxic agent to specificity of action.

Perhaps the best way to explain this approach is by describing experiments in our own laboratory and in a number of others. Several years ago we gave rabbits bovine serum albumin (BSA) as an antigen and then treated them with 6-MP for two-week periods. A month later we challenged the rabbits with both BSA and bovine gamma globulin (BGG). The rabbits failed to respond to the BSA but had a normal immunologic response to the BGG. It should be stressed that at the time of rechallenge with BSA the animals were not receiving any drug treatment. Although they were able to respond normally to an antigen not given during the period of drug treatment (BGG), they had lost their ability to respond to the antigen administered with the immunosuppressant

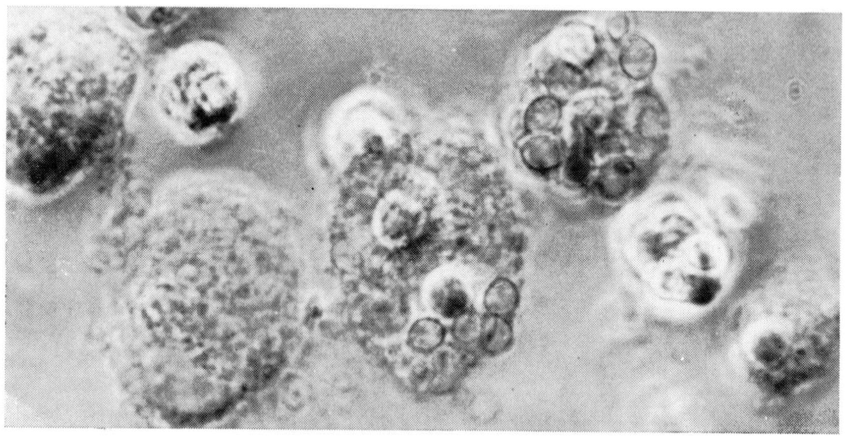

Macrophage ingestion of antigen is shown by phase microscopy. In this slide large numbers of sheep erythrocytes can be seen within the phagocytic cells.

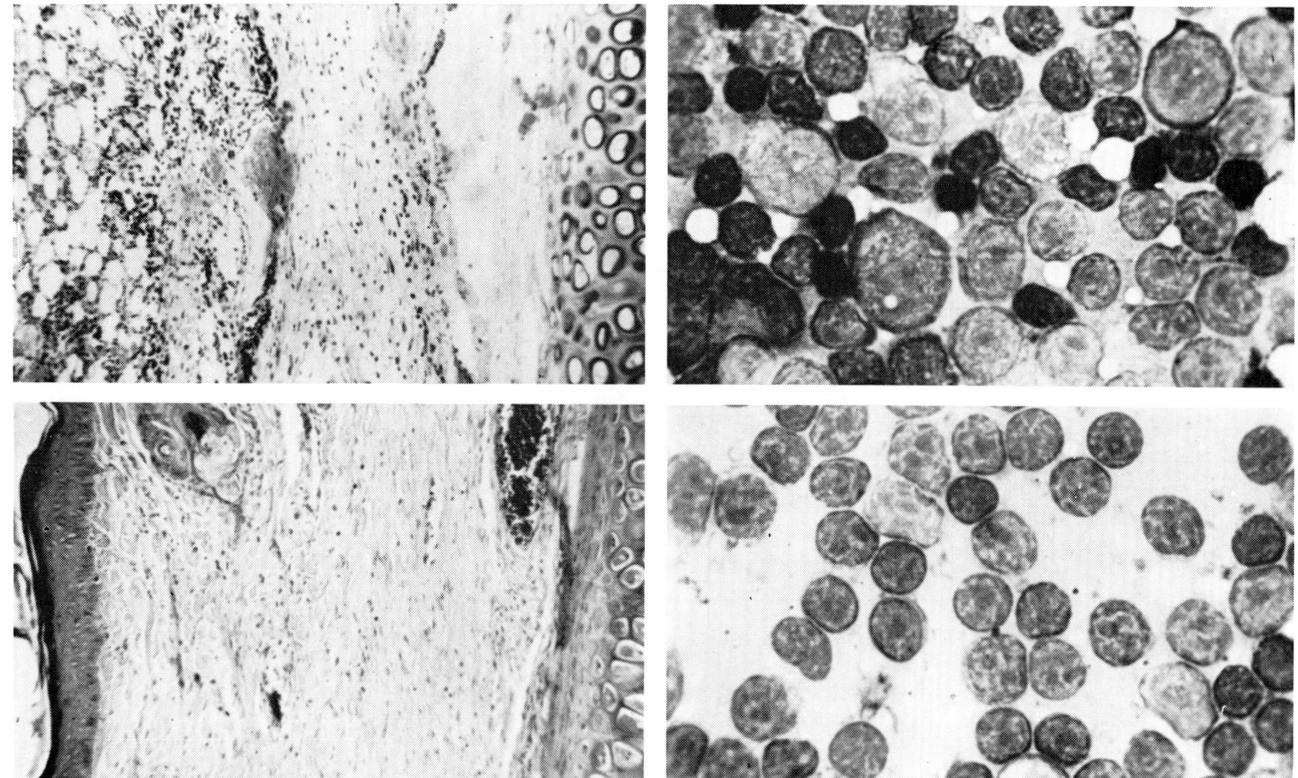

Effect of 6-MP on skin grafts in the rabbit is shown histologically. Untreated graft (top l. and r.) is being rejected; the lymphocyte population contains many activated large lymphocytes. Drug-treated graft is being accepted; only small lymphocytes are visible.

drug. The drug had induced tolerance in adult animals analogous to the tolerance produced in newborn animals in Medawar's classic experiments.

Since these early experiments other investigators have elaborated on the concept. A particularly intriguing application was made by Salvin, now at the University of Pittsburgh, in which he was able to prevent the development of autoimmune thyroiditis. He injected thyroglobulin into guinea pigs, a maneuver that normally results in thyroiditis. However, by giving a short course of treatment with cyclophosphamide Salvin not only blocked the development of the autoimmune disease but also showed that these animals were refractory to repeated challenges with thyroglobulin mixed in an adjuvant. In short, these animals lost their ability to form antithyroid antibodies and became tolerant of thyroglobulin antigen. He has repeated this experiment successfully in a number of other systems, in all of which tolerance was induced by a very brief course of cyclophosphamide. Patterson at the University of Chicago has done essentially the same thing, using as his model system experimental allergic encephalomyelitis. Again the drug was cyclophosphamide.

In current studies largely supported by the National Institutes of Health, we are working with a system that we find very intriguing, the response of mice to sheep erythrocytes. Normally, a mouse will make a very good antibody response to just a single injection of the erythrocytes. But it can be made tolerant of sheep red cells with just one injection of cyclophosphamide. The dose, incidentally, is only about 100 mg/kg of body weight, well below the LD_{50} of 250 mg. This basic experiment has been done by Frisch at the University of Oregon, Aisenberg at Massachusetts General Hospital, and Dietrich of Basel. The tolerance produced is extremely specific, since these mice will respond perfectly normally to horse erythrocytes. One of the most promising aspects of this system has been our ability to maintain this tolerance for many months after administering one dose of cyclophosphamide. Tolerance must be maintained by repeated doses of antigen, but the animals grow normally, show no signs of toxicity, and are immunologically completely competent except for the single deletion of responsiveness to sheep erythrocytes.

What we believe we're doing in these experiments is greatly increasing the selectivity of cyclophosphamide activity. In other words, we are employing the antigen to select a group of cells highly sensitive to the cytotoxic effect of the immunosuppressive drug. These cells are therefore eliminated and with this elimination we are abolishing the ability to make antibody to sheep erythrocytes. In short, what has been achieved is the specific deletion of immunologic activity against a selected or defined antigenic configuration; i.e., tolerance.

More recently, the nature of the antigen-activated cell eliminated by cyclophosphamide has been elucidated. It is a thymus-dependent lymphocyte, which, interestingly, has also been identified as the target cell for ALS. Perhaps the thymus-dependent lymphocyte is the point of leverage for many other immunosuppressants. This speculation has an optimistic implication for the prospects of tolerance induction by immunosuppressants, since current evidence indicates that, of all

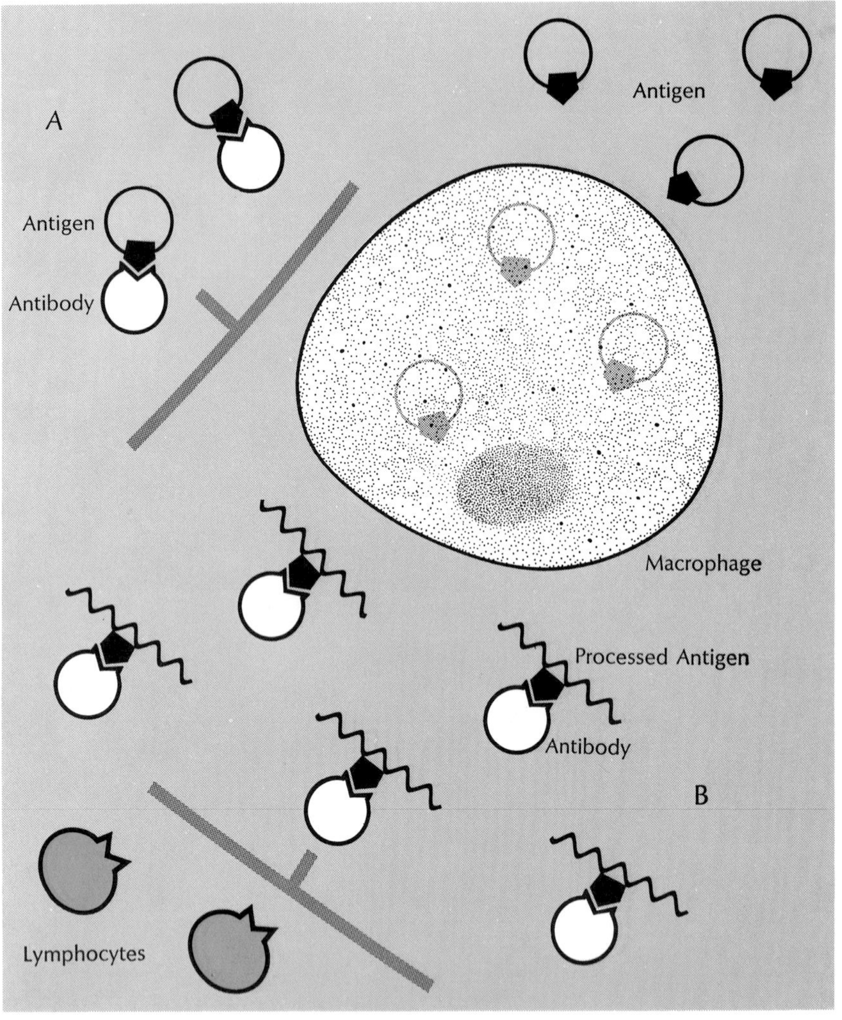

Antibody may prove to be the ideal immunosuppressant because of its inherent specificity. It could interrupt the chain of immunobiologic events by binding to the antigen before processing by the macrophage (A), or by combining with the processed antigen and in this way preventing sensitization of the lymphocyte (B). Alternatively, in homograft reactions (below) humoral antibody might cover the combining sites on the graft itself and block access to the lymphocytes.

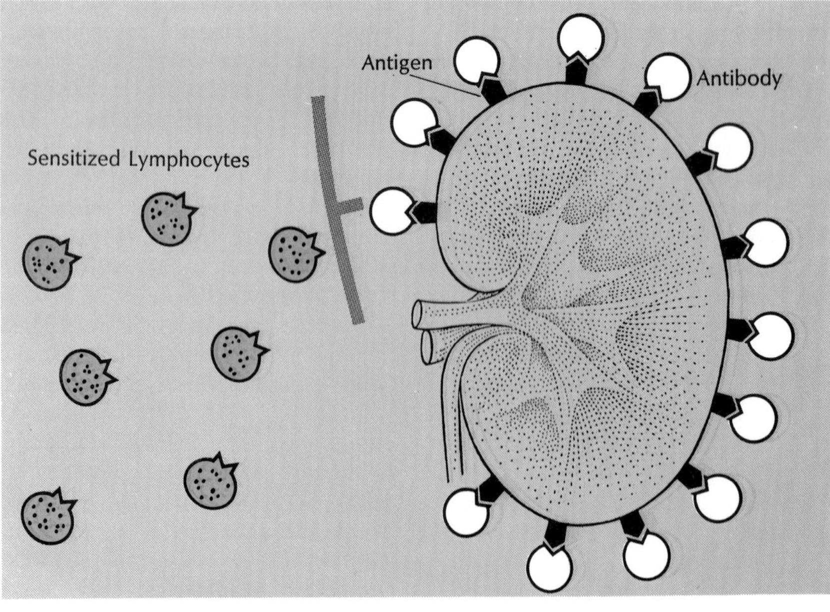

lymphocytes, the thymus-dependent lymphocyte bears immunologically specific information.

By defining tolerance we also define the goal for any immunosuppressive agent. In this context our present clinical methods are only expedients because as yet we have no convincing evidence that tolerance has been induced in man. Now it is highly possible that tolerance has actually been produced in many cases but that for a number of reasons we haven't been able to demonstrate it. Such a demonstration would probably necessitate that immunosuppressive therapy be stopped after the initial course while antigenic stimulation was continued, since such stimulation has been necessary to maintain tolerance in animal systems. It is not difficult to understand why clinicians doing kidney transplants, for example, have been reluctant to stop giving immunosuppressants to their patients to see whether they will retain their grafts. This has been done in dogs. In some instances the animal was tolerant of its grafted kidney, as judged by the failure of the dog to reject the transplant after the chemotherapy was stopped. As for the continuing supply of antigen, it is possible that the graft itself might provide it, but again this remains to be shown.

A third factor that would be needed before tolerance in man could be demonstrated and employed, at least with regard to transplants, is an improved system for typing donors and recipients. It is abundantly evident from animal work that the closer the histocompatibility between donor and recipient the easier it is to suppress the immune response and to induce tolerance. With a strong histocompatibility difference, induction of tolerance becomes either extremely difficult or impossible. Needed in addition to an improved typing system is a drug that can be given as a single pulse and a purified antigen that can be administered both with the therapeutic agent and subsequently over a prolonged period (to maintain tolerance).

It will be recalled that earlier, in the discussion of corticosteroids, the possibility was raised that the value of these drugs in transplantation and in autoimmune disease may be related to their anti-inflammatory action rather than to immunosuppression. It

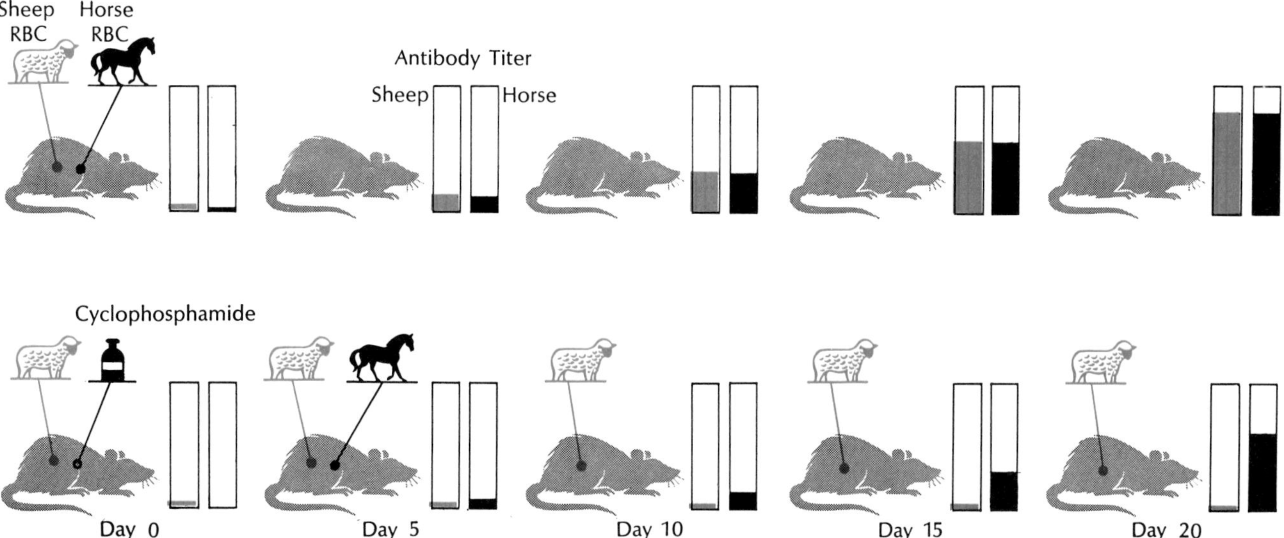

The ability of a cytotoxic drug to induce specific tolerance has been demonstrated in experiments in which horse and sheep erythrocytes are injected into mice. When no drug is used (top), the normal response is continuously rising antibody titers to both antigens. But when cyclophosphamide is injected simultaneously with the sheep RBC, the mouse will lose its capacity to respond to this antigen if subsequent injections of sheep cells are given to maintain tolerance. However, the same animal will show a completely normal response to horse erythrocytes administered five days after the single injection of the drug.

should now be noted that other immunosuppressive drugs have anti-inflammatory activity too and that their value in autoimmune diseases may also be a concomitant of this capacity. We have some clinical evidence that strongly supports this possibility. A number of lupus patients being treated with azathioprine and methotrexate were immunized with a test antigen. We were surprised to find that some of these patients had perfectly normal antibody responses. Moreover, the very patients who were making antibody were getting an excellent clinical effect from the drugs. On the basis of these experiments, we have been conservative in the dosages of immunosuppressants we give to lupus patients and to patients with a number of other autoimmune diseases. Our observation has been that they may get along just as well on low dosages as on higher ones. Perhaps there is a lesson in this experience for the transplanters, who may be losing some patients to infection because of overuse of immunosuppressants.

While we are on the subject of autoimmune disease, it is worthwhile to suggest that it may one day be possible to reestablish tolerance to the offending antigens in these patients. This might be much more difficult than in transplantation situations, for the patient with autoimmune disease comes to treatment already sensitized, while the transplant patient in effect is waiting to be challenged with the antigen. However, Good at the University of Minnesota has shown that rabbits already sensitized to an antigen (BSA) can be rendered tolerant to that antigen by treatment with 6-MP. This offers a ray of hope that sensitization does not preclude the induction of tolerance.

Similar hope is offered by work originally done by Burnet's group in Australia and abundantly confirmed by other investigators. They have shown that hybridized New Zealand mice spontaneously developing autoimmune renal disease will have a marked reduction in the incidence of this disease when cyclophospamide is administered. Burnet has interpreted this to mean that the drug produces an ablation of the forbidden clone in these animals. Although there is no solid evidence that a forbidden clone can be ablated in man, we have seen a number of patients with lupus, autoimmune hemolytic anemia, and ulcerative colitis who, after treatment with antimetabolites, have gone into remission. In these cases the drug has been stopped but the remission has persisted, in some instances now for as long as two or three years. Obviously, we cannot exclude the possibility of spontaneous remission in these patients, but one can also dare to hope that we may be approaching a state of induced tolerance in man.

To me, incidentally, the potential offered by induction of tolerance in autoimmune diseases is even more exciting than its potential in facilitating homotransplantation. I believe this for two reasons: 1) because there are far more patients with these conditions than there are transplant cases, 2) because in many instances, notably the kidney, the need for a transplant only arises because the organ has been destroyed by an immune process. The requirement for a transplant in a sense thus represents a failure – a failure in our knowledge of the causes of and the therapy for the condition that destroyed the patient's organ. Would it not be far better to treat the original disease effectively and eliminate the eventual necessity for a transplant? The results in the long run would be less spectacular than transplantation but far more satisfying.

In voicing the hope that we may achieve induction of tolerance in man, I recognize that there are many gaps to be filled and no guarantees that we can fill them. On the other hand, there is no immunologic reason to doubt that what has been accomplished in mice cannot be achieved in a species so immunologically similar – man.

Chapter 25

Antilymphocytic Serum: Its Properties and Potential

EUGENE M. LANCE
Cornell University
and
PETER B. MEDAWAR
National Institute for Medical Research, London

The current surge of interest in antilymphocytic serum undoubtedly dates from the report by M. F. A. Woodruff and N. Anderson of Edinburgh University in 1963 that administration of ALS greatly prolonged the survival of skin homografts in rats. Coming as it did when the clinical applicability of organ transplantation was expanding, this short report in *Nature*, followed soon after by the important pathfinding work of P. S. Russell and A. P. Monaco at the Massachusetts General Hospital, fired the imagination of researchers and led investigators everywhere to study the preparation, properties, and potentials of ALS.

The novelty of this interest has led many to think of ALS as a very modern immunosuppressive agent. In point of fact, it can be regarded as one of the oldest, if not the oldest, in the immunologic repertoire. An antilymphocytic serum was first devised by the great Russian zoologist Elie Metchnikoff just before the turn of the century. In the next 60 years a number of distinguished pathologists, including Drs. Simon Flexner and A. M. Pappenheimer Sr., studied and described the properties of ALS. Its first use as an immunosuppressant can probably be credited to Dr. John Humphrey working at the National Institute for Medical Research in 1956.

No matter how long ALS has taken in coming, it has now arrived. ALS has a distinctive combination of functional properties which should make it of the utmost value in transplantation surgery and in the control of autoimmune disease. They are properties, moreover, that make ALS a specially useful tool in immunologic research. Before I turn to these it will be useful to say something of its preparation and of how it works.

Antilymphocytic serum, as its name implies, is an antiserum raised in one species against the lymphocytes of another. Thus an ALS for use in human subjects can be made by injecting human lymphoid cells into a horse or for use in mice by injecting murine lymphoid cells into rabbits. The antiserum produced by the injection of whole lymphoid cells contains a complex of antibodies that differ in their antigenic specificity. Those antibodies that are directed against specific lymphocyte antigens are essential to the action of antilymphocytic serum and their removal (by absorption, for instance) eliminates the immunosuppressive effect. Other antibodies arise, however, that can react with other cell types such as erythrocytes or platelets, for example, either as a consequence of shared antigens between lymphocytes and other cell types or owing to contaminating cells in the material used for immunization. These antibodies are not only irrelevant to the action of antilymphocytic serum but are potentially toxic and should be removed by selective absorption procedures. An alternative to the removal by absorption of potentially noxious antibodies has been the search for better antigenic preparations to use for immunization. It now seems likely that the extraction from lymphocyte suspensions of the subcellular membrane and microsome fraction may provide a way to increase the antigenic specificity and reduce the production of unwanted and undesirable antibodies.

Another way in which the antibodies in ALS differ is in respect to gamma globulin class. The reports from many laboratories now make it quite clear that the active principle of ALS resides wholly within the IgG fraction. Antibodies of the IgM class are without effect in vivo. Therefore, the raw antiserum may be purified to derive and administer only the IgG fraction, thereby eliminating an unnecessary load of foreign protein.

We routinely assay the potency of antilymphocytic serum by measuring its ability to prolong the survival of skin allografts in vivo. This test provides a critical and direct assessment of that property of ALS in which we are most interested. Nonetheless, it would be a great advantage, especially in the context of clinical use, if a reliable in vitro test of potency were available. While a variety of in vitro methods have been explored, e.g.,

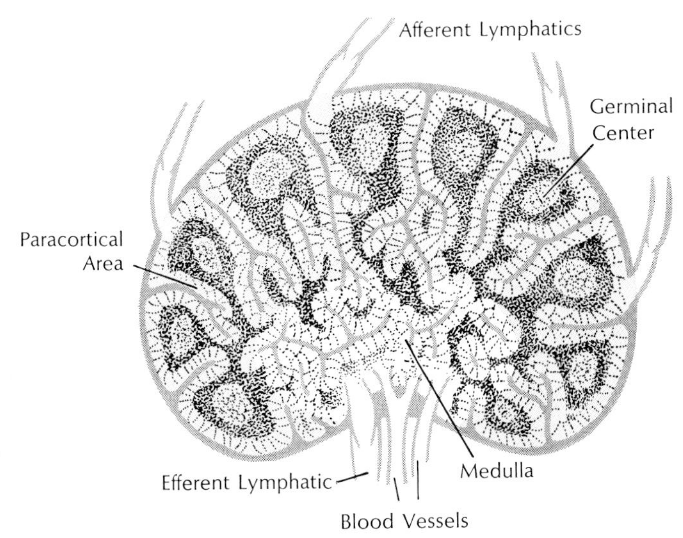

Effects of ALS on immunologic response are schematized on this page. Smaller drawing at the left represents the anatomy of the lymph node. The germinal centers are the areas in cells capable of giving rise to humoral antibodies and are relatively impregnable to ALS. The paracortical areas contain the system through which small lymphocytes, the mediators of cell-bound antibody reactions, pass from the blood to the lymphatic circulation. This concept of recirculation is shown below. When ALS is injected, its antibodies are able to reach the lymphocytes while they are in the circulation. As a result both complexing and cell disruption take place in the presence of complement. The ALS-lymphocyte-complement complexes are made vulnerable to phagocytosis, which, in this diagram, is depicted as occurring in the Kupffer cells of the liver.

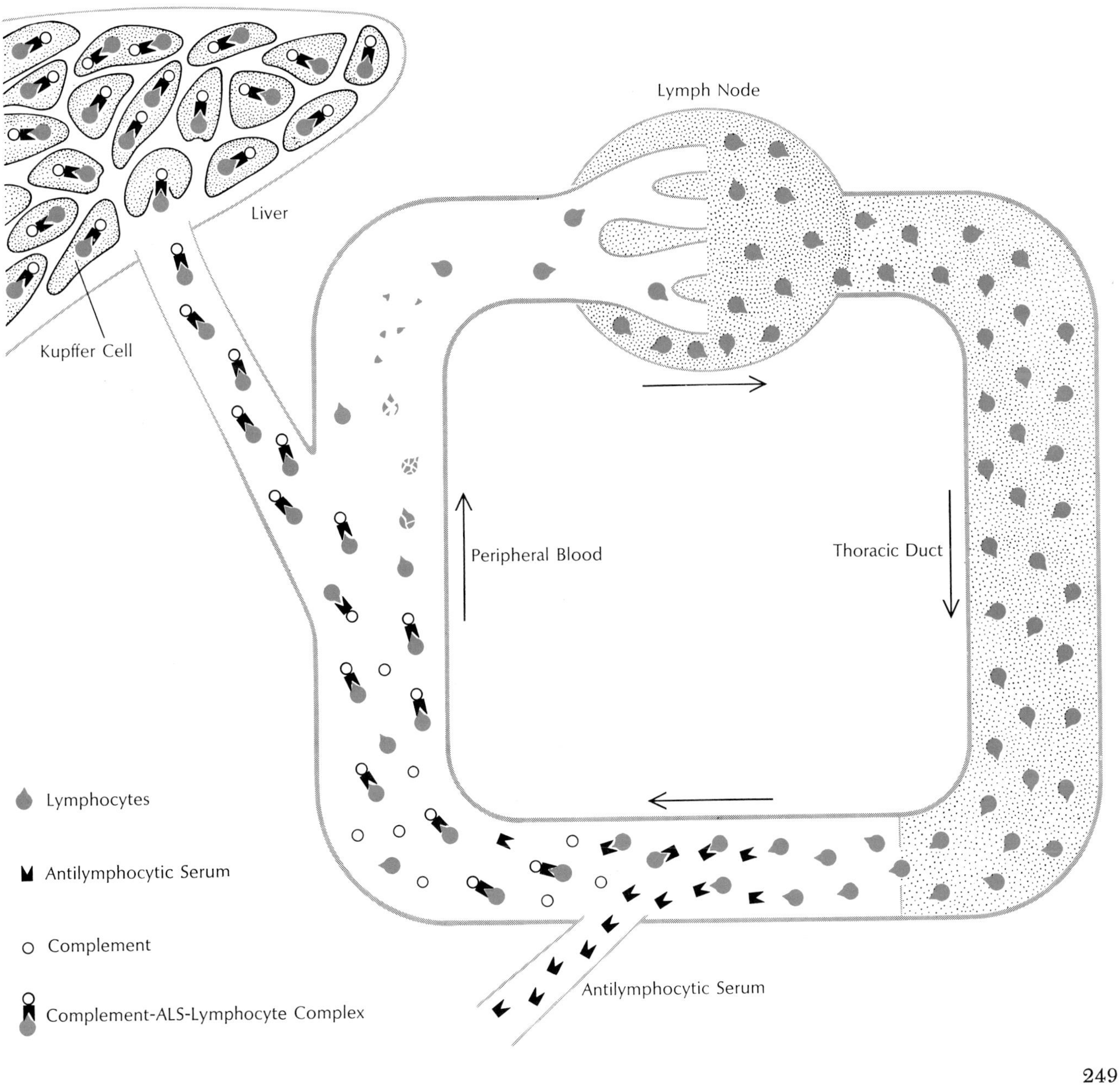

Lymph Node
Liver
Kupffer Cell
Peripheral Blood
Thoracic Duct
Antilymphocytic Serum

Lymphocytes
Antilymphocytic Serum
Complement
Complement-ALS-Lymphocyte Complex

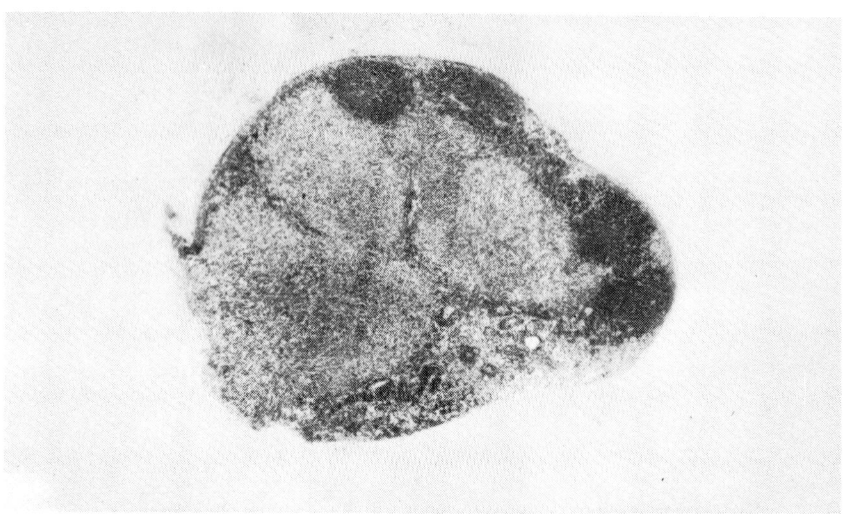

Brachial lymph node of CBA mouse 48 hours after ALS injection: Lymphocytes are depleted in paracortical areas; cortical and primary follicular zones are spared.

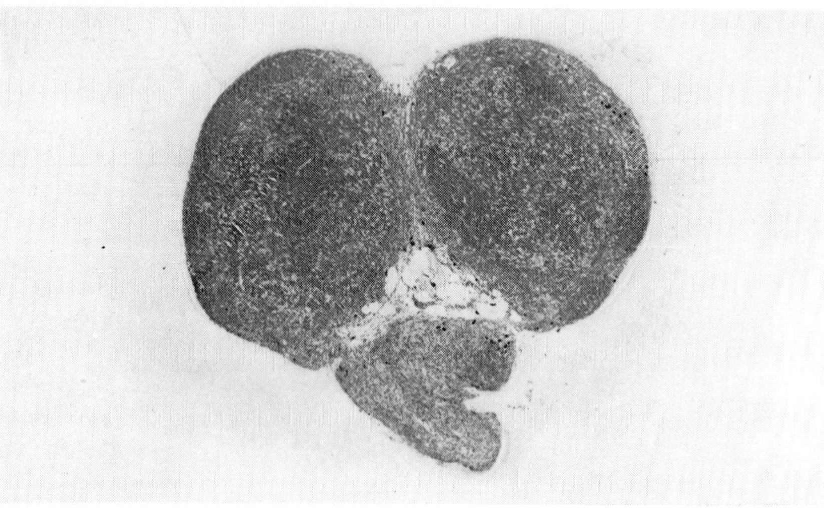

Brachial node in control mouse (injected with normal rabbit serum) does not show any significant reduction of lymphocyte population in the paracortical areas.

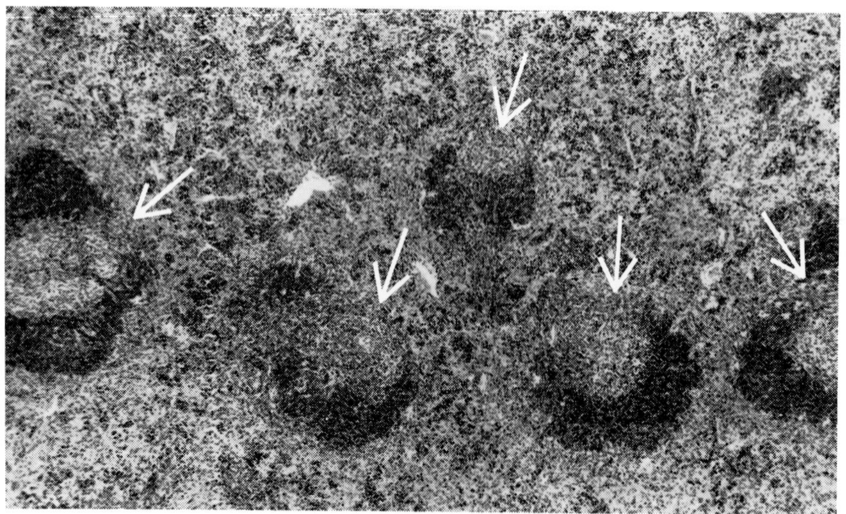

Mouse spleen week after course of ALS shows "punched-out" lesions (arrows) due to depletion of small lymphocytes from lymphoid follicles (all above, Taub and Lance).

cytotoxicity, agglutination, opsonization, lymphocyte transformation, and rosette inhibition, none of these, with the possible exception of the rosette-inhibition test, at present correlates well enough with the in vivo results to justify placing complete reliance upon it.

Because ALS is produced across species lines it is itself highly immunogenic, raising antibodies against itself, and until recently many people believed that this immunogenicity underlay its mode of action. Perhaps, it was reasoned, ALS acts as an obligative antigen, forcing all available lymphoid cells to respond to it and so usurping the immunologic capabilities of the recipient. Studies at Mill Hill by one of us (E.M.L.) and D. W. Dresser have now shown that this is not the case. They have made mice completely unreactive to rabbit immunoglobulin as such. These immunologically paralyzed mice are as responsive to rabbit ALS as are normal mice, but they can no longer react to ALS as an antigen.

The immunogenicity of ALS (we speak here also of the IgG subfraction) has several undesirable consequences. The antibodies that the host elaborates in response to this foreign protein form complexes that neutralize the ability to combine with lymphocytes. Therefore, once immunization has taken place subsequent doses of ALS will be progressively less immunosuppressive. A second undesirable aspect is that serum sickness will ensue, with all of its possible consequences including immune complex nephritis, representing yet another hazard to the recipient.

The question of how ALS works has now been settled to the satisfaction of most workers. There is general agreement that it acts primarily on peripheral lymphocytes, i.e., on the lymphocytes that circulate between the lymphatic and vascular systems, as opposed to those that are housed in central lymphoid tissues such as lymph nodes or spleen. In due course, however, ALS will extend its action to the central lymphoid organs, because the cells they issue into the circulation and would normally recapture from it are progressively destroyed. This generalization is derived from three lines of investigation: the study of normal lymphocyte transfer reactions in guinea pigs; observations on the induction of tolerance by the injection of lymphoid cells; and the more recent studies by Drs. Lance and R. N. Taub at the National Institute for Medical Research on lymphocytes labeled with radioactive chromium. These studies have shown that peripheral lymphocytes are removed from the circulation if they are injected within a few hours of the injection of ALS, but are protected from its action if they are given time to lodge in the central lymphoid organs before the antilymphocytic serum is administered.

The question of what ALS actually does to the lymphocytes was at first controversial. Partly because the lymphopenia produced by ALS is transient, R. H. Levey and I were at first reluctant to believe that ALS actually kills the lymphocytes upon which it acts. We thought it possible that ALS might coat lymphocytes and "blindfold" them in such a way that they are unable to recognize antigen; or, alternatively, that ALS activates immunologically competent cells nonspecifically (as phytohemagglutinin does), so causing them to be removed from the potentially reactive pool of the organism. However, present findings clearly favor the theory that ALS acts through the complement system to destroy lymphocytes or to cause them to be phagocytosed. Indeed, there is definite evidence that the action of ALS is complement dependent. All antilymphocytic sera that are active in the sense of being able to prolong homograft survival have been found to be cytotoxic in vitro in systems containing the complement of the recipient species, and antilymphocytic sera lacking this cytotoxicity have no immunosuppressive activity.

The concept of the mode of action of ALS that is now coming to be widely accepted was first formulated by Dr. Lance in 1967, and confirmatory evidence, much of it arrived at independently, has come from many other quarters, especially from the Medical Research Council's Rheumatology Research Unit, the Chester Beatty Research Institute, and the Hall Institute in Melbourne. ALS acts primarily on lymphocytes belonging to the long-lived, thymus-dependent, recirculating pool, i.e., on the cell population generally considered to be responsible for homograft rejection and other cell-mediated immunities. There is now direct evidence that the lymphocyte population of animals chronically exposed to ALS is essentially short-lived, the long-lived cells having been depleted or eliminated, and it is especially satisfactory that Dr. N. B. Everett of Seattle, to whom we are indebted for the distinction between long-lived and short-lived lymphocytes, should have found direct evidence of this mode of action of ALS. Taub and Lance have confirmed that

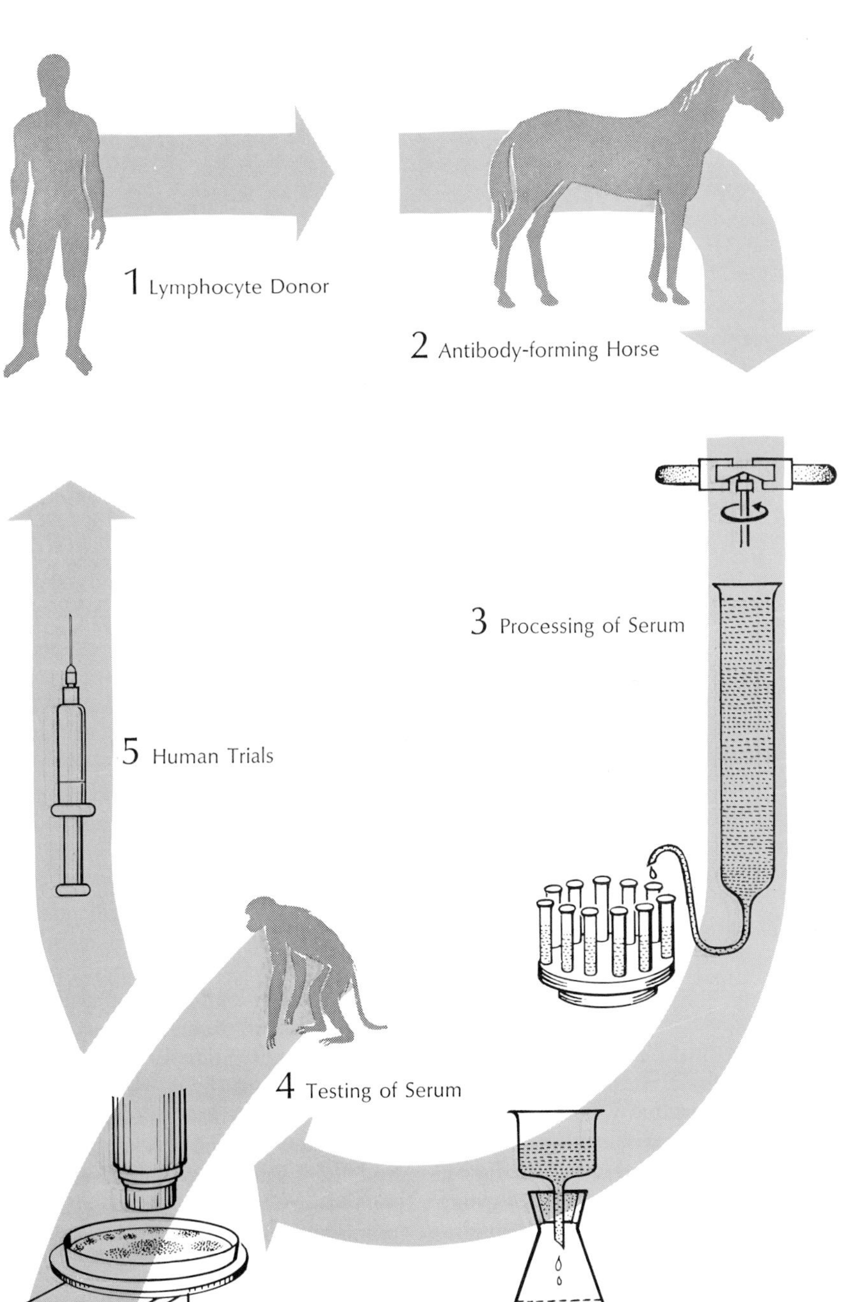

The preparation of ALS begins with the drawing of serum containing thymocytes, peripheral blood cells, and thoracic duct lymphocytes from human donor (1). This is injected into horse to raise antiserum (2). After appropriate time, blood is drawn, the serum separated, heated to 56° C, and fractionated on a sephadex column to recover immunoglobulins (3). Sterilization by filtration completes the preparation process. The resultant material is then subjected to tests for cytotoxic and opsonification capacity on human lymphocytes in presence of complement and is tested for animal toxicity in monkeys (4). If ALS passes all tests it is then considered ready for human trials.

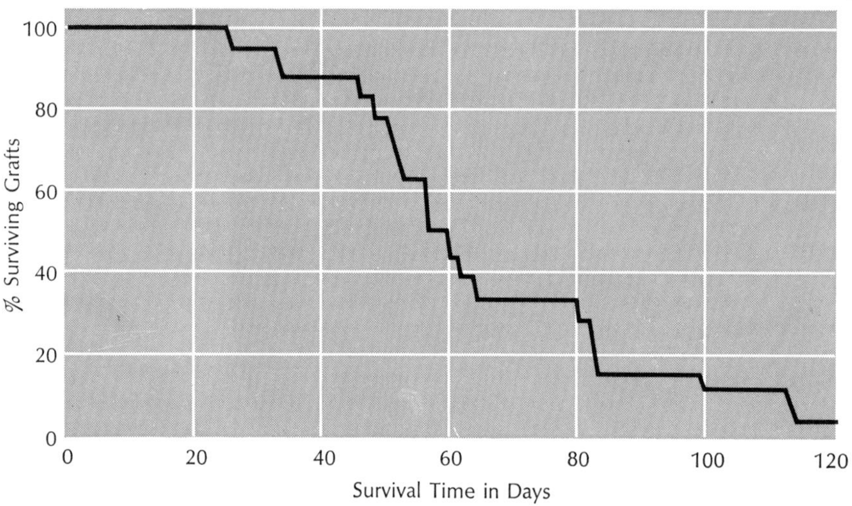

Finite duration of immunosuppressive action of ALS is shown by survival curve of A strain skin grafts in CBA mice once ALS administration (minimum of 100 days in recipient animals) was terminated. Mean homograft survival time was 75 days (Lance).

the changes produced in the lymph nodes and other lymphoid organs by purified ALS are just those that would be expected if the antiserum selectively removes the thymus-dependent moiety of the lymphocyte population, for it is the thymus-dependent areas, defined by Dr. Delphine Parrott and her colleagues and by Dr. J. L. Turk, that are characteristically affected by ALS.

Having described the mode of action of ALS so far as we understand it, let us turn to those functional properties of ALS that relate to its present and potential clinical applications. The first of these, already mentioned in passing, is the impermanence of its immunosuppressive effect. Its action is manifest during the injection of ALS and for a limited period thereafter. In mice this does not exceed an average of about 50 days after the course of ALS administration is completed. We have no doubt that this 50-day period represents the mean turnover time of the animal's lymphoid population, that is to say, the mean time it takes for a new lymphoid population to regenerate and so restore immunologic competence to its original level.

Levey and I showed that the effect of ALS is prolonged by hydrocortisone, which seems to retard recruitment or peripheral release of lymphocytes and is shortened by agents or treatments that accelerate the turnover of the lymphocyte population. Of particular significance is the effect of thymectomy on the duration of ALS-induced immunosuppression, an effect first described by Russell and Monaco. Thymectomy greatly prolongs the immunosuppressive action of ALS. There is no reason to doubt that this occurs because of the now well-known ability of thymectomy to retard the recruitment of immunologically competent lymphocytes, even in adult animals. After ALS has eliminated thymus-dependent lymphoid cells, their regeneration will be extremely slow, and so will be the return of cell-dependent immune competence in the thymectomized animal.

Interactions between ALS and treatments that affect the duration of its activity, though interesting in themselves, do not differentiate ALS from more conventional immunosuppressive agents. Three properties of ALS do in fact set it apart. The first has already been mentioned: the selective activity of ALS against cell-dependent immune responses. In this respect it is exactly the opposite of conventional immunosuppressive agents – x-rays, DNA base analogs and substituents, alkylating agents, antifolics, toxic antibiotics. These agents have all been borrowed from cancer chemotherapy, where they were devised or chosen for their antiproliferative activity. Being antiproliferative, they necessarily inhibit the humoral antibody response, because in the formation of antibodies there is always an episode of cell proliferation between the activation of antibody-forming cells and the production of humoral antibodies in effective quantities. Because they are inhibitors of the humoral antibody response, the conventional immunosuppressants weaken the ordinary protective immunity that operates against bacteria and viruses.

Our realization that ALS acts differentially upon cell-mediated responses grew out of "clinical observation" (if that is not too pompous an expression when the patients are merely mice). It was noted that when given in doses large enough to suppress the homograft reaction ALS did not at the same time lay its recipients open to infectious disease. Thus ALS could be employed at dose levels which would have been impractical with other immunosuppressants simply because they would lay prostrate the entire immunologic defense system of the treated animals.

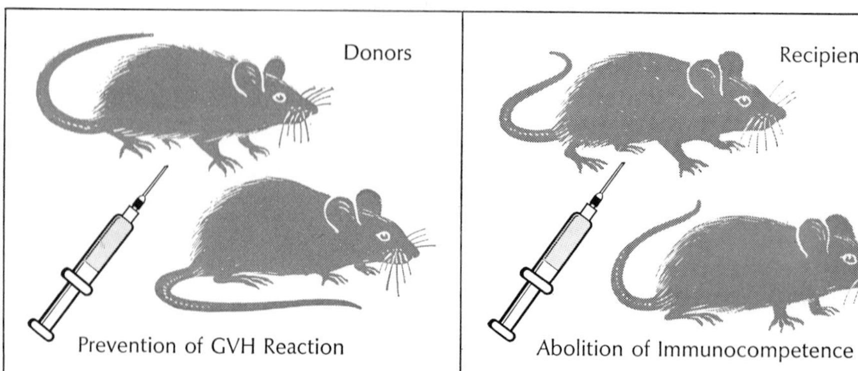

In this schematic representation of the induction of tolerance with ALS, the first step is the injection of ALS into donor animals to forestall graft-vs-host reaction. ALS is also injected into recipient animals to abolish immunocompetence. Then 25 million

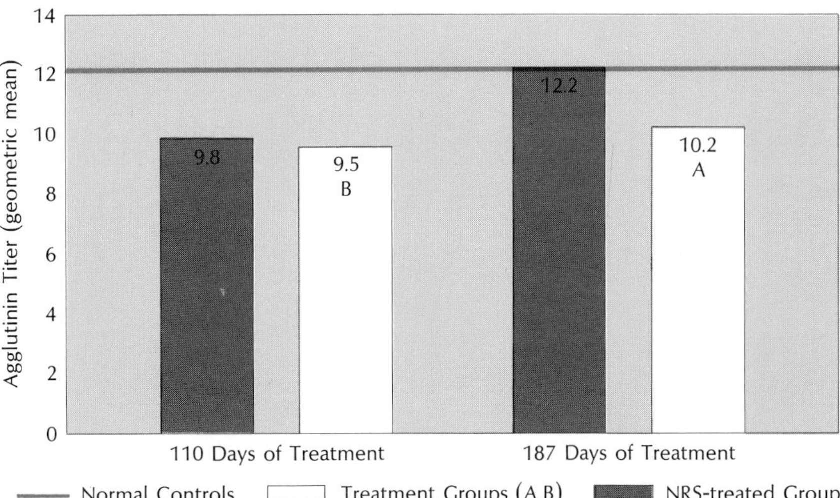

Selectivity of ALS in inhibiting only cell-mediated immunity is demonstrated by fact that ALS-treated mice (groups A and B) have essentially the same antibody response to salmonella antigens as untreated or normal-rabbit-serum-treated animals.

Although ALS is differentially more effective in opposing cell-mediated immunities, it is not without effect on the primary antibody response to a variety of antigens. Recent experimental evidence suggests that the antibody response to many antigens is at least partially thymus dependent in that the development of the full response requires an interaction between a thymus-derived lymphocyte and a bone marrow–derived lymphocyte. When ALS is given prior to immunization in dosages that drastically reduce the numbers of thymus-derived lymphocytes, then a marked inhibition of the antibody response to "thymus-dependent" antigens can occur. However, because of the different requirements for thymus-derived cells in cellular and humoral immunities, it is possible to devise a dosage regimen that will completely abrogate cellular immunity while producing only minor alterations in humoral responsiveness. Moreover, antilymphocytic serum is largely ineffective in opposing the secondary humoral response.

A second singular property of ALS is its ability to produce what Dr. Levey and I have described as "erasure of memory" in homograft systems. The work of Monaco and Russell had established the fact that the injection of ALS weakens the "second set" response through which an animal rapidly and violently rejects a second homograft when it has had prior experience of a first. Erasure of immunologic memory is, however, more than the weakening of this preexisting sensitivity. It means that ALS has the power to restore an animal to a state of virgin reactivity, a state in which it behaves as if it had never met with or reacted against homograft antigens before. Obviously this property of ALS has considerable promise for such a clinical application as the treatment of autoimmune disease. If autoimmune disease represents a reaction to self-constituents which behave as if they were foreign antigens, then any agent capable of abolishing recognition of endogenous antigens could provide the basis for cure instead of treatment that is merely symptomatic or palliative.

The third major distinctive property of ALS is its relative insensitivity to antigenic differences between the homograft donor and its recipient. Ordinary immunosuppressive agents work comparatively well – sometimes better than ALS – when donor and recipient are closely related. But when the genetically determined histocompatibility barrier between them is a strong one, conventional immunosuppression usually fails. With ALS it makes comparatively little difference whether or not the donor and recipient are well matched. Indeed, the use of ALS is now making it possible to transplant grafts across species barriers, i.e., to transplant heterografts or xenografts.

In our laboratory we have grown human skin on ALS-treated mice for periods of two months or more without seeing any evidence of specific immunologic reaction. In this experiment, incidentally, one does not encounter the problem of graft-vs-host reaction because mammalian skin does

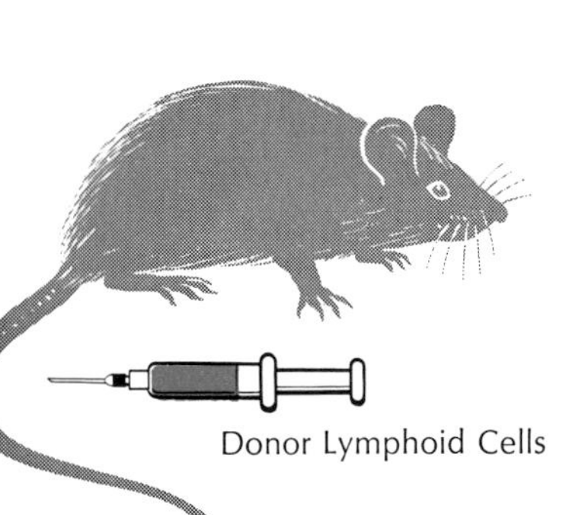

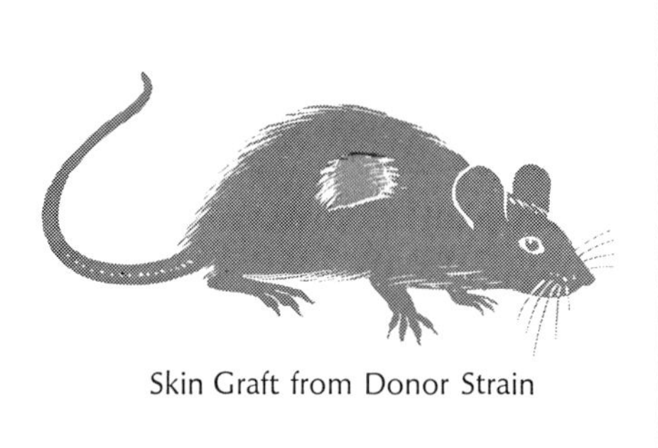

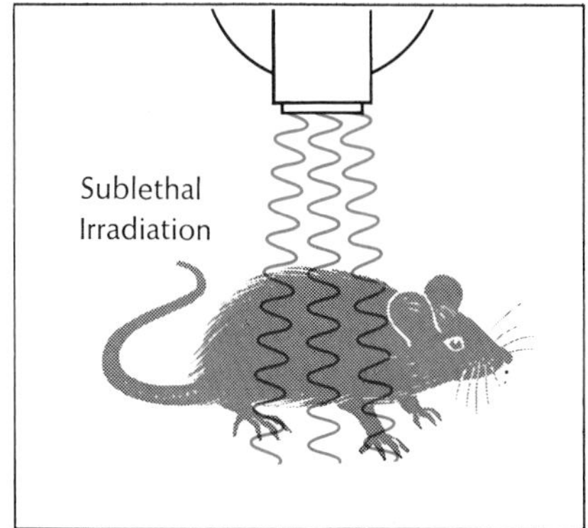

donor lymphoid cells are injected intravenously into the recipient. This is followed (or preceded) by a skin graft. Graft will survive 75 to 150 days, but if recipient is irradiated with 450r (far right) before injection of lymphoid cells it may live indefinitely, possibly because x-rays destroy recipient lymphocytes and give donor cells room to proliferate (Lance and Medawar).

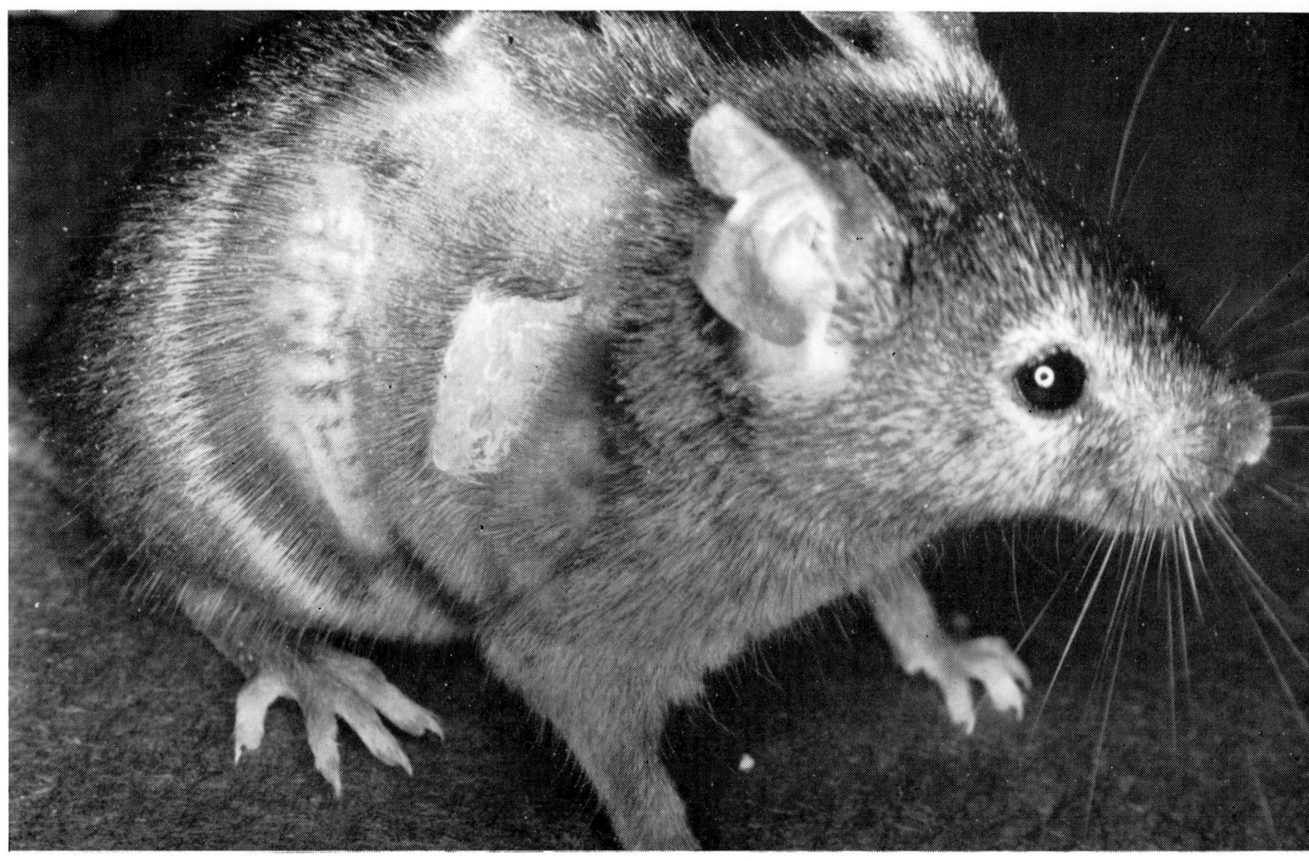

Antilymphocytic serum can be used to permit grafts across species lines. The mouse above was treated with ALS for eight weeks and carries a human skin heterograft. Histologic section of a similar graft shows a reasonably normal connective tissue struc-

not contain any significant number of immunologically competent cells.

A note of caution here: The success of this experiment should not tempt people to believe that the era of xenografting is at hand. There are a great many reasons why xenografts might fail after transplantation, and they are by no means all immunologic. The kind of opposition a xenograft may elicit is likely to vary not merely from species to species but also from organ to organ. We already have clear evidence, for example, that humoral antibodies are far more significant in the rejection of xenografts than they are in the rejection of homografts. It seems quite logical that a liver transplant, say from chimpanzee to human, should raise problems quite different from and much graver than those raised by a skin transplant from man or rat to mouse.

Having discussed the three important ways ALS differs from conventional immunosuppressive agents, we should mention one significant way in which it behaves like them. ALS can also be used to induce immunologic tolerance [Chapter 24, "Immunosuppression: The Challenge of Selectivity" Robert S. Schwartz]. The ability to induce tolerance may provide a way around the one great obstacle that blocks the general clinical use of ALS, namely, that the immunosuppressive action of ALS lasts only as long injections are actually being given and for a finite period thereafter. If the immunosuppressive action of ALS is to be made permanent, we are obliged to follow one of a very limited number of approaches.

The first is to inject the antiserum throughout the life of the patient. This is intrinsically objectionable, particularly in light of our knowledge of the immunogenicity of ALS. Alternatively, one could consider potentiating the action of ALS by administration of corticosteroids or by thymectomy. Thymectomy is a procedure one would not voluntarily use except as a last resort. As for corticosteroids, a major attraction of ALS has been that it offers the hope of dispensing with the use of toxic doses of corticosteroids, with all their well-known side effects. The alternatives are thus not very satisfactory.

We are left, then, with the possibility of using ALS to promote the inception of immunologic tolerance, that is to say, to bring about a state of specific nonreactivity towards particular homograft antigens, as opposed to the general nonreactivity in respect to all cell-mediated immune responses. The induction of immunologic tolerance to homografts with ALS has already been achieved experimentally. Monaco and Russell did this first by combining the administration of ALS with the injection of very high doses of donor-specific antigen in thymectomized mice. More recently, Lance and I found that tolerance can be induced without thymectomy and with very much lower doses of donor antigen. Unfortunately the tolerance was by no means permanent, lasting on the average for from three to six months after the injections of ALS had ceased.

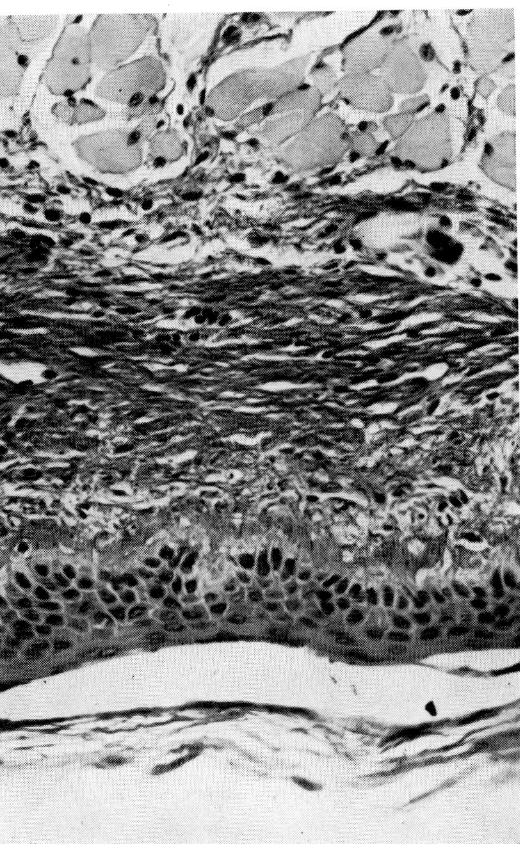

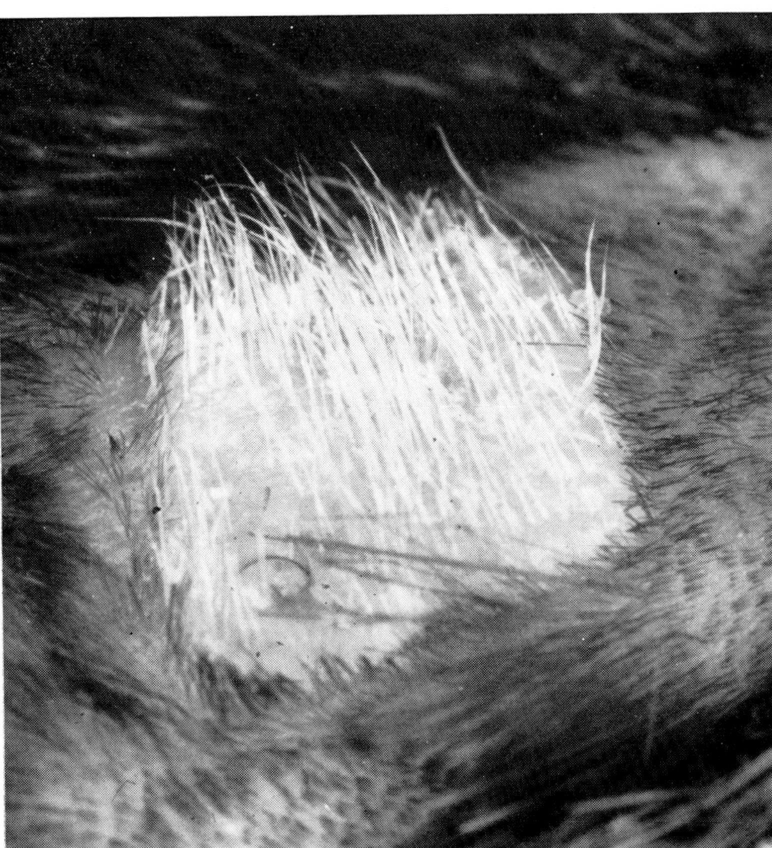

ture, with no pathologic reaction (Lance and Medawar). At right: a rat-tail heterograft is thriving three months after transplantation to a mouse which was made tolerant through administration of ALS (Lance, Levey, Medawar, and M. Ruszkiewicz).

The reasons for the relatively short duration of tolerance are not all clear, but the presumption is that the procedures we were using did not prevent the ultimate regeneration of the host's own immunologically competent cells. Further experiments indicate that this difficulty can be circumvented, for example, by combining ALS with low doses of conventional immunosuppressive agents. Using this approach, Lance and I have achieved *mean* homograft survival in mice exceeding a year from the end of ALS treatment, and have kept skin heterografts from rats alive for upwards of four months.

The induction of tolerance to rat grafts on mice illustrates a principle of great importance. The essence of the procedure is to inject high doses of rat lymphoid cells into mice incapacitated by high doses of ALS. But why do not the rat lymphoid cells kill the mice almost instantaneously by a graft-vs-host reaction? The reason is that the rat cell donors have themselves been treated with ALS before the cell transfer, so that they contain no immunologically competent cells (see illustration on pages 252 and 253).

In this description of research on tolerance all references have been to skin transplants. It will probably be much easier, in an immunologic sense, to induce lasting tolerance with complex organs such as liver or kidney than with skin. One possible reason for this is that large organs maintain the chronic antigenic input that is essential if tolerance is to be maintained. Organ homografts are in any event less exacting than skin grafts immunologically, in spite of the great surgical and physiological difficulties that attend their transplantation.

Let us now try to evaluate the clinical and experimental potentialities of ALS. To start with the most obvious application, ALS holds out the promise of bringing the homograft reaction under genuinely complete control. Certainly ALS is now the only agent that could broaden the base of transplantation surgery to include the use of heterografts. Beyond this, ALS makes it possible in principle to correct all autoimmune disorders that depend on a cell-mediated, homograft-like mechanism.

There has been a growing clinical experience with use of antilymphocytic serum since such studies were inaugurated by Dr. Thomas Starzl and his group at the University of Colorado. The wider application of antilymphocytic serum has been retarded chiefly by two limitations. Serious difficulties have been posed in the scaling up of laboratory production of ALS sufficiently to assure an adequate and safe supply for clinical use. The technical problems associated with this mass production are now in the course of solution and large quantities of ALS produced through commercial sources should soon become available. The demonstration by Najarian and his colleagues that cultured human lymphoblasts can be used to raise an antihuman ALS that is safe to apply in patients represents a great stride forward in this direction.

The problem of measuring potency of ALS for human use remains very much with us. Some investigators have used human volunteers to demonstrate the effectiveness of ALS in prolonging human skin allografts. This is, however, an obviously impractical solution. A compromise that appears of clinical utility has been the testing of antihuman ALS in subhuman primates. Such antisera can be screened in this way both for potential toxicity and for potency in promoting allograft survival. In the meantime, the search for a suitable in vitro assay continues, with several promising methods under current study.

As clinical investigators begin to apply the fruits of experimental research to the clinical trials, the results steadily improve. Most clinical centers have adopted the procedure of administering only the IgG fraction of ALS and a number have demonstrated the feasibility of inducing tolerance to IgG to prevent the undesirable consequences of immunization spoken of above. Now that ALS of documented potency and purity is being given in therapeutic doses, the advantages of this agent are becoming apparent. The need for adjunctive immunosuppression, such as corticosteroids, has been reduced and, moreover, the results in poorly matched renal transplants have greatly improved. The early experience in the use of ALS to treat clinical autoimmune diseases reported by Dr. Brendel and his colleagues in Munich is also encouraging. It seems a safe prediction that antilymphocytic serum will constitute an important contribution to the clinical armamentarium.

There is no known property that precludes the clinical use of ALS. However there is still an important question mark over the clinical use of ALS: What will be the secondary consequences of a total abrogation of cell-mediated immunity? The implied charge against ALS is exactly analogous to that which is brought against the conventional immunosuppressive agents, except that it relates to the cellular, not the humoral, response. Briefly, we appear to depend on a cellular mechanism for immunity to mycobacteria, to some viruses – and perhaps to malignant growth, for many people now believe that there exists a natural mechanism of defense against tumors which is cognate with the homograft reaction. Are there then not great dangers in the clinical use of ALS?

Only the use of ALS itself can resolve this question. If it is true that the natural immunologic defenses against tumors are closely akin to homograft reactivity, then prolonged administration of ALS should cause tumors to spring up in all parts of the body. This would be highly discouraging to those of us who have high hopes of ALS in the control of graft rejection and of autoimmune disease, though in compensation it would yield a most important generalization about the mechanisms of oncogenesis. An experimental answer is now being sought to this vital question by maintaining mice from birth until death on a regimen of continuous ALS administration.

Just as ALS may help elucidate the role of immunologic defenses in cancer, so it may provide the experimenter with the key to a better understanding of cell-mediated responses of all kinds. Having now for the first time at our disposal a differential inhibitor of cell-mediated immune responses, we should be able to achieve a deeper understanding of the role of these responses in bacterial, mycobacterial, and virus infections and in autoimmune diseases.

Even if ALS receives a security clearance for special clinical use, it is still not the final answer to the problems we seek to solve. To inject into human beings substances as complex, as imperfectly defined, as variable in composition, and as difficult to prepare as antilymphocytic sera is fundamentally unsatisfactory. Our hope is that the existence of ALS as a differential inhibitor of the cell-mediated immune response – and, as such, an improvement over the immunosuppressants derived from cancer chemotherapy – will stimulate chemists and pharmacologists into developing relatively simple chemical compounds possessing similar selective properties. If ALS opens the way to such a development, it will have played an important part in the history of medical research.

Chapter 26

Interferon and Interferon Inducers: The Clinical Outlook

THOMAS C. MERIGAN JR.
Stanford University

Ever since Alick Isaacs and Jean Lindenmann discovered the potent antiviral protein interferon in 1957, researchers have had growing hopes that this substance might some day take its place in the clinical armamentarium. It has not yet come into use because of serious technical problems. In the last two years, however, certain of the difficulties have been resolved.

Important experiments reported very recently have demonstrated that sufficiently high levels of interferon can be induced in animals to combat a variety of infections, even after disease has progressed far enough to become manifest clinically. Initial clinical trials seem very likely within the next year or so unless unexpected complications arise.

Today we still have to work with our hands tied when it comes to dealing with virus infections. Antibiotics enable us to control most significant bacterial infections, but we have to face the viruses with little more than we had two decades ago. Of course, vaccination will prevent many serious infections. But we must vaccinate against one disease, and usually one strain, at a time. In most cases vaccination is useless after the patient has been exposed. Furthermore, there are many diseases for which we have

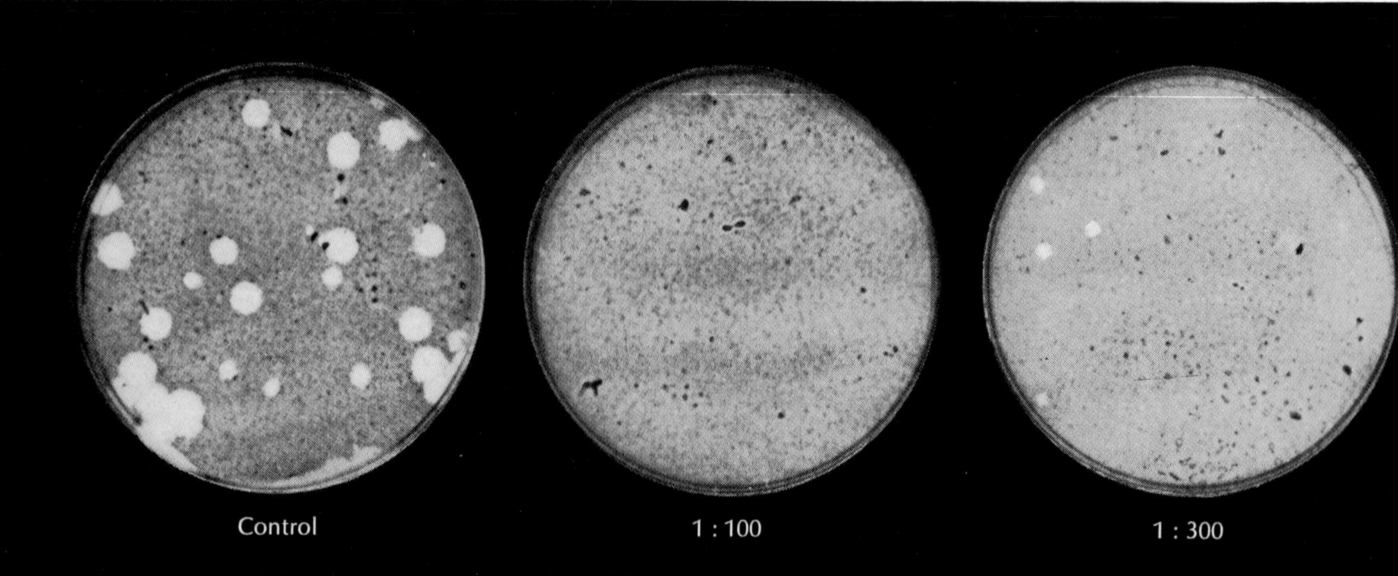

Tissue culture assay in chick embryo fibroblasts demonstrates antiviral activity of interferon: plaque formation is totally inhibited by dilution of 1:100, with inhibition progressively diminishing as interferon dilution is increased. At 1:100,000 the

no vaccines at this time.

What we need is a substance that can be administered or induced in the body to block viruses with the same efficiency that antibiotics destroy bacteria. In theory, at least, interferon is such a substance. Most researchers in the field accept the evidence indicating that interferon is part of nature's first line of defense for fighting off virus infection in higher animals. Our objective with interferon therapy will be to strengthen this natural defense system to prevent as much virus replication and tissue damage as possible.

Interferon's most appealing property as an antiviral agent is its broad spectrum of action. Only a minority of viruses are resistant, and we have little reason to suspect that resistance will increase if interferon is widely used. This is because interferon is found naturally in animals. The viruses have all been exposed to it for thousands of years, and all but a few are still susceptible.

This failure to evoke resistance will be particularly useful in an antiviral agent. A large number of viruses produce the same initial symptoms. This is particularly true for the commonest virus infections, those of the respiratory and gastrointestinal tract, as well as those that involve the central nervous system. Accordingly, treatment could be started before the specific virus strain involved has been identified.

As a naturally occurring substance, interferon is also apparently harmless to the cells of the animal in which it is made. It is very active in blocking virus replication within a cell, but does not interfere with the host's own cellular activities. Its level of antiviral activity is extremely high, in fact. Molecule for molecule, it is as active as the most active antibiotics are against sensitive bacteria.

One serious limitation on clinical potential is that interferon is most active prophylactically or early in infection, before the bulk of virus replication and consequent tissue destruction have occurred. In addition, the protective effect is transient, unlike antibody protection, which usually lasts a lifetime. There seem to be two reasons why this is so. First, interferon has a short halflife in the circulatory system. Second, the protection induced by interferon treatment declines rapidly in the cells themselves. This limitation means that continued protection from infection will have to be maintained by regular administration of interferon or, more likely, regular restimulation of natural interferon production.

Unfortunately, interferon's high level of activity has produced some difficulties in the laboratory. Only small amounts of the protein are available in nature, and this has restricted determination of physical and chemical properties, mechanism of action, and biologic role.

There is no question that the antiviral activity is associated with a protein, or rather a family of proteins. Trypsin digestion destroys the activity, which is not, however, affected by ribonuclease or desoxyribonuclease. Three general classes of interferon have been identified on the basis of molecular weights, but there does not appear to be any difference in their biologic activity. The three classes have these molecular weights: 20,000 to 30,000, 40,000 to 60,000, and 90,000 to 160,000.

Other physical characteristics of the molecule have been difficult to determine. Precise electrophoresis and CM sephadex chromatography applied to chick interferon have demonstrated a continuum in the charge and size of the molecules.

Chemical information about interferon is even more scanty. A protein must be an essential part of the active

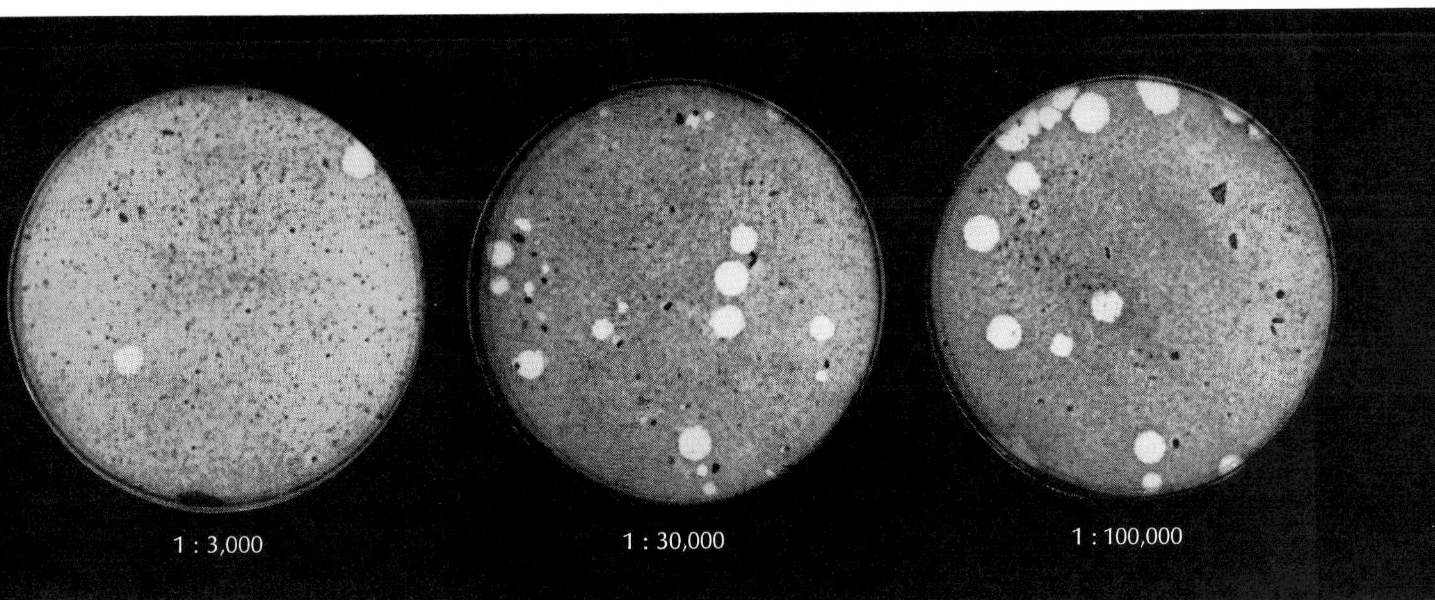

number of plaques formed (16) is about 80% of the control culture. Virus used in this demonstration was that of bovine vesicular stomatitis. The titer of this sample of interferon that would inhibit plaque formation by 50% would be 1:20,000.

molecule. Japanese investigators have separated a carbohydrate cofactor from the protein in rabbit interferon and demonstrated the former's antiviral activity, but the implications of this work are unclear. No sugar or polysaccharide moiety has been found in chick interferon. Even after 14 years of work we must admit that the chemical nature of interferon is still a mystery.

Undoubtedly we will some day have a more detailed understanding of this chemistry, and this could have important clinical implications. It is conceivable that a small polypeptide factor or prosthetic group could be the active unit, and that this unit might even be amenable to synthesis.

Inferferon's high potency is probably related to its mechanism of action. The protective effect is blocked by substances that inhibit formation of ribonucleic acid (RNA) and protein. Accordingly, the present hypothesis is that interferon induces synthesis of a second, highly specific antiviral protein. In this way the effect of a single interferon molecule could be amplified many times over, perhaps even enough to affect all of the thousands of ribosomes in the cell. A model for this mechanism, devised by Phillip I. Marcus and Jesse M. Salb of Albert Einstein School of Medicine, is shown in illustration on pages 262-263.

This second protein is presumed to be directly responsible for protecting the interferon-treated cell. Marcus and Salb proposed that the second protein inhibits translation of virus messenger RNA into virus protein by the cell's ribosomes. But this protein does not interfere with the ribosomes' ability to recognize and therefore translate host messenger RNA. Although infection by some viruses can kill the cell, even if it is interferon-protected, the virus cannot replicate and infection therefore cannot spread to other cells in the body.

Interferon has been identified in vertebrates from fish to man. Interferon obtained from one species will be most active in that species. It may have limited activity in cells from animals that are closely related phylogenetically, and will have little or no effect when the animals are very distantly related. Chick interferon, for example, acts only on chick cells but not on human or mouse cells. Mouse interferon, on the other hand, will retain about 5% of its activity in hamster cells. At present, only human and monkey interferon have been shown to have any significant effect in man.

Some investigators have questioned the role of interferon as a major defense mechanism against virus infections. Nevertheless, the evidence is strongly in favor of this view, if not completely convincing in all cases. Circulating interferon can be detected early in the course of an infection – while viremia is increasing but before gross pathological changes occur. Dr. Samuel Baron of the National Institute of Allergy and Infectious Diseases has shown in animals that clinical improvement begins when interferon can first be detected circulating in the blood. Antibodies, on the other hand, do not appear for several days after that. In certain infections Dr. Baron has demonstrated that interferon is present at the correct time and in sufficient quantities to increase natural resistance and promote recovery. It is found under these circumstances either at the place where the virus entered the host or in the tissues of the target organ.

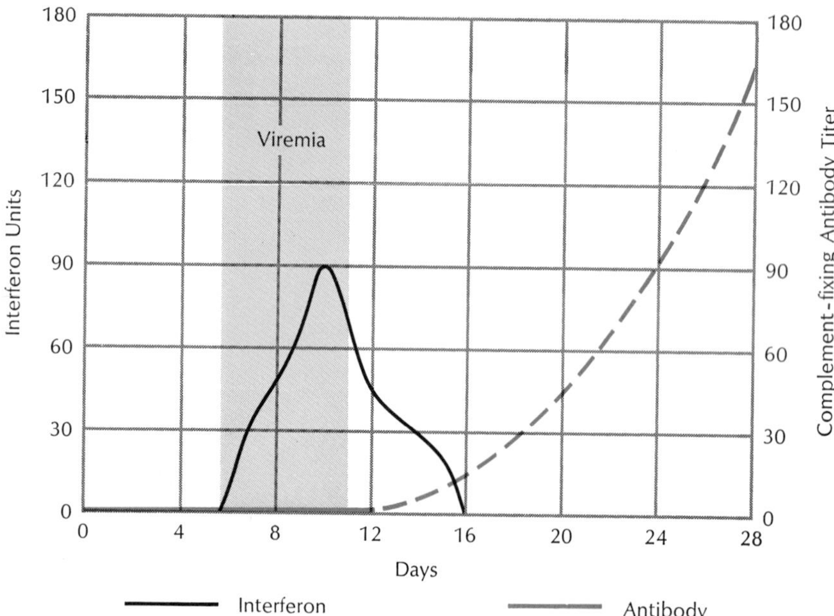

Interferon peaks early in the course of an infection – the example given is from the author's study of primary measles vaccination in infants – when almost no antibody can be detected. By the time the antibody titer reaches a significant level, interferon is gone. Viremia-interferon sequence is based on studies in monkeys.

From all this it is clear that we do not know all we would like to know about interferon and how it works. But the indications to date are that the viral protective mechanism could have an important future in clinical medicine. Now we need to ask how interferon has been used against natural and experimental infections and what this experience suggests in the way of future applications.

There are two basic ways interferon can be used in the prevention or treatment of virus infection. The first is direct administration of the protein, obtained from tissue culture. The second is stimulation of natural interferon production by the host's own cells. The latter can be carried out either locally at the sites of virus invasion or growth, or systemically where widespread infection has occurred or in situations when local therapy cannot be instituted.

Both French and Russian investigators have administered human interferon systemically to patients in clinical trials. The protein was produced by cultured leukocytes. Monkey interferon, collected from cultured kidney cells, has been used by British researchers as local therapy for infections of the cornea and skin. The results of such experiments were favorable, but the procedure required to produce interferon for administration is so cumbersome it does not seem to have much future for widespread application. Tissue culture is a tedious and expensive process, and the interferon requires careful purification.

Stimulation or induction of interferon by the treated host is a much more practical approach. For instance, in our laboratory in 1964 we used the highly attenuated virus employed for primary measles vaccination in infants to induce interferon production. We stimulated enough interferon to protect the children against infection by a second, unrelated virus – the vaccinia virus given to them for protection against smallpox.

Russian workers are already claiming clinical value for a virus inducer. They utilize ultraviolet-irradiated Semliki Forest virus that has been killed but still stimulates interferon production. They report this is active against viral infections in the eye, respiratory tract, and skin. Local treatment with the inducer has been used against herpes simplex in the eye and influenza in the respiratory tract. Chickenpox and herpes zoster infections of the skin, on the other hand, are treated systemically.

The initial Russian studies were controlled, but recent investigations have only been compared retrospectively with past experience using other forms of therapy. This is because their clinicians feel they cannot withhold effective therapy from any patient. Unfortunately, these experiments have not been described in English in sufficient detail to allow us to evaluate their findings.

Viruses are not the only agents that will induce interferon and produce protection. Intracellular parasites higher up the phylogenetic scale, such as bacteria and protozoa, will also do this. But the use of infectious agents for induction has several disadvantages. They may be contaminated with more dangerous adventitious agents, or they may not behave benignly in all hosts. In particular, they will often cause disease in the individuals we would most like to protect – those whose defenses against infection are already deficient.

Even nonliving extracts of intracellular parasites are active in interferon stimulation. Examples include endotoxin, phytohemagglutinin, and the antibiotic cycloheximide. But these substances all have toxic effects at the

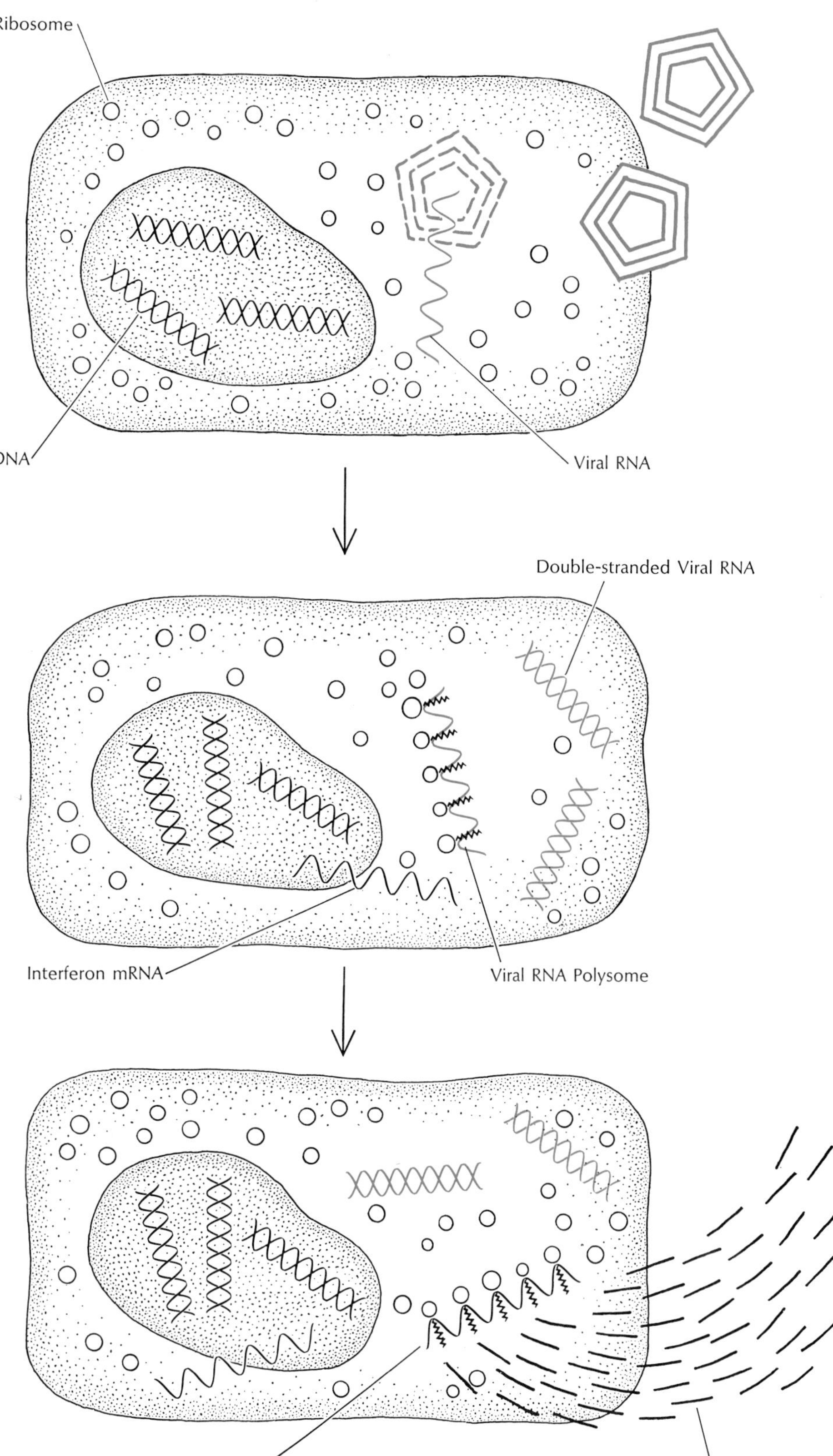

Model for the induction of interferon begins with cell penetration by a virus, followed by its uncoating and the release of a single strand of RNA. In the second stage, the viral RNA has replicated, and one strand has attached to host cell ribosomes; the former event, still hypothetical, may serve as the trigger for the derepression of a host cell DNA cistron, followed by the formation of interferon messenger RNA. In the third stage of induction, polysomes incorporating the interferon mRNA produce and release interferon. Succeeding events are depicted on the next two pages.

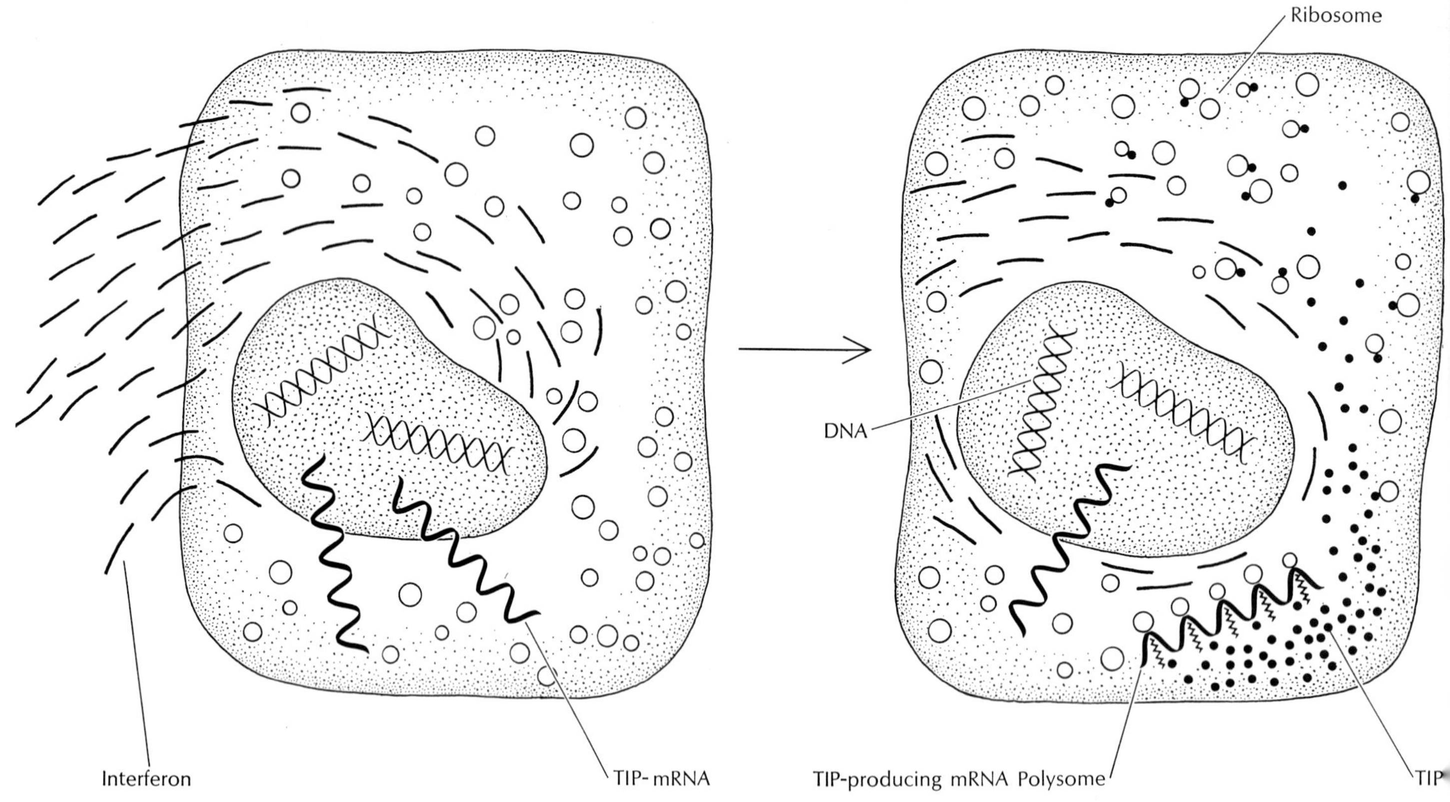

How Marcus and Salb suggest interferon may work to protect the cell is schematized above: As interferon enters an uninfected cell it derepresses a host DNA cistron to form "translation inhibitory protein" messenger RNA (left). This TIP-mRNA binds to ribosomes, leading to the synthesis of TIP and the contribution of TIP molecules to the ribosomal pool (center). Now, when

levels required to trigger sufficient production.

Despite the drawbacks of each of the methods of induction mentioned so far, investigation has not been discouraged. The availability of a large number of inducers suggests that eventually a safe and relatively inexpensive one can be found.

Four years ago a new lead on this problem produced exciting results with the discovery of a whole group of materials that may meet these criteria. These materials are double-stranded ribonucleic acids. They can be obtained from many sources, including certain fungal, bacterial, and animal viruses. In addition, synthetic double-stranded RNA made in a test tube can serve as a very effective interferon inducer.

There is an interesting story behind discovery of the RNA inducers. Several years ago Dr. Maurice Hilleman and his associates at the Merck Institute for Research in West Point, Pa., obtained patents on a fungus that had antiviral effects when injected into animals. Then, in 1964, Dr. Walter Kleinschmidt and his group at Lilly Research Laboratories in Indianapolis, Ind., published a report about a similar fungus that was active against viruses only through its ability to stimulate interferon production. Both research teams pursued this further and discovered that the fungus itself was not active but that it harbored a mycophage, or fungal virus, which was the critical factor in producing interferon.

Hilleman's group learned that the fungal virus contained a double-stranded RNA. This went along with their empirical discovery that almost all types of double-stranded RNA are active interferon inducers. These researchers even made RNA synthetically, producing a double-stranded homopolymer (with a single nucleotide repeated throughout each strand) that stimulated production too.

These findings have been widely confirmed and it has now been demonstrated that the RNA inducers work against many experimental animal infections. Several laboratories have major efforts under way to evaluate these compounds. Preliminary tests of toxicity are being undertaken prior to clinical studies. Studies are also in progress to determine the best route of administration, most effective time for injection, length of action, and methods for potentiating the inducers' action. One method of potentiation, for instance, involves treating cells with polycations. Dr. Fernando Dianzani of Siena University in Italy has shown that these materials promote the action of the inducer on the cells.

Three recent reports have further encouraged those of us involved in this field. All three have depended upon the synthetic homopolymer polyinosinic-polycytidylic acid, which is abbreviated as PI:C. The first report was from Dr. John H. Park of New York Medical College and Dr. Baron late in 1968. They demonstrated the therapeutic effect of PI:C in severe rabbit keratoconjunctivitis. Treatment promoted recovery even when it was begun as late as three days after herpes simplex virus was applied to the animals' eyes.

As the researchers wrote in *Science*, "The present findings demonstrate that the interferon mechanism can be applied to enhance recovery from a

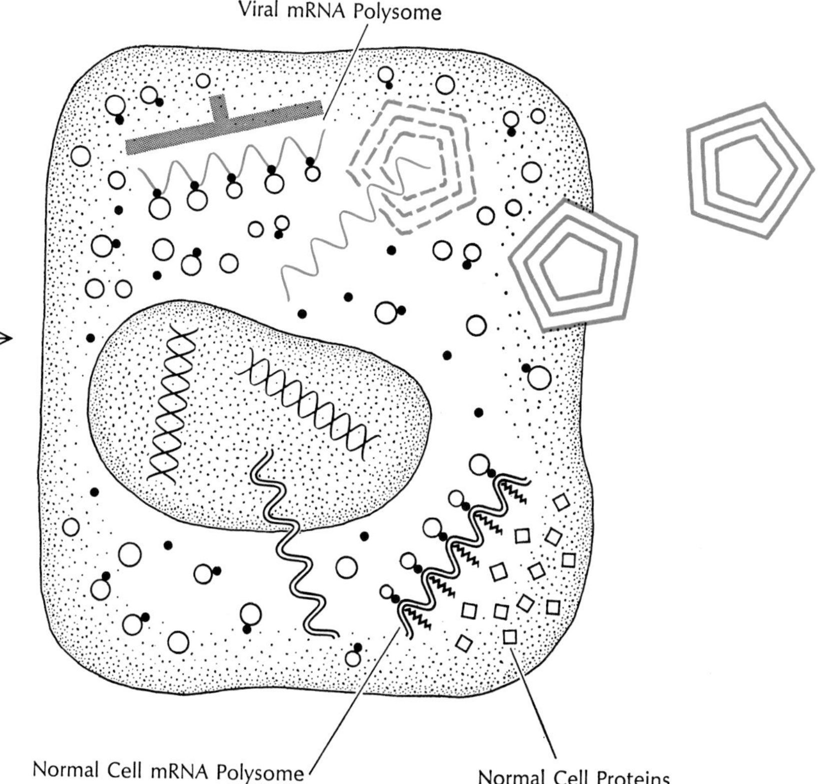

a virus penetrates the cell, TIP's association with the ribosomes prevents the takeover of the latter by the viral RNA. Viral capability for replication is blocked but normal cell mRNA continues to be translated to form normal cell proteins.

fully established acute viral infection." Park and Baron went on to predict further extensions of their therapeutic findings "because herpes simplex virus is only moderately sensitive to the antiviral action of interferon in rabbit cells. Since there are many viruses that are more sensitive to the antiviral effect of interferon, it seems possible that effective therapy of these infections will be demonstrated."

Just a month later Dr. Ralph Pollikoff of Temple University School of Medicine reported confirming the herpes simplex results and achieving similar results with a very different virus, that causing vesicular stomatitis, which previously had not been associated with a corneal lesion.

Early in 1969 Dr. Hilton Levy of the National Institute of Allergy and Infectious Diseases and Drs. Lloyd Law and Alan Rabson of the National Cancer Institute revealed that daily injections of PI:C produced regressions of eight types of transplanted tumors in mice. The most striking effect was against a slowly growing tumor. Such tumors are usually very resistant to drugs. All control animals with this tumor were dead in six weeks. Treated animals all survived that period of time; one third were still alive two months later and showed no signs of cancer. These dramatic experiments will undoubtedly lead to similar studies in man very shortly.

The authors admit that they are by no means sure that the antitumor effects are due solely to interferon induction. The effects of PI:C in the whole animal are multiple; it increases the activity of both the reticuloendothelial system and the delayed hypersensitivity mechanism. Recent findings of Dr. Ion Gresser suggest, however, that even partially purified interferon preparations also have an antitumor effect in the whole animal. Dr. Gresser is with the Institut de Recherches Scientifiques sur le Cancer, at Villejuif, France.

There may be no absolute necessity that the RNA inducer contain two complementary strands. It may be that the two-strand form is more resistant to degradation by nucleases in the cell than single-stranded RNA. In both our laboratory and Baron's it has been shown that activity can be demonstrated with a single homopolymer type (polyinosinic or polycytidylic acid) when sensitive systems for measuring interferon production are used.

Even compounds that do not contain ribonucleotides but only grossly resemble RNA can serve as inducers. Collaborating with Dr. William Regelson of the Medical College of Virginia, we have demonstrated the interferon-inducing effects of the plastic pyran in both animals and man. Pyran is a random copolymer of maleic acid and divinyl ether. A group of Belgian workers, led by Drs. Pierre De Somer and Eric De Clercq of the University of Leuven, have studied a closely related plastic, polyacrylic acid.

In order for a plastic to induce interferon production it must have three characteristics. First, it must have a polymeric backbone which is hard to break down. Second, there should be a high density of negative charges; carboxylates serve here instead of the phosphates in RNA. Third, the molecular weight should be high, on the order of that found in RNA.

Our initial studies with plastics in man have unfortunately demonstrated that these compounds have some undesirable side effects. They produce transient thrombocytopenia, although there are no hemorrhagic sequelae. They also persist in the reticuloendothelial system for long periods of time. We do not have experience with other componds that persist this way, and we do not know what the consequences may be.

On the other hand, the plastics do provide extended protection against certain virus infections, sometimes lasting for months after a single injection. This may be attributable to prolonged induction of low levels of interferon. If this is the case, reticuloendothelial persistence may not be such a handicap.

The plastics do not stimulate as wide a variety of cells as the ribonucleic acids, and accordingly bring about distinctly lower levels of circulating interferon. This may prove to be an additional shortcoming with these compounds. A possible explanation for this is that the plastics only penetrate cells with a high assimilative capacity material – macrophages, in other words.

Because of their persistence in the

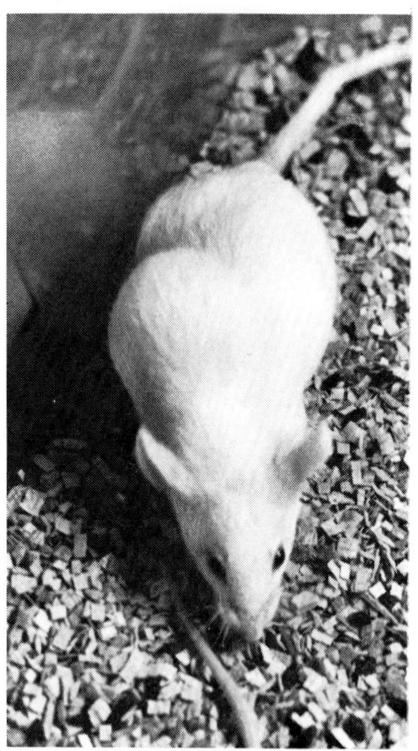

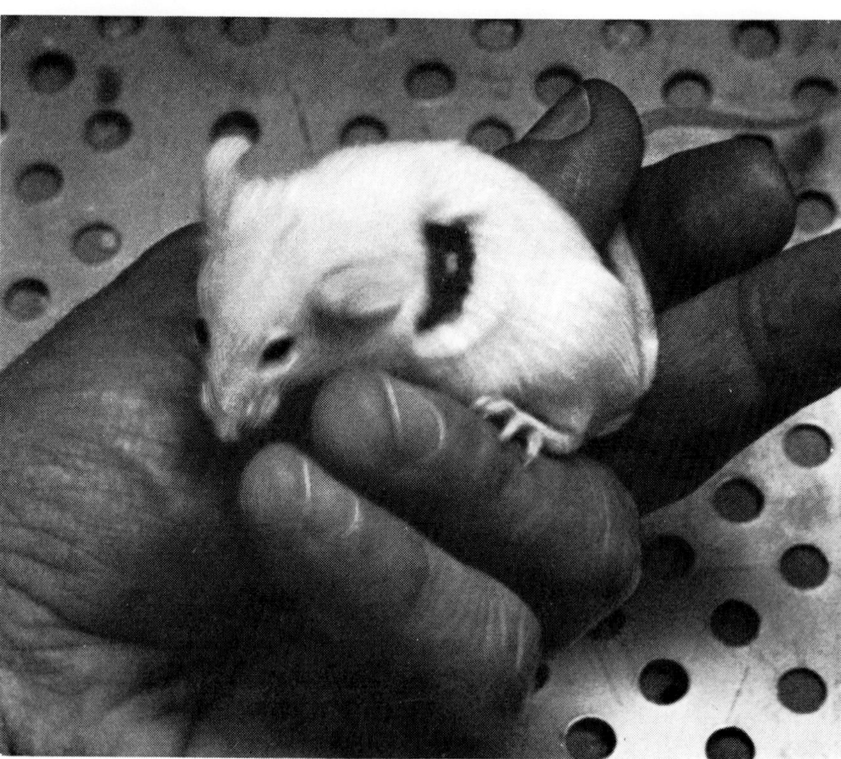

Tumor induced by human adenovirus 12(MT_1) and implanted in BalbC mouse (left) is invariably lethal; if mouse is treated with PI:C, as Dr. Hilton Levy and other investigators at NIH reported recently, massive destruction and sloughing of tumor tissue occurs (right). Similar regressions of eight different types of transplanted tumors have been observed in PI:C-treated mice.

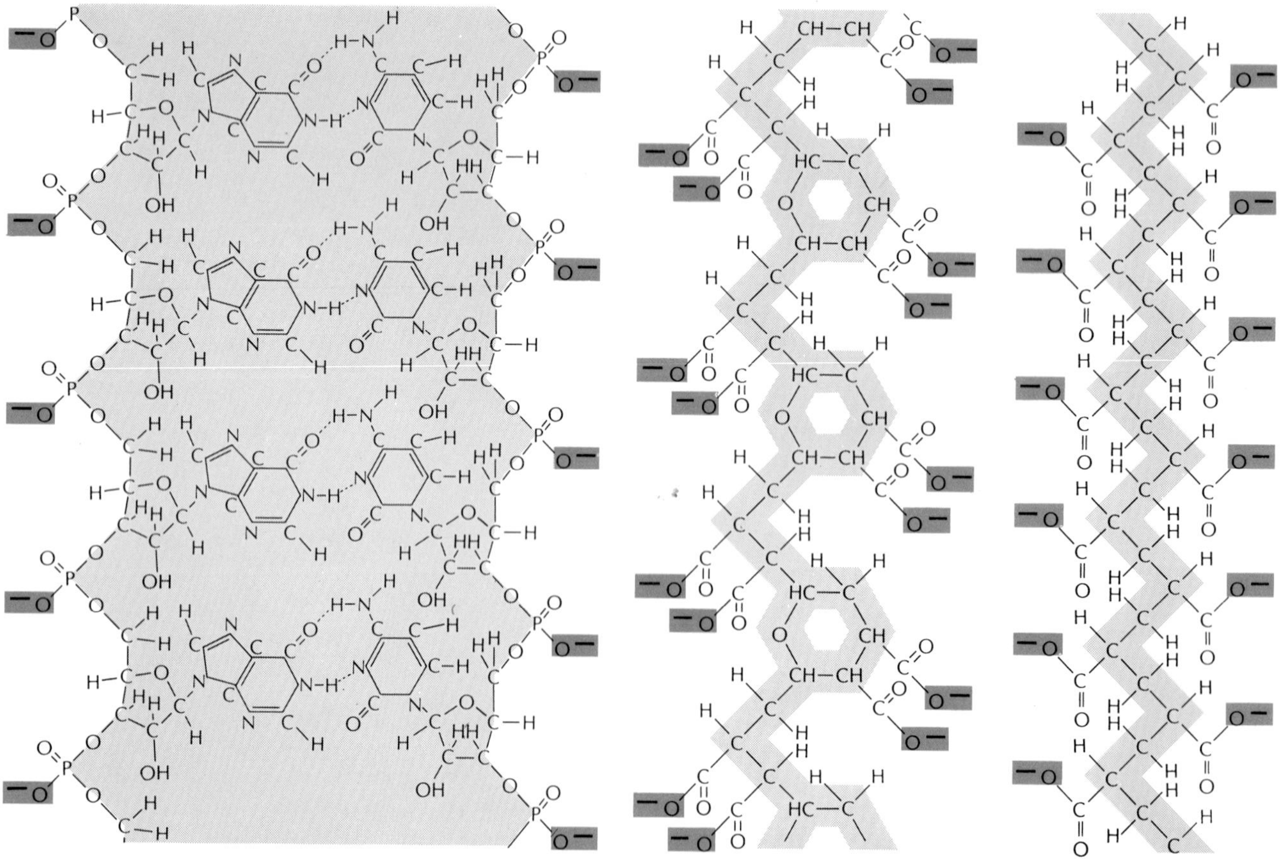

Molecular structure of the interferon inducer PI:C is compared with those of two plastics having interferon-inducing properties, pyran (center) and polyacrylic acid (right). In all three the stable polymeric backbone believed necessary to antiviral activity is shown in color as are the essential negative charges which give these polymers their anionic nature.

body, it seems likely that the synthetic plastic inducers will come into use initially in veterinary practice. Many virus diseases in animals are economically important and also serve as models for human conditions. Suitable diseases for testing might include Aleutian disease in mink, chicken leukosis, shipping fever and hoof-and-mouth disease in cattle, and distemper in dogs. Temporary protection from any one of these ailments would be useful while subtle, long-term toxicities were being investigated. Exploratory studies are already under way in several veterinary units.

Just as infectious agents more complex than viruses can spur cells to produce interferon, interferon inducers are also probably effective against intracellular parasites other than viruses. Dr. René Jahiel and his associates at New York University School of Medicine have utilized the fungal mycophage statolon, PI:C, and Newcastle disease virus as inducers in mice to protect them against the malarial parasite *Plasmodium berghei.*

Research in our laboratory, conducted in cooperation with two other groups of investigators, has independently demonstrated that interferon itself is active against agents other than viruses. With Drs. Levelle Hanna and Ernest Jawetz of the University of California School of Medicine in San Francisco, we found that mouse interferon applied to mouse cells in tissue culture was effective against the trachoma agents. These agents more nearly resemble bacteria than viruses – they replicate differently, contain RNA, DNA, and certain enzymes, and are susceptible to certain antibiotics. In collaboration with Dr. Jack Remington here at Stanford, we found that chick and mouse interferon also protect their respective cells from the intracellular protozoan *Toxoplasma gondii.*

These findings could prove very useful in improving our understanding of diseases caused by these parasites. It is conceivable that the cyclical, relapsing course of these infections is a result of the interferon mechanism. The parasites may induce interferon production, respond to it, but then persist in some latent form, only to cause a subsequent outbreak and patient relapse at another time. If such is the case, we might eventually learn to manipulate the host's interferon production to keep the disease under control.

Despite the encouraging results with inducers so far, we must accept the possibility that they may have noxious side effects – or, on the other hand, valuable immunologic effects – of which we are not yet aware. One problem with inducers is that animals seem to become less reactive to them when they are given repeatedly. This could ultimately limit their effectiveness, particularly in providing sustained protection during an epidemic, or their usefulness in patients with chronic infection or weakened immunologic defenses.

There are also some puzzling questions raised by the materials that inhibit the interferon mechanism. Two of these are virus-induced proteins, "stimulon" and "enhancer," that curb interferon's protective activity and accordingly promote virus replication. The first of these was recognized by Dr. Charles Chany of Hôpital St.-Vincent-de-Paul in Paris, France. Another substance reduces interferon production, but does not alter its action. This material is known as "blocker." It is possible that these substances could seriously limit the effectiveness of interferon prophylaxis or therapy, but our experience with animal models for human disease suggests this will not be the case.

At present I feel there are enough unresolved problems with systemic induction of interferon to limit initial human experiments to patients with severe infections carrying a high morbidity or mortality. Diseases in this category would include encephalitis, hepatitis, and overwhelming vaccinia, variola, varicella, or herpes zoster. Under such circumstances patients would have much to gain, and the benefit would outweigh any possible danger from the inducer. If such tests showed that the inducer was safe to administer, then the approach could be extended to more benign ailments of the respiratory tract or gut.

Patients with tumors, neurological diseases, or autoimmune conditions that may be of viral etiology could also be early candidates for interferon therapy. One of the earliest clues to the potential value of such an approach against malignant disease was provided by Drs. Fred Wheelock and John Dingle at Case Western Reserve University School of Medicine. Several years ago they reported that the course of a patient with acute leukemia improved on several occasions with systemic induction of interferon by different live viruses. One difficulty here is that interferon is only active against the DNA tumor viruses in tissue culture when it is used before the virus has caused malignant transformation.

Recently, however, Dr. Chany reported that prolonged interferon treatment reversed the transformed state of cells infected with the Moloney sarcoma virus in tissue culture. In addition, Drs. Gresser and Wheelock each independently showed that interferon was effective against virus-induced mouse leukemia in vivo.

Findings such as these have led Maurice Hilleman to suggest that we may want to interrupt the vertical transmission of yet-to-be-proven human tumor viruses through the use of interferon inducers. They might be administered early in childhood, or even to the mother to prevent virus transmission to the fetus. Obviously such an approach would require complete confidence in the safety of the inducer as well as clear evidence that some human cancer has a viral etiology.

My experience leads me to be cautious in predicting the immediate clinical future for interferon treatment. Nevertheless, the latest findings are more encouraging than any of us had expected. Limited clinical trials will probably be under way within the next year or two. They should make important contributions to our understanding of the role of the interferon mechanism in human disease.

Chapter 27

The Control of Rh Disease

VINCENT J. FREDA
Columbia University

A generation ago exchange transfusion was added to the weapons available for combating erythroblastosis fetalis. The technique markedly reduced postnatal deaths caused by the disease, as well as its nonfatal sequelae.

Over the past 10 years a further reduction in both postnatal and prenatal deaths has been achieved. Thanks, in the main, to diagnostic advances, mortality has been reduced by about two thirds during this period. And today, even newer — and still experimental — approaches give promise of wiping out the disease entirely in the foreseeable future.

When exchange transfusion was first applied in the 1940's it quickly proved its efficacy in reducing the postnatal sequelae of erythroblastosis fetalis. Provided the infant survived delivery and the hazards of transfusion, his chances for avoiding neurologic damage were great.

But something like 30 percent of the infants did not survive, about two thirds of these deaths occurring in utero from anemia coupled with heart failure. The casualties, almost without exception, were victims of Rh incompatibility (ABO blood incompatibilities are hardly ever significant in prenatal life). It was suspected that a substantial proportion of this fetal wastage could be prevented by early delivery. Unfortunately, there were no good criteria for deciding when to do this.

On the assumption that a sharp rise in antibody titer reflected increased fetal jeopardy, obstetricians at that time guided themselves, as best they could, by the level of Rh antibodies in the mother's blood. Experience soon showed, however, that only about one third of all Rh-incompatible fetuses caused a rise in maternal antibodies. In the most severe cases, in fact, the titer remained stable throughout pregnancy four times out of five. It became clear that antibody tests, measuring events in the mother's bloodstream, were but feeble indicators of any clinically significant changes in the fetus. As a result, the obstetrician was faced with the alternative of early delivery in all suspected cases — with resulting heavy loss from prematurity — or, more often, of crossing his fingers and letting the pregnancies go to term, with equally heavy losses from erythroblastosis.

In 1952, Dr. D. C. A. Bevis of Manchester, England, suggested that spectrophotometric analysis of amnionic fluid could provide valuable information in Rh pregnancies. Such an assay, he pointed out, would provide evidence on the concentration of pigments, chiefly bilirubin, produced by hemolysis in the fetal bloodstream and it would therefore be a fairly sensitive indicator of the degree to which fetal survival was compromised.

Bevis' suggestion proved exceedingly fertile, and within a few years amniocentesis and spectrophotometric assay of the fluid sample had come into wide use in England, Australia, and the U. S. At Presbyterian Hospital we have carried out more than 8,000 of these procedures, with no mortality or morbidity in either mother or fetus, and have found them invaluable in the management of Rh pregnancies. They enable us to say, with considerable assurance, when the fetus is in no danger, when danger threatens but is not immediate, when hemolysis is producing significant circulatory distress and when the threat of death is so severe as to make some sort of intervention obligatory.

Our own criteria for undertaking amniocentesis are partly based on the mother's obstetric history but chiefly on her antibody level. This may sound like something of a contradiction. But antibody titers, although they cannot identify the fetus that is in danger, can consistently point out the fetus that is not. Our own clinical records show that where the antiglobulin titer was 1:16 or less 10 days prior to delivery, there were virtually no stillbirths or neonatal deaths due to Rh. Accordingly, we do not perform amniocentesis unless the antibody titer is in excess of that level.

It should be emphasized, however, that because of minor differences in titration techniques among laboratories, the figure of 1:16 cannot be taken as a "standard"; each hospital must evolve its own serologic criteria based on its own experience. Given a suspicious titer (1:32 or higher), we then undertake amniocentesis immediately. Until quite recently we employed radioisotope injection and/or thermography to locate the placenta, so as to avoid piercing it with the sampling needle. We have now found, however, that simply by performing the puncture lower down on the abdomen—at the suprapubic site—we can consistently miss the placenta. A bimanual examination can localize the fetus, and elevation of the presenting part can prevent fetal trauma.

When the sampled fluid is scanned and charted by spectrophotometry, abnormal amounts of hemolysis pigments show up as a "hump" in the normally smooth slope of the curve. Interpretation of the curves is rather too complex to describe here in detail; briefly, we classify them, depending on the height of the hump, on an arbitrary scale ranging from "normal" to "4+ abnormal."

With a normal reading, the only follow-up required is a repeat test two weeks later, since no reading can safely prognosticate beyond that period. A 1+ curve is interpreted in much the same way, except that the follow-up should be delayed for no more than 10 days. Experience shows that a 1+ can rise quite rapidly to 3+ or even 4+.

With a 2+ curve, we know unequivocally that the fetus is Rh positive and is affected by some degree of hemolysis. We also know that it is in no immediate danger, but now the test must be repeated weekly. This reading is therefore not an indicator for premature delivery, that is, before 37 weeks, unless there has been a previous affected pregnancy. In that case, data for the earlier pregnancy should be reviewed in an effort to determine the optimum time for delivery.

A 3+ reading indicates that the fetus is in distress. We believe the rise in pigment concentration does not necessarily reflect more energetic hemolysis but is caused by the beginning of circulatory impairment. As a result the pig-

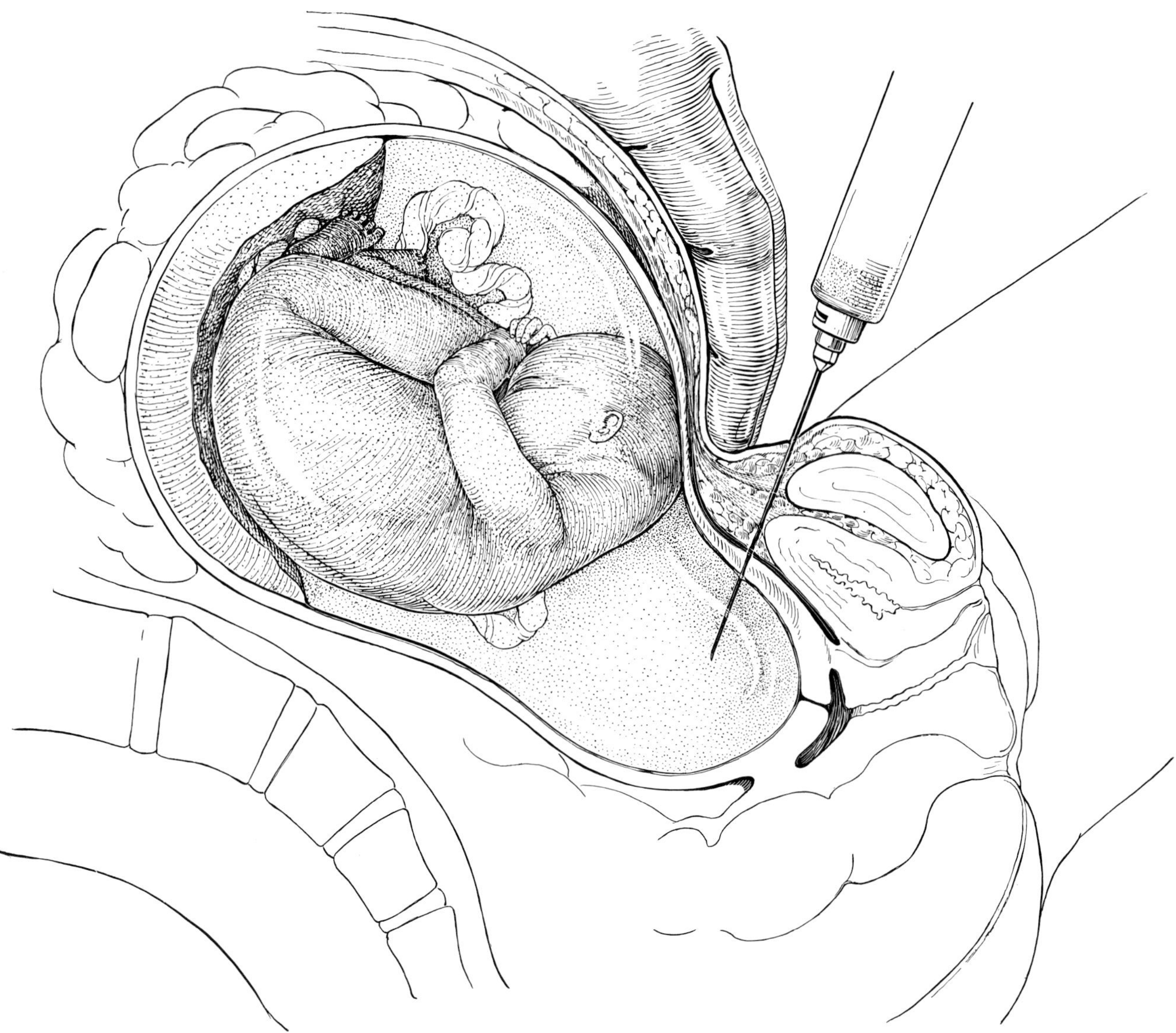

Amniocentesis to obtain fluid sample for spectrophotometric analysis is basic technique that has cut mortality in Rh disease. Normally it is carried out at suprapubic site after localization and manual elevation of the fetus.

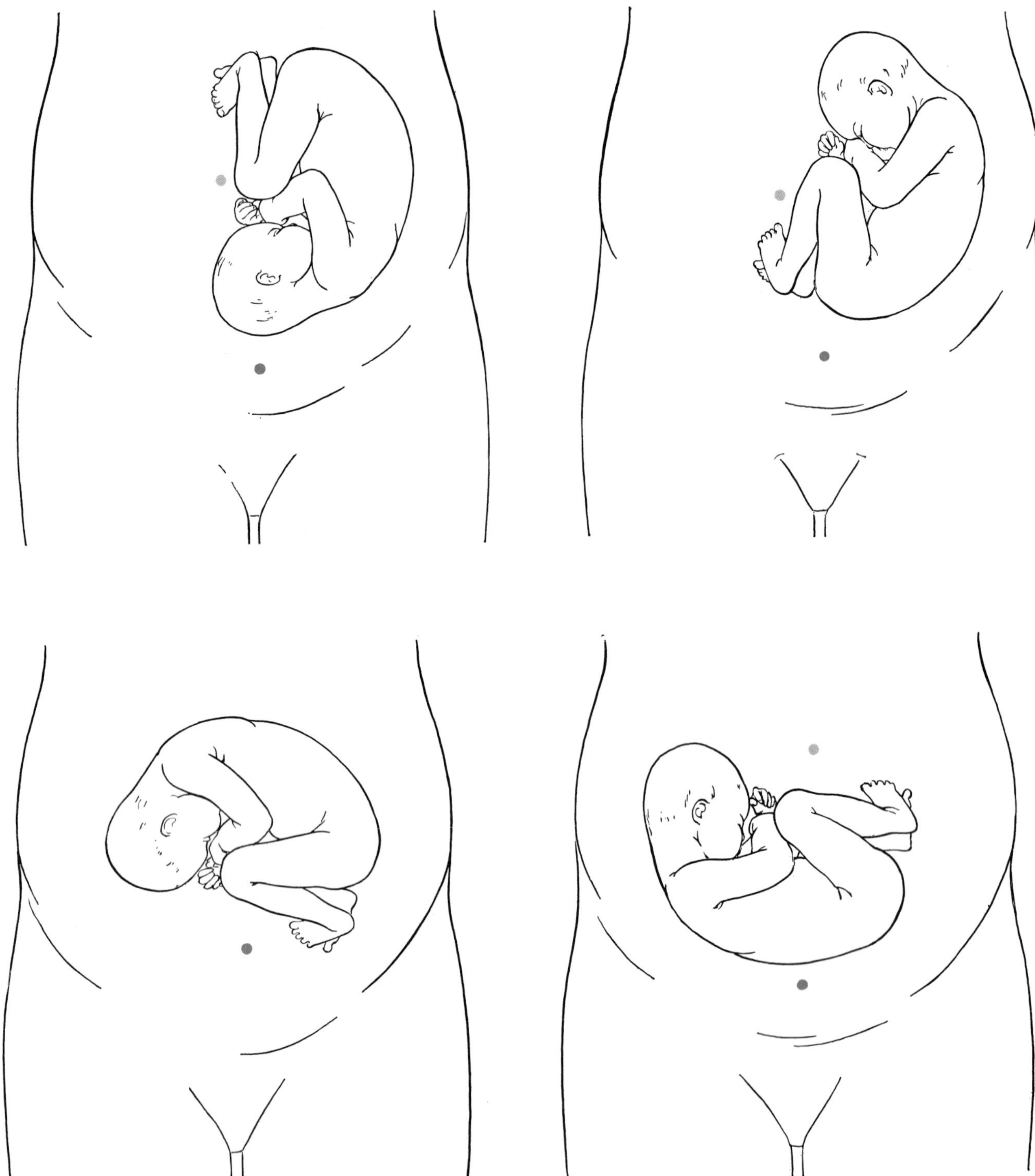

Unless fetal position makes it impracticable, suprapubic area (colored dots) is preferred for amniocentesis. Alternative sites (shown as tinted dots) require that the placenta be located by x-ray or thermographic techniques.

ments are less effectively cleared from the blood via the placenta and tend to be excreted more copiously into the amnionic fluid by one or more pathways. A 3+ curve is also clear evidence that the fetus' course will inevitably continue to deteriorate. If pregnancy has reached at least the 32nd week, delivery should be undertaken with little delay — if possible by induced labor, otherwise by section. A 4+ reading indicates that fetal death is imminent, so that delivery should be undertaken immediately, though the prognosis in these cases is poor in any event.

It is worth stressing that spectrophotometric analysis of the fluid samples is essential. Visual examination is not only inherently inaccurate but can be thrown off, in a "false positive" direction, by various contaminants. Spectrophotometry, however, can usually distinguish the color abnormalities produced by contaminants from those indicating hemolysis. One important exception is that of meconium contamination, when an accurate reading is sometimes impossible. In early pregnancy, this type of contamination is fortunately rare; when it is unrelated to the Rh problem it usually clears up within a few weeks. After 35 weeks, however, meconium contamination may in itself be an indicator of impending fetal demise. This then calls for immediate delivery. Curiously enough, detailed analysis of several hundred cases revealed that the spectrophotometric readings, especially those in the "normal" to "2+ abnormal" range, show a rather poor correlation with such conventional postnatal measurements as cord hemoglobin and cord bilirubin. They show a very high correlation, however, with the clinical outcome, in terms of fetal and neonatal survival.

Amniocentesis, simply by providing the obstetrician with clear criteria for premature induction of labor, has cut mortality in Rh pregnancies from around 30 percent to 10 percent. By itself, however, it offers no hope for the fetus in acute distress prior to 32 weeks — i.e., the time before which it would have only a slight chance of survival if delivered immediately. A partial solution to this problem has come through the work of Dr. A. W. Liley of Aukland, New Zealand, one of the pioneers in developing spectrophotometric amniocentesis.

Liley's success with the diagnostic technique encouraged him to undertake a procedure that if undertaken "blind" would have seemed prohibitively risky: transfusion in utero. His first case, in 1963, was successful. Since then the procedure has been carried out hundreds of times in various institutions.

As generally performed, it begins with localization of the fetal viscera using injections of special contrast media into the amnionic fluid, followed by x-ray of the uterus. A needle is then passed through the mother's uterine and abdominal walls into the peritoneal space of the fetus. Through this needle, packed erythrocytes are injected. The procedure can be repeated as needed at 14-day intervals until the fetus has attained sufficient maturity to allow premature delivery.

While the Liley technique represents a major gain in management of Rh pregnancies, it is only a partial

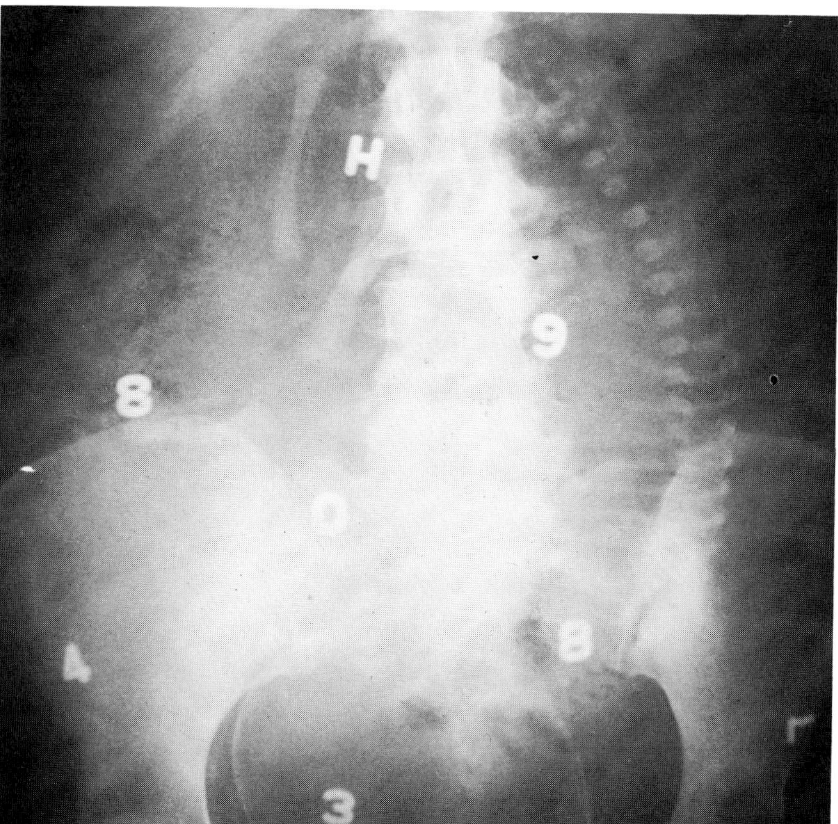

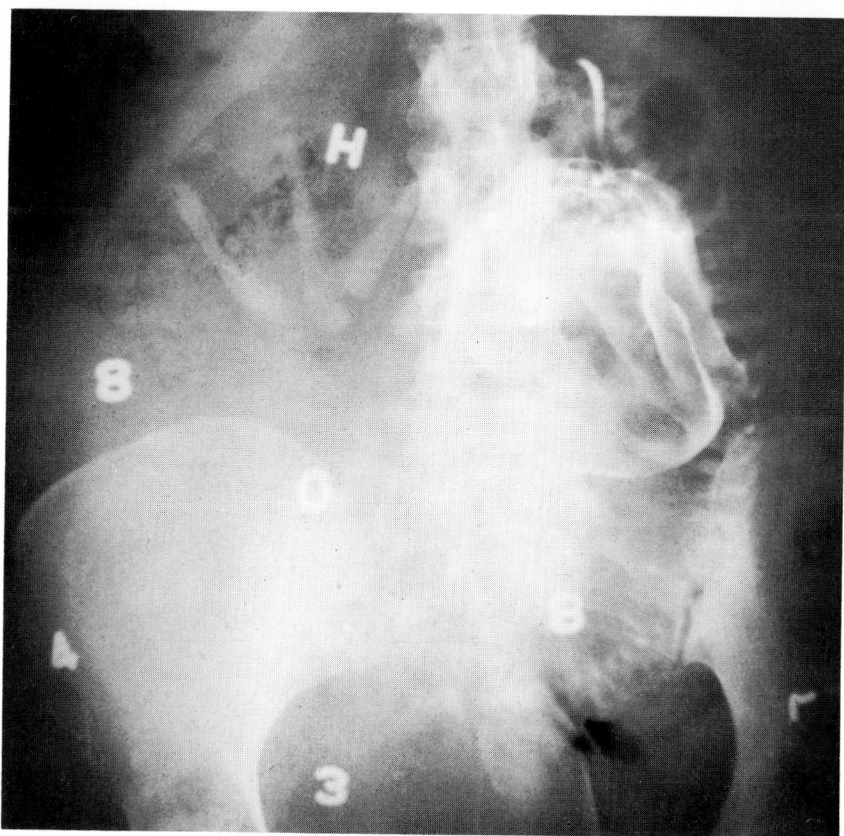

"Closed" transfusion requires injection of dye into amnionic cavity 24 hours prior to the procedure. The dye is then concentrated in the alimentary canal of the fetus (top) and is the target for the needle. A catheter is threaded through the needle, which is then removed, and dye is injected through the catheter to outline the peritoneal cavity of the baby (bottom) and thus confirm correct placement of the needle.

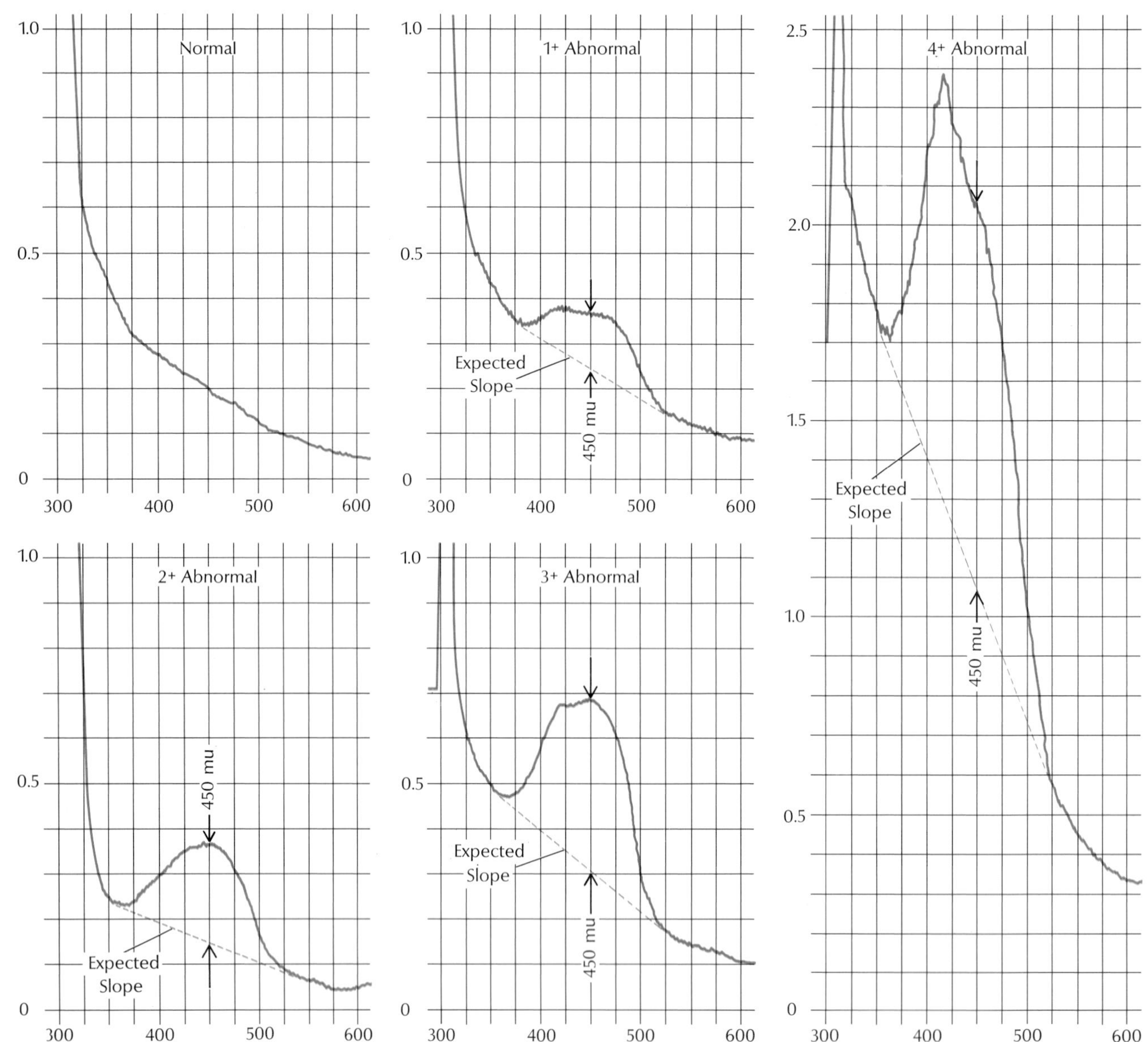

Spectrophotometric curves graph absorption of light by sample of amnionic fluid at various wavelengths. Broad "hump" centered about 450 mμ shows fetal hemolysis; its height indicates the degree and immediacy of danger, as explained more fully in text. Shift to peak at 420 mμ, incipient in 3+ curves, is invariably well marked in 4+ curves.

answer, for the most severe Rh cases are still not being salvaged. Various reports have described the technique as successful in from 30 to 50 percent of the "nonhydropic" cases. My own feeling is that the lower figure is probably the significant one, assuming one excludes cases in which the procedure was in fact unnecessary — for example, if the spectrophotometric reading was no worse than 2+. It is important to bear in mind that all of these reports exclude the already hydropic fetuses, that is, those in which abnormally rapid circulatory decline has made transfusion a forlorn hope at best. Transfusions of this type are likely to prove most useful in cases where the fetus is not in severe distress before about 28 weeks and can be tided over by transfusion until it can be delivered with a fair chance of survival.

Before 25 weeks, Liley's "closed" transfusion approach has yielded discouraging results. Because of the rapid increase in fetal blood volume, repeated transfusions are always required. The fetus at that age is a small, moving target, and the chance of injuring it — assuming, of course, that the target is hit at all — is prohibitively great.

The limitations of this closed approach have led us, and other clinicians, to attempt more radical transfusion techniques. In most cases these have involved hysterotomy and the insertion of an indwelling catheter into the fetus, through which it can be transfused repeatedly. In some cases, this "open" technique has kept the fetus alive as long as two months. A compilation of case reports thus far shows only two fetal survivals out of 15 surgical attempts. It should be noted, however, that six of the fetuses that died were severely hydropic to begin with. Thus the "true" survival figure is something like 22 percent; this, while obviously unsatisfactory, is not grossly different from our own results (in 40 older fetuses) with the closed technique.

Whether technical improvements can better the results of either the closed or open approach is questionable. In any event, any surgical approach would seem to be a stopgap measure at best. A far more satisfactory solution would be to devise a safe and effective method of neutralizing the maternal Rh antibodies or of controlling the mother's immune response. This would provide a simple, safe therapy for all Rh-immunized pregnancies.

Though no method of this sort is now in the offing, a number of theoretical approaches to it are worth exploring. For example, it is conceivable that interference with the mother's physiologic "feedback" mechanisms might do the job. I for one have always believed that even where active immunity has been established, the actual production of antibodies may be controlled by feedback — in basically the same way as endocrine production is known to be controlled. Since the thyroid gland, for instance, can be inhibited from producing thyroxin by giving endogenous thyroid, it seems reasonable to suppose that the mother's production of Rh antibody could be blocked by administration of exogenous antibody during pregnancy. A major problem here, however, is that the exogenous substance would have to be unable to pass the placenta (to avoid iatrogenic damage to the fetus) yet be sufficiently specific in structure to be "recognized" by the mother's immunologic mechanisms, thereby suppressing them.

Interestingly, and perhaps significantly, a somewhat similar immunologic approach has been applied — and far more productively — to the still more basic problem of preventing Rh disease entirely. This involves blocking immunization in the mother; it is based on an established concept, dating from as early as 1909, that passive immunity can block active immunity.

Around 1960, it occurred to Dr. John G. Gorman, director of our hospital blood bank, Dr. William Pollack of the Ortho Research Foundation,

Critical Cut-Off Points for the Spectral Estimation of Clinical Severity

Freda's Classification	*Clinical Interpretation*	*Net Absorptivity at 450 mμ*
1+	Normal or possibly affected	<0.20
2+	Affected, but not in jeopardy	0.20-0.34
3+	Distressed and probably in failure	0.35-0.70
4+	Impending fetal death	>0.70

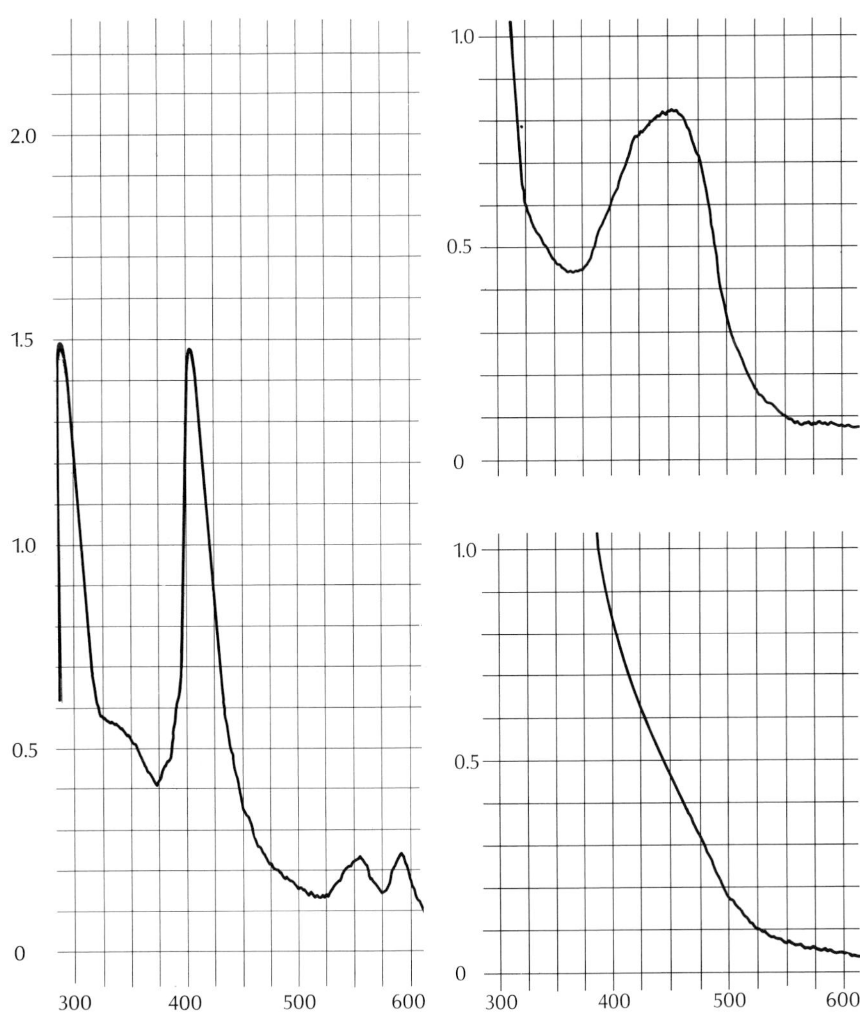

Hemoglobin contamination of sample produces a sharp peak at 415 mμ as well as small secondary peaks (left). All are easily distinguished from the "hump" characteristic of erythroblastosis. Visual rating of samples can be misleading. Curves of fluid (top right) and maternal urine (bottom right) are markedly different, yet color seemed identical.

and me that mothers could be protected against Rh immunization by giving them exogenous Rh antibody shortly after delivery of the first Rh-positive child. The antibody obviously could not affect the child, yet should protect the mother against sensitization since it was generally thought that this occurred during labor and delivery rather than in earlier stages of pregnancy. The same idea occurred quite independently to another group, headed by Dr. R. Finn, in Liverpool. The British researchers had begun working with raw plasma from already immunized women, but we ruled this out because of the danger of hepatitis and serum reactions. Instead, we favored a pure gamma G globulin with a high anti-Rh titer that could produce a satisfactory circulating titer when injected in small doses intramuscularly.

Through Dr. Pollack we were able to obtain such a preparation and immediately set to work testing it on male volunteers at Sing Sing Prison. Over a four-year period we proved that it actually suppresses Rh antibody production following IV injections of Rh-positive cells. In patients heavily stimulated by Rh-positive cells, the Rh immunoglobulin gave 100% protection, with no side effects, even when given three days after the cell injection. It can be given as long as 72 hours after the red cells and still provide a complete effect. The Liverpool group, and others, subsequently

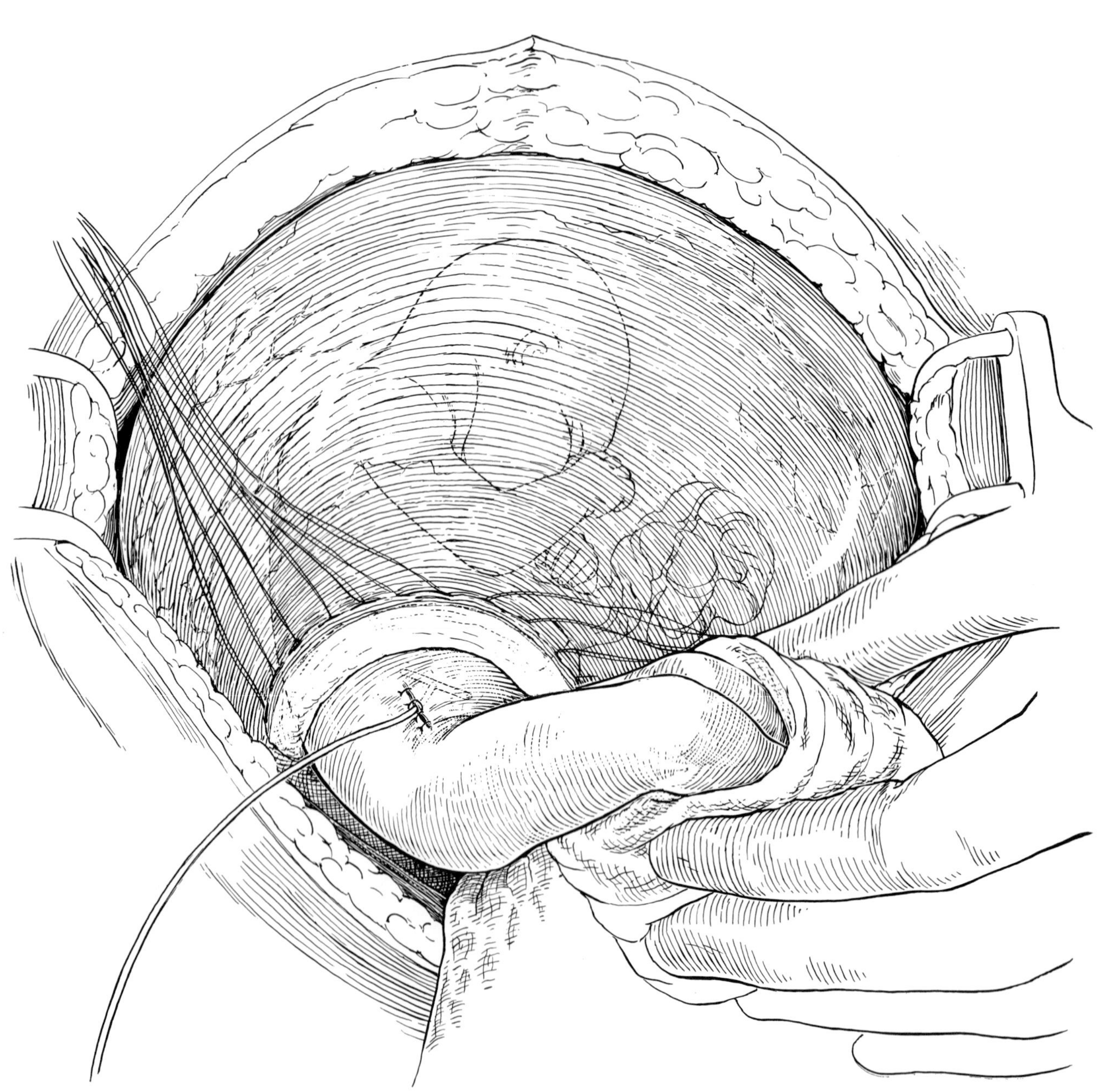

"Open" procedure for fetal transfusion involves hysterotomy, partial extraction of fetus, and insertion of T-tube into its abdominal cavity. After all incisions are closed, indwelling catheter permits repeated transfusions. Few of these infants survive to birth, but the operation is performed only where survivals could not otherwise be expected.

learned of this specialized preparation and adopted it in their own clinical trials.

Because of the encouraging findings, we felt confident enough of this material to begin a trial in Rh-negative mothers.

The first trial in mothers was begun by our group at Columbia-Presbyterian Medical Center in April 1964. In this trial, Rh immunoglobulin was injected intramuscularly into nonimmunized Rh-negative mothers within 72 hours of delivery of an ABO-compatible, Rh-positive baby. These mothers and noninjected controls were then followed at intervals with antibody screening. In this study the postpartum presence of fetal cells in the maternal circulation had no influence on whether a mother was admitted to the study; all mothers at risk were included.

Additional clinical trials using our preparation were then established in various centers around the world. The combined data from these studies were overwhelmingly impressive and far better than we had anticipated. The combined results clearly indicated that the Rh immunoglobulin preparation worked exceedingly well and was virtually completely effective in suppressing the primary immune response in all of the cases studied. The final proof of the complete efficacy of this preparation was obtained and confirmed after the results from a significant number of subsequent Rh-positive pregnancies had become known.

[A survey of world experience with controlled studies on the efficacy of Rh immunoglobulin treatment, in which the results of treatment were determined six months or more following delivery, shows that of 2,523 women treated, only four became sensitized. In subsequent pregnancies, these women were delivered of 303 infants, only two of whom had Rh disease. Among 2,299 women in control groups, 160 were sensitized; these women subsequently gave birth to 351 children, 48 of whom were affected.]

The patient, i.e., the mother who is a candidate for Rh immunoglobulin, should of course be Rh negative with plasma shown to be free of Rh antibodies. Her infant must be Rh positive and demonstrate a negative direct Coombs test. Since this preparation is in some respects similar to a unit of blood, it is recommended that the laboratory perform in vitro tests to ensure that the mother receives a compatible dose. Because it has been strongly suspected that a miscarriage may also cause sensitization to the Rh factor, it has been suggested that Rh immunoglobulin be administered after a miscarriage.

This author has already accumulated sufficient data to incriminate miscarriage as a significant source of Rh sensitization. The more advanced the pregnancy at the time of miscarriage, the greater the risk of sensitization. The risk of sensitization following miscarriage apparently lies somewhere between two and nine percent depending on the length of gestation. It appears to be virtually negligible at one month, definitely appreciable at two months, and very significant at three months and beyond. Consequently, all Rh-negative unsensitized mothers who have a miscarriage at two months or beyond should also receive Rh immunoglobulin whenever and wherever possible. The burden of this responsibility falls solely and squarely upon the attending obstetrician just as it does in the case of term pregnancies.

In the last analysis, it is the obstetrician who will and *must* play a key role in the ultimate eradication of this disease. How quickly it disappears clinically depends entirely on how well the obstetrician discharges his responsibility to the Rh-negative mother. The ultimate conquest of Rh disease of the newborn (or any other disease for that matter) has always depended on the development of effective prophylactic techniques – as any conquest must. Rh immunoglobulin is an extremely effective prophylactic treatment. Thus, the conquest of Rh disease is now a reality.

Chapter 28

To Vaccinate or Not?

C. HENRY KEMPE
University of Colorado

Smallpox vaccination, the first immunizing procedure employed by medicine, is also unquestionably the most successful. It has eradicated the disease in North America and (except for cases from exotic sources) in Europe, and has markedly reduced inroads of the disease elsewhere in the world. But in medicine, as in other fields of human activity, success breeds problems of its own. Ironically, the very achievements of vaccination have focused attention on the price, in terms of mortality and morbidity, at which these achievements are currently being purchased. Indeed, they have raised the question of whether, in this country, vaccination should be discontinued as a routine and quasi-universal public health measure.

My own view of the matter is that it should be: first, because I consider the protection mass vaccination now provides against smallpox outbreaks in America to be largely imaginary; second, because the price of this rather dubious protection is in fact higher than is often realized. But quite apart from this fundamental question, a fresh look at vaccination seems to me in order because it may lead to a better understanding of its complications, their sources and treatment, which could markedly reduce their incidence and severity.

Worldwide, variola major is estimated to strike some 100,000 people each year, of whom about a third die. Most cases are concentrated in Africa and Asia (primarily India and Pakistan); though smallpox is still endemic in some South American countries, it is predominantly of the far less dangerous alastrim, or variola minor, type, with a mortality of less than 1%.

In the United States, there has not been a death from smallpox for 20 years. But the reason is not that our population, being vaccinated, is solidly immune to the disease. It is well known that immunity falls off fairly rapidly following primary vaccination. Within the first postvaccination year, susceptibility to the disease is estimated at about one thousandth that of the unvaccinated individual, but in another 15 years or so this has risen to one half, and by 20 years after vaccination protection is essentially gone. Thus we find, for example, that among 18-year-old inductees, all of whom are routinely revaccinated, up to 85% show major reactions, indicating low immunity levels. Also, in Central Europe, where populations are at least as well vaccinated as our own, exotic cases introduced several years ago nonetheless produced secondary and tertiary cases.

The absence of smallpox in this country must be credited not to continued vaccination but to our very efficient quarantine regulations, which require a recent vaccination certificate from anyone entering or reentering the country, to the fact that relatively few people enter the U. S. from smallpox-endemic areas, and to plain luck. Should our luck run out and an exotic case somehow slip by the quarantine — which is likely to happen sooner or later — we must assume that from 20 to 100 secondary cases will result, and perhaps tertiary cases as well. The only way to prevent this would be by routine revaccination of the entire U. S. population at regular intervals of three to five years — a project whose magnitude and expense rule it out of consideration.

Thus mass vaccination according to any practicable schedule holds little promise of performing its presumed positive function — that of preventing smallpox outbreaks due to accidentally introduced cases. At the same time, vaccination itself produces negative results of considerable extent.

It is difficult to estimate the incidence of complications following vaccination (e.g., postvaccinal encephalitis, eczema vaccinatum, generalized vaccinia), since in the past, few were reported routinely. A national study of 1963 data by John M. Neff, formerly of the PHS Communicable Disease Center, and associates found a rate of 52.9 complications per million primary vaccinations. Of these, more than half required hospitalization. The death rate was about one per million. Infants up to one year old experienced by far the highest morbidity rate, 146.8 complications per

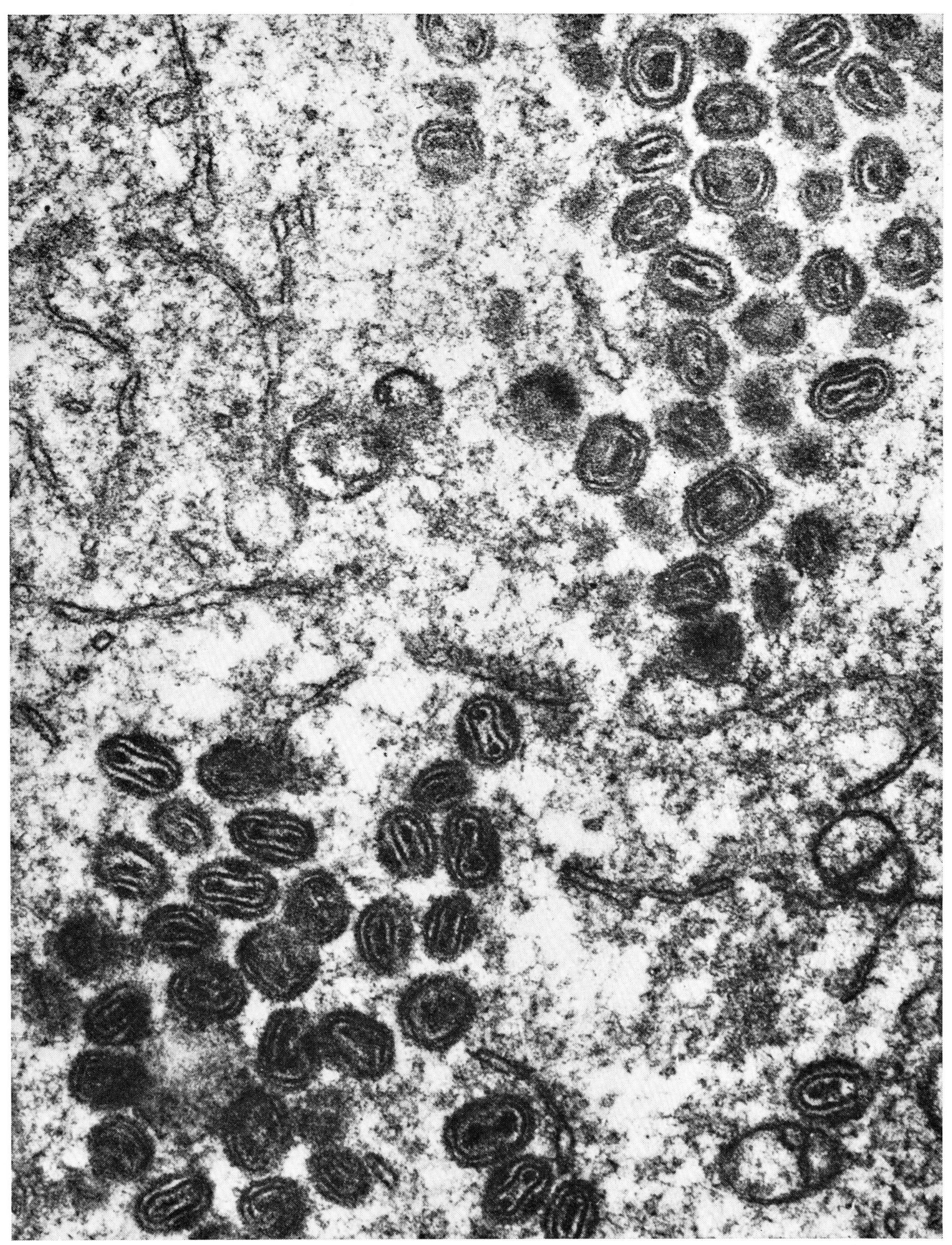

Electronmicrograph shows an ultrathin section through a cell infected with vaccinia virus. This virus is structurally identical to the smallpox virus. It consists of a core in the shape of a biconcave disc, a thin membrane, and a dense coat. The variation in appearance reflects the angle at which the particles were sectioned. Electronmicrograph was made at 45,000x.

million. Complications following revaccinations were few, 2.2 per million, with no deaths.

Other studies, including replies to a questionnaire sent to nearly 20,000 physicians, suggest that these figures are minimal. I believe that primary vaccinations are responsible for from 12 to 18 deaths a year, or at least 240 deaths since the last U. S. smallpox death in 1948. Taking the mortality of smallpox at 33%, we would have had to have had more than 700 smallpox cases during that period to produce the same number of deaths.

Admittedly, many of the complications — up to two thirds — were preventable, a subject on which I shall have more to say later. But the quickest and simplest way of preventing nearly all future vaccination complications is to stop routine vaccination. In smallpox prevention, as in no other field of medicine, we have conspicuously failed to relate the risk of doing something to the risk of doing nothing. But, it will be asked, can we accept the risk of doing nothing? I believe we can, for several reasons.

In the first place, it should be emphasized that we are not talking about *the* risk but the *added* risk. For the reasons already mentioned, the fact of having been vaccinated at one time or another does not mean permanent immunity to smallpox. I know of no comprehensive studies of immunity in the U. S., but given the known rate of drop-off following vaccination, I would estimate that at any given time as much as half of our population will not be protected. Moreover, solid immunity is almost certainly highest among those who would need it least in the event of an outbreak — i.e., infants and young children whose potentially infectious contacts are largely limited to their immediate families.

A second point is that smallpox, while unquestionably infectious, is considerably less so than such diseases as measles, rubella, influenza, and chickenpox. Thus while cases imported into smallpox-free regions almost invariably produce some secondary cases, regardless of the extent of vaccination, they do not rapidly produce major epidemics even in inadequately protected countries.

The reason for this has been worked out experimentally. The smallpox virus is one of the largest known (about 250 μ); moreover, what might be called the infectious unit does not seem to be a single virus particle but a group of many that are probably enclosed in a protein coat. Thus the virus does not seem to spread through aerosols, e.g., through coughing and sneezing, but, like beta streptococcus in dust, settles out of the air relatively rapidly. We find that among known intimate contacts of smallpox cases, the infection rate is much less than 100%, unlike that of the diseases previously mentioned.

My final reason for minimizing the risk of ending mass vaccination is that a drug now exists that can prevent smallpox among the contacts of an imported case: methisazone. Clinical trials have shown that this drug provides good protection against smallpox even after exposure. It is also interesting in itself, being one of the very few chemotherapeutic agents useful in viral disease. It is effective against both the variola and the vaccinia virus, the latter property making it useful in treating complications of vaccination.

Methisazone is one of a class of drugs, the thiosemicarbazones, discovered by Gerhard Domagk, discoverer of the sulfa drugs. One of this group is still being used in parts of Africa as an antituberculosis agent — not a very good one, but very cheap. It was Dorothy Hamre of the Squibb Institute who first showed that some of the thiosemicarbazones possessed antiviral activity — specifically, against neurovaccinia. Later work by Bauer and Sadler, two British investigators, established that methisazone and a very close chemical relative were the most pharmacologically active against variola-vaccinia.

Methisazone is available in England and a number of other countries, but has not been approved by our FDA. It is clinically useful against variola and some other viruses; for this reason the number of cases in which it has been used experimentally here is insufficient to meet FDA regulations for release. Moreover, its potential domestic market is so small that no manufacturer seems interested at present in spending the money needed to comply with FDA procedures, let alone the research sums that would be required to produce a modified and improved version of the drug.

For methisazone is far from perfect. It is an all-too-effective emetic and is

Age in years	*Generalized vaccinia*
Under 1	52
1-4	46
5-9	24
10 and over	12
Totals	134

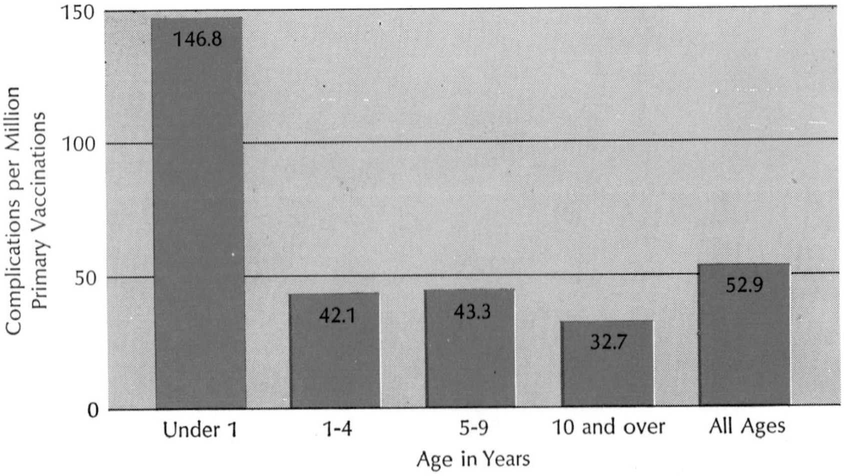

Neff study showed that children under a year old have more than three times the risk of experiencing a complication after primary vaccination than all other age groups. With revaccination, complications rate is a low 2.2 per million overall.

Complications of Vaccination, 1963

Postvaccinal encephalitis	*Vaccinia necrosum*	*Eczema vaccinatum*	*Accidental infections*	*Others*	*Totals*
1	1	24	10	20	108
2 (1)	2	55 (2)	50	17	172 (3)
7 (3)	4	20	34	8	97 (3)
2 (1)	2	12	21	7	56 (1)
12 (5)	9	111 (2)	115	52	433 (7)

Includes complications arising from primary vaccination, revaccination, and contact. Figures in parentheses represent deaths.

poorly absorbed. (Incidentally, with ingestion of alcohol, methisazone produces the same effects as disulfiram.) Despite these pronounced deficiencies, its prophylactic effects against smallpox are marked. The largest study with it was done by Bauer, Downie, St. Vincent, and me in Madras, India, in 1963, during a variola outbreak. We made a concerted effort to track down intimate contacts of hospitalized patients and carried out prophylaxis among more than 5,000 of them, usually within one or two days after admission of the index case. All the contacts were vaccinated, and about half of them were also given methisazone in various doses and on different schedules. In the drug-plus-vaccination group, 0.7% developed smallpox within two weeks after prophylaxis; in the control (vaccination only) group, the attack rate was nearly six times as high (4.1%), a very significant difference. The data were inadequate to support any firm conclusions on the optimum dosage regimen. The most effective seemed to be two doses of 3 gm, eight hours apart, but even a single 3-gm dose gave considerable protection. Similar results were obtained during a variola minor outbreak in South America.

Thus in my view the most rational way of heading off a smallpox outbreak, in the event an accidental importation should get into this country, would be the tracing of contacts and their treatment with vaccination and methisazone, precisely as we did in Madras. True, the drug is not generally available, but it is available as an experimental drug, and it would be readily accessible in the event of a threatened outbreak. (Physicians wishing to use methisazone either to treat smallpox contact cases or patients with vaccination complications may contact either the manufacturer, Burroughs Wellcome Co., Medical Department, Tuckahoe, N. Y., or the Center for Disease Control in Atlanta, Ga.) There is, indeed, every reason why supplies of the drug should be stockpiled in the health departments of each of the 50 states as well as at major ports of entry.

In addition, high-risk groups should be routinely revaccinated according to a regular schedule. These include hospital personnel, who accounted for a large proportion of the cases in the Central European outbreaks, and persons who come into regular contact with travelers — customs officials, airline personnel, and the like. These measures, I am convinced, would enable us to discontinue universal vaccination with no more risk of smallpox outbreaks than exists at present.

Vaccination would not be discontinued entirely, of course. In addition to the high-risk groups, it would be necessary for anyone planning travel to a smallpox-endemic area and would probably be desirable for anyone planning travel abroad. (Under present regulations, it is required for anyone planning to return to the U. S., except from Canada, Mexico, and the Caribbean islands.) But taking all these groups together, vaccination — and its inevitable proportion of complications — would still apply to only a tiny fraction of the U. S. population.

Such a revision of present practices implies that most people would receive their primary vaccination in their teens or later, instead of in infancy or early childhood. This immediately raises certain concerns with respect to complications. Most of these show no increase as the age at which primary vaccinations are given goes up; if anything, their incidence seems to decrease. This is not true, however, of the most serious complication — postvaccinal encephalitis — which seems to become somewhat more frequent, though less likely to be fatal, when the primary vaccination is given at age five or above. Its incidence is still not high in that age group — perhaps three to five per million — but certainly higher than is comfortable.

An immediate solution to this problem is to administer vaccinia hyperimmune gamma globulin in conjunction with the vaccination. This, it has been shown, can reduce the incidence of postvaccinal encephalitis to "normal," i.e., childhood, levels. A better solution, and one that could be arrived at quite rapidly, would be the use of a "prevaccine" — an attenuated vaccinia strain that would give almost complete protection against any complications of the vaccination itself. Such strains are under active study and could be made available to physicians.

There have been a number of experiments, here and abroad, with killed vaccinia, either as a primary vaccine or as a prevaccine, but the results have been poor. Far more promising, I believe, is an attenuated strain. Such a strain was developed in the early 30's by the late Thomas Rivers, but he stopped work on it when he found that it apparently produced only low immunity levels. This was reason-

Vaccinations in the United States, 1963

Age in years	*Primary vaccinations*	*Revaccinations*	*Total vaccinations*
Under 1	654,000	0	654,000
1-4	2,973,000	311,000	3,284,000
5-9	1,847,000	1,572,000	3,419,000
10 and over	765,000	5,892,000	6,657,000
Totals	6,239,000	7,775,000	14,014,000

able enough given the objective of building lasting smallpox immunity with the primary vaccination; now, however, the rationale for such a vaccine would be protection, not against smallpox but against vaccination.

My associates and I have been working with a further attenuated (78th passage) version of the Rivers strain. We have used it experimentally in 2,000 children suffering from eczema — a high-risk group so far as complications are concerned. Many of these children were subsequently vaccinated with the regular strain. There was not a single case of inoculation eczema vaccinatum from either the first or second vaccination, though we would have expected at least 20.

An attenuated prevaccine, either CVI-78 or some other strain, would also provide a fundamental answer to the question of whether and when to vaccinate. It, rather than the present needlessly virulent vaccinia strain, could be used for routine vaccination in early childhood. Subsequently, individuals could be revaccinated with the standard strain at whatever time circumstances made it appropriate. It is worth noting that this attenuated strain is now being produced and is approved for new drug evaluation.

However, abandonment of mass vaccination with the needlessly virulent standard strain is obviously not going to come immediately. And since conventional vaccination, and its complications, will be with us for a while yet, let us consider how these complications can best be minimized.

The simplest step concerns merely the age at which primary vaccination is given. The Neff study showed clearly that every one of the common complications (excluding encephalitis and vaccinia necrosum) was markedly more frequent among infants under one year old. My own feeling is that the safest age for primary vaccination under present requirements is between two and four. There is every reason to believe that observance of this limitation would obviate a sizable proportion of complications (in the Neff study, the group under one year old constituted only 10% of the total vaccinations, but accounted for nearly 30% of the complications; see graph on page 276).

Apart from this simple chronological contraindication, there are a number of medical contraindications as well. The most obvious of these is eczema, either in the patient or in the immediate family, which can lead to eczema vaccinatum, a very serious condition. This is essentially a widespread surface infection of individuals with multiple minor skin defects, in which hundreds or even thousands of simultaneous "takes" occur all over the body. The clinical picture is analogous to that of a severe dermal burn, and supportive therapy is very similar. Mortality in this condition was formerly high — in infants under one year, as much as 30% — and even with modern treatment it must still be considered a life-threatening disease.

The standard treatment is administration of vaccinia hyperimmune gamma globulin. This should be supplemented with methisazone. I have used the drug in seven cases (three children, four adults) of progressive eczema vaccinatum in which, even after more than a month of massive gamma globulin therapy, the old lesions continued to extend and new ones to develop. The patients were given methisazone orally — 200 mg/kg to start, then 50 mg/kg *qid* for three days. All seven showed prompt clinical response, with eventual full recovery.

It is estimated that of some five million children who each year become candidates for routine vaccination, about 90,000 have specific dermal contraindications. Few of them are vaccinated (none of them should be) but this in itself creates problems. They must present letters from their physicians to the appropriate public health and educational authorities, and even then the administrative machine sometimes finds it difficult to adjust to their presence. If the family for some reason wants to go abroad, either for pleasure or because of an overseas job or military assignment, the administrative difficulties can become insuperable. And in any case the eczematous, nonvaccinated child remains at risk of contamination from just-vaccinated schoolmates or siblings (in the Neff study, the only deaths from eczema vaccinatum were among contacts, not vaccinees). The problems faced by these 90,000 children and their families, it seems to me, are in themselves a strong argument for ending routine vaccination or making generally available an attenuated prevaccine, or both.

Other contraindications to vaccination can be summed up roughly as serious disorders of the immune mechanisms, whether natural or iatrogenic. These would include athymia, agammaglobulinemia of either the Bruton or Swiss type, leukemia, lymphoma, Hodgkin's disease, systemic lupus erythematosus, and any recent treatment with immunosuppressive agents, radiation, or systemic corticosteroids.

Though all these contraindications should be observed, not all are equally serious. By all odds the most dangerous are those (such as the Swiss-type agammaglobulinemia) involving a deficiency of the small lymphocytes, leading to an absence of the delayed hypersensitivity mechanism. It is this absence, I believe, rather than a deficiency in leukocytes or in the neutralizing antibodies produced by the plasma cells, that permits the vaccinia virus to spread from the primary lesion, producing the very dangerous condition of vaccinia gangrenosa.

Obviously it is impossible to perform blood studies on all children who are candidates for vaccination. Two very useful screens exist, however. One is a simple failure to thrive, which not infrequently indicates the presence of some immune disorder. Even more specific is a history of persistent moniliasis of the skin or mouth with a negative skin reaction to candida antigens, which is almost pathognomonic of a depressed delayed hypersensitivity reaction. Children showing any of these signs should have blood studies done; it is important, by the way, that the slide be examined by someone who is really competent in distinguishing large lymphocytes from small ones, since the former may well be present despite dangerous deficiency of the latter.

In general, complications stemming from immunologic disorders, as well as the considerably larger number that are idiosyncratic, are treated in much the same manner as eczema vaccinatum—with vaccinia hyperimmune gamma globulin which is available through the Red Cross (see adjoining list of consultants). If there is insufficient response, methisazone might well be tried if available, though there is not yet sufficient clinical experience to assay its benefits in most complications. If all other measures fail, transfusions of immunologically competent blood are sometimes lifesaving. It should be emphasized, however, that blood transfusion is absolutely contraindicated in patients with small lymphocyte deficiency. Because these individuals are tolerant hosts they will not reject the transfused lymphocytes, but the lymphocytes will eventually produce a graft-versus-host reaction which can itself produce a fatal outcome. A possible alternative in such cases is to attempt to graft a thymus, using material obtained from aborted fetuses, or to transfuse lymphocytes obtained from the livers or spleens of such fetuses provided they are not more than 12 weeks old.

A final word should be said on complications in adults. Because individuals reentering the country are normally required to have a recent vaccination certificate, not a few persons suffering from lymphoma or Hodgkin's disease or receiving immunosuppressant therapy have undergone routine revaccination — and developed vaccinia gangrenosa. In fact, revaccination is not necessary if such an individual is returning from a smallpox-free country. A letter from his physician, explaining the circumstances and attached to the international vaccination form, is accepted by the quarantine officers at U. S. ports of entry; I know of no recent instance where anyone with a verified medical contraindication has been denied admittance, or forcibly vaccinated, or quarantined. However, such people are often, and rightly, asked to check in with the public health authorities daily for 12 days after arrival.

Distribution of Vaccinia Immune Globulin

The following is a list of American Red Cross volunteer consultants and alternates through whom vaccinia immune globulin may be obtained:

CALIFORNIA

Dr. Paul F. Wehrle (*alternates*, Dr. John M. Leedom, Dr. Allen W. Mathies Jr.), Los Angeles County General Hospital, 1200 North State Street, Los Angeles 90033.

Dr. Moses Grossman, University of California Service, Ward 83, San Francisco General Hospital, 1001 Potrero Avenue, San Francisco 94110.

COLORADO

Dr. C. Henry Kempe, University of Colorado School of Medicine, 4200 East Ninth Avenue, Denver 80220.

DISTRICT OF COLUMBIA

(For the Armed Forces) Col. Edward L. Buescher (*alternate*, Dr. M. S. Artenstein), Walter Reed Army Institute, Washington 20012.

Dr. Allan S. Chrisman, American National Red Cross, 17th and D Streets N.W., Washington 20006; (*alternate*, Dr. Robert H. Parrott, Children's Hospital, 2125 13th Street N.W., Washington 20009).

GEORGIA

Dr. Andre J. Nahmias, Emory University School of Medicine, 69 Butler Street S.E., Atlanta 30303; (*alternate*, Dr. J. Michael Lane, Center for Disease Control, Atlanta 30303).

HAWAII

Dr. Sharon J. Bintliff (*alternate*, Dr. Harry C. Shirkey), Kauikeolani Children's Hospital, 226 North Kuakini Street, Honolulu 96817.

ILLINOIS

Dr. Irving Schulman, University of Illinois College of Medicine, 840 South Wood Street, Chicago 60612.

LOUISIANA

Dr. Margaret H. D. Smith (*alternate*, Dr. Mark A. Belsey), Tulane University School of Medicine, 1430 Tulane Avenue, New Orleans 70112.

MARYLAND

Dr. John M. Neff, Johns Hopkins Hospital, Baltimore 21205.

NEW YORK

Dr. Horace L. Hodes (*alternate*, Dr. Eugene Ainbender), Mount Sinai School of Medicine, Fifth Avenue and 100th Street, New York City 10029; (*alternate*, Dr. Julian B. Schorr, American Red Cross, 150 Amsterdam Avenue, New York City 10023).

Vaccinia immune globulin may also be purchased through Hyland Division of Travenol Labs, Inc., 3300 Hyland Avenue, Costa Mesa, Calif. 92626.

Chapter 29

Uses and Abuses of Gamma Globulin

MICHAEL E. MILLER
University of Pennsylvania

In surveying certain "horrible examples" of inept and unnecessary gamma globulin therapy, one is tempted to write an article entitled "The Case Against GG." Yet such an emphasis, though tempting, would be unduly negative.

Gamma globulin therapy *is* on occasion instituted for the wrong reasons. It frequently has no effect on the patient apart from the discomfort and inconvenience of the injection; too often it is sustained not because of any beneficial effects but by the need of the family and the physician to "do something." Yet, with all this, there certainly is a place for GG therapy in specific cases. Moreover, there are indications that it may eventually prove useful in areas – such as certain cases of chronic upper respiratory infection – where its use today is dubious in the extreme.

To understand the present limitations and future potentials of GG therapy, we must begin by saying something about the laboratory methods used to establish immunoglobulin deficiencies. Before doing so, however, it is worth noting that where such deficiencies are suspected the practitioner should not feel compelled to rush to the nearest immunology laboratory for consultation – which in most cases will tell him little that he cannot surmise clinically. The immune diseases are not so esoteric that the nonspecialist is helpless; for example, the Bruton type of congenital agammaglobulinemia can almost always be diagnosed by the astute clinician.

Nevertheless, the physician confronted by an unfamiliar disease may well want consultation to confirm a diagnosis. Given the confirmation, he should have no trouble in determining when GG therapy can be applied fruitfully. The following summary of key points on immunoglobulin assay, available GG preparations, and the uses and misuses of GG therapy may help him in his deliberations.

Measurement: The key to appropriate GG therapy is obviously accurate knowledge of the extent of the deficiency. Thus, a quantitative assay is required; "semiquantitative" methods – serum electrophoresis is increasingly unreliable the farther the value departs from the normal range, immunoelectrophoresis is at best only semiquantitative – cannot provide the necessary accuracy.

Several true quantitative methods are available, however. One is the radial diffusion method originally devised by Mancini, and this or an equivalent method is likely to be in use at a laboratory accustomed to doing both qualitative and quantitative determinations, especially those at medical centers and those accredited by the College of American Pathologists. The physician at a remote location can send specimens safely through the mails, since antibodies are fairly stable, and the results can be discussed by telephone.

At a minimum, a laboratory report should show: 1) immunoelectrophoretic patterns, with information on the individual appearance of the IgM, IgG, and IgA bands and any indications of abnormal protein, and 2) some accurate quantitative measurement of IgA, IgG, and IgM groups – along with a table of normal values *by age* or a statement that the measured values are normal or abnormal for age (see the scale of normal values by age on page 282).

The need to be certain that the laboratory is using age-adjusted standards cannot be overstressed. The commonest cause of avoidable pediatric referral, we have found, involves GG levels interpreted as "borderline low" by adult standards but which, had age been taken into account, would have been seen to be within the normal range.

It should also be recognized that, in rare situations, antibody deficiency can be present even in the face of normal concentrations of immunoglobulins. As a general rule, however, the physician is usually on safe grounds in assuming that the IgG, IgM, and IgA values are fair reflections of functional antibody competence.

Preparations: Commercial supplies of GG are available from 15 or 20 different sources. For a number of reasons these preparations are by no means as rigidly standardized as are most drugs. Typically, the protein content of the fraction accounting for all GG activity will vary from 12.5% to 16.5%. Heiner and Evans at the University of Utah conducted an analysis of 27 lots of gamma globulin produced by 10 manufacturers. They found the samples roughly similar in amounts of IgG, variable in amounts of IgA, IgM, and other serum proteins. Thus the physician deludes himself if he believes his patient is receiving an identical amount of GG in each administration of the same fluid volume.

It is a mistake, then, to administer a "minimum" dose, even in the praiseworthy attempt to hold down the cost and the side reactions produced by the intramuscular injection. In view of the variations in GG content, such a "conservative" approach is likely to be self-defeating, assuming the treatment is really needed.

To achieve truly adequate blood concentrations of GG there is no alternative to giving large fluid volumes. In adults and in heavier children, this will inevitably produce considerable discomfort and local pain. It will also involve a rise in antibody formation against heterologous GG, especially if administration is chronic. Both these side reactions are good arguments against unnecessary use of the substance, and another is that GG supplies are limited and should be conserved for genuine needs.

Uses: Expanding clinical experience and advances in active immunization have notably narrowed the usefulness of GG. Thus, in viral prophylaxis it is worth while only in rather special cases, such as for the patient on corticosteroids who is faced with a risk of chickenpox. In certain serious diseases, where active immunization cannot or has not been achieved, it is also useful, as in the attenuation of hepatitis. The rubella vaccine, now in development, probably will end any application of GG preparations in this disease, and medicine may be the better for it inasmuch as GG preparations cannot be wholly relied on to protect the fetus of an exposed mother. It should be noted that in almost any viral condition the timing of injection after exposure is crucial, and the right moment often is missed, so that the best that can be hoped for is attenuation rather than prevention of the disease (see table on page 285).

Congenital hypogammaglobulinemia usually becomes apparent only as maternal antibodies disappear in the infant after third or fourth month of life. Gamma globulin

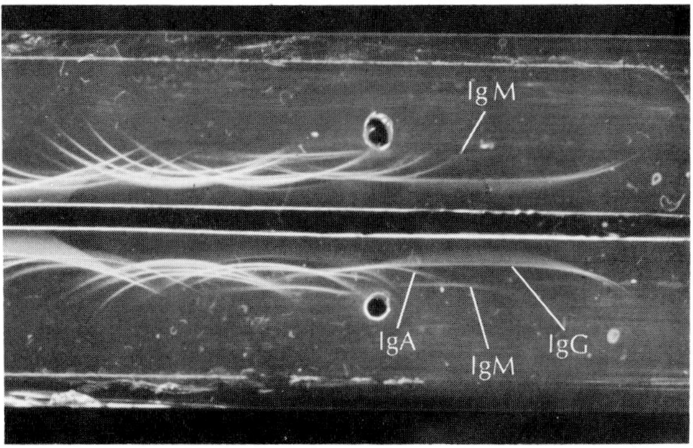

Semiquantitative nature of immunoelectrophoresis may be source of error in diagnosing GG deficiency. Above: the lower pattern is a control obtained with normal serum; three well-defined Ig arcs can be seen. Top pattern was obtained with serum of four-year-old child suspected of GG deficiency; poor visualization of IgM seems confirmatory. But when accurate quantitations were performed, completely normal, age-matched values of each immunoglobulin were found to be present.

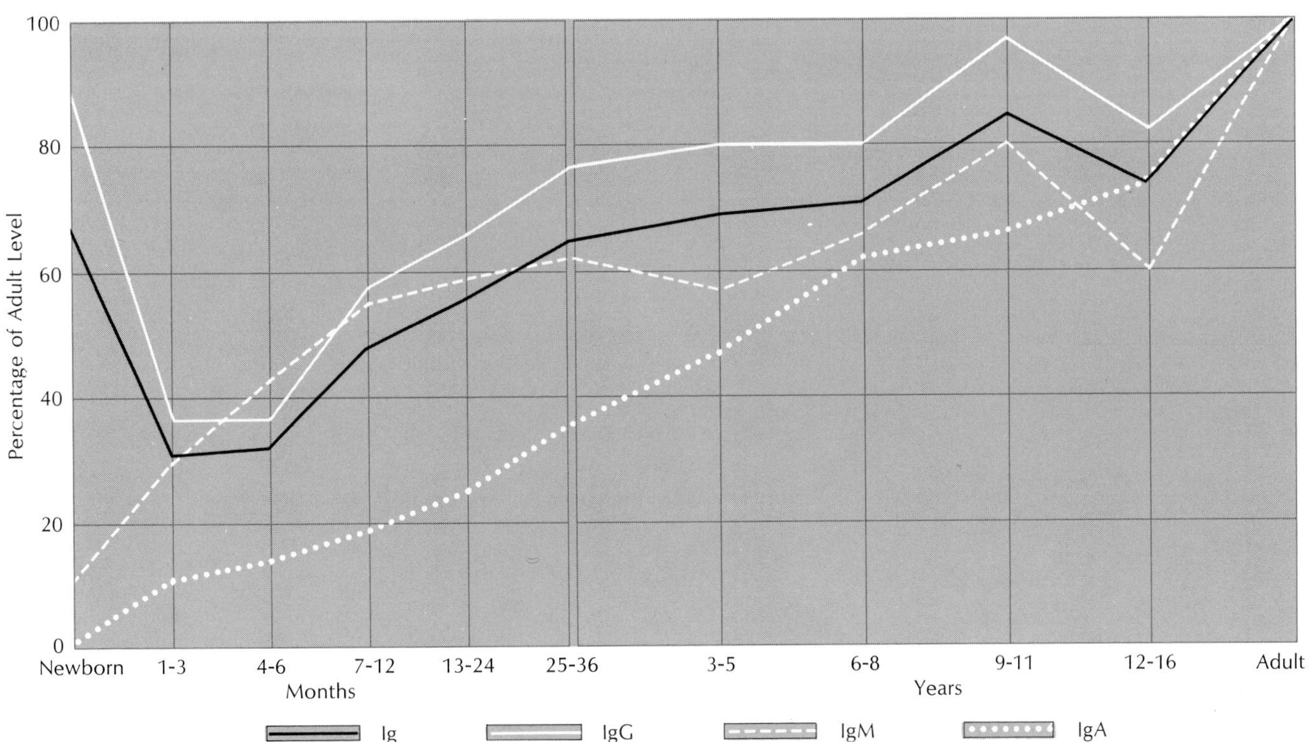

As graph shows, normal pediatric values for immunoglobulins are always (if variably) lower than adult norms. Failure to take these age differences into account may lead to interpretation of laboratory results within normal range as borderline or low.

therapy is dramatically effective in a few, but by no means all, immunological diseases. Although his condition is not completely curable, the child with congenital hypogammaglobulinemia will do fairly well, though a tendency to infection persists. Once such a child develops chronic pulmonary disease, he responds poorly to therapy but should nonetheless receive it. The same advice holds for the "acquired hypogammaglobulinemic" child, in whom therapy will at least minimize bacterial infection.

For unknown reasons some infants do not begin to produce IgG demonstrably until nine, 10, or 11 months of age, or occasionally later. Hence, the child with *transient hypogammaglobulinemia* is unprotected for the five months or so between the time maternal antibody levels become inadequate and the time his own IgG levels are measurable. During the interim, with quantitative evidence that IgG values are at hazardously low levels, gamma globulin therapy certainly is indicated.

One study found diminished IgG values at two or three months of age in some premature infants who weighed 1,000 to 1,500 gm at birth. Such infants, it was suggested, might benefit from GG therapy starting at birth, in effect compensating for supposedly low stores of maternal IgG. Whether or not this recommendation is valid remains to be seen; I have seen no corroborative evidence. In our own studies, dangerously low IgG levels have not yet shown up among such premature infants, but we have yet to compare their IgG values at birth with values at one, two, or three months.

The child with an immune deficiency condition involving a defective thymus and inability to reject skin grafts is unlikely to benefit from GG therapy no matter how massive or continuous. Thus, a child with the Swiss type of agammaglobulinemia will sustain continual and unavoidable viral, fungal, and bacterial infection. In a few such patients we have given almost continuous infusions of gamma globulin without achieving any change in the course of disease.

Nor is GG therapy useful for most *functional dysgammaglobulinemias*. In these diseases immunoglobulin values are normal but specific antibody may be lacking. An example is the individual who is unable to make antibody to staphylococcus but whose IgG value is in the normal range. In this case GG therapy will only be effective if the preparation contains the specific antibody lacked by the patient. Another and far more common type involves a diffuse immune defect, with one, two, or all of the major immunoglobulins at abnormal values. The collagenoses may represent one of these conditions. It has been suggested that GG therapy might be useful for a disease like rheumatoid arthritis, in which, although the level is adequate, IgG is presumed to be either nonfunctional or poorly functioning. At the moment, however, data supporting the presumption are sketchy and debatable, and no agreement exists that GG therapy is indeed useful in this group of diseases.

More recently, the treatment of Rh-negative mothers with anti-Rh^D gamma globulin at the time of delivery appears to prevent sensitization and possible erythroblastosis in future pregnancies. Although the dosage is not yet standardized, the use of gamma globulin for this purpose seems well justified.

Levels of Immune Globulins in Sera of Normal Subjects, By Age

Age	IgG		IgM		IgA		Total Immunoglobulin	
	mg/100 ml	*% of Adult Level*	*mg/100 ml*	*% of Adult Level*	*mg/100 ml*	*% of Adult Level*	*mg/100 ml*	*% of Adult Level*
Newborn	1,031 ± 200	89 ± 17	11 ± 5	11 ± 5	2 ± 3	1 ± 2	1,044 ± 201	67 ± 13
1-3 mo	430 ± 119	37 ± 10	30 ± 11	30 ± 11	21 ± 13	11 ± 7	481 ± 127	31 ± 9
4-6 mo	427 ± 186	37 ± 16	43 ± 17	43 ± 17	28 ± 18	14 ± 9	498 ± 204	32 ± 13
7-12 mo	661 ± 219	58 ± 19	54 ± 23	55 ± 23	37 ± 18	19 ± 9	752 ± 242	48 ± 15
13-24 mo	762 ± 209	66 ± 18	58 ± 23	59 ± 23	50 ± 24	25 ± 12	870 ± 258	56 ± 16
25-36 mo	892 ± 183	77 ± 16	61 ± 19	62 ± 19	71 ± 37	36 ± 19	1,024 ± 205	65 ± 14
3-5 yr	929 ± 228	80 ± 20	56 ± 18	57 ± 18	93 ± 27	47 ± 14	1,078 ± 245	69 ± 17
6-8 yr	923 ± 256	80 ± 22	65 ± 25	66 ± 25	124 ± 45	62 ± 23	1,112 ± 293	71 ± 20
9-11 yr	1,124 ± 235	97 ± 20	79 ± 33	80 ± 33	131 ± 60	66 ± 30	1,334 ± 254	85 ± 17
12-16 yr	946 ± 124	82 ± 11	59 ± 20	60 ± 20	148 ± 63	74 ± 32	1,153 ± 169	74 ± 12
Adults	1,158 ± 305	100 ± 26	99 ± 27	100 ± 27	200 ± 61	100 ± 31	1,457 ± 353	100 ± 24

Values shown above were derived by Drs. E. R. Stiehm and H. H. Fudenberg from measurements made in 296 normal children and 30 adults. Levels were determined by radial diffusion plate method using specific rabbit antisera to human immunoglobulins.

In summary, GG therapy is useful in attenuating some viral diseases in individuals for whom vaccination is not advisable or where vaccines have not been developed. For immune deficiency states in general, GG therapy is successful only in a few well-described entities, and it is to these that I believe treatment should be limited at the present time.

Misuses: The use of GG preparations in *protein deficiency conditions* is almost always mistaken. Even kwashiorkor, probably the most profound protein deficiency known in man, is unlikely to produce low IgG levels. If anything, in fact, children with kwashiorkor are likely to have high levels, for IgG seems to be one of the last serum protein fractions to be depleted in these patients.

Another misuse is in cases of *massive blood loss.* Such a patient usually receives replacement blood, plasma, or both — which, since blood loss producing dangerously low serum GG levels would probably be incompatible with survival, makes it probable that intramuscular injections of gamma globulin would be superfluous. *Fluid loss* through skin trauma (e.g., burns) also is unlikely to reduce GG levels to the point where supplementation is necessary. *Diarrhea* is rarely so severe as to require it, even in elderly persons or neonates. So-called IgA-deficient steatorrhea, with severe loss through the GI tract, might represent a genuine need — but no one knows how to deliver the immunoglobulin to the proper site in usable form.

Happily, the idea is disappearing that *newborns* need GG therapy in the nursery to ward off bacterial infection, a fad that persisted for several years. Three lines of evidence now argue against it: 1) Virtually all of the newborn's immunoglobulin is IgG acquired from the mother, is protective, and is at a par with or higher than that of the adult and older child. Injections of commercial gamma globulin provide only IgG in appreciable amounts, and there is no reason to believe that additional IgG is going to be of any use. 2) While newborns are admittedly susceptible to infection by coliform and gram-negative bacteria, the major portion of antibody activity against these organisms lies in the IgM fraction. Thus commercial GG preparations, which do not contain much of this fraction, are therapeutically irrelevant. 3) There is accumulating evidence that hypersusceptibility to infection, where it exists, may reflect immature mobilization of inflammatory responses as much as it does immunoglobulin deficiency.

In addition, it is now clear that the newborn has immune function of his own and that immunity is not entirely acquired from the mother. Silverstein has shown that the well-challenged fetal lamb shows an immune response both in antibody output and cellular immunity. The child with congenital rubella or cytomegalovirus exposure shows high IgM values at birth — presumably as a response to the intrauterine infection.

The fact that IgM, which confers resistance to gram-negative organisms, does not cross the placenta is often cited in texts as the reason why neonates have trouble with these infections. But a good deal of evidence suggests that IgM deficiency is not solely responsible.

Inability to handle gram-negative organisms may stem, at least in part, from deficiencies of other plasma factors, such as the complement system. Treated by heat, in a way that will not alter the IgM, adult plasma can be rendered as ineffective as newborn plasma in capacity to opsonize gram-negative bacteria. (Deficiency of a heat-labile substance in newborn plasma contributes to its ineffectiveness, several studies have shown.) Again, our laboratory has found that the polymorphonuclear leukocyte of the newborn is not as good a phagocyte as that of the adult; preliminary evidence indicates that the newborn leukocyte is deficient chemotactically, presumably because of immaturity.

Along with the heat-labile plasma factor and deficient phagocytic functions, a thorough explanation may have to encompass a finding by Cohen and Norrins that the IgG of newborns has significant activity against gram-negative bacteria. Why then is this defensive wall breached? One may speculate that the infant's defensive capacity is overtaxed by the leakage of enterotoxins through the highly permeable wall of the newborn gut, so newly and richly colonized with gram-negative organisms. But in any event, these explanations and speculations emphasize that we are dealing with an immature being, many of whose infection problems will be "cured" with growth and development.

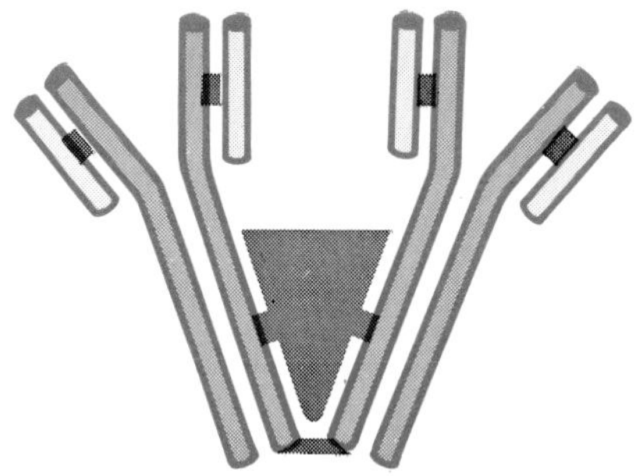

If IgA deficiency is involved in susceptibility to respiratory infection, it is probably a deficiency of secretory IgA with "piece" (diagrammed above) and not of serum IgA.

Apart from these theoretical considerations, little clinical evidence supports the efficacy of GG therapy in the newborn. The few studies contradicting this conclusion are, on close examination, open to question. Thus Amer and colleagues suggested that GG therapy reduced the incidence of low-grade (not life-threatening) respiratory infection in the nursery, but the size of their sample made the conclusion debatable. In addition, their newborns, divided at random into GG-receiving and control groups, were observed for distribution and kinds of infection — but immunoglobulin levels were not measured systematically.

Observations: Most misuses of GG might be avoided if the physician takes a careful history and makes a thorough physical examination. For example, a child with recurrent URI beginning in the first week of life is probably not hypogammaglobulinemic, for the child with congenital hypogammaglobulinemia usually has sufficient maternal antibody for several months, and his infections invariably are bacterial. Moreover, his peripheral lymphoid tissue is hard to detect. You don't see tonsils. You don't feel lymph nodes. If you do, congenital hypogammaglobulinemia is not likely to be the diagnosis, and GG therapy is unnecessary. The clinician, then, is in a good position to make a preliminary judgment that an esoteric condition does *not* exist, though, as noted, in supporting his judgment with a laboratory determination he must be alert to the kind of measurement the laboratory is making and the use of the proper table of normal values.

The biggest cause of misuse of GG therapy lies with a common — and controversial — diagnosis: the URI syndrome. Too often, physicians tend to jump at the prospect of a "workable" therapy for chronic URI, which forms so much of their caseload. The repeated low-grade infections characterize the child, in the parents' eyes, as a victim of "severe" disease, so that they harass the physician to provide a "specific treatment," thereby reflecting the common outlook in American society that every malady must be treatable. Yet, in fact, the physician fails in his obligation to the family when he employs GG therapy as a placebo or psychological crutch. He must try to convince them that the child is normal, will outgrow the susceptibility to infection, and does not suffer from a true GG deficiency.

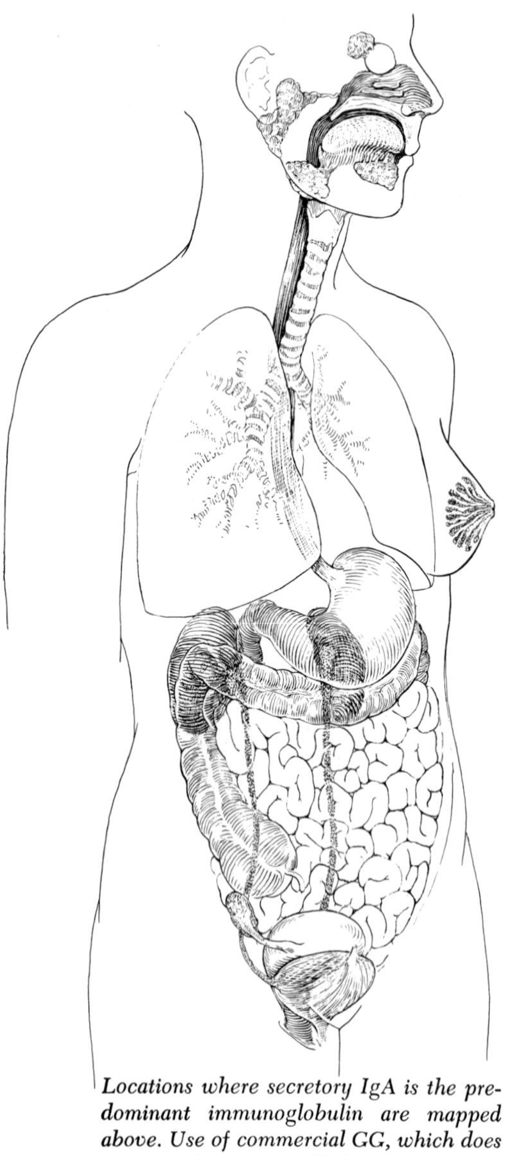

Locations where secretory IgA is the predominant immunoglobulin are mapped above. Use of commercial GG, which does not contain secretory IgA, to treat infections at these sites is probably futile.

I am well aware that some physicians do not share my own belief that GG amounts to a placebo in such cases, yet the evidence for its efficacy can be criticized on both theoretical and practical grounds.

Although the question is still debated, the generally accepted position is that resistance to respiratory infection may depend in part on IgA produced in the respiratory mucosa, and that recurrent URI — if it involves immunoglobulin deficiency at all — probably stems from a deficiency of this "local" IgA, whose status is not adequately represented by even the most careful serum IgA measurements. (Some studies show no correlation between absence of serum IgA and high incidence of respiratory disease.) Thus, addition of IgA to the serum will not help the patient. (A study by Buser and associates has recently been cited as evidence that low *serum* IgA values are associated with recurrent respiratory infection and that GG therapy can benefit patients. But the study was criticized for using immunoelectrophoretic assay instead of a true quantitative method. Moreover, the authors acknowledged that establishing a valid control group in such studies is difficult and the group in their investigation might not be considered adequate as a control. An editorial in the *Journal of Pediatrics*, which published the study, provided a critical perspective on it — but a surprising number of physicians read only the report, not the editorial.)

There are also grounds for doubting that serum IgA, even if assumed to reach the respiratory mucosa, could be protective there. "Local" IgA produced in the mucosa has attached to its molecule a secretory, or transport, piece that may protect it against proteolytic enzymes at the tissue site — and this piece is missing from serum IgA molecules [see "The Gamma A Globulins: First Line of Defense" by Thomas B. Tomasi, which is Chapter 8 of this book]. Thus, even if serum IgA — the only type of IgA in GG preparations — were delivered directly to tissue sites by, say, aerosol, the instillation would be in vain.

Potential uses: After what I have just said, it may seem eccentric to suggest that GG ultimately could be found useful in treating chronic URI. Yet I believe it might be — provided we are able to develop much more refined methods for defining and assaying immunoglobulin deficiencies, plus the ability to deliver the right globulin in the right form to the right place.

More is being learned each day about the gamma globulin groups. IgG, for example, is now known to have subgroups, much as erythrocytes do. Thus the possibility exists that an individual with normal or slightly low IgG levels by the usual parameters could still have a large subgroup deficit critical to protection against an infecting agent. I hesitate to dwell on this possibility for fear of encouraging the use of pooled gamma globulin in the hope of blindly hitting a subgroup deficit in a refractory case. Yet I, and other clinicians, have had the experience of making use of gamma globulin in desperation, even though the patient lacks demonstrable deficiency on repeated measurement — and obtaining a dramatic improvement. The experience is not so rare that it can be dismissed out of hand. Possibly by sheer luck a unit of pooled gamma globulin happened to compensate for a subgroup deficiency.

The future may hold a reliable means of picking up the few children whose recurrent otitis media or respiratory infection can benefit from specific subgroup therapy. Hopes for such therapy for both the ear and respiratory tract have some anatomical justification. If the respiratory tract produces IgA, its extensions — the eustachian canal and middle ear — could do likewise. Viral infections that underlie recurrent otitis are similar to those in the respiratory tract proper. And though recurrent ear infections have been explained by chronic allergic and respiratory infections that block the eustachian canal and cause hydrodynamic changes, the evidence is against this. I suspect the true explanation could prove to be an IgA deficiency throughout the respiratory tract and its extensions, producing shared infections and shared response to infections.

Granting this, however, I believe the efficacy of treatment is still going

Gamma Globulin Therapy: A Selective Approach

Clinical Presentation	*Indications*	*Dosage**	*Efficacy*
Rubeola Prevention	Exposure of nonimmune infants under age of two; of all nonimmune children with severe concomitant illness	0.25/ml/kg of body weight IM within 6 days of exposure	Effective only if given within appropriate interval following exposure
Modification	Exposure of all other nonimmune children and adults	0.05 ml/kg IM within 6 days of exposure	
Infectious Hepatitis	Exposure of all children and adults	0.022 to 0.044 ml/kg IM within 1 week of exposure	Disease not entirely prevented but may be modified considerably clinically; may be necessary to repeat in 4 to 5 months if exposure is continuous
	In pregnant women or if exposure has been prolonged	0.06 to 0.09 ml/kg	
Rubella	Not indicated for children; exposure of pregnant women in first trimester	0.25 to 0.44 ml/kg	Highly questionable; may mask clinical symptoms
Varicella	Not indicated except in life-threatening situations (rare)	0.44 to 1.3 ml/kg within 3 days of exposure	
Agammaglobulinemia or Hypogammaglobulinemia	For prevention of bacterial infections through maintenance of serum levels between 100 and 300 mg/ml	Initial dose: 1.5 ml/kg; thereafter: 0.77 ml/kg every 3 to 4 weeks	Quite variable in different conditions; see text
Rh-negative mothers with Rh-positive fetus	For prevention of sensitization and possible erythroblastosis in future pregnancies	Anti-Rh^D 1 to 1.5 ml/kg 15% solution (dosage not yet standardized)	Probably quite effective

** of Immune Serum Globulin (Human) U.S.P. or Poliomyelitis Immune Globulin (Human)*

to depend on our ability to engineer IgA resembling the form occurring naturally at the site (i.e., including the transport or secretory piece) and on our ability to deliver it to the site. The engineered molecule could in theory be delivered through aerosols or snuff powders, but these vehicles do not yet seem reliable, and other possibilities may have to be tried. The goal, of course, justifies further research and development to help the many children with recurrent URI.

Some of the discomfort and side reactions associated with intramuscular GG administration may be overcome by preparations that can be given intravenously. The problem has been that such preparations tend to form aggregates that cause thrombus formation on vessel walls or produce a quasi-allergic or anaphylactic-like reaction. Furthermore, modification of the molecules to prevent such reactions is associated with sharply reduced halflife — while the conventional intramuscular preparation has a halflife of about three weeks, the halflife of the intravenous materials generally is much less than a day.

Recently, however, a new plasmin-digest preparation was described by investigators at Boston Children's Hospital: It apparently has a halflife equal to that of intramuscular preparations, without vascular toxicity. The long-term clinical effectiveness of this preparation remains to be demonstrated. Like all GG preparations, it does not preclude the possible formation of antibodies against heterologous gamma globulin. Such an intravenous product would best be used for the child or adult with an immune deficiency disease who needs gamma globulin every three or four weeks to keep free of bacterial infection.

An era of clumsiness and over-eagerness in the use of gamma globulin is, I believe, ending. In the future, gamma globulin may well be used less often yet it will be used more effectively, with preparations tailored to an individual's precise need. For that kind of job we will need highly capable laboratories to characterize and measure the immunoglobulins and subgroups, clinicians schooled in sophisticated diagnosis and the application of new preparations, and systems for delivering the preparations in the appropriate form to the site where they are needed.

Chapter 30

Radioimmunoassay: A Status Report

SOLOMON A. BERSON *and* ROSALYN S. YALOW
Mount Sinai School of Medicine

Although radioimmunoassay came into being almost by accident, its application has been purposeful and extensive in the decade since its first development. The physiologist has found it invaluable in delineating the mechanisms and patterns of hormone regulation, and the clinician has often availed himself of its diagnostic usefulness in the evaluation of various endocrine abnormalities associated with under- or over-secretion. Originally applied to the measurement of insulin in plasma, radioimmunoassay is presently being utilized or developed for the study of at least 20 peptide hormones and at least one nonhormonal peptide. In addition, the technique has been extended to nonpeptide hormones and other biologically active substances in nonimmune systems.

Current research and clinical interest in radioimmunoassay are not surprising when one considers that prior to its development no uniform technique was available for measuring the peptide hormones in plasma. Whereas the thyroid and steroid hormones have attributes of structure and solubility that make them amenable to direct chemical measurement, the peptide hormones are not sufficiently unique in these respects to permit their ready distinction from other serum proteins by classical chemical procedures. Moreover, the very low concentrations of the peptide hormones in blood and urine create still further difficulties.

Prior to immunoassay the only available method was bioassay. In this technique, a specific hormonal effect of plasma is tested on a living system, in vivo or in vitro, and the response is compared with that produced by a known standardized preparation of hormone. Thus, due to the intrinsic nature of the bioassay, it is necessary to design an entirely separate system for each hormone. Moreover, it appears that few available bioassays combine adequate specificity with sensitivity keen enough to measure the low concentrations of peptide hormones as generally found in plasma. For example, the bioassay for plasma ACTH, which depends on the release of corticosterone from the rat adrenal, is highly specific, but it usually requires large amounts of plasma because its sensitivity is limited. On the other hand, the bioassays for plasma insulin are reasonably sensitive but are not absolutely specific for that hormone. For many of the peptide hormones no bioassay is available.

These two essential requisites — a high degree of specificity and exquisite sensitivity — are combined in radioimmunoassay, a technique based on competition between labeled and unlabeled hormone for binding to specific antibody. It is possible to measure as little as one micromicrogram or less of a specific hormone in the presence of a several billionfold higher concentration of other plasma proteins. This sensitivity is far greater than that generally obtained through bioassay.

From a practical standpoint, radioimmunoassay provides an in vitro determination that can be carried out on several hundred to a thousand samples simultaneously in any laboratory equipped for measurement of radioactivity. However, possibly the most far-reaching advantage of radioimmunoassay is that it offers a single approach to the evaluation of all the peptide hormones and, by extension, of a variety of other biologically important substances, both antigenic and nonantigenic.

An explanation of the rationale and methodology of radioimmunoassay might begin with a description of its origin, which, as indicated, came about as an offshoot of another line of investigation. About 15 years ago we were interested in evaluating whether diabetics destroyed insulin more rapidly or more slowly than normal subjects. It had been recognized that not all diabetes is associated with an absolute deficiency of insulin, and Dr. Arthur

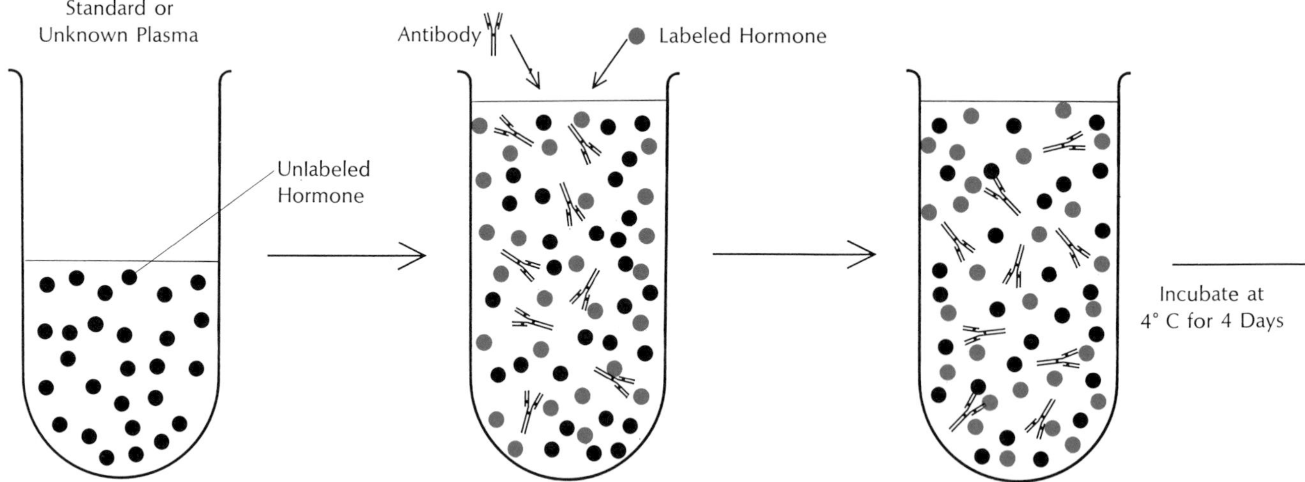

The steps in competitive radioimmunoassay as applied to the measurement of circulating insulin are represented above. One starts with solutions of unlabeled hormone derived from a standard preparation and with the plasma samples to be assayed. To all of these, identical quantities of radioiodine-labeled hormone and of specific antibody (in the form of diluted antiserum) are added. The mixtures are incubated at 4° C. During this period, the unlabeled hormone will compete (in approximate proportion to its concentration in the complete mixture) against labeled hormone for binding to antibody. Next, separation of bound and

Mirsky, now at the University of Pittsburgh, suggested that this phenomenon might be traceable to an overly active insulin destroying enzyme, insulinase. To test this hypothesis, we injected radiolabeled insulin intravenously and determined the rates of disappearance and degradation of the tagged hormone. Surprisingly, we found that insulin did not disappear more rapidly from the circulation of the diabetics but was retained in the plasma for longer periods than in the normal subjects. However, it turned out that this slow disappearance rate was not directly related to the presence of diabetes. Rather, it was because the diabetics had anti-insulin antibodies that complexed with the hormone in the plasma, thus preventing the insulin molecule from passing through the capillary walls.

This finding, significant in itself, also helped account for the insulin resistance observed in a small percentage of insulin-treated patients. But if all treated patients developed antibodies, why did only a small fraction show resistance to insulin? We suspected the answer was related to the amount of antibody that was present, and this suspicion was confirmed by quantitative studies of the binding of insulin to its antibodies. Most treated diabetics had only small concentrations of antibody; those who were resistant had very high titers.

During the course of these studies we found it convenient to use radiolabeled insulin as a tracer, giving increasing amounts of unlabeled hormone in order to quantitate the insulin-binding capacity of the plasma antibodies. It was evident that the labeled and unlabeled insulins were competing for antibody combining sites and that the extent of this competition could serve as the basis for

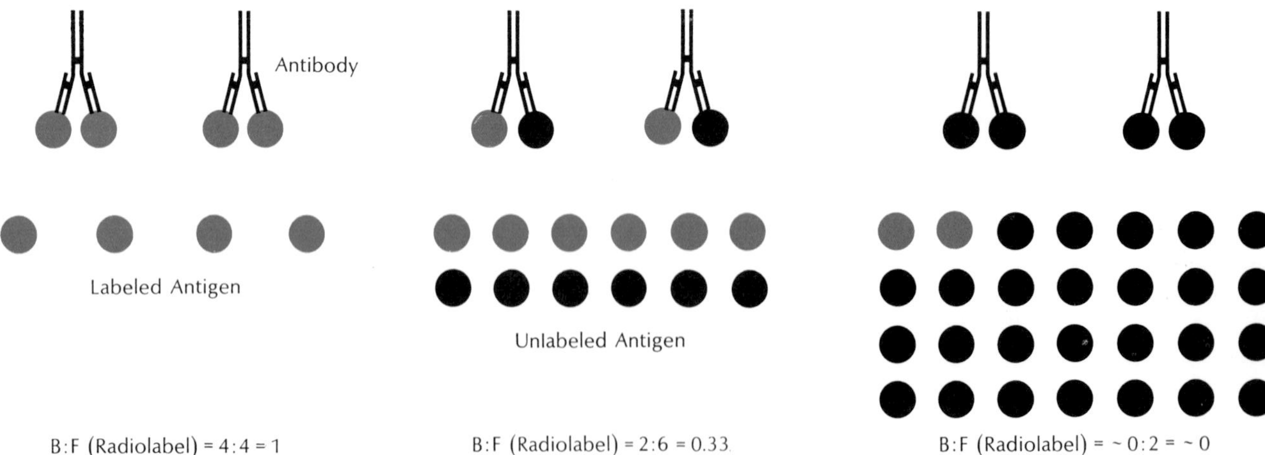

This schematization of competitive immunoassay presupposes a fixed amount of antibody. In the first situation, there is no unlabeled antigen, and the amount of labeled antigen that is bound equals that which remains free (B:F = 1). When sufficient unlabeled antigen is added to compete equally with the labeled hormone, the B:F ratio goes down to 0.33. If the sample being assayed is rich enough in unlabeled hormone so that the labeled hormone is "shut out," B:F approaches zero.

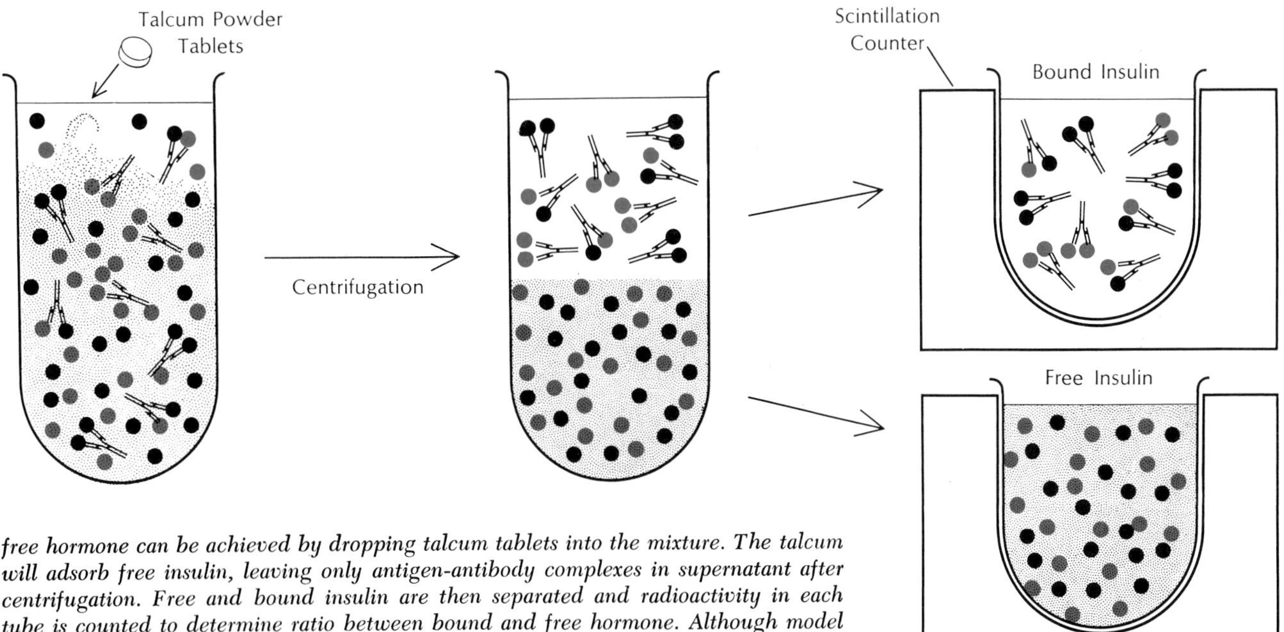

free hormone can be achieved by dropping talcum tablets into the mixture. The talcum will adsorb free insulin, leaving only antigen-antibody complexes in supernatant after centrifugation. Free and bound insulin are then separated and radioactivity in each tube is counted to determine ratio between bound and free hormone. Although model shows talc and supernatant volumes as equal, actually talc is only small precipitate.

an assay of insulin. We also found that the affinity of the antibodies for insulin was extremely variable among our human antisera, and a high affinity was absolutely required to measure low concentrations of the hormone in plasma. Immunization of several animal species indicated that guinea pigs produced insulin antibodies of suitably high affinity. Thus, although classical chemical procedures were not very suitable for detecting and measuring individual peptide hormones in plasma, immunochemical reagents, produced biosynthetically in the form of antibodies, served admirably.

It had long been recognized that antibodies, by virtue of structural complementarity, are quite specifically reactive with the antigen (in this case a hormone) that stimulates their production. The combination of immunologic specificity with the exquisite sensitivity inherent in properly selected antisera of high affinity for the antigens made it possible to measure plasma hormones.

In brief, radioimmunoassay exploits the ability of unlabeled hormone in plasma or other solutions to compete with labeled hormone for antibody and thereby to inhibit the binding of labeled hormone. As a result of this competitive inhibition, the ratio of antibody-bound (B) to free (F) labeled hormone, denoted B:F, is diminished as the concentration of unlabeled hormone is increased. The concentration in an unknown sample is obtained by comparing the inhibition observed in that sample with that produced by standard solutions containing known amounts of hormone.

A typical radioimmunoassay begins with the simultaneous preparation of a series of standard and unknown mixtures in test tubes. Usually there are about a dozen standards and as many as 1,000 unknowns, all of which are set up in buffered solutions and contain identical concentrations of labeled hormone and antiserum. Increasing known amounts of hormone are added to the standards; only plasma (or other biologic fluid) is added to the unknown tubes. After a few days of incubation, the bound and free fractions of the labeled hormone are separated by one of several techniques — paper chromatoelectrophoresis, double antibody precipitation, or adsorption of the free hormone to charcoal or talcum powder. The B:F ratios in the standards are plotted against hormone concentration to obtain a "standard curve." The concentration of hormone in an unknown sample is determined by comparing the observed B:F ratio with the standard curve.

The rationale of radioimmunoassay has been extended to nonimmune systems, in which the assay technique is more accurately designated "competitive radioassay." One such application, developed simultaneously by Dr. Sheldon Rothenberg in our own laboratory and by Dr. Roger Eakins in London, has been in the measurement of vitamin B_{12} in plasma. Here the specific reactor is intrinsic factor, a protein whose particular function is to bind vitamin B_{12}. Dr. Rothenberg has also carried out measurements of folic acid using the enzyme folic acid reductase as the specific reactor. Again, the rationale is similar to that of radioimmunoassay; labeled and unlabeled folic acid molecules compete for a specifically adapted enzyme, and the degree of competitive inhibition observed is a measure of the concentration of unlabeled folic acid.

The principle of competitive radioassay has been widely applied in

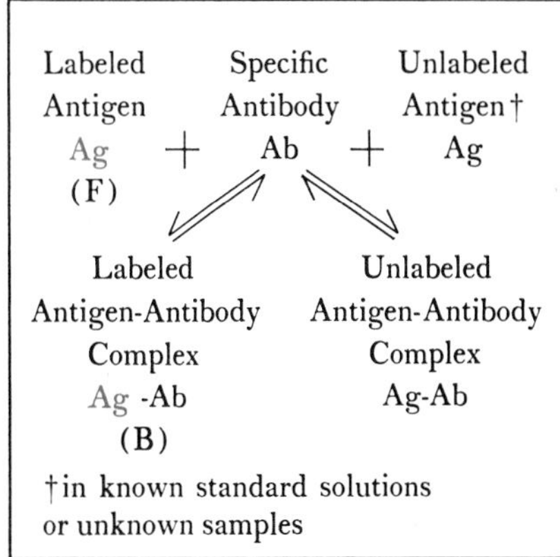

Principles of competitive immunoassay are summarized in competing equations above.

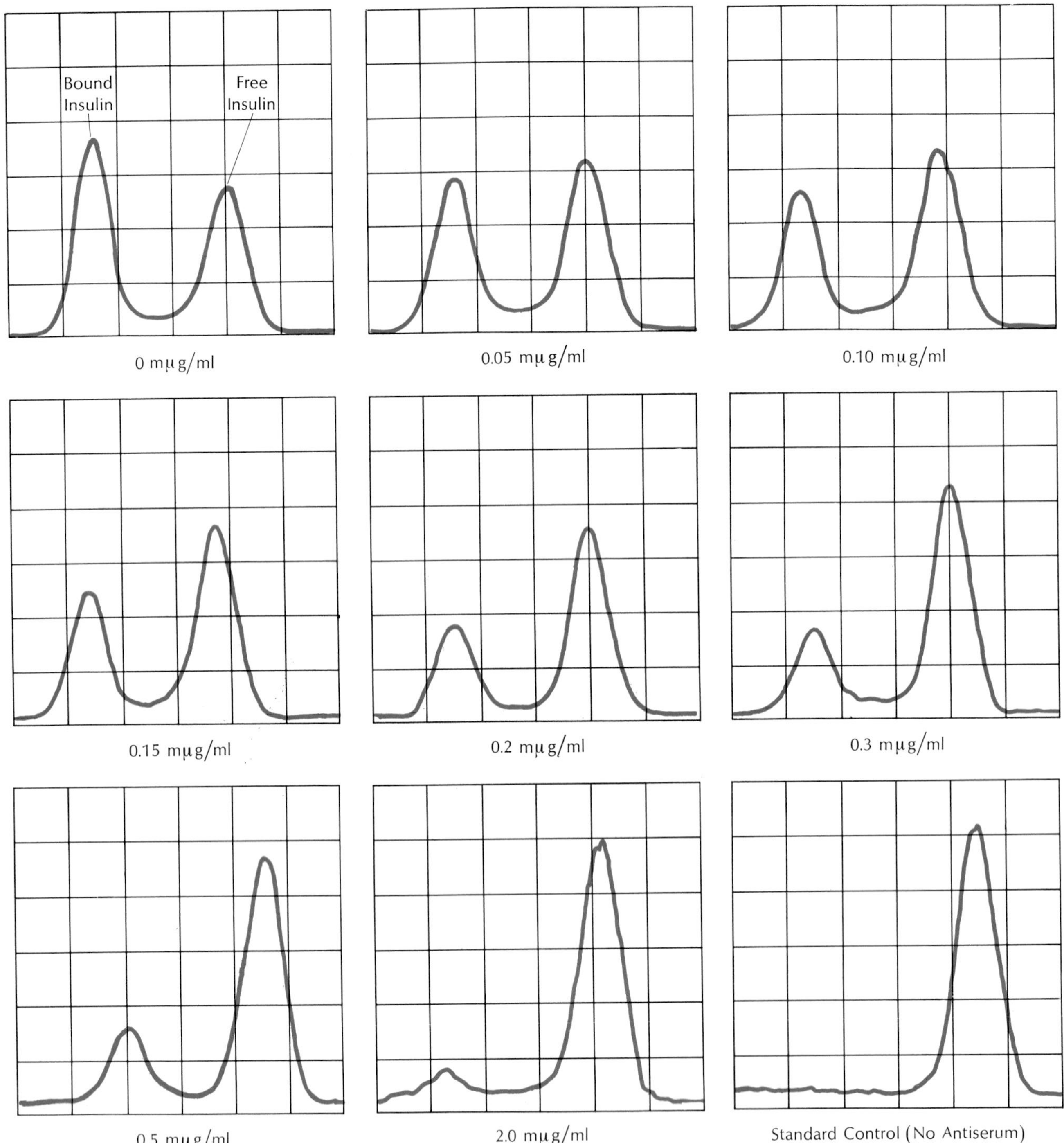

In this experiment, antibody-bound and free labeled insulin were separated by paper strip chromatoelectrophoresis and scanned automatically. The series of scans shows how B:F ratios are used to derive a standard curve for human insulin. Labeled insulin's binding to antibody is diminished as the concentration of unlabeled insulin in sample to be assayed is increased. In the absence of unlabeled insulin (to left), the amount of bound labeled insulin is maximal and the B:F ratio highest for the antiserum dilution employed. As the amount of unlabeled insulin rises, the bound labeled insulin and B:F ratio fall.

another area – measurement of nonpeptide hormones, which do not readily stimulate the formation of antibodies, namely, thyroxin and various adrenocortical and gonadal steroids. Dr. B. E. P. Murphy of Queen Mary Veterans Hospital in Montreal has worked out methods for a large number of these hormones, using as specific reactors particular hormone binding proteins of the plasma. A still further and more recent application has been in the measurement of messenger RNA, which utilizes as specific reactor the complementary DNA; the hybridization of RNA and DNA serves as the counterpart of antigen-antibody complex formation.

Radioimmunoassay itself has been applied (see table on page 293) to such widely different substances as drugs (digitalis glycosides, morphine), vitamins (folic acid), cyclic nucleotides, enzymes, serum proteins, and viruses

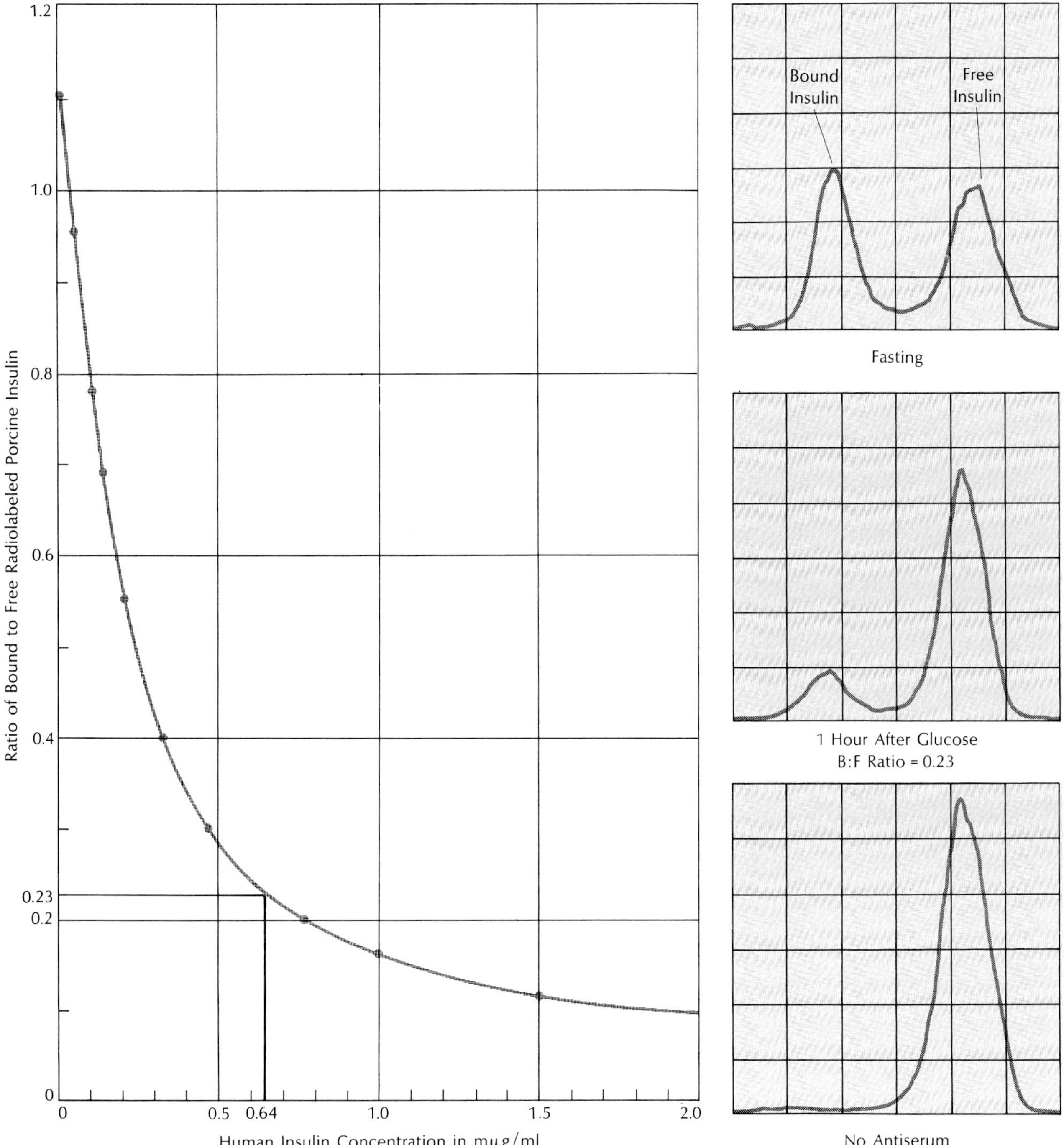

From the known standards at the left, an overall curve can be derived, and this curve can be employed to determine the human insulin concentration in an unknown sample. In this case, two plasma samples were assayed (right), one fasting and another an hour after glucose load. In addition, a sample was processed in absence of antibody and, of course, all radioactivity was found in the "free" fraction. In the postglucose sample, B:F was 0.23. By setting this ratio on the standard curve, the actual insulin concentration in the sample could be determined as 0.64 mμg/ml. Insulin was almost absent in the fasting sample.

(Australia antigen).

Many of these assays have been developed only within the past five or six years. While pertinent data are beginning to emerge from assays of nonimmune systems, the immune systems already have been most revealing. As a result of the application of radioimmunoassay to the physiology of the endocrine glands, new information of interest has been reported in many fields. Let us focus on a few of those assays that are valuable clinically.

An early diagnostic application of radioimmunoassay was in measuring plasma insulin in patients with islet cell adenoma and in patients with idiopathic hypoglycemia of childhood.

Patients with functioning islet cell tumors frequently have normal or high plasma insulin concentrations even when the blood sugar concentration is below normal, an association that indicates an autonomous secretion of insulin that is not responding appropriately to the normally suppressive influence of hypoglycemia. It had previously been observed by others that hypoglycemic attacks were often precipitated by leucine feeding in children with idiopathic hypoglycemia. Radioimmunoassay of plasma insulin revealed that leucine was singularly potent in stimulating insulin secretion not only in children with this disorder but also frequently in patients with islet cell adenomas. Measurement of plasma insulin before and after leucine stimulation is therefore useful diagnostically in these conditions.

Another diagnostic application of radioimmunoassay is in determining under- or over-secretion of human growth hormone. Prior to the advent of radioimmunoassay, very little was known about the secretion of this hormone, and considerable mystery existed regarding its role in adults. We were first beginning to measure growth hormone by radioimmunoassay when Drs. Seymour Glick and Jesse Roth came as Fellows to our laboratory. They subsequently contributed greatly to our present knowledge of the secretory regulation of growth hormone. Their studies showed that levels of plasma growth hormone rise during fasting periods, then drop abruptly after feeding of a carbohydrate meal.

On further investigation, it was found that growth hormone secretion could be stimulated abruptly by the induction of hypoglycemia with insulin. It was also shown that neither epinephrine nor glucagon could produce this rapid secretory stimulation, that growth hormone levels are generally high in hypoglycemia even when unrelated to insulin, and that administration of glucose to fasting patients was followed by a fall in growth hormone concentration.

The diagnostic applicability of these physiologic findings is fairly apparent. Through immunoassays of the output of growth hormone in response to insulin-induced hypoglycemia, it is possible to demonstrate whether a dwarfed child has any mobilizable endogenous hormone. Pituitary dwarfs have little or no growth hormone in their plasma and evidence little response to insulin stimulus, while children of short stature due to other causes show a marked and rapid secretory increase following administration of small amounts of insulin.

In addition to its role in establishing hypopituitarism, radioimmunoassay has been helpful in diagnosing certain conditions, such as acromegaly, that are caused by oversecretion of growth hormone. Although acromegaly is often clinically obvious, many early cases are questionable in the absence of laboratory evaluation. One certainly wants a definitive diagnosis before embarking on pituitary ablation therapy with surgery or irradiation. As noted, administration of glucose suppresses the secretion of growth hormone in normal subjects. Acromegalic patients rarely show a marked secretory suppression in response to glucose, and this observation, along with the demonstration of high concentrations of growth hormone in the plasma, permits a secure diagnosis of hyperpituitarism.

Diagnostic immunoassays have also been developed for the following:

Parathyroid: Here the most obvious need for hormone assay is in patients suspected of having a parathyroid adenoma. Most such patients have high concentrations of plasma hormone. Although we occasionally get normal values even when adenoma is present, the concomitant presence of hypercalcemia (which normally suppresses parathyroid secretion) and normal plasma parathyroid hormone concentrations raises the index of suspicion.

Radioimmunoassay has revealed that extraordinarily high levels of parathyroid hormone may be present in patients with chronic renal disease. Because of the serious sequelae (bone disease and metastatic calcification) of severe secondary hyperparathyroidism, total or nearly total parathyroidectomy may be advisable in this disorder. Measurement of plasma hormone levels can serve as a useful guide not only in determining when parathyroidectomy is first indicated but also in monitoring the completeness of parathyroid removal and in detecting significant regrowth.

ACTH: The distinction between bilateral adrenal hyperplasia and primary adrenal tumor as the cause of Cushing's syndrome can usually be made by means other than radioimmunoassay. However, in doubtful cases, a high plasma level of ACTH or an absence of circadian periodicity aids in implicating bilateral adrenal hyperplasia rather than adrenal adenoma or carcinoma.

Chorionic gonadotropin: Choriocarcinoma is a relatively rare malignancy. Once uniformly fatal, it is now frequently curable through administration of methotrexate. Radioimmunoassay and other immunoassays of chorionic gonadotropin in urine have proved useful in evaluating therapy.

Follicle stimulating hormone: Although diagnostic usefulness of the FSH assay is not yet clearly defined, current interest in this hormone would indicate that such application is imminent. It would appear that accurate measurements of FSH could provide valuable clues to the mechanisms of the newer antiovulatory drugs and thereby refine their usage.

Radioimmunoassay has been used by Dr. Philip Gold and his associates in Montreal to determine the presence of carcinoembryonic antigen, a protein-polysaccharide complex that frequently finds its way into the circulation in patients with carcinoma of the colon and rectum. Its disappearance after successful therapy and its reappearance with recurrence of the tumor serve as helpful guides in diagnosis and management. Since other malignancies are likely to be associated with similar phenomena, the application of radioimmunoassay to nonendocrine tumor diagnosis is expected to be increasingly useful.

Very recently, Dr. John Walsh in our laboratory has developed a radioimmunoassay for Australia antigen (Au). At least 100-fold more sensitive than complement fixation techniques, the radioimmunoassay procedure may permit more efficient detection of Au carriers and of potentially infective units of blood scheduled for transfusion.

Recent studies on radioimmunoassay of the antral hormone, gastrin, have led to the discovery of two forms of the hormone in plasma. Further investigations revealed that the two forms are also present in extracts of antrum, duodenum, and jejunum, as well as of Zollinger-Ellison tumors, which characteristically produce large amounts of the hormone. The presence of these tumors can readily be diagnosed by the finding of very high immunoreactive plasma gastrin levels in association with high rates of HCl production by the stomach.

In discussing the testing advantages and diagnostic applicability of radioimmunoassay, we want to avoid the impression that there are no difficulties connected with its use. One major problem has been acquisition of suitably sensitive antisera for each specific hormone. Antiserum is used in immunoassays at dilutions as great as 1:4,000,000, and a satisfactory blood sample taken from a single animal may be enough for 10 million assays or more. However, scores of animals may have to be immunized over a period of a year or longer before a highly sensitive antiserum is obtained. Still another problem has been the relative unavailability of adequately purified synthetic hormones. These difficulties are mainly technical and will yield with time.

More interesting and potentially more fruitful than diagnostic accuracy is the increased knowledge of physiology that has stemmed from radioimmunoassay. Heretofore unsuspected stimuli and suppressants of hormonal secretion and mechanisms of secretory regulation are finally being elucidated through precise measurement of plasma hormone levels. Patterns of hormone synthesis and pathways of metabolic degradation of the peptide hormones have become more amenable to study through radioimmunoassay.

Newer chemical techniques have provided powerful tools for the purification, analysis, and synthesis of the peptide hormones. The parallel development of radioimmunoassay in the same era is permitting a synergistic approach to a fuller understanding of the roles and behavior of these life-sustaining molecules.

Substances Now Measured by Competitive Radioassay

Immune Systems (Antibody Is the Specific Reactor)

PEPTIDE HORMONES		NONHORMONAL SUBSTANCES	NONPEPTIDAL HORMONES
Insulin	Vasopressin	Intrinsic factor	Testosterone
Growth hormone	Angiotensin	Digoxin	Estradiol
ACTH	Oxytocin	Digitoxin	Aldosterone
Parathyroid hormone	Bradykinin	cAMP, cGMP, cIMP, cUMP	Estrone
Glucagon	Thyroglobulin	Australia antigen	Dihydrotestosterone
TSH	αMSH	C_1 esterase	
HCG	βMSH	Fructose -1, 6-diphosphatase	
FSH	Gastrin	Carcinoembryonic antigen	
LH	Calcitonin	Rheumatoid factor	
Placental lactogen	Proinsulin C-peptide	Human IgG	
Proinsulin	PZ-CCK	Folic acid	
Secretin		Neurophysin	
		TBG	
		Morphine	

Nonimmune Systems

HORMONES	SPECIFIC REACTOR
Thyroxine	Specific binding proteins in plasma
Cortisol	Specific binding proteins in plasma
Corticosterone	Specific binding proteins in plasma
Cortisone	Specific binding proteins in plasma
11-desoxycortisol	Specific binding proteins in plasma
Progesterone	Specific binding proteins in plasma
Testosterone	Specific binding proteins in plasma
ACTH	Adrenal receptor sites

NONHORMONAL SUBSTANCES	SPECIFIC REACTOR
Vitamin B_{12}	Intrinsic factor
Folic acid	FA reductase
Cyclic AMP, GMP	Phosphodiesterases
Messenger RNA	Complementary DNA (competition-annealing)

Selected References

Chapter 1

The Thymus in Immunobiology. Good RA, Gabrielsen AE, Eds. Harper & Row, New York, 1964

A compendium of the papers presented at the first thymus conference held following discovery of the essential role of the thymus in developmental immunobiology.

Miller JF: Immunological function of the thymus. Lancet 2:748, 1961

Good RA, Dalmasso AP, Martinez C, et al: The role of the thymus in development of immunologic capacity in rabbits and mice. J Exp Med 116:773, 1962

Glick B, Chang TS, Jaap RG: The bursa of Fabricius and antibody production. Poult Sci 35:224, 1956

Warner, NL, Szenberg A, Burnet FM: The immunological role of different lymphoid organs in the chicken. I. Dissociation of immunological responsiveness. Aust J Exp Biol Med Sci 40:373, 1962

Cooper MD, Peterson RD, Good RA: Delineation of the thymic and bursal lymphoid systems in the chicken. Nature (London) 205:143, 1965

Cooper MD, Raymond DA, South MA, Good RA: The functions of the thymus system and the bursa system in the chicken. J Exp Med 123:75, 1966

Good RA, Papermaster BW: Ontogeny and phylogeny of adaptive immunity. Advances Immun 4:1, 1964

Kincade PW, Lawton AR, Bockman DE, et al: Suppression of immunoglobulin G synthesis as a result of antibody-mediated suppression of immunoglobulin M synthesis in chickens. Proc Nat Acad Sci USA 67:1918, 1970

Bruton OC: Agammaglobulinemia. Pediatrics 9:722, 1952

Good RA: Morphological basis of the immune response and hypersensitivity. Host Parasite Relationships in Living Cells. A symposium sponsored by the James W McLaughlin Fellowship Program. Felton M, et al, Eds. Charles C Thomas, Springfield, Ill, 1957, p 68

Gitlin D, Gross PAM, Janeway CA: Gamma globulins and their clinical significance. I. Chemistry, immunology and metabolism. New Eng J Med 260:21, 1959

Hitzig WH, Willi H: Hereditäre lymphoplasmocytäre Dysgenesis. (Alymphocytose mit Agammaglobulinemie.) Schweiz Med Wschr 91:1625, 1961

Von Tobler R, Cottier H: Familiäre Lymphopenie mit Agammaglobulinemie und schwerer Moniliasis. Die "essentielle Lymphocytophthise" als besondere Form der frühkindlichen Agammaglobulinemie. Helv Paediat Acta 13:313, 1958

Peterson RD, Cooper MD, Good RA: The pathogenesis of immunologic deficiency diseases. Amer J Med 38:579, 1965

Immunologic Deficiency Diseases in Man. Birth Defects Original Article Series. Vol 4, No. 1. Bergsma D, Good RA, Eds. The National Foundation, New York, 1968

Fudenberg HH, Good RA, Hitzig W, et al: Classification of the primary immune deficiencies: WHO recommendation. New Eng J Med 283:656, 1970

Merler E, Rosen FS: The gamma globulins. I. Structure and synthesis of the immunoglobulins. New Eng J Med 275:480, 536, 1966

Alper CA, Rosen FS, Janeway CA: The gamma globulins. II. Hypergammaglobulinemia. New Eng J Med 275:591, 652, 1966

Rosen FS, Janeway CA: The gamma globulins. III. The antibody deficiency syndromes. New Eng J Med 275:709, 769, 1966

Janeway CA, Rosen FS: The gamma globulins. IV. Therapeutic uses of gamma globulin. New Eng J Med 275:826, 1966

Chapter 2

Symposium on la circulation lymphocytaire chez l'homme. Société Française d'Hématologie. Nouv Rev Franc Hemat 8:33-758, 1968

Everett NB, Tyler RW: Lymphopoiesis in the thymus and other tissues: functional implications. Int Rev Cytol 22:205, 1967

Ford WL, Gowans JL: The traffic of lymphocytes. Seminars Hemat 6:67, 1969

Gowans JL: Lymphocytes. Harvey Lect 64:87, 1968-69

Gowans JL, Knight EJ: The route of re-circulation of lymphocytes in the rat. Proc Roy Soc (Biol) 159:257, 1964

Gowans JL, McGregor DD: The immunological activities of lymphocytes. Progr Allerg 9:1, 1965

Antigen Sensitive Cells. Their Source and Differentiation. Möller G, Ed. Transpl Rev 1:3, 1969

Wilson DB, Billingham RE: Lymphocytes and transplantation immunity. Advances Immun 7:189, 1967

Chapter 3

Uhr JW: Delayed hypersensitivity. Physiol Rev 46:359, 1966

Turk JL: Delayed Hypersensitivity. John Wiley and Sons, New York, 1967

General reviews, with descriptions of variety of lesions mediated by delayed hypersensitivity.

Waksman BH: A comparative histopathologic study of delayed hypersensitive reactions. Ciba Symposium on Cellular Aspects of Immunity. JA Churchill, London, 1960, p. 280

Flax MH, Caulfield JB: Cellular and vascular components of allergic contact dermatitis. Amer J Path 43:1031, 1963

Description of histologic and ultrastructural features of this group of lesions.

Kosunen TU, Waksman BH, Flax MH, et al: Radio autographic study of cellular mechanisms in delayed hypersensitivity. I. Delayed reactions to tuberculin and purified proteins in the rat and guinea-pig. Immunology 6:276, 1963

Use of isotopic cell labeling to identify origin of cells in lesions.

Bloom BR, Chase MW: Transfer of delayed-type hypersensitivity. A critical review and experimental study in the guinea pig. Progr Allerg 10:151, 1967

Lubaroff DM, Waksman BH: Bone marrow as source of cells in reactions of cellular hypersensitivity. I. Passive transfer of tuberculin sensitivity in syngeneic systems; II. Identification of allogeneic or hybrid cells by immunofluorescence in passively transferred tuberculin reactions. J Exp Med 128:1425, 1437, 1968

Use of adoptive transfer of living lymphoid and other cells to identify specific and nonspecific components of delayed reactions.

Intersociety Symposium on In Vitro Correlates of Delayed Hypersensitivity, 51st Annual Meeting of the Federation of American Societies for Experimental Biology, Chicago. Fed Proc 27:3, 1968

Description of several newer in vitro techniques for measuring delayed hypersensitivity.

Greaves MF, Torrigiani G, Roitt IM: Blocking of the lymphocyte receptor site for cell mediated hypersensitivity and transplantation reactions by anti-light chain sera. Nature 222: 885, 1969

First attempt to identify "antibody" responsible for specificity of sensitized lymphocytes in delayed hypersensitivity.

Rocklin RE, Meyers OL, David JR: An in vitro assay for cellular hypersensitivity in man. J Immun 104:95, 1970

Application of macrophage migration-inhibition test to measurement of human sensitivity.

Chapter 4

De Duve C, Wattiaux R: Functions of lysosomes. Ann Rev Physiol 28:435, 1966

Good general review of lysosomal physiology.

Lysosomes in Biology and Pathology. Dingle JT, Fell HB, Eds. John Wiley and Sons, New York, 1969

Extensive treatise by many authors.

Weissmann G, Dukor P: The role of lysosomes in immune responses. Advances Immun 12:283, 1970

Review directed towards immunology.

Weissmann G: Effect on lysosomes of drugs useful in connective tissue disease. Biological Council Symposium on the Interaction of Drugs and Subcellular Components in Animal Cells. Vol 2. Campbell PN, Ed. Little, Brown & Co, Boston, 1968, p 203

Review of pharmacologic agents: steroids, chloroquine, etc., with extensive discussions by Allison, deDuve, Seeman.

Weissmann G, Spilberg I, Krakauer K: Arthritis induced in rabbits by lysates of granulocyte lysosomes. Arthritis Rheum 12:103, 1969

Experimental arthritis and lysosomes.

Hirschhorn R, Brittinger G, Hirschhorn K, Weissmann G: Studies on lysosomes. XII. Redistribution of acid hydrolases in human lymphocytes stimulated by phytohemagglutinin. J Cell Biol 37:412, 1968

Documenting the role of lysosomes in lymphocyte transformation.

Chapter 5

Cohn ZA: The structure and function of monocytes and macrophages. Advances Immun 9:163, 1968

Dannenberg AM Jr: Cellular hypersensitivity and cellular immunity in the pathogenesis of tuberculosis: Specificity, systemic and local nature, and associated macrophage enzymes. Bact Rev 32:85, 1968

Mediators of Cellular Immunity. Proceedings of an International Conference, Augusta, Mich. Lawrence HS, Landy M, Eds. Academic Press, New York, 1969

Mackaness GB: Resistance to intracellular infection. J Infect Dis 123:439, 1971

Mackaness GB, Blanden RV: Cellular immunity. Progr Allerg 11:89, 1967

Nelson DS: Macrophages and Immunity. Frontiers of Biology. Vol 11. John Wiley & Sons, New York, 1969

Mononuclear Phagocytes. van Furth R, Ed. F. A. Davis Co, Philadelphia, 1970

Chapter 6

Baehner RL, Karnovsky ML: Deficiency of reduced nicotinamide-adenine dinucleotide oxidase in chronic granulomatous disease. Science 162:1277, 1968

Bellanti JA, Cantz BE, Schlegel RJ: Accelerated decay of glucose 6-phosphate dehydrogenase activity in chronic granulomatous disease. Pediat Res 4:405, 1970

Douglas SD: Analytic review: Disorders of phagocyte function. Blood 35:851, 1970

Good RA, Quie PG, Windhorst DB, et al: Fatal (chronic) granulomatous disease of childhood: A hereditary defect of leukocyte function. Seminars Hemat 5:215, 254, 1968

Holmes B, Park BH, Good RA, et al: Chronic granulomatous disease in females. A deficiency of leukocyte glutathione peroxidase. New Eng J Med 283:217, 221, 1970

Karnovsky ML: The metabolism of leukocytes. Seminars Hemat 5: 156, 1968

Klebanoff SJ: Myeloperoxidase: Contribution to the microbicidal activity of intact leukocytes. Science 169:1095, 1970

Lehrer RI, Cline MJ: Leukocyte myeloperoxidase deficiency and disseminated candidiasis: The role of myeloperoxidase in resistance to Candida infection. J Clin Invest 48:1478, 1969

Reed PW: Glutathione and the hexose monophosphate shunt in phagocytizing and hydrogen peroxide-treated rat leukocytes. J Biol Chem 244:2459, 1969

Strauss RR, Paul BB, Jacobs AA, et al: The role of the phagocyte in host-parasite interactions. XIX. Leukocytic glutathione reductase and its involvement in phagocytosis. Arch Biochem 135:265, 271, 1969

Chapter 7

Nisonoff A, Inman FP: Structural basis of the specificity of antibodies. Reproduction: Molecular, Subcellular and Cellular. Society for the Study of Developmental Biology – 24th Symposium. Locke M, Ed. Academic Press, New York, 1965, p 39

Lennox, ES, Cohn M: Immunoglobulins. Ann Rev Biochem 36:365, 1967

Cohen S, Milstein C: Structure and biological properties of immunoglobulins. Advances Immun 7:1, 1967

Edelman GM, Gall WE: The antibody problem. Ann Rev Biochem 38:415, 1969

Putnam FW: Immunoglobulin structure: variability and homology. Science 163:633, 1969

Hood L, Talmage DW: Mechanism of antibody diversity: germ line basis for variability. Science 168:325, 1970

Each of the articles above is a review emphasizing structural aspects of the immunoglobulins. The first paper listed describes the dissociation of immunoglobulins into subunits and fragments. The other reviews are largely concerned with properties of immunoglobulins from various species and the relationship of amino acid sequences to genetic theories of antibody formation.

Chapter 8

Tomasi TB Jr, Bienenstock J: Secretory immunoglobulins. Advances Immun 9:1, 1968

Tomasi TB: Distribution and synthesis of human secretory components. Conference on Secretory Immune System, Vero Beach, Fla, Dec 10-13, 1969 (in press)

Heremans JF, Crabbé PA: Immunohistochemical studies in exocrine IgA. Nobel Symposium – Third – Sodergarn – Sweden – 1967 on Gamma Globulins. Killander J, Ed. John Wiley and Sons, New York, 1967

General reviews.

Tomasi TB Jr, Tan EM, Solomon A, et al: Characteristics of an immune system common to certain external secretions. J Exp Med 121:101, 1965

Cebra JJ, Small PA Jr: Polypeptide chain structure of rabbit immunoglobulins. 3. Secretory gamma-A-immunoglobulin from colostrum. Biochemistry 6:503, 1967

Chemistry of secretory immunoglobulins.

Crabbé PA, Heremans JF: The distribution of immunoglobulin-containing cells along the human gastrointestinal tract. Gastroenterology 51:305, 1966

Tourville DR, Adler RH, Bienenstock J, Tomasi TB Jr: The human secretory immunoglobulin system: immunohistological localization of gamma A, secretory "piece" and loctoferrin in normal human tissues. J Exp Med 129:411, 1969

Synthesis of secretory immunoglobulins.

Waldman RH: Respiratory secretion antibody mediates protection in viral respiratory tract infections. Arch Environ Health 19:1, 1969

Ogra PL, Karzon DT: Poliovirus antibody response in serum and nasal secretions following intranasal inoculation with inactivated poliovaccine. J Immun 102:15, 1969

Ogra PL, Karzon DT: Distribution of poliovirus antibody in serum, nasopharynx and alimentary tract following segmental immunization of lower alimentary tract with poliovaccine. J Immun 102:1423, 1969

Tomasi TB Jr, DeCoteau E: Mucosal antibodies in respiratory and gastrointestinal disease. Advances Intern Med, 16:401, 1970

Secretory immunoglobulins in human diseases.

Chapter 9

Ishizaka T, Ishizaka K, Johansson SG, et al: Histamine release from human leukocytes by anti-gamma E antibodies. J Immun 102:884, 1969

Ishizaka T, Ishizaka K, Orange RP, et al: Release of histamine and slow reacting substance of anaphylaxis (SRS-A) by γE system from sensitized monkey lung. J Allerg 43:168, 1969

Ishizaka K, Ishizaka T: Immune mechanisms of reversed type reaginic hypersensitivity. J Immun 103:588, 1969

Ishizaka K, Ishizaka T, Hornbrook MM: Physicochemical properties of reaginic antibody. V. Correlation of reaginic activity with γE globulin antibody. J Immun 97:840, 1966

Detection of γE antibody by radioimmunodiffusion and successful absorption of reaginic activity with anti-γE. Similarities between γE antibody and reaginic antibody with respect to physicochemical properties are noted.

Ishizaka K, Ishizaka T, Hornbrook MM: Allergen-binding activity of γE, γG, and γA antibodies in sera from atopic patients: in vitro measurements of reaginic antibody. J Immun 98:490, 1967

Correlation between γE antibody concentration, as measured by antigen-binding activity, and skin-sensitizing activity in whole patients' sera was observed. The minimum dose of γE antibody required for a positive PK reaction was estimated.

Ishizaka K, Ishizaka T: Identification of gamma-E-antibodies as a carrier of reaginic activity. J Immun 99:1187, 1967

The γE fraction was obtained from ragweed-sensitive serum. The fraction contained γE antibody but no antibody belonging to the other immunoglobulin class and had a high skin-sensitizing activity. The activity in the fraction was removed by anti-γE.

Johansson SG, Bennich H: Immunological studies of an atypical (myeloma) immunoglobulin. Immunology 13:381, 1967

Physicochemical properties and antigenic structure of an atypical myeloma protein are described. The protein was later proved to be E myeloma. (Bennich H, Ishizaka K, Ishizaka T, et al: A comparative antigenic study of gamma E-globulin and myeloma-IgND. J Immun 102:826, 1969).

Bennich H, Johansson SG: Studies on a new class of human immunoglobulin. II. Chemical and physical properties. Nobel Symposium – Third – Sodergarn – Sweden – 1967 on Gamma Globulins. Killander J, Ed. John Wiley and Sons, New York, 1967

Physicochemical properties and four chain structures of E myeloma protein are described. Both papain and pepsin fragments of the myeloma protein were isolated.

Ishizaka K, Ishizaka T: Human reaginic antibodies and immunoglobulin E. J Allerg 42:330, 1968

Review article including information on immunochemical properties of γE antibodies.

Johansson SG, Bennich H, Berg T, et al: Some factors influencing the serum IgE levels in atopic diseases. Clin Exp Immun 6:43, 1970

Patients with asthma and atopic dermatitis have raised IgE level. Effect of hyposensitization treatment, steroid and disodium cromoglycate, on IgE level is discussed.

Ishizaka K, Ishizaka T: Biologic function of γE antibodies and mechanisms of reaginic hypersensitivity. Clin Exp Immun 6:25, 1970

Review article including immunochemical properties, immune mechanisms of reaginic hypersensitivity, and site of IgE formation.

Ishizaka T, Ishizaka K, Orange RP, et al: The capacity of human immunoglobulin E to mediate the release of histamine and slow reacting substance of anaphylaxis (SRS-A) from monkey lung. J Immun 104:335, 1970

Evidence is described showing that IgE antibody mediates the antigen-induced release of both histamine and SRS-A from primate lung tissues.

Ishizaka K, Ishizaka T, Lee EH: Biologic function of the Fc fragments of E myeloma protein. Immunochemistry (in press)
The Fc fragments of E myeloma protein obtained by papain digestion sensitize human and monkey skin, human leukocytes, and monkey lung for reversed-type (anti-IgE-induced) reactions. Nonspecifically aggregated Fc fragments induce erythema-wheal reactions in the skin, release histamine from human leukocytes and both histamine and SRS-A *from monkey lung.*

Chapter 10

Gewurz H, Pickering RJ, Clark DS, et al: The complement system in the prevention, mediation and diagnosis of disease and its usefulness in the determination of immunopathogenetic mechanisms. Immunologic Deficiency Diseases in Man. Birth Defects Original Articles Series. Vol 4, No. 1. Bergsma D, Good RA, Eds. The National Foundation, New York 1968, p 396

Gewurz H, Shin HS, Pickering RJ, et al: Interactions of the complement system with endotoxic lipopolysaccharides: Complement-membrane interactions and endotoxin-induced inflammation. Cellular Recognition. Smith R, Good RA, Eds. Appleton-Century-Crofts, New York, 1969, p 305

Humphrey JH, Dourmashkin RR: The lesions in cell membranes caused by complement. Advances Immun 11:75, 1969

Lepow IH: Serum complement and properdin. Immunological Diseases. Samter M, Alexander HL, Eds. JA Churchill, London, 1965, p 188

Mayer M: Mechanism of hemolysis by complement. Ciba Foundation Symposium on Complement. Wolstenholme GEW, Knight J, Eds. Little, Brown & Co, Boston, 1965, p 4

Müller-Eberhard HJ: Chemistry and reaction mechanisms of complement. Advances Immun 8:1, 1968

Nelson RA Jr: The role of complement in immune phenomena. The Inflammatory Process. Zweifach BW, et al, Eds. Academic Press, New York, 1965, p 819

Osler AG: Functions of the complement system. Advances Immun 1:131, 1961

Chapter 11

Lawrence HS: Transfer factor. Advances Immun 11:195, 1969

Lawrence HS, Valentine FT: Transfer factor in delayed hypersensitivity. Ann NY Acad Sci 169:269, 1970

Mediators of Cellular Immunity. Proceedings of an International Conference, Augusta, Mich. Lawrence HS, Landy M, Eds. Academic Press, New York, 1969

Lawrence HS: Transfer factor and cellular immune deficiency disease. New Eng J Med 283:411, 1970

Lawrence HS, Valentine FT: Transfer factor and other mediators of cellular immunity. Amer J Path 60:437, 1970

Burnet, Sir FM: Self and Cellular Immunology. Book I. Cambridge University Press, New York, 1969

Bloom BR, Chase MW: Transfer of delayed-type hypersensitivity. A critical review and experimental study in the guinea pig. Progr Allerg 10:151, 1967

Delayed Hypersensitivity: Specific Cell-Mediated Immunity. Brit Med Bull 23:1, 1967

Uhr JW: Delayed hypersensitivity. Physiol Rev 46:359, 1966

Gowans JL, McGregor DD: The immunological activities of lymphocytes. Progr Allerg 9:1, 1965

Levin AS, Spitler LE, Stites DP, et al: Wiskott-Aldrich syndrome, a genetically determined cellular immunologic deficiency: Clinical and laboratory responses to therapy with transfer factor. Proc Nat Acad Sci USA 67:821, 1970

Rocklin RE, Chilgren RA, Hong R, et al: Transfer of cellular hypersensitivity in chronic mucocutaneous candidiasis monitored *in vivo* and *in vitro*. Cellular Immun 1:290, 1970

Chapter 12

Austen KF, Humphrey JH: In vitro studies of the mechanism of anaphylaxis. Advances Immun 3:1, 1963

Becker EL, Austen KF: Mechanisms of immunologic injury of rat peritoneal mast cells. The effect of phosphonate inhibitors on the homocytotropic antibody-mediated histamine release and the first component of rat complement. J Exp Med 124:379, 1966

Orange RP, Austen KF: Slow reacting substance of anaphylaxis. Advances Immun 10:105, 1969

Ishizaka T, Ishizaka K, Orange RP, Austen KF: The capacity of human immunoglobulin E to mediate the release of histamine and slow reacting substance of anaphylaxis (SRS-A) from monkey lung. J Immun 104:335, 1970

Orange RP, Stechschulte DJ, Austen KF: Immunochemical and biologic properties of rat IgE. II. Capacity to mediate the immunologic release of histamine and slow-reacting substance of anaphylaxis (SRS-A). J Immun 105:1087, 1970

Chapter 13

Claman HN, Chaperon EA: Immunological complementation between thymus and marrow cells–a model for the two-cell theory of immunocompetence. Transpl Rev 1:92, 1969

Miller JF, Mitchell GF: Thymus and antigen-reactive cells. Transpl Rev 1:3, 1969

Chiller JM, Habicht GS, Weigle WO: Kinetic differences in unresponsiveness of thymus and bone marrow cells. Science 171:813, 1971

Weigle WO: Natural and Acquired Immunologic Unresponsiveness. World Publishing Co., Cleveland, 1967

Dresser DW, Mitchison NA: The mechanism of immunological paralysis. Advances Immun 8:129, 1968

Immunological Tolerance. Perspectives in Immunology: Series of Publications Based on Symposia. Vol 1. M Landy, W Braun, Eds. Academic Press, New York, 1969

Pearsall NN, Weiser RS: The Macrophage. Lea and Febiger, Philadelphia, 1970

Chapter 14

Ratnoff OD: Some relationships among hemostasis, fibrinolytic phenomena, immunity, and the inflammatory response. Advances Immun 10:145, 1969

Kellermeyer RW, Graham RC Jr: Kinins – possible physiologic and pathologic roles in man. New Eng J Med 279:754, 802, 859, 1968

Donaldson VH: Blood coagulation and related plasma enzymes in inflammation. Aspects of Inflammation. Series Haematologica. Vol 3, 1970, p 39

Austen KF: Inborn and acquired abnormalities of the complement system of man. Trans Ass Amer Physicians 83:49, 1970

Chapter 15

Lawrence HS, Landy M: Mediators of Cellular Immunity. Proceedings of an International Conference, Augusta, Mich. Lawrence HS, Landy M, Eds. Academic Press, New York, 1969

Intersociety Symposium on In Vitro Correlates of Delayed Hypersensitivity, 51st Annual Meeting of the Federation of American Societies for Experimental Biology, Chicago. Fed Proc 27:3, 1968

World Health Organization: Cell-Mediated Immune Responses. Report of a WHO Study Group. WHO Tech Rep, Ser 423, WHO, Geneva, 1969; Int Arch Allerg 36 (No. 6): 7, 1969

David JR: Cellular hypersensitivity and immunity; inhibition of macrophage migration and the lymphocytic mediators. Progr Allerg (in press)

Chapter 16

Dixon FJ: The role of antigen-antibody complexes in disease. Harvey Lect 58:21, 1962-63

Cochrane CG, Koffler D: Immune complex disease. Advances Immun Vol 14 (in press)

Cochrane CG, Dixon FJ: Cell and tissue damage through antigen-antibody complexes. Calif Med 111:99, 1969

Dixon FJ: Pathogenesis of immune complex glomerulonephritis of New Zealand mice. J Exp Med. Vol 134 (in press)

Unanue ER, Dixon FJ: Experimental glomerulonephritis: Immunological events and pathogenetic mechanisms. Advances Immun 6:1, 1967

Chapter 17

Lerner RA, Glassock RJ, Dixon FJ: The role of anti-glómerular basement membrane antibody in the pathogenesis of human glomerulonephritis. J Exp Med 126:989, 1967

Dixon FJ, Feldman JD, Vazquez JJ: Experimental glomerulonephritis. The pathogenesis of a laboratory model resembling the spectrum of human glomerulonephritis. J Exp Med 113: 899, 1961

Dixon FJ: Pathogenesis of glomerulonephritis (editorial). Amer J Med 44:493, 1968

Treser G, Semar M, Ty A, et al: Partial characterization of antigenic streptococcal plasma membrane components in acute glomerulonephritis. J Clin Invest 49:762, 1970

Koffler D, Schur PH, Kunkel HG: Immunological studies concerning the nephritis of systemic lupus erythematosus. J Exp Med 126:607, 1967

McPhaul JJ, Dixon FJ: Immunoreactive basement membrane antigens in normal human urine and serum. J Exp Med 130: 1395, 1969

Chapter 18

Fong S, Fudenberg HH, Perlmann P: Ulcerative colitis with anti-erythrocyte antibodies. Vox Sang 8:668, 1963

Fudenberg HH: Immunologic deficiency, autoimmune disease, and lymphoma: observations, implications, and speculations. Arthritis Rheum 9:464, 1966

Kamin RM, Fudenberg HH, Douglas SD: A genetic defect in "acquired" agammaglobulinemia. Proc Nat Acad Sci USA 60: 881, 1968

Fudenberg HH, Franklin EC: Rheumatoid factors and the etiology of rheumatoid arthritis. Ann NY Acad Sci 124:884, 1965

Guttman PH, Davis WC, Fudenberg HH, et al: Effect of interferon on the course of spontaneous and radiation-induced renal lesions in the RF/Un mouse. Vox Sang 17:279, 1969

Douglas SD, Goldberg LS, Fudenberg HH, et al: Agammaglobulinaemia and co-existent pernicious anaemia. Clin Exp Immun 6: 181, 1970

Wuepper KD, Wegienka LC, Fudenberg HH: Immunologic aspects of adrenocortical insufficiency. Amer J Med 46:206, 1969

Conn, HO, Binder H, Burns B: Pernicious anemia and immunologic deficiency. Ann Intern Med 68:603, 1968

Hotchin J, Collins DN: Glomerulonephritis and late onset disease of mice following neonatal virus infection. Nature 203: 1357, 1964

Oldstone MB, Dixon FJ: Lymphocytic choriomeningitis: production of antibody by "tolerant" infected mice. Science 158: 1193, 1967

McDevitt HO, Sela M: Genetic control of the antibody response. I. Demonstration of determinant-specific differences in response to synthetic polypeptide antigens in two strains of inbred mice. J Exp Med 122:517, 1965

McDevitt HO, Benacerraf B: Genetic control of specific immune responses. Advances Immun 11:31, 1969

Chapter 19

Hume DM: Immunological consequences of organ homotransplantation in man. Harvey Lect 64:261, 1968-69

Hume DM, Sterling WA, Weymouth RJ, et al: Glomerulonephritis in human renal homotransplants. Transpl Proc 2:361, 1970

Penn I, Hammond W, Brettschneider L, et al: Malignant lymphomas in transplantation patients. Transpl Proc 1:106, 1969

Starzl TE: Experience in Hepatic Transplantation, WB Saunders Company, Philadelphia, 1969, p 415

Williams GM, DePlanque B, Lower R, Hume DM: Antibodies and human transplant rejection. Ann Surg 170:603, 1969

Williams GM, Rolley RT, Hume DM: A comparison of lymphocyte and kidney cell typing in eleven patients. Surg Forum 19:209, 1968

Wolf JS, Fawley JC, Hume DM: In vitro interaction of specifically-sensitized and non-sensitized lymphocytes with kidney cells from human renal homografts. Transpl Proc 1:328, 1969

Chapter 20

Starzl TE, Brettschneider L, Penn I, et al: Clinical liver transplantation. Transplant Rev 2:3, 1969

The entire issue of this journal is concerned with liver transplantation. Among other articles, it contains accounts by R. Calne, A. C. Birtch, and F. D. Moore about the clinical experience with liver transplantation at Cambridge and Harvard universities.

Fortner JG, Beattie EJ Jr, Shiu MH: Orthotopic and heterotopic liver homografts in man. Ann Surg 172:23, 1970

Starzl TE: Experience in Renal Transplantation. WB Saunders Company, Philadelphia, 1964

Starzl TE: Experience in Hepatic Transplantation. WB Saunders Company, Philadelphia, 1969

Chapter 21

Alexander P: Immunotherapy of cancer: experiments with primary tumours and syngeneic tumour grafts. Progr Exp Tumor Res 10:22, 1968

Bubenik J, Perlmann P, Helmstein K, et al: Immune response to urinary bladder tumours in man. Int J Cancer 5:39, 1970

Gold P, Freedman SO: Specific carcinoembryonic antigens of the human digestive system. J Exp Med 122:467, 1965

Good RA, Finstad J: Essential relationship between the lymphoid system, immunity, and malignancy. Symposium on Neoplasms and Related Disorders of Invertebrate and Lower Vertebrate Animals. Nat Cancer Inst Monog 31:41, 1969

Hellström KE, Hellström I: Cellular immunity against tumor antigens. Advances Cancer Res 12:167, 1969

Hellström KE, Hellström I: Immunological enhancement as studied by cell culture techniques. Ann Rev Microbiol 24:373, 1970

Hellström I, Hellström KE, Evans CA, et al: Serum-mediated protection of neoplastic cells from inhibition by lymphocytes immune to their tumor-specific antigens. Proc Nat Acad Sci USA 62:362, 1969

Hellström I, Hellström KE, Pierce GE, et al: Demonstration of cell-bound and humoral immunity against neuroblastoma cells. Proc Nat Acad Sci USA 60:1231, 1968

Hellström I, Hellström KE, Pierce GE, et al: Studies on immunity to autochthonous mouse tumors. Transpl Proc 1:90, 1969

Hellström I, Hellström KE, Pierce GE, et al: Cellular and humoral immunity to different types of human neoplasms. Nature 220:1352, 1968

Heppner GH: Studies on serum-mediated inhibition of cellular immunity to spontaneous mouse mammary tumors. Int J Cancer 4:608, 1969

Huebner RJ, Todaro GJ: Oncogenes of RNA tumor viruses as determinants of cancer. Proc Nat Acad Sci USA 64:1087, 1969

Klein G: Tumor antigens. Ann Rev Microbiol 20:223, 1966

Klein G, Clifford P, Klein E, et al: Search for tumor-specific immune reactions in Burkitt lymphoma patients by the membrane immunofluorescence reaction. Proc Nat Acad Sci USA 55:1628, 1966

Morton DL, Malmgren RA: Human osteosarcomas: Immunologic evidence suggesting an associated infectious agent. Science 162:1279, 1968

Old LJ, Boyse EA: Immunology of experimental tumors. Ann Rev Med 15:167, 1964

Sjögren HO: Transplantation methods as a tool for detection of tumor-specific antigens. Progr Exp Tumor Res 6:289, 1965

Chapter 23

Das Antikörpermangelsyndrom. Barandun S, Cottier H, et al, Eds. Benno Schwabe, Basel, 1959

DiGeorge AM: Congenital absence of the thymus and its immunologic consequences: Concurrence with congenital hypoparathyroidism. Immunologic Deficiency Diseases in Man. Birth Defects Original Article Series. Vol 4, No 1. Bergsma D, Good RA, Eds. The National Foundation, New York, 1968, p 116

Cleveland WW, Fogel BJ, Brown WT, et al: Foetal thymic transplant in a case of DiGeorge's syndrome. Lancet 2:1211, 1968

August CS, Rosen FS, Filler RM, et al: Implantation of a foetal thymus, restoring immunological competence in a patient with thymic aplasia (DiGeorge's syndrome). Lancet 2:1210, 1968

Gatti RA, Meuwissen HJ, Good RA, et al: Immunological reconstitution of sex-linked lymphopenic immunological deficiency. Lancet 2:1366, 1968

Lischner HW, DiGeorge AM: Role of the thymus in humoral immunity; observations in complete or partial congenital absence of the thymus. Lancet 2:1044, 1969

Good RA: Progress toward a cellular engineering. JAMA 214:1289, 1970

Ford CE: Traffic of lymphoid cells in the body. The Thymus: Experimental and Clinical Studies. Ciba Foundation Symposium. Wolstenholme GEW, Porter R, Eds. Williams & Wilkins Company, Baltimore, 1966, p 131

Parrott DV, de Sousa MA, East J: Thymus-dependent areas in the lymphoid organs of neonatally thymectomized mice. J Exp Med 123:191, 1966

Immunology in Clinical Medicine. Turk JL, Ed. Appleton-Century-Crofts, New York, 1969

Till JE, McCulloch EA: Early repair processes in marrow cells irradiated and proliferating in vivo. Radiat Res 18:96, 1963

Stutman O, Yunis EJ, Good RA: Studies on thymus function. I and II. Cooperative effect of thymic function and lymphohemopoietic cells in restoration of neonatally thymectomized mice; cooperative effect of newborn and embryonic hemopoietic liver cells with thymus function. J Exp Med 132:583, 601, 1970

Chapter 24

Gabrielsen AE, Good RA: Chemical suppression of adaptive immunity. Advances Immun 6:92, 1967

Schwartz RS: Immunosuppressive drug therapy. Human Transplantation. Rapaport FT, Dausset J, Eds. Grune & Stratton, New York, 1968, p 440

Many A, Schwartz RS: On the mechanism of immunological tolerance in cyclophosphamide-treated mice. Clin Exp Immun 6:87, 1970

Borel Y, Faueconnet M, Miescher PA: Effect of 6-mercaptopurine (6-MP) on different classes of antibody. J Exp Med 122:263, 1965

Miller JF, Mitchell GF: Cell to cell interaction in the immune response. V. Target cells for tolerance induction. J Exp Med 131:675, 1970

Chapter 25

Lance EM: The selective action of antilymphocyte serum on recirculating lymphocytes: A review of the evidence and alternatives. Clin Exp Immun 6:789, 1970

Medawar PB: Biological effects of heterologous antilymphocyte sera. Human Transplantation. Rapaport FT, Dausset J, Eds. Grune & Stratton, New York, 1968, p 501

Proceedings of International Symposium on Antilymphocyte Sera. Symposia Series on Immunobiological Standardization. Vol 16. Bach JF, et al, Eds. S. Karger, Basel, 1970

Proceedings of the Conference on Antilymphocyte Serum (held at Brook Lodge, Augusta, Mich. May 2-3, 1969). Fed Proc 29:97, 1970

Sell S: Antilymphocytic antibody: Effects in experimental animals and problems in human use. Ann Int Med 71:177, 1969

Antilymphocytic Serum. Ciba Foundation Study Group #29. Wolstenholme GEW, O'Connor M, Eds. JA Churchill, London, 1967

Taub RN: Biological effects of heterologous antilymphocyte serum. Progr Allerg, 14:208, 1970

Chapter 26

Vilcek J: Interferon. Virology Monographs Vol 6. Springer-Verlag, New York, 1969

A single author presents a monograph-type review of this whole field.

Hilleman MR: Prospects for the use of double-stranded ribonucleic acid (poly 1:C) inducers in man. J Infect Dis 121: 196, 1970

A leading worker reviews perspectives and the accomplishments of his group.

De Clercq E, Merigan TC: Current concepts of interferon and interferon induction. Ann Rev Med 21:17, 1970

An interpretive review of recent progress in this area.

Interferon. Ciba Foundation Symposium. Wolstenholme GEW, O'Connor M, Eds. Little, Brown and Co, Boston, 1968

A group of well-edited contributions by active workers in this area, with interesting discussions following each article.

The Interferons: An International Symposium. Rita G, Ed. Academic Press, New York, 1968

Another group of symposium presentations by leading authorities.

Symposium on Interferon and Host Response to Virus Infection. Merigan TC, Ed. AMA Arch Int Med 126:49, 1970

A series of clinically oriented invited discussions by established workers.

Interferon, Proceedings of a Symposium Sponsored by the New York Heart Association. Vilcek J, Ed. J Gen Physiol 56 (No 1, Pt 2), July, 1970

A selected set of workers review the important areas of contemporary work in relationship to findings in their own laboratories.

Interferons. Finter NB, Ed. WB Saunders Company, Philadelphia, 1966

Interferons, 2nd Ed. Finter NB, Ed. North Holland, Amsterdam (in press)

A well-edited, integrated, and up-to-date series of monographs that cover the present status of work in this field.

Finkelstein MS, Merigan TC, et al: Interferon – 1968. Calif Med 109:24, 1968

Hilleman, MR: Interferon induction and utilization. J Cell Physiol 71:43, 1968

Chapter 27

Liley AW: Liquor amnii analysis in the management of the pregnancy complicated by rhesus sensitization. Amer J Obstet Gynec 82:1359, 1961

Freda VJ, Gorman JG, Pollack W: Successful prevention of experimental Rh sensitization in man with an anti-Rh gamma$_2$ globulin antibody preparation: A preliminary report. Transfusion 4:26, 1964

Freda VJ: The Rh problem in obstetrics and a new concept of its management using amniocentesis and spectrophotometric scanning of amniotic fluid. Amer J Obstet Gynec 92:341, 1965

Freda VJ: Antepartum management of the Rh problem. Progr Hemat 5:266, 1969

Queenan JT: Modern Management of the Rh Problem. Harper & Row, New York, 1967

Freda VJ, Gorman JG, Pollack W: Suppression of the primary Rh immune response with passive Rh IgG immunoglobulin. New Eng J Med 277:1022, 1967

Pollack W, Gorman JG, Freda VJ: Prevention of Rh hemolytic disease. Progr Hemat 6:121, 1969

Chapter 28

Kempe CH: Studies on smallpox and complications of smallpox vaccination. Pediatrics 27:176, 1960

Kempe CH, Fulginiti V, Minamitani M, et al: Smallpox vaccination of eczema patients with a strain of attenuated live vaccinia (CVI-78). Pediatrics 42:980, 1968

Lane JM, Ruben FL, Abrutyn E, et al: Deaths attributable to smallpox vaccination, 1959 to 1966, and 1968. JAMA 212:441, 1970

Lane JM, Millar JD: Routine childhood vaccination against smallpox reconsidered. New Eng J Med 281:1220, 1969

Neff JM, Lane JM, Pert JH, et al: Complications of smallpox vaccination. I. National survey in the United States, 1963. New Eng J Med 276:125, 1967

Bauer DJ, St. Vincent L, Kempe CH, et al: Prophylaxis of smallpox with methisazone. Amer J Epidem 90:130, 1969

Kempe CH, Benenson AS: Smallpox immunization in the United States. JAMA 194:161, 1965

Fulginiti VA, et al: Progressive vaccinia in immunologically deficient individuals. Immunologic Deficiency Diseases in Man. Birth Defects Original Article Series. Vol 4, No 1. Bergsma D, Good RA, Eds. The National Foundation, New York, 1968

Chapter 29

Dossett JH, Williams RC Jr, Quie PG: Studies on interaction of bacteria, serum factors and polymorphonuclear leukocytes in mothers and newborns. Pediatrics 44:49, 1969

Demonstration that antibodies in 19S serum fractions (IgM) are efficient opsonins for Escherichia coli; *however, complement is necessary to demonstrate their opsonic potential.*

Fulginiti VA, Sieber OF Jr, Claman HN, et al: Serum immunoglobulin measurement during the first year of life and in immunoglobulin-deficiency states. J Pediat 68:723, 1966

Serum immunoglobulin levels at different age intervals and for selected immunologic deficiency states are measured by a capillary immunoprecipitation technique.

Heiner DC, Evans L: Immunoglobulins and other proteins in commercial preparations of gamma globulin. J Pediat 70:820, 1967

Immunoglobulin composition of various commercial gamma globulin preparations determined. Several differences among these are documented and discussed.

Henney CS, Ellis EF: Antibody production to aggregated human gamma-G-globulin in acquired hypogammaglobulinemia. New Eng J Med 278: 1144, 1968

A patient with acquired hypogammaglobulinemia who suffered "anaphylactic shock" following intramuscular administration of commercial gamma globulin is shown to have precipitating antibody specific for gamma globulin aggregates.

Miller ME: Deficiency of chemotactic function in the human neonate: A previously unrecognized defect of the inflammatory response; humoral and cellular factors. Pediat Res 3:497, 1969 (full manuscript in press)

Cellular and humoral deficiencies in the neonatal chemotactic response are defined.

Miller ME: Phagocytosis in the newborn infant: humoral and cellular factors. J Pediat 74:255, 1969

Humoral and cellular deficiencies are defined in the neonatal phagocytic response.

Stiehm ER, Fudenberg HH: Serum levels of immune globulins in health and disease: a survey. Pediatrics 37:715, 1966

Immunoglobulin levels in sera of normal persons of various ages are quantitated by a radial diffusion technique. In addition, levels are measured in patients with a variety of conditions, including mongolism, gonadal dysgenesis, hypergammaglobulinemia, and immunologic deficiency diseases.

West CD: Comment on IgA deficiency and susceptibility to infection. J Pediat 72:153, 1968

Pertinent comments on the possible association of serum IgA deficiency with recurrent upper respiratory infections.

Chapter 30

Berson SA, Yalow RS: Immunoassay of protein hormones. The Hormones: Physiology, Chemistry and Applications. Vol 4. Pincus G, et al, Eds. Academic Press, New York, 1964, p 557

Glick SM, Roth J, Yalow RS, Berson SA: The regulation of growth hormone secretion. Recent Progr Hormone Res 21: 241, 1965

Yalow RS, Berson SA: Labeling of proteins – problems and practice. Trans NY Acad Sci 28:1033, 1966

Berson SA, Yalow RS: Peptide hormones in plasma. Harvey Lect 62:107, 1966-67

Yalow RS, Berson SA: Size and charge distinctions between endogenous human plasma gastrin in peripheral blood and heptadecapeptide gastrins. Gastroenterology 58:609, 1970

Walsh JH, Yalow RS, Berson SA: Detection of Australia antigen and antibody by means of radioimmunoassay techniques. J Infect Dis 121:550, 1970

Thomson DM, Krupey J, Freedman SO, et al: The radioimmunoassay of circulating carcinoembryonic antigen of the human digestive system. Proc Nat Acad Sci USA 64:161, 1969

Index

T

V

W-Z